Hip and Knee Reconstructive and Replacement Surgery

Hip and Knee Reconstructive and Replacement Surgery

Oscar Hazel

AMERICAN
MEDICAL PUBLISHERS
www.americanmedicalpublishers.com

AMERICAN
MEDICAL PUBLISHERS
www.americanmedicalpublishers.com

Cataloging-in-publication Data

Hip and knee reconstructive and replacement surgery / Oscar Hazel.
p. cm.
Includes bibliographical references and index.
ISBN 979-8-88740-183-6
1. Hip joint--Surgery. 2. Knee--Surgery. 3. Surgery, Plastic. 4. Total hip replacement.
5. Total knee replacement. 6. Orthopedic surgery. I. Hazel, Oscar.
RD549 .H56 2023
617.581 059 2--dc23

American Medical Publishers,
41 Flatbush Avenue,
1st Floor, New York,
NY 11217, USA

ISBN 979-8-88740-183-6 (Hardback)

Contents

Preface

Hip replacement, also known as hip arthroplasty, is a surgery in which a prosthetic implant, often known as a hip prosthesis, replaces the hip joint. A whole hip replacement or hemi (half) replacements are two options for hip replacement surgery. Total hip replacement surgery may be prescribed in cases of joint failure caused by osteoarthritis, rheumatoid arthritis, avascular necrosis, traumatic arthritis, protrusio acetabuli, certain hip fractures, benign and malignant bone tumors, etc. Knee replacement or knee arthroplasty, is a surgical method that replaces the weight-bearing surfaces of the knee joint to reduce pain and impairment. This type of surgery is mostly recommended when conservative measures fail to relieve joint discomfort, as well as for other knee disorders such as rheumatoid arthritis and psoriatic arthritis. Infections, blood clot, a fracture during or after surgery, nerve damage, and continued pain or stiffness are some possible complications associated with hip and knee replacement surgery. This book consists of contributions made by international experts. There has been rapid progress in this area of orthopedic surgery. Doctors and students actively engaged in hip and knee arthroplasty will find this book full of crucial and unexplored concepts.

Significant researches are present in this book. Intensive efforts have been employed by authors to make this book an outstanding discourse. This book contains the enlightening chapters which have been written on the basis of significant researches done by the experts.

Finally, I would also like to thank all the members involved in this book for being a team and meeting all the deadlines for the submission of their respective works. I would also like to thank my friends and family for being supportive in my efforts.

Oscar Hazel

1

Coexistence of EBM and Personalized Medicine

Kim Madden and Mohit Bhandari

1.1 What Is Evidence-Based Medicine?

Evidence-based medicine (EBM) is a philosophy of healthcare that aims to ensure that healthcare interventions are applied based on the best available evidence, combined with clinical expertise and patient values [1]. This is in contrast to the philosophy of "eminence-based" medicine, which is characterized by a paternalistic view that expert clinicians know what is best for their patients by virtue of their clinical experience. The term EBM was coined by Professor Gordon Guyatt in 1990 and further developed by academic physicians such as Professor David Sackett. Sackett described EBM as having three integrated key components: best available evidence, clinical expertise, and patient values [1]. Here, we discuss each of these three components in more detail.

1.1.1 Best Available Evidence

It makes intuitive sense that healthcare professionals should be reasonably sure that a treatment works and that the benefits outweigh the harms before wide implementation of the intervention. It is important to question unsubstantiated claims about treatments, diagnostic tools, and other aspects of healthcare so that we do not widely use treatments that are ineffective or do more harm than good. Using systematic and scientific methodology, EBM gives us the tools to evaluate healthcare interventions and determine how strong and convincing the evidence is for those interventions, and therefore whether we should believe claims of their efficacy. The phrase "best available evidence" implies that some evidence is better than other evidence. This brings us to one of the key principles of EBM: the hierarchy of evidence. Many healthcare professionals are aware of the "evidence pyramid" that places high-quality evidence on the top of the pyramid and low-quality evidence on the bottom of the pyramid [2]. EBM helps us to sort out which studies are high quality and which studies are low quality. However, this categorization is not binary; quality of evidence is a continuum. In general, the highest quality of evidence for questions about treatment efficacy comes from randomized controlled trials (RCTs) and systematic reviews of RCTs. The reason for this is that, when done correctly, the process of randomization should balance the known and unknown prognostic factors across treatment groups, with the only difference between groups being the treatment of interest. RCTs are not always at the top of the hierarchy of evidence. EBM also

K. Madden · M. Bhandari (✉)
Department of Surgery, McMaster University, Hamilton, ON, Canada
e-mail: maddenk@mcmaster.ca; bhandam@mcmaster.ca

encourages downgrading evidence in the presence of substantial methodological flaws [3]. For example, if a study is too small to properly balance prognostic factors across groups, that could lead to the study being downgraded from the top level of evidence. Prospective cohort studies are often at the second tier of evidence (Level II evidence) because they lack the randomization process that aims to balance prognostic factors. They are therefore more biased and of lower quality. Retrospective studies are Level III evidence because they are subject to even more bias than prospective studies, for example, recall bias. Case series are Level IV evidence because they lack a control group. We therefore cannot be sure whether apparent treatment effects can actually be attributed to the treatment or some other effect such as time. Expert opinion is Level V evidence because opinions can easily be biased by personal views, conflicts of interest, and other factors such as confirmation bias. By applying a critical lens to studies, we can practice "enlightened scepticism" to be reasonably sure that the treatments that we choose to use are effective.

1.1.2 Clinical Expertise

Critics of EBM often protest that EBM downplays the role of the clinician's expertise in favor of a cold, calculating style of medicine based only on evidence [4]. This is not the case. Evidence is not a substitute for clinical training and experience. Evidence alone is never enough to make a clinical decision. The proper application of EBM requires the integration of expertise and evidence. The JAMA series on the Users Guides to the Medical Literature, a key EBM resource, gives guidance on how to evaluate whether particular evidence is applicable to specific patients [5]. It teaches clinicians to ask "Were the study patients similar to the patient in my practice?" To answer this question, clinicians must use their diagnostic expertise and judgment. For example, surgeons may decide that a study that included mostly elderly female patients with comorbidities would not necessarily apply to an elite male athlete, even if the evidence is of very high quality.

1.1.3 Patient Values

The third major component of EBM is the integration of patient values [6, 7]. Although this point is the most often forgotten, it has been written into formal definitions of EBM since the 1990s [1]. Along with the best available evidence and the clinician's expertise, we must take into account the patient's preferences. For example, an active, newly retired man with hip osteoarthritis may place more value on implant longevity than a very elderly man. Similarly, a young tradeswoman with moderate knee arthritis may value whichever treatment option can get her back to work faster. This principle particularly emphasizes that EBM is not a set of rigid rules, nor is it a one-size-fits-all approach to treating patients.

1.2 Are There any Drawbacks to EBM?

EBM is not perfect and is ever-evolving. A major practical challenge is that performing EBM properly requires a lot of practice and skill. However, this is the same for any other skill, for example, arthroplasty surgeons train for a decade or more to become experts at joint replacement. Sometimes, feasibility issues arise in EBM, for example, to get the highest quality evidence (i.e., RCTs), it can take years and cost millions of dollars to do it correctly. However, there are quicker and cheaper designs that can be done if an RCT is not feasible. For example, one could conduct retrospective chart reviews with matched controls or statistical adjustments based on propensity scores. This design is not as strong as an RCT but can efficiently provide better evidence than anecdote alone. One of the biggest challenges of EBM is that sometimes policymakers and clinicians forget that evidence alone is not sufficient, and they create overly strict policies that they say are evidence based. There needs to be integration of clinical judgment and patient values, which is in harmony with the principles of personalized medicine. Another perceived drawback of EBM is the misconception that results from trials can never apply to individual patients; they only apply to the "average patient." However, EBM books [5] and workshops [8] give explicit guidance on how to apply EBM to individual patients.

1.3 What Is Personalized Medicine?

Personalized medicine is a philosophy of treatment that arose from genomics, with particular applications in cancer treatment. The idea is that patients can be stratified into risk groups (e.g., biomarker present vs. absent) and provided with personalized treatment based on that risk factor [9]. This philosophy has clear applications in orthopedics, particularly in arthroplasty where many patients are not satisfied with their replaced joint despite a lack of major complications [10]. Kinematic alignment techniques that restore individual joint anatomy and soft-tissue balance, custom implants that can more accurately mimic the natural joint, robotic surgery for more precise cuts, and 3D printing are all innovations that can benefit the field of orthopedics by individualizing particular aspects of patient care. This intuitively sounds like a good idea. However, custom implants and technological innovations can drive up costs of surgery. We need evidence that these interventions are worth the additional money.

1.4 Are EBM and Personalized Medicine at Odds?

When Professor Gordon Guyatt was asked this question, he responded with "we find this somewhat amusing" [11]. The idea that personalized medicine is the opposite of EBM, or that they are somehow at odds, stems from a fundamental misunderstanding of what EBM is and is not. Particularly, the misconceptions that EBM is dogmatic, do not take into account patient values or differences between patients, there is no room for clinical judgment, that only randomized trials matter, and that EBM is a static set of rules, are misconceptions that contribute to the divide between personalized medicine and EBM. Let us address these misconceptions.

- *EBM is dogmatic.* EBM is not dogma; it is a set of guidelines that helps us decide whether a healthcare intervention is effective and safe and whether the evidence applies to our patients. Individual expertise, decision making, and judgment come into play at every stage of EBM.
- *EBM does not take into account patient values.* One of the three basic principles of EBM is that patient values and differences between patients should be taken into account when choosing a treatment. There is a whole field dedicated to how this can best be achieved, for example, with the use of patient decision aids and shared decision making [12]. Additionally, EBM is beginning to involve patients as collaborators when designing research and selecting outcomes for studies [13].
- *EBM does not take into account differences between patients.* EBM gives guidance on subgroup analyses to take into account differences between patients [14] Subgroups allow us to draw different conclusions for different groups of patients by categorizing them by a prognostic variable of interest, just like "stratified medicine." For example, in the SRINT trial investigating reamed versus unreamed intramedullary nailing for tibia fractures, the treatment effects varied for patients with open fractures versus closed fractures [15].
- *There is no room for clinical judgment.* One of the three basic principles of EBM is that clinical judgment cannot be replaced by evidence alone. Clinical expertise is still required to decide whether the evidence can be applied to a specific patient.
- *Only randomized trials matter.* EBM acknowledges that there are many ways to obtain evidence. The existence of the hierarchy of evidence proves this. Sometimes, patients cannot be randomized for ethical or feasibility reasons. In this case, EBM would say that an RCT is not the best available evidence. EBM has also always had an option for an N-of-1 trial, which is a trial where a single patient is their own control group [16]. This N-of-1 approach allows clinicians to determine whether a treatment works for that specific

patient and provides better evidence than anecdote alone.

- *EBM is a static set of rules.* EBM is not a set of rules (see point 1), and EBM is constantly evolving. Some of the newer innovations in EBM include better methods of disseminating evidence (e.g., OrthoEvidence; myorthoevidence.com), extending EBM concepts to diagnostic and prognostic studies as well as interventions (e.g., the work of the Grading of Recommendations, Assessment, Development and Evaluation (GRADE) group) [17], methods of synthesizing information quickly (e.g., BMJ Rapid Recommendations; bmj.com/rapid-recommendations), and ever-evolving methods of analyzing data, particularly non-RCT data.

1.5 So, Can EBM and Personalized Medicine Coexist?

Not only *can* EBM and personalized medicine coexist, they *should* coexist. Personalized medicine-based interventions contribute to the growing number of innovations in orthopedics and other fields. However, these interventions still need to be evaluated for effectiveness, cost-effectiveness, and safety before they are widely adopted, just as standard approaches need to be evaluated with a critical lens. For example, one could randomize patients to receive conventional unicompartmental knee arthroplasty (UKA) versus custom UKA. Such a study would combine the best of both worlds and promote innovation in our field. There is no reason that the philosophies of EBM and personalized medicine cannot work together.

References

1. Sackett DL, Rosenberg WM, Gray JA, Haynes RB, Richardson WS. Evidence based medicine: what it is and what it isn't. BMJ. 1996;312(7023):71–2.
2. Panesar SS, Philippon MJ, Bhandari M. Principles of evidence-based medicine. Orthop Clin North Am. 2010;41(2):131–8.
3. Guyatt GH, Oxman AD, Kunz R, Vist GE, Falck-Ytter Y, Schünemann HJ, GRADE Working Group. What is "quality of evidence" and why is it important to clinicians? BMJ. 2008;336(7651):995–8.
4. Wilson K. Evidence-based medicine. The good the bad and the ugly. A clinician's perspective. J Eval Clin Pract. 2010;16(2):398–400.
5. Guyatt GH, Haynes RB, Jaeschke RZ, et al. Users' guides to the medical literature: XXV. Evidence-based medicine: principles for applying the Users' guides to patient care. Evidence-based medicine working group. JAMA. 2000;284:290–6.
6. Kelly MP, Heath I, Howick J, Greenhalgh T. The importance of values in evidence-based medicine. BMC Med Ethics. 2015;16(1):69.
7. Guyatt G, Montori V, Devereaux PJ, Schünemann H, Bhandari M. Patients at the center: in our practice, and in our use of language. ACP J Club. 2004;140(1):A11–2.
8. McMaster Evidence-Based Clinical Practice Workshops. https://ebm.mcmaster.ca/.
9. Academy of Medical Sciences. Stratified, personalised or P4 medicine: a new direction for placing the patient at the centre of healthcare and health education (Technical report). 2015. https://acmedsci.ac.uk/download?f=file&i=32644.
10. Gunaratne R, Pratt DN, Banda J, Fick DP, Khan RJK, Robertson BW. Patient dissatisfaction following total knee arthroplasty: a systematic review of the literature. J Arthroplast. 2017;32(12):3854–60.
11. Guyatt G, Jaeschke R. Evolution of EBM. Part 1: EBM and personalized medicine. Are they different? 2018. https://empendium.com/mcmtextbook/interviews/perspective/197445,evolution-of-ebm-part-1-ebm-and-personalized-medicine-are-they-different.
12. Montori VM, Breslin M, Maleska M, Weymiller AJ. Creating a conversation: insights from the development of a decision aid. PLoS Med. 2007;4(8):e233.
13. Sacristán JA, Aguarón A, Avendaño-Solá C, Garrido P, Carrión J, Gutiérrez A, Kroes R, Flores A. Patient involvement in clinical research: why, when, and how. Patient Prefer Adherence. 2016;10:631–40.
14. Sun X, Ioannidis JP, Agoritsas T, Alba AC, Guyatt G. How to use a subgroup analysis: users' guide to the medical literature. JAMA. 2014;311(4):405–11.
15. SPRINT Investigators, Sun X, Heels-Ansdell D, Walter SD, Guyatt G, Sprague S, Bhandari M, Sanders D, Schemitsch E, Tornetta P 3rd, Swiontkowski M. Is a subgroup claim believable? A user's guide to subgroup analyses in the surgical literature. J Bone Joint Surg Am. 2011;93(3):e8.
16. Guyatt G, Jaeschke R, McGinn TPART. 2B1: therapy and validity. N-of-1 randomized controlled trials. In: Guyatt G, Rennie D, Meade MO, Cook DJ, editors. Users' guides to the medical literature. New York: McGraw-Hill: American Medical Association; 2002. p. 275e90.
17. Iorio A, Spencer FA, Falavigna M, Alba C, Lang E, Burnand B, McGinn T, Hayden J, Williams K, Shea B, Wolff R, Kujpers T, Perel P, Vandvik PO, Glasziou P, Schunemann H, Guyatt G. Use of GRADE for assessment of evidence about prognosis: rating confidence in estimates of event rates in broad categories of patients. BMJ. 2015;350:h870.

Part I

Personalized Hip Replacement

2

Anatomy and Biomechanics of the Hip

Romain Galmiche, Henri Migaud,
and Paul-E. Beaulé

Key Points

- Surgeons have to cope with many variations in anatomy depending on gender, geographic area, or specific diseases.
- Surgeons have to either adapt their surgical technique and/or implant positioning to deal with all anatomies or use custom-made implants.
- Implant positioning needs to be accurate as error(s) in the position of component(s) can modify essential biomechanical parameters and thus jeopardize the clinical result.
- A better understanding of the dynamic/functional orientation of articular anatomical structures and the femoro-acetabular prosthetic interplay will benefit hip arthroplasty and feed future innovations.

R. Galmiche · H. Migaud
Service d'orthopédie C, Hopital Salengro, Centre Hospitalier Universitaire de Lille, Lille, France
e-mail: hemigaud@nordnet.fr

P.-E. Beaulé (✉)
Orthopaedic Department, The Ottawa Hospital, Ottawa, ON, Canada
e-mail: pbeaule@ottawahospital.on.ca

Modern total hip replacement and hip resurfacing have been shown to generate good long-term clinical outcomes. Advances in materials, engineering, and improved knowledge in joint anatomy and biomechanics, have enabled this success. Successful hip prosthetic surgery relies on a proper understanding of the hip anatomy and its biomechanics. In this chapter, we will review these essential points.

2.1 Normal Hip Biomechanics

Understanding of the human gait has progressed since the early methods of chronophotography by Etienne-Jules Marey, which enabled capture of human movement. Expansion on this through advancement in technology, such as infrared cameras, electromyographs, and force platforms, has led to a greater understanding not only of human locomotion, but also the effects our surgery has. The importance of hip biomechanics has become more and more prominent with the development of gait laboratories giving us a more accurate, but also more complex, view of the hip's in vivo function.

2.1.1 Kinematics

Hip motion is allowed in three planes (sagittal, frontal, and transverse) due to its **ball-and-socket**

configuration. Nevertheless, some authors have described the femoral head with a conchoid (or ellipsoid) shape [1]. This particular shape makes the joint less likely to sublux when compared to a true ball-and-socket joint. Moreover, this shape may contribute to generation of the optimal stress magnitude and distribution [2]. In the same manner, the horseshoe geometry of the acetabular cartilage has been shown to optimize the contact stress distribution. Thus, through the acknowledgment of these anatomic features, we immediately understand that allowing mobility while maintaining stability is the first challenge a prosthetic spherical implant faces.

The sagittal plane portrays the greatest **passive range of motion**: flexion, on average, can reach 100° (extended knee) and 140° (flexed knee, due to the hamstring release). Extension is 15°–20°. In the frontal plane, the range of abduction is from 10° to 45°, whereas the range of adduction is 10°–30°. The external rotation reaches 60° and the internal rotation 30°, but it can go further when the hip joint is flexed due to the release of the soft tissues (up to 90° for external and 60° for internal rotation). However, these figures are subject to interindividual variation. Gender, age, individual patient anatomy (femoral neck angle, femoral neck offset, acetabulum version …), and level of physical activity are features that can alter the hip range of motion. For example, a subject with a coxa valga tends to exhibit a better abduction peak angle than a coxa vara subject, due to the delayed impingement between the femoral neck and the acetabular labrum.

As an orthopedic surgeon, it is important to know the **values of hip motion involved in activities of daily living**. For example, tying shoe laces with feet on the floor will require up to 125° hip flexion, 19° external rotation, and 15° of abduction; ascending stairs will require a mean hip flexion of 70°, whereas descending them needs 35°. **Gait** is characteristic of the human species. This is a succession of imbalance phases that is actually much more complex than the human eye can see. Measurements in the sagittal plane (Fig. 2.1) show that the hip joint is maximally flexed (35°–45°) during the late swing phase of gait, as the limb moves forward for heel strike. Then, the hip extends as the body moves forward, and the extension peak is reached at heel-off. The frontal and transverse planes are also involved. Abduction occurs during the swing phase of gait and reaches a maximum just after toe-off. At heel strike, the hip joint reverses into adduction and keeps it during the entire stance phase. The hip joint is externally rotated during the swing phase and, to provide a fitted angle for the foot strike, the hip rotates internally. This internal rotation is gradually lost as the contralateral hip moves forward. One should also consider the motion of the pelvis (in sagittal, axial, and frontal planes) during the walking sequence. Pelvic motion is highly variable between individuals and its amplitude depends on multiple parameters, such as walking speed, pelvic and hip anatomy (e.g., width of pelvis), flexibility of the spine and the hips, etc. This pelvic motion probably has a significant influence on the hip biomechanics and the risk of degeneration. One must acknowledge that the pelvis undergoes axial rotation (about 8°) as the leg moves forward. There is a heightening of the hemi-pelvis before toe-off as well (corresponding to a 5° rotation in the frontal plane), introducing the concept of "pelvic vertebra" asserted by Jean Dubousset. These motions require further investigation, given they are highly variable between individuals and may produce deleterious effects on bearing components (edge loading, impingement) in dynamic situations [3].

2.1.2 Kinetics

Joint reaction forces are the forces generated within the joint in reaction to forces acting on the joint. For the hip, it is the result of the need to balance the moment arms of the body weight and abductor tension in order to keep a leveled pelvis. The hip contact forces are then a combination of ground reaction force to body weight, and of internal muscle contraction forces. The resultant hip reaction forces can be calculated either in vivo, by strained-gauged prosthesis, or by analytical approaches (2D models or more sophisticated 3D

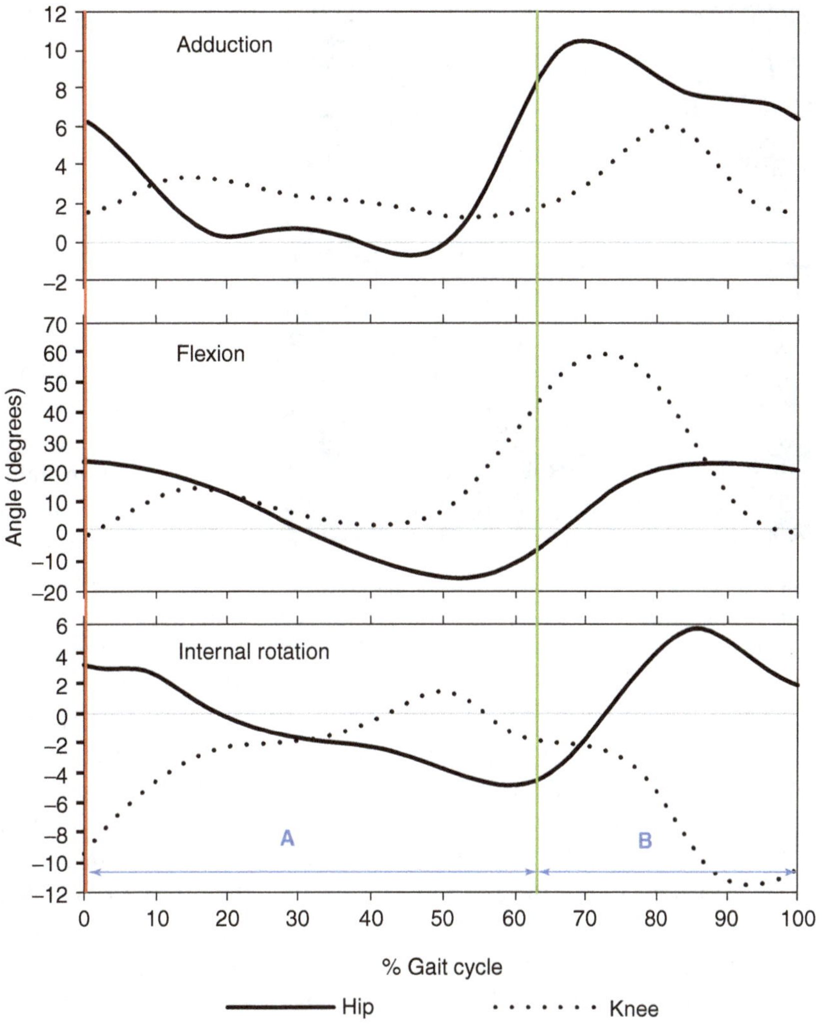

Fig. 2.1 Hip's movements in the three dimensions during a normal gait cycle. Red vertical line represents heel-strike and green vertical line is toe-off. *A* Stance phase, *B* Swing phase

models). In a simple 2D model, when both legs support the weight of the body equally, in a standing position, the weight force vector is centered between the two hips. As a result, each femoral head supports one-half of the body weight. Indeed, in this model the pelvis is stable and there is no muscle reaction force to add in. During a single-legged stance, five-sixths of the body weight act on the femoral head in charge; its vector is vertical. In parallel, the abductor muscle force is oriented medially and superiorly at an assumed 30° angle from the vertical line. The lever arm of both body weight and abductor muscles can be determined on an AP pelvis radiograph (Fig. 2.2). Thus, the abductor muscles' force multiplied by their lever arm (external moment) has to be equal to the bodyweight force multiplied by its lever arm (internal moment), in order to keep a poised pelvis. Since the effective lever arm of abductor muscles is considerably shorter than the effective lever arm of body weight, the combined force of abductors must be a multiple of body weight. It ensues peak hip joint forces can reach 1.8 to 4.3 times body weight during gait [4]. These numbers could rise to eight times body weight for activities like running or skiing. This highlights how these forces will play a first rank role in the selection of components, implantation, wear, and durability. On the femoral head, maximum contact pressures occur at the supero-anterior area during walking, whereas for the acetabulum, the supero-posterior zone is more exposed to constrain. When moving from standing to sitting position or from sitting to standing position, the contact pressure is higher

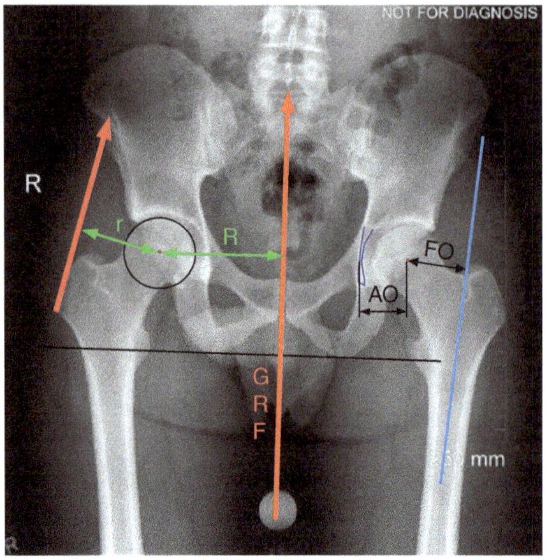

Fig. 2.2 AP pelvis X-rays. *Fabd* Abductor muscle force, *GRF* Ground Reaction Force, *FO* Femoral Offset, *AO* Acetabular Offset, *r* Abductor lever arm, *R* Body weight lever arm

mainly due to the smaller contact area at the edge of the posterior horn of the acetabulum. Indeed, as the hip is flexed, the contact area moves posteriorly. There are typically two hip resultant force peaks during the stance phase: a first one in early stance and a second one in late stance. One should also consider forces in the horizontal plane, which have been barely investigated. These forces may jeopardize efforts to optimize bearing components' behavior, as their influence is not fully understood.

Many parameters influence the intensity and repartition of the resultant hip joint contact forces. From a mechanical point of view, the **abductor lever arm** (tied to the neck-shaft angle and neck length) and the body-weight lever arm (tied to pelvis width) are two important parameters, particularly because they can easily be modified by THR surgery. The magnitude of **body weight** is also significantly influential. An increase in the abductor lever arm will lead to a decrease of the abductor's force needed to maintain a horizontal pelvis. It will tend to decrease the hip joint reaction forces. In the same way, a wider pelvis increases the **body weight lever arm,** and so will increase the joint contact forces during the one-legged stance. All of this is true in reverse, and applicable to prosthetic hips as well. As we suggested at the beginning of this chapter, the native hip joint is actually more complex than a simple ball-and-socket model. **Cartilage and bone elasticity**, a **slight lack of congruency** due to acetabular deformation the more the hip is loaded, the **conchoid femoral head shape,** as well as the **acetabular and femoral neck orientation** are parameters playing intricate roles in the hip contact forces' magnitude and repartition. Nonspherical shapes allow rolling movements in addition to sliding movements, which are logically the only ones found in a perfect ball-and-socket model. Thus, studies showed these conchoid or ellipsoid shapes contributed to optimal stress magnitude and repartition. In the same manner, cartilage elasticity, which is lost in an arthroplasty surgery, optimizes load transfer. In vitro, a decrease in acetabular anteversion leads to a dramatic increase in the hip's load, as reported by Sanchez Egea. A similar result is observed when decreasing femoral anteversion or neck-shaft angle [5]. However, one should consider the in vivo interaction between the femoral and acetabular anteversion–inclination. Indeed, it is more relevant to look at the interplay between acetabulum and proximal femur orientation. It introduces the concept of combined version, which recommends that the sum of the stem and cup anteversion values approximates 37 ° [6]. Accurate combined anteversion is more likely to result in a harmonious interaction between the femoral head and the cup, with no impingement throughout the entire range of body positions.

In the prosthetic joint, the **femoral head diameter, articular clearance, and cup orientation** are other important parameters influencing the head/acetabulum contact area (or contact patch), and therefore the hip joint contact forces. For a bigger head diameter, one would expect a larger contact patch between head and cup. However, the contact patch size is closely tied to the inner diameter of the cup, as well as defining the clearance. Thus, too high a clearance will reduce the contact patch area, potentially leading to a high wear rate. On the other hand, low clearance hips have a more conformal contact and a larger contact patch, which decreases the distance between the edge of the contact patch and the rim of the cup, thereby increasing the risk of edge loading and wear. Edge loading occurs when the contact patch between the head and cup extends over the cup rim, which results in a large increase in local pressure, disruption of the lubrication mechanism, and increased wear. Clearance is now known to be an important factor in edge loading phenomenon [7]. This consideration is of high importance specifically for large diameter MoM bearings. A cup abduction angle of 45° or less is recommended to avoid excessive wear. It is of particular importance for MoM resurfacing in order to avoid edge-loading phenomenon. The effect of cup anteversion on wear is less straightforward and should be considered alongside the femoral version [8]. Nevertheless, modifying the cup inclination and/or anteversion will influence both the anterosuperior and the posteroinferior cup-head contact areas in opposite ways. For hard on smooth bearing couples, liner wear rates for 22, 28 or 32 mm heads do not vary significantly. Nevertheless, volumetric wear increases with head size, as it impacts the sliding distance between bearing components.

2.2 Variability in Hip Anatomy

In order to restore physiological hip biomechanics, THR surgery often aims to respect the patient's individual anatomy. However, hip anatomy is subject to a high interindividual variability. Immediately we understand the surgical difficulties related to this, in particular our capacity to restore the infinite natural variation with prosthetic implants.

Are there gender differences? In addition to the age, weight, and height, which play a major role in interindividual differences, there are other elements linked to anatomical variation. Gender is the first parameter associated with anatomical variability [9–13], with the pelvis exhibiting specific characteristics depending on gender; in females the pelvis is wider and the acetabulum generally deeper with greater anteversion when compared to males: 18° vs. 21° [14] and inclination 38.5° vs. 36° [15] (Fig. 2.3). These differences are partially explained by the developmental

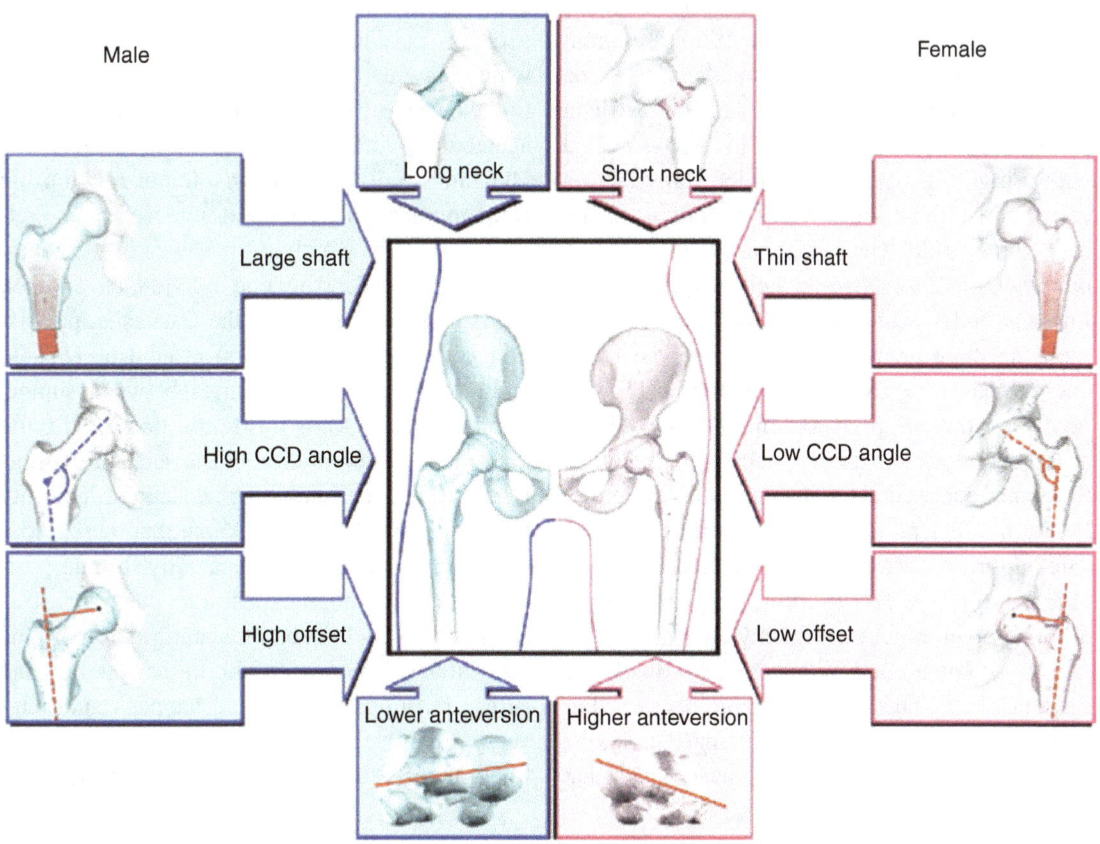

Fig. 2.3 Main gender differences regarding hip morphology [14]

response to the need to give birth, where the birth canal is wider. However, with the broader pelvis, the body-weight lever arm is increased, which is associated with a deeper acetabulum (up to coxa profunda), thus reducing the body-weight lever arm. On the femoral side, females have a smaller femoral head diameter (adjusted for height and weight), a greater femoral anteversion, thinner femoral shaft, and a lower femoral shaft-neck angle with an associated smaller femoral offset when compared to men: 48 mm vs. 55 mm. Another key difference is the lower bone mineral density seen in females, especially after menopause, increasing the risk of peri-prosthetic fracture. These anatomical differences and their impact on joint replacement were quite evident with metal-on-metal hip resurfacing, where the smaller head size and acetabular orientation lead to a higher risk of failure. Differences are also found in the range of motion: women exhibit a greater peak hip flexion and internal rotation (hip at 90° flexion), whereas men show greater peak hip extension and external rotation.

Are there racial/ethnical variants? A number of studies, mainly from the 1950s, reported wider pelvises (both pelvic inlet and outlet) in the Caucasian population compared to the African population. This was thought to be associated with a higher geographic latitude. Many factors can explain these differences in pelvic shape around the world. The climate adaptation theory, which claims that narrower pelvises are seen in lower latitudes, while wider pelvises are seen in more northern areas in order to save heat and energy, has recently gained attention [16]. It questions the original, and until now, widely accepted theory that pelvic shape is the result of the evolutionary compromise (obstetric dilemma) between efficient bipedal locomotion and the safe parturition of a neonate. In reality, it is probable that multiple factors influence pelvic shape, and that environment and lifestyle (e.g., alimentation, activities) are likely to be equally as responsible as ethnical/geographic factors. For example, with regard to the neck-shaft angle, the activity level is a strong determinant, given that the neck tends to become more varus as the activity level increases [9, 10]. Finally, racial differences in sacral geometry and spino-pelvic alignment have already been reported [17] in addition to gender differences [18].

Is there a "normal" hip? Independent of gender or ethnic origin, some constitutional variations are found among us, and they sometimes lead to a pathological process. Acetabular retroversion on plain X-ray can affect 6% of hips in a healthy population and up to 20% and 42% in osteoarthritis and Legg–Perthes–Calve cohorts, respectively [19, 20]. Coxa profunda may affect 5–20% of the whole population [21]. Acetabular retroversion represents a particular form of hip dysplasia, characterized by abnormal posterolateral orientation of the acetabulum. This pathophysiology predisposes the individual to subsequent anterior impingement of the femoral neck upon the anterior acetabular margin and fibrous labrum. Similarly, developmental hip dysplasia has a prevalence of 3.6–4.3% in the healthy adult population [22]. These pathologies can present a technical challenge for prosthetic surgery, particularly in their extreme states, which may involve a combination of hip dislocation, leg length discrepancy, posterior–superior acetabulum defect, and acetabulum retroversion. Dynamic study of the pelvis–femur relationship can complicate the notion of anteversion and retroversion. Firstly, pelvic tilt values in the standing position differ from one individual to another, with an average of 12° in the Caucasian population with standard deviation around 6° [17]. In addition, the pelvic tilt varies between supine, standing, and sitting positions, thus modifying the functional orientation of the acetabulum; this is enabled by the lumbar spine sagittal flexibility [23–25]. Thus, one has to know that these variations cannot be ignored, especially for cup positioning: in the supine position, the pelvis tilts anteriorly, which decreases anteversion of the acetabular component, while in the standing and sitting positions, the reverse happens and anteversion is increased [24, 26]. With regard to the femoral neck-shaft angle, Boese et al. reported in a review article that the interindividual differences in the healthy population can range from 98° to 160° and from 115° to 155° in the osteoarthritic population [27]. This in turn affects the femoral offset, which is directly linked to the neck-shaft angle and femoral neck length. Similarly, femoral torsion can also vary, resulting in anteversion or retroversion of >40°; this may justify the need for 3D templating given regular AP pelvis radiographs are less accurate in assessing femoral torsion and medial offset. In addition to these key reconstruction parameters, the endofemoral canal can take the form of several different shapes, as measured by the femoral flare index and the cortico-medullary index (Fig. 2.4) [28]. This is of particular relevance in cementless fixation, where the need for a close bone–prosthesis interface is essential. One may favor hip resurfacing in some of these more complex situations (Fig. 2.5). In addition, anatomical variations exist in the vascularization of the femoral head, particularly the role of the inferior gluteal and medial femoral circumflex arteries, which are important to consider in hip resurfacing arthroplasty [29]. Each hip is therefore defined by an infinite combination of anatomical and geometric parameters, in addition to its functional capacity.

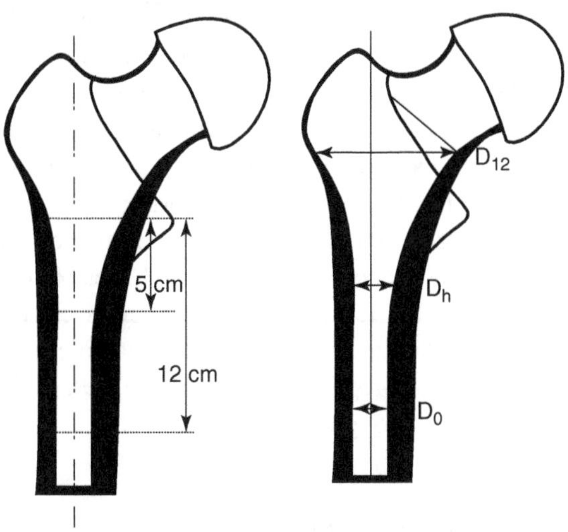

Fig. 2.4 Femoral Flare Index = D0/D12; Cortico-medullary Index = Medial + Lateral cortical thickness/D0

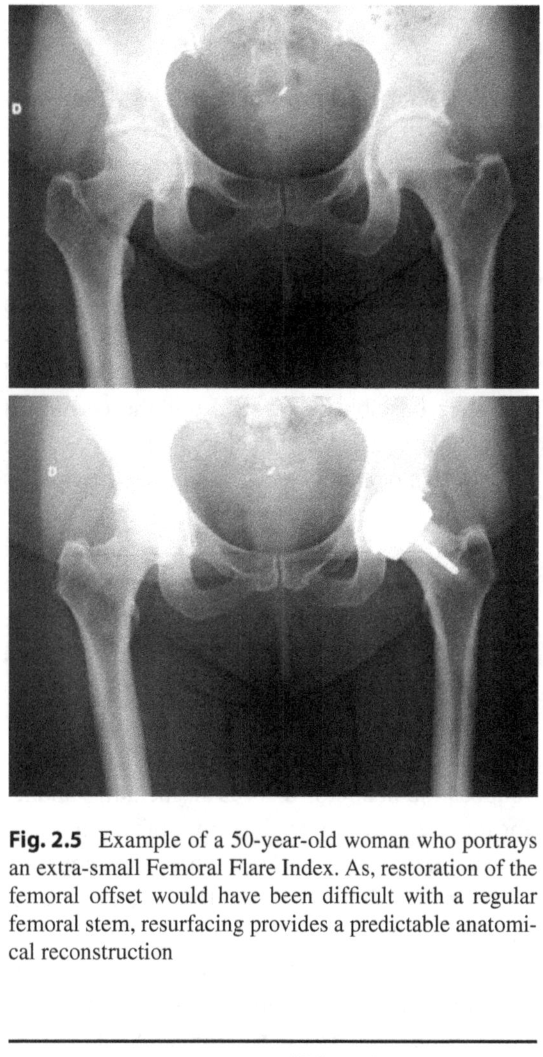

Fig. 2.5 Example of a 50-year-old woman who portrays an extra-small Femoral Flare Index. As, restoration of the femoral offset would have been difficult with a regular femoral stem, resurfacing provides a predictable anatomical reconstruction

2.3 Anatomy Modifications Affecting Clinical Results

2.3.1 Relative to Components' Positioning

Hip replacement and resurfacing aim to achieve sustainable restoration of hip mobility without pain. Component positioning plays a role in every aspect of the clinical outcomes: function, wear rate, occurrence of complication, and components' life span.

Center of rotation. In the frontal plan, the acetabular offset defines the mediolateral location of the center of rotation (Fig. 2.2). By medializing the acetabular component, one reduces the body moment arm, thus decreasing the amount of force generated by the abductors resulting in a decrease in the joint reaction force. However, if done excessively, this can reduce abductor muscle tension, which may need to be adjusted with the femoral offset. Thus, in order to restore the global offset (or the sum of the acetabular and femoral offset) in order to maintain adequate abductor muscle tension, you have to increase the femoral offset [30]. If the global offset decreases, the abductors' tension drops and becomes unstable. Conversely, if the combined offset increases, the abductors' tension will be excessive, potentially yielding more trochanteric pain, and there will be more torque force on the femoral stem, potentially leading to loosening [31] and peri-prosthetic fracture issues. When the center of rotation is lateralized compared to the native one, the femoral offset has to be reduced in order to conserve the original relationship between the greater trochanter and the pelvis. However, reduction of the femoral offset directly reduces the abductor lever arm, meaning abductor muscles have to produce more force in order to stabilize the pelvis. This consequently increases the joint reaction forces and wear at bearing surfaces. A geometric technique has been described to find the theoretical center of rotation by using the U landmark; a constant ratio has been observed between lateral position and height of the center of rotation and pelvis' width and height. Thus, it can be useful in cases where both sides are pathological [32].

Cup orientation. Hip prosthetic surgery entails removing the labrum and decreasing the head size for a THA case. Given this, the hip stability cannot remain the same. The native acetabulum covers the femoral head at 170°, whereas a prosthetic acetabular cup portrays a 180° design (170° or less for resurfacing cups). Thus, cup positioning has to consider stability and avoid prosthetic impingement. Cup positioning must also take into account the influence on wear. Two parameters have to be considered for the position of the cup around its own center of rotation: its inclination and its anteversion. The **cup inclination** will play a role in the edge-loading phenomenon by influencing the CPCR (contact patch center to rim distance) and CPER (contact patch edge to rim distance). The less inclined the cup is, the greater CPCR is in order to avoid edge loading. In addition, edge loading affects the lubrication regime and behavior of synovial fluid, which will further increase wear rates. With regard to **cup anteversion**, it is a major feature for prosthesis' stability, as a more anteverted cup will tend to avoid posterior dislocation. Having said that, cup version is not the only determinant of hip stability, as other factors (e.g., surgical approach, prosthetic design, head diameter, prosthetic neck anteversion) play a major role. Several methods have been described to position the cup during surgery and used either intra- (posterior and anterior rim, transverse acetabular ligament) and/or extra- (anterior pelvic plane) articular anatomical landmarks. Lewinnek initially described the safe cup implantation zone in order to reduce the risk of dislocation. It was defined as a 15° ± 10° anteversion and a 40° ± 10° lateral opening. However, better understanding of the lumbo-pelvic sagittal kinematics and the functional acetabular orientation has challenged the value of the Lewinnek safe zone when compared to a more personalized individual "safe zone" [33, 34]. Arthroplasty is progressively switching from a systematic to a patient-specific approach [33, 34].

Femoral stem positioning. Error in the implantation of the femoral stem will alter the restoration of the native hip anatomy and biomechanics. It's positioning in varus or valgus may either increase or decrease the femoral offset and abductor lever arm and potentially hinder optimal clinical outcomes. In the same manner, error in adjusting the stem version will modify the lever arms, potentially induce impingement, and affect the location of the contact patch between the head and acetabulum. Above all, the leg length discrepancy is clearly directly linked to the femoral stem cranio-caudal positioning and represents the second highest cause of litigation among US surgeons [35].

2.3.2 Relative to Components' Features

As aforementioned, component positioning can modify the native anatomy and biomechanics, but in addition, the components themselves differ from the native anatomy features. On the femoral side, switching from a conchoid shape to a completely spherical shape changes anatomy. It has been shown that this special conchoid shape makes the joint less likely to sublux when compared to a true ball-and-socket joint. Furthermore, these shapes may contribute to the optimal stress magnitude and distribution. Adding to that the fact that the labrum is removed in prosthetic hip surgery, this emphasizes how anatomical concepts can be modified during hip surgery. In normal hip joint biomechanics, the labrum is crucial in retaining a layer of pressurized intra-articular fluid for joint lubrication and load support/distribution. Its seal around the femoral head is further regarded as a contributing factor to hip stability through its suction effect [36]. It is important in increasing the contact area, thereby reducing contact stress as well. For the head diameter, usual prosthetic head size ranges from 22 to 36 mm, whereas the native average head size is 49 mm for women and 53 mm for men. The main drawback of this size reduction is the stability impairment. It is well known nowadays the dislocation rates decrease when the femoral head size increases. Reduction of the femoral head size could also have a negative impact on proprioception. Another point is the head–neck offset modification; its main impacts are on the range of motion and the prosthetic impingement risk (additionally influenced by both cup positioning and femoral stem anteversion). Prosthetic impingement could lead to cup loosening (by increasing torque on the cup), prosthetic instability, increased wear, and liner fracture. A larger femoral head will offer a better head–neck offset and thus will reduce the risk of prosthetic impingement, in addition to facilitate a better range of motion. Several authors showed that this risk becomes negligible with a prosthetic femoral head ≥32 mm [37, 38]. The medial femoral offset is dictated by the femoral stem design, and its restoration is intimately tied to the prosthetic portfolio available. Another element to consider is the modification of Young's modulus of elasticity inside the femoral shaft by using a 15–20 cm length titanium or CoCr alloy stem. It raises questions about proprioception modifications and above all, introduces the stress-shielding concept. Mini-stem designs and resurfacing could lead to better proprioception by enabling natural femoral shaft deformation and elasticity, primarily for patients practicing impact sports (running). Nevertheless, scientific ways to evaluate that kind of hypothesis are limited. Moreover, using a conventional femoral stem, a part of the stress force is directly transferred to the femoral shaft, bypassing the metaphysis area. Nonnatural bone remodeling phenomenon is subsequently involved, modifying the initial bone architecture. Hip resurfacing avoids these drawbacks by preserving a close to natural stress distribution.

2.4 When Is it Safe to Recreate the Constitutional Hip Anatomy?

Osteoarthritis can be primary or secondary. In primary cases, the patient's anatomy is deemed as normal and may be reproduced, whereas for some cases of secondary osteoarthritis, the patient's hip anatomy is considered abnormal, with articular cartilage damage being a consequence of impaired hip biomechanics. As Karimi et al. [39] mentioned, we have to be even more careful with the younger population as the percentage of secondary arthritis is higher among this group. The answer to the question "which constitutional hip anatomies may safely be restored when performing hip replacement?" still remains elusive.

It is important to be aware that most abnormal hip anatomies (CAM effect, abnormal combined anteversion causing pincer femoro-acetabular impingement, roof insufficiency) responsible for hip degeneration are automatically corrected when anatomically implanting modern component designs. Nonetheless, severely abnormal hip anatomy (e.g., atypical femoral and/or acetabular anteversion, protrusio acetabulum) may need to be corrected as they are potentially biomechanically inferior. For individuals with abnormal femur and/or acetabulum anteversion, one should: (1) assess the individual spine–hip relationship to understand the functional acetabular orientation and (2) perform 3D planning with simulated hip ROM, in order to predict the optimal implant positioning and design. For a protrusio acetabuli or a dysplastic acetabulum with roof deficiency, an appropriate center of rotation will have to be reconstructed, which will diverge from the constitutional one. Whatever the severity of the protrusio, the ilio-ischial line remains a good landmark for reconstructing the center of rotation; the goal is to lateralize the hip center in order to avoid instability and prosthetic neck–bone impingement. Any severe defect of the acetabular roof should be corrected by either bone grafting or metallic augmentation, plus or minus a reinforcement ring.

The proximal femoral anatomy is highly variable between individuals. Coxa vara and coxa valga, as well as unusual femoral offset, are anatomic features that generally have to be respected. Aside from cases of developmental hip disease, any modifications of the proximal femur anatomy are likely to hinder optimal clinical outcomes [40]. The surgical solutions to restore these parameters when facing extreme values are detailed below in this chapter. Nevertheless, hip resurfacing appears to be the best means of keeping the natural hip anatomy with regard to the femoral side, although it is technically strenuous. When performing hip resurfacing, special attention must be paid to the constitutional head-to-neck offset of hips, which have degenerated due to cam-type impingement. In order to obtain good and steady results in these cases, surgical correction of this bone impingement is required alongside resurfacing. This is achieved by maximizing and/or moving anteriorly the femoral component, plus or minus osteoplasty of the anterosuperior part of the neck.

Hip osteoarthritis often leads to a true leg length discrepancy due to articular surface wear. One should not ignore the possibility of an additional functional leg length discrepancy from a fixed pelvis obliquity and/or hip stiffness. A sound understanding of these mechanisms is essential to avoid any errors in reestablishing the correct leg length. The length of the femur is a parameter that can be reliability restored by adjusting the craniocaudal positioning of the stem and the head neck length. Nonetheless, we have to bear in mind that our surgery can sometimes lead to functional leg length discrepancy by lengthening the hip (voluntary in case of high-grade dysplasia) or by increasing the global offset (voluntary in case of protrusio). These functional discrepancies are often resolved within a year after surgery as soft tissues progressively remodel.

2.5 Limitations of Implants in Restoring Native Hip Anatomy

There are two kinds of limitations for prosthetic implants. Firstly, there is the compulsory limit set by the **portfolio size**. The size scale is globally limited to the values represented within the 90% in the center of the bell curve. For most femoral stems, the femoral offset increases with the size of the implant; an issue can arise when the patient displays a mismatch between the femoral canal width and the femoral offset (Fig. 2.6). Nevertheless, modularity, especially modular-neck

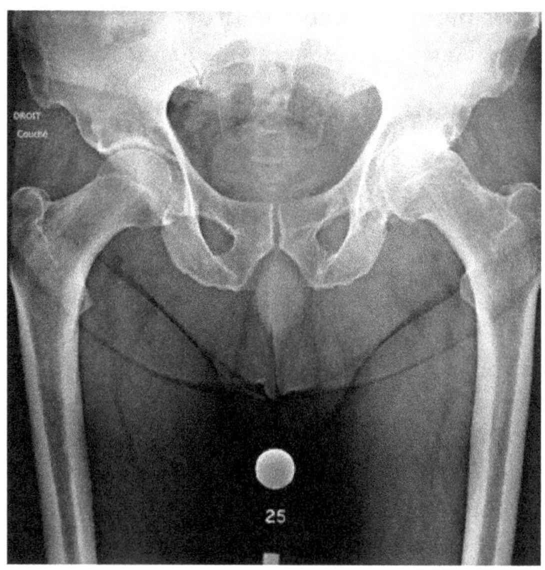

Fig. 2.6 In this case, the patient, a male of 72 years old, portrays an out-of-the-range femoral offset and neck's length whereas he depicts a very narrow femoral canal. Without templating, the error would be to try putting on a regular stem: the chosen size would be necessarily a small one because press fit would be quickly acquired in the femoral canal. In consequence, the femoral offset, tied to the size of the femoral stem would not be restored, as it should. Decision to use a custom femoral implant has been taken (Fig. 2.7)

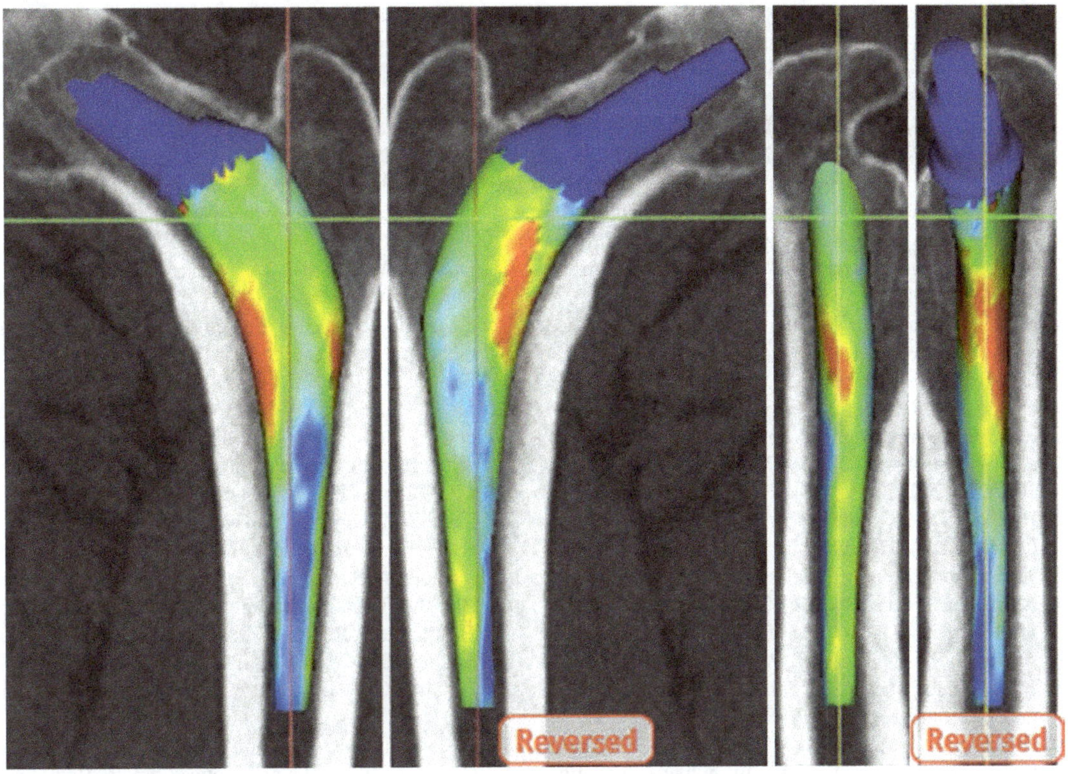

Fig. 2.7 Custom femoral implant designed for patient in Fig. 2.5

femoral stems, has provided a solution in some cases over the last few decades. Secondly, there is an engineering limitation: **excessively long femoral neck**, for example, cannot be safely reproduced by a manufactured implant due to the risk of prosthetic neck fracture. This means that even custom implants can encounter difficulties when dealing with extreme anatomies. As represented in Fig. 2.7, custom implants sometimes enable us to deal with abnormal anatomy, such as extreme coxa vara. However, the cementless fixation mode remains the same (even if the implant design fits the endo-femoral canal), while the torque that the femoral stem has to tolerate becomes higher. Perhaps we should monitor the long-term life span of custom implants made for this kind of use.

2.6 Conclusion

With the technical possibilities currently offered by materials and prosthesis engineering, the need to consider interindividual variation in hip anatomy is gaining recognition among the orthopedic community. There are more and more technical solutions to suit all femoral and acetabular shapes. In parallel, the recent understanding of hip biomechanics, with regard to the dynamic relationship between the femur and acetabulum, has altered our classic view of the anatomy. These concepts present a challenge for each orthopedic surgeon and should be a central point in our future research.

References

1. Menschik F. The hip joint as a conchoid shape. J Biomech. 1997;30(9):971–3.
2. Gu D-Y, Hu F, Wei J-H, Dai K-R, Chen Y-Z. Contributions of non-spherical hip joint cartilage surface to hip joint contact stress. Conf Proc IEEE Eng Med Biol Soc. 2011;2011:8166–9.
3. Dujardin F, Selva O, Mejjad O, Pasero D, Piraux JL, Thomine JM. Intra and interindividual variations of pelvic mobility in normal adult walk. Rev Chir Orthop Reparatrice Appar Mot. 1995;81(7):592–600.

4. Bergmann G, Deuretzbacher G, Heller M, Graichen F, Rohlmann A, Strauss J, et al. Hip contact forces and gait patterns from routine activities. J Biomech. 2001;34(7):859–71.
5. Sánchez Egea AJ, Valera M, Parraga Quiroga JM, Proubasta I, Noailly J, Lacroix D. Impact of hip anatomical variations on the cartilage stress: a finite element analysis towards the biomechanical exploration of the factors that may explain primary hip arthritis in morphologically normal subjects. Clin Biomech. 2014;29(4):444–50.
6. Dorr LD, Malik A, Dastane M, Wan Z. Combined anteversion technique for total hip arthroplasty. Clin Orthop. 2009;467(1):119–27.
7. Underwood RJ, Zografos A, Sayles RS, Hart A, Cann P. Edge loading in metal-on-metal hips: low clearance is a new risk factor. Proc Inst Mech Eng H. 2012;226(3):217.
8. Hart AJ, Ilo K, Underwood R, Cann P, Henckel J, Lewis A, et al. The relationship between the angle of version and rate of wear of retrieved metal-on-metal resurfacings: a prospective, CT-based study. J Bone Joint Surg Br. 2011;93(3):315–20.
9. Anderson JY, Trinkaus E. Patterns of sexual, bilateral and interpopulational variation in human femoral neck-shaft angles. J Anat. 1998;192(Pt 2):279–85.
10. Gilligan I, Chandraphak S, Mahakkanukrauh P. Femoral neck-shaft angle in humans: variation relating to climate, clothing, lifestyle, sex, age and side. J Anat. 2013;223(2):133–51.
11. Milligan DJ, O'Brien S, Bennett D, Hill JC, Beverland DE. The effects of age and gender on the diameter of the femoral canal in patients who undergo total hip replacement. Bone Jt J. 2013;95-B(3):339–42.
12. Tannenbaum E, Kopydlowski N, Smith M, Bedi A, Sekiya JK. Gender and racial differences in focal and global acetabular version. J Arthroplast. 2014;29(2):373–6.
13. Wang SC, Brede C, Lange D, Poster CS, Lange AW, Kohoyda-Inglis C, et al. Gender differences in hip anatomy: possible implications for injury tolerance in frontal collisions. Annu Proc Assoc Adv Automot Med. 2004;48:287.
14. Nakahara I, Takao M, Sakai T, Nishii T, Yoshikawa H, Sugano N. Gender differences in 3D morphology and bony impingement of human hips. J Orthop Res Off Publ Orthop Res Soc. 2011;29(3):333–9.
15. Traina F, De Clerico M, Biondi F, Pilla F, Tassinari E, Toni A. Sex differences in hip morphology: is stem modularity effective for total hip replacement? J Bone Joint Surg Am. 2009;91(Suppl 6):121–8.
16. DeSilva JM, Rosenberg KR. Anatomy, development, and function of the human pelvis. Anat Rec Hoboken NJ. 2017;300(4):628–32.
17. Endo K, Suzuki H, Nishimura H, Tanaka H, Shishido T, Yamamoto K. Characteristics of sagittal spinopelvic alignment in Japanese young adults. Asian Spine J. 2014;8(5):599.
18. Legaye J, Duval-Beaupère G, Hecquet J, Marty C. Pelvic incidence: a fundamental pelvic parameter for three-dimensional regulation of spinal sagittal curves. Eur Spine J. 1998;7(2):99–103.
19. Wassilew GI, Heller MO, Janz V, Perka C, Müller M, Renner L. High prevalence of acetabular retroversion in asymptomatic adults: a 3D CT-based study. Bone Jt J. 2017;99-B(12):1584–9.
20. Krebs V, Incavo SJ, Shields WH. The anatomy of the acetabulum: what is normal? Clin Orthop. 2009;467(4):868.
21. Diesel CV, Ribeiro TA, Coussirat C, Scheidt RB, Macedo CA, Galia CR. Coxa profunda in the diagnosis of pincer-type femoroacetabular impingement and its prevalence in asymptomatic subjects. Bone Jt J. 2015;97-B(4):478–83.
22. Tian F-D, Zhao D-W, Wang W, Guo L, Tian S-M, Feng A, et al. Prevalence of developmental dysplasia of the hip in Chinese adults: a cross-sectional survey. Chin Med J. 2017;130(11):1261–8.
23. Shon WY, Gupta S, Biswal S, Hur CY, Jajodia N, Hong SJ, et al. Validation of a simple radiographic method to determine variations in pelvic and acetabular cup sagittal plane alignment after total hip arthroplasty. Skelet Radiol. 2008;37(12):1119–27.
24. Eddine TA, Migaud H, Chantelot C, Cotten A, Fontaine C, Duquennoy A. Variations of pelvic anteversion in the lying and standing positions: analysis of 24 control subjects and implications for CT measurement of position of a prosthetic cup. Surg Radiol Anat SRA. 2001;23(2):105–10.
25. Lazennec J-Y, Rousseau M-A, Brusson A, Folinais D, Amel M, Clarke I, et al. Total hip prostheses in standing, sitting and squatting positions: an overview of our 8 years practice using the EOS imaging technology. Open Orthop J. 2015;9:26–44.
26. Grammatopoulos G, Gofton W, Cochran M, Dobransky J, Carli A, Abdelbary H, et al. Pelvic positioning in the supine position leads to more consistent orientation of the acetabular component after total hip arthroplasty. Bone Jt J. 2018;100-B(10): 1280–8.
27. Boese CK, Dargel J, Oppermann J, Eysel P, Scheyerer MJ, Bredow J, et al. The femoral neck-shaft angle on plain radiographs: a systematic review. Skelet Radiol. 2016;45(1):19–28.
28. Fessy MH, Seutin B, Béjui J. Anatomical basis for the choice of the femoral implant in the total hip arthroplasty. Surg Radiol Anat. 1997;19(5):283–6.
29. Beaulé PE, Campbell P, Lu Z, Leunig-Ganz K, Beck M, Leunig M, et al. Vascularity of the arthritic femoral head and hip resurfacing. J Bone Joint Surg Am. 2006;88(Suppl 4):85–96.
30. Scheerlinck T. Cup positioning in total hip arthroplasty. Acta Orthop Belg. 2014;80(3):336–47.
31. Lecerf G, Fessy MH, Philippot R, Massin P, Giraud F, Flecher X, et al. Femoral offset: anatomical concept, definition, assessment, implications for preoperative templating and hip arthroplasty. Orthop Traumatol Surg Res. 2009;95(3):210–9.
32. Pierchon F, Migaud H, Duquennoy A, Fontaine C. Radiologic evaluation of the rotation center of

the hip. Rev Chir Orthop Reparatrice Appar Mot. 1993;79(4):281–4.

33. Rivière C, Lazennec J-Y, Van Der Straeten C, Auvinet E, Cobb J, Muirhead-Allwood S. The influence of spine-hip relations on total hip replacement: a systematic review. Orthop Traumatol Surg Res. 2017;103(4):559–68.
34. Murphy WS, Yun HH, Hayden B, Kowal JH, Murphy SB. The safe zone range for cup anteversion is narrower than for inclination in THA. Clin Orthop. 2018;476(2):325–35.
35. Upadhyay A, York S, Macaulay W, McGrory B, Robbennolt J, Bal BS. Medical malpractice in hip and knee arthroplasty. J Arthroplast. 2007;22(6 Suppl):2–7.e4.
36. Bsat S, Frei H, Beaulé PE. The acetabular labrum: a review of its function. Bone Jt J. 2016;98-B(6):730–5.
37. Crowninshield RD, Maloney WJ, Wentz DH, Humphrey SM, Blanchard CR. Biomechanics of large femoral heads: what they do and don't do. Clin Orthop. 2004;429:102–7.
38. Matsushita I, Morita Y, Ito Y, Gejo R, Kimura T. Activities of daily living after total hip arthroplasty. Is a 32-mm femoral head superior to a 26-mm head for improving daily activities? Int Orthop. 2011;35(1):25–9.
39. Karimi D, Kallemose T, Troelsen A, Klit J. Hip malformation is a very common finding in young patients scheduled for total hip arthroplasty. Arch Orthop Trauma Surg. 2018;138(4):581–9.
40. Fottner A, Peter CV, Schmidutz F, Wanke-Jellinek L, Schröder C, Mazoochian F, et al. Biomechanical evaluation of different offset versions of a cementless hip prosthesis by 3-dimensional measurement of micromotions. Clin Biomech Bristol Avon. 2011;26(8):830–5.

3

Advancements and Future of Hip Arthroplasty

Charles Rivière, Ciara Harman, Kartik Logishetty, and Catherine Van Der Straeten

Key Points

- Improvements in implant design and surgical techniques have dramatically reduced the risk of complications, thus reducing the risk of revision surgery while enabling a return to high level of function.
- Complications related to poor components' interaction remain with traditional alignment techniques, despite the more precise implantation of components facilitated by technological assistance.
- Complications related to poor components' interaction are poorly predicted by the radiographic appearance of implant position but have been shown to be correlated with the patient's spinopelvic mobility.
- Personalized strategies for hip arthroplasty taking into account lumbopelvic kinematics and constitutional hip anatomy are under investigation.
- By generating a physiological prosthetic hip (from anatomical restoration of the native) and by optimizing the components interaction during activities of daily living (from selecting a cup orientation that fits the spine flexibility), the kinematic alignment technique for hip replacement may perfect clinical outcomes of prosthetic hip.

C. Rivière (✉)
The MSK Lab-Imperial College London, White City Campus, London, UK

South West London Elective Orthopaedic Centre, Epsom, UK

C. Harman
South West London Elective Orthopaedic Centre, Epsom, UK

K. Logishetty
The MSK Lab-Imperial College London, White City Campus, London, UK
e-mail: k.logishetty@imperial.ac.uk

C. Van Der Straeten
Ghent University Hospital, Corneel Heymanslaan 10, Ghent, Belgium

3.1 Evolution of Hip Implant Designs

There have been significant developments since the first attempts to treat degenerated hips with tissue interpositional arthroplasty (with materials such as fascia lata and pig's bladder) or hemi-resurfacing using glass molds by Smith-Peterson in 1937 [1]. While the first total hip replacement has been attributed to Wiles in 1938, it was considered a failure—its success and widespread adoption only occurred in the 1960s when Sir John Charnley introduced "low-friction arthroplasty" using acrylic cement for fixation. This early age of hip arthroplasty has been followed by decades of incremental development directed at reducing failure (including that related to loosening, instability, implant wear, and osteolysis) while accommodating the high-activity profile and increased longevity of the modern patient [1].

Cemented stem designs were progressively refined with distinction between the *taper slip and composite beam* concepts [2]. Modern techniques for cementing were developed with the use of pulsatile lavage, retrograde femoral canal cement filling, and cement pressurization, but also an appreciation that both the *English and French cementing techniques* can deliver excellent results [3]. The French technique consists of completely emptying the medullary canal of cancellous bone and implanting a canal-filling femoral component for line-to-line fit, with a thin cement mantle mainly acting as a void filler. This principle—termed the "French paradox"—runs contrary to the perceived wisdom that cement mantles should have a minimal thickness of 2–4 mm and should be complete (English cementation technique). Yet, it is a user-friendly technique that has led to reproducible good long-term clinical outcomes with Charnley-Kerboull and Ceraver Osteal type stems [3].

Uncemented implant designs were developed to solve the issue of osteolysis that was initially but wrongly attributed to cement debris (so-called "cement disease"). Early cementless stem designs were suboptimal because they were excessively stiff (cylindrical shape and chrome-cobalt alloy) and prone to diaphyseal fixation due to extensive coating. A high rate of mid-thigh pain and proximal bone loss from stress shielding were therefore observed [4]. Subsequent stem designs were designed to be *more flexible* (non-cylindrical shape and titanium-based alloy) and many are partially coated for greater *proximal fixation* and load transfer [4]. Contemporary uncemented stems are either *tapered, cylindrical, or anatomical*. This latter group of anatomic design stems closely fill the metaphysis; this promotes physiological load distribution but does not allow intraoperative adjustment of femoral anteversion (Fig. 3.1).

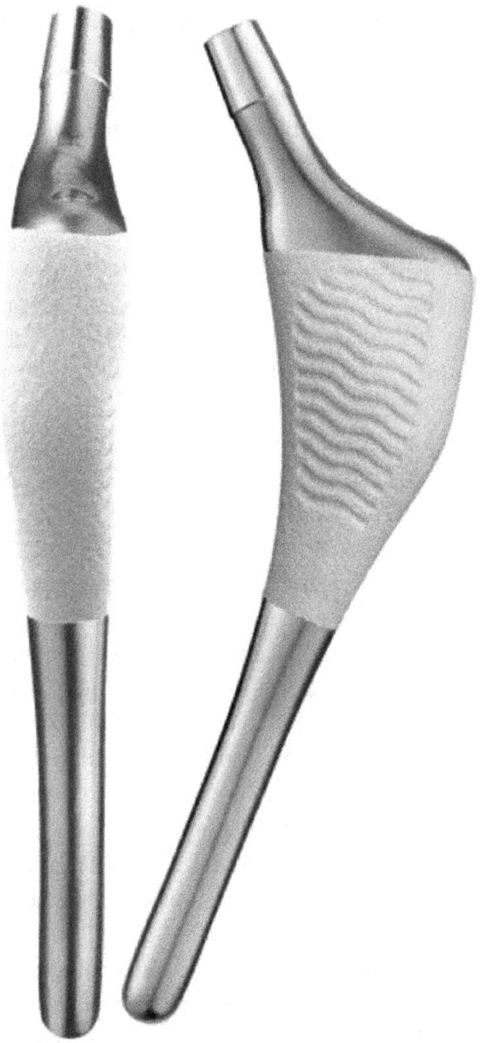

Fig. 3.1 Anatomical femoral stem

Similar to the evolution of cementless stems, first-generation uncemented cups were poorly designed and had a high rate of failure. A suboptimal locking mechanism design permitted excessive micromotion between the liner and the metal back. This generated a high amount of polyethylene debris and subsequent osteolysis and aseptic loosening [1]. At revision, it was noted that early component designs had a significant amount of fibrous tissue at the bone–implant interface. *Hydroxyapatite* coating was therefore introduced to cementless cups to enhance bone ingrowth and stimulate bony gap closure [5].

In the 1980s, the realization that osteolysis was caused by a host reaction against polyethylene wear particles and not cement debris shifted the focus to reducing bearing surface wear [1]. First-generation ultrahigh molecular weight polyethylene (UHMWPE) had a low abrasive wear resistance and was therefore vulnerable to volumetric wear. The generated debris was responsible for triggering a macrophagic response in periprosthetic tissue, and bone resorption by activated osteoclasts. Low-wear *highly cross-linked polyethylene* have since been introduced alongside *alternative bearings* either made of ceramic or metal (cobalt chromium) or, more recently, in Oxinium™—a ceramicized metal alloy [1]. After decades of developments—including four generations of ceramic—modern bearing couples of metal-on-highly X-linked polyethylene, ceramic-on-highly X-linked polyethylene, and ceramic-on-ceramic are now recognized as the most reliable options [1, 6, 7].

Increasing the femoral head diameter improves the interaction between the head and cup components by increasing jump distance and stability and reducing the risk of microseparation, edge loading, prosthetic impingement, and dislocation [8, 9]. This increase in contact surface area is tolerated by modern bearing couples as they are resistant to abrasive wear, while with first-generation UHMWPE abrasive wear was higher with larger diameter femoral heads. When used with total hip implants, recent designs of metal-on-metal large-diameter bearings have been shown to result in high torque and excessive fretting corrosion at the head–neck junction (trunnionosis) with subsequent clinically deleterious adverse reactions to metal debris [1]. When used for hip resurfacing, the same metal-on-metal bearings were demonstrated to be safe in well-designed and well-positioned implants, i.e., avoiding edge loading [1, 6, 7]. In order to prevent the risk of ceramic liner fracture and promote ceramic-on-ceramic large-diameter bearings for total hip replacement, *monoblock ceramic cups* with a pre-assembled ceramic liner housed within a metal back were developed (Fig. 3.2). These have good midterm clinical outcomes despite frequent noise generation (squeaking), which have a negligible clinical impact [10–12].

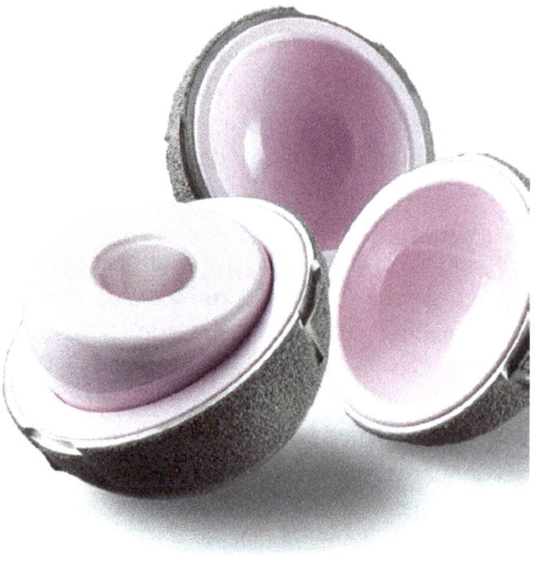

Fig. 3.2 Monoblock ceramic acetabular cup

Another innovation designed to reduce the risk of dislocation is the dual mobility cup design (Fig. 3.3) [13]. Bousquet and Rambert posited that by introducing a mobile articulation between the cup and head, patients could have a higher range of impingement-free movement. Emerging clinical results suggest that dual mobility cups can reduce the incidence of dislocation in primary and revision hip arthroplasty and may be useful in primary total hip arthroplasty in patients with limited spino-pelvic mobility, neuromuscular disease, or soft tissue problems [14, 15].

Finally, femoral neck preserving short stem designs (Fig. 3.4) [16], which favor preservation of proximal femur anatomy and bone stock, and minimally invasive surgery have also shown good midterm outcomes since the turn of the century. The expected benefits of more physiological metaphyseal loading, faster recovery, reduced late periprosthetic fracture, easier revision, when compared to conventional stem design, remain to be proven [16].

All of these developments have contributed to the success of hip replacement surgery and its qualification as the "operation of the century" [1]. Return to normal function and satisfaction are generally obtained, with implants survival of 95% at 14 years reported in the National Joint

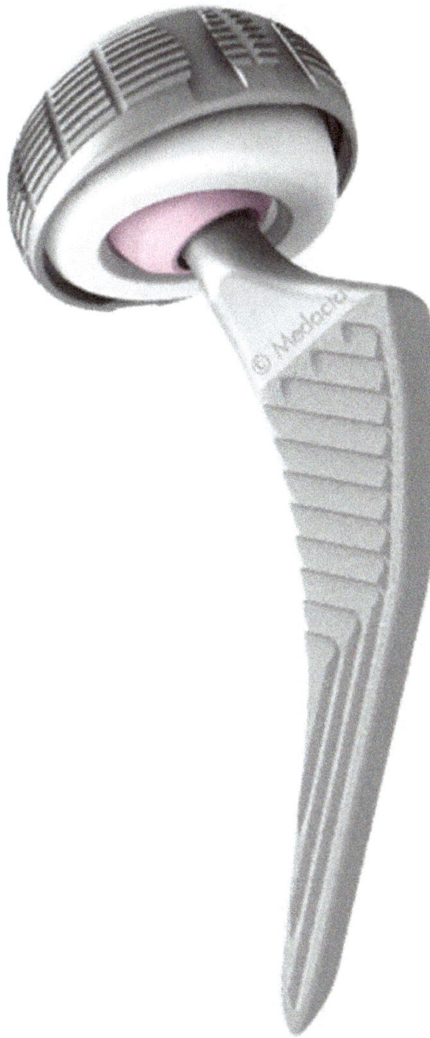

Fig. 3.3 A dual-mobility cup articulating with a ceramic head inserted on a cementless stem

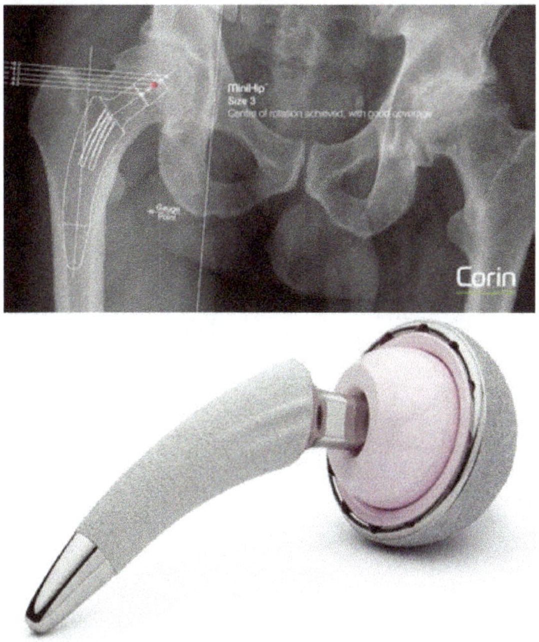

Fig. 3.4 A short femoral stem which loads only proximal bone by fixation in the femoral neck and metaphysis

Registry, regardless of the type of fixation and bearing (the exception being for certain large metal on metal bearings) [6, 7].

3.2 Evolution of Instrumentation for Implanting Hip Components

The precise orientation of implants has traditionally been dependent on a surgeon's visuospatial ability, with the help of basic instruments like alignment rods. Technological assistance could enable surgeons to increase reproducibility for positioning components, restoring constitutional hip biomechanics and impingement-free range of motion, and thus improving patient outcomes. Computer navigation systems, patient-specific instrumentation (Fig. 3.5), and robotics have been successively introduced with this goal in mind [1, 6]. Patient-specific instrumentation (PSI) requires preoperative 3D imaging and computer-aided design (CAD) planning to create patient-specific cutting guides so that the surgeon can precisely size and position components to the preoperative plan. In contrast, computer navigation systems and robotics assist implantation through intraoperative 3D planning and then either guiding the position of the cutting blocks (computer navigation) or performing the cut (robotics). Slight displacement of the cutting blocks can occur when they are fixed to the bone with pins or during the bone cut by the saw. Robotics are thus considered to be more precise than computer navigation systems as they typically do not use cutting blocks; instead, power to the saw, reamer, or burr is terminated when placed in an orientation or position outside of the surgical plan. While

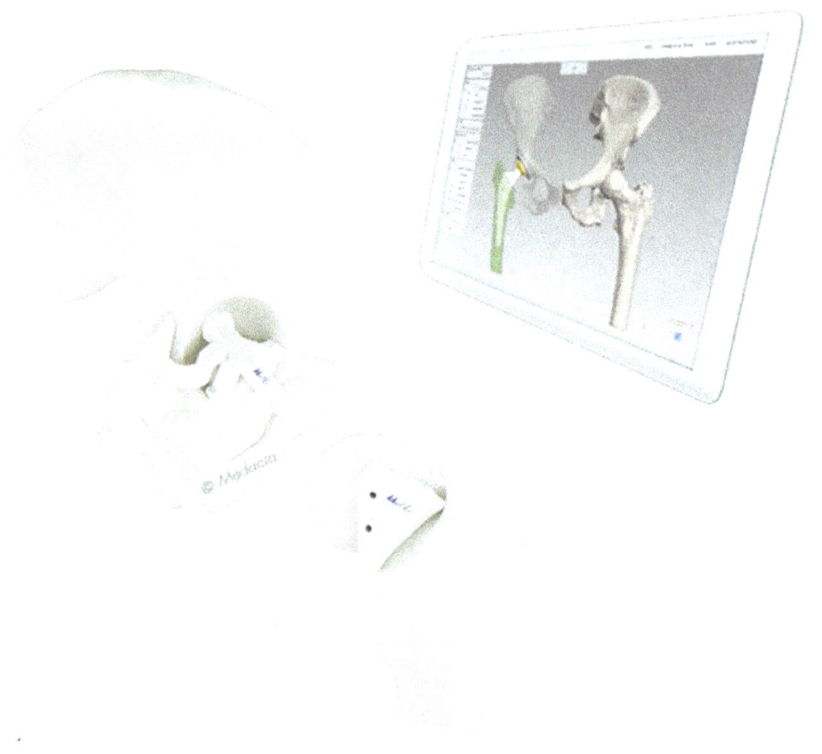

Fig. 3.5 Patient-specific instrumentation—this cutting guide is 3D printed to match the patient's anatomy and deliver a planned cup orientation and femoral neck osteotomy

there is little doubt that these technologies improve surgical precision, their clinical benefit is yet to be proven compared to manual techniques for implanting components [6].

3.3 Evolution of Hip Approaches

The hip may be accessed through multiple anatomical routes to perform arthroplasty, typically via posterior, lateral, superior, or anterior surgical approaches. Access, by definition, disrupts the integrity of periarticular soft tissues, which in turn slows recovery after joint replacement and may sometimes be directly responsible for complications (e.g., instability, residual limp, pain, and heterotopic ossification). Minimally invasive surgical approaches such as the mini-posterior or the muscle-sparing approaches (including the Direct Anterior, Rottinger, SupraPath) were developed to reduce these issues (Fig. 3.6) [1, 17]. Their execution has been facilitated by the development of specific instrumentation and short femoral stem designs [16]. Compared to traditional approaches, minimally invasive surgical

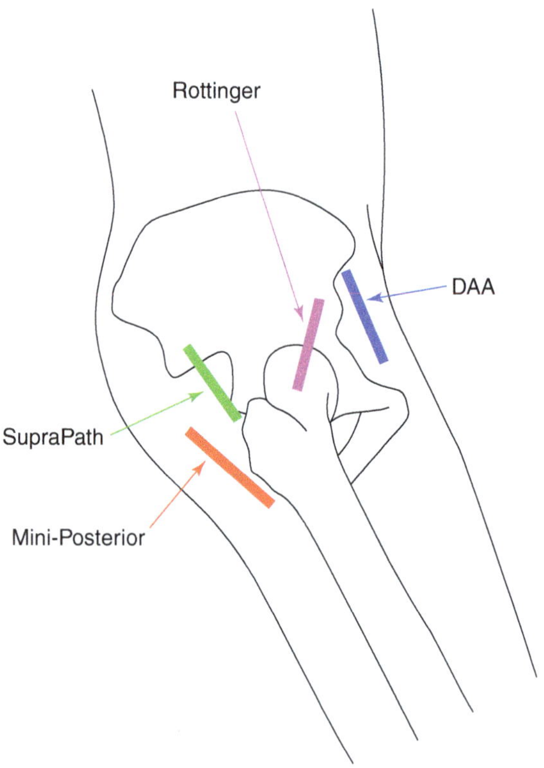

Fig. 3.6 Common minimally invasive surgical approaches to perform a hip replacement. *DAA* Direct anterior approach

approaches have shown to be more technically demanding with subsequent longer learning curves, but can speedup recovery while keeping the dislocation rate similarly low [6, 17, 18].

3.4 Evolution of Techniques for Aligning Hip Components

The **'mechanical alignment' technique** (Fig. 3.7), defined half a century ago, is considered to be the gold standard technique for implanting total hip components [19, 20]. It focuses on achieving a set biomechanical goal, while disregarding individual patient anatomy [19, 21]. The hip's center of rotation is medialized to reduce stress on implants, and components are systematically oriented in universal "safe zones." The goal is to obtain a 15° and 40° radiographic cup anteversion and inclination, respectively, and to position the femoral stem with a 10° to 15° anteversion relative to the posterior condylar line [19–21]. Technological assistance has increased the reproducibility in positioning the cup, by defining the anterior pelvic plane and considering its tilt in either the supine or the standing positions; in this way, the concept of *functional cup positioning* was born [20, 22, 23].

Alternative concepts of combined anteversion [20, 24] and anatomical implantation [25–30] have gained relevance since the increased uptake of cementless femoral component. Cementless stems must obtain a stable press fit to obtain bone fixation, and thus adapt to the highly variable proximal femoral canal geometry. Therefore, unlike during implantation of cemented stems, there is limited ability to adjust femoral anteversion, and a greater risk of prosthetic impingement if the cup is systematically placed [7, 8, 31–33]. An increased awareness of this dynamic interplay between the acetabular and femoral components

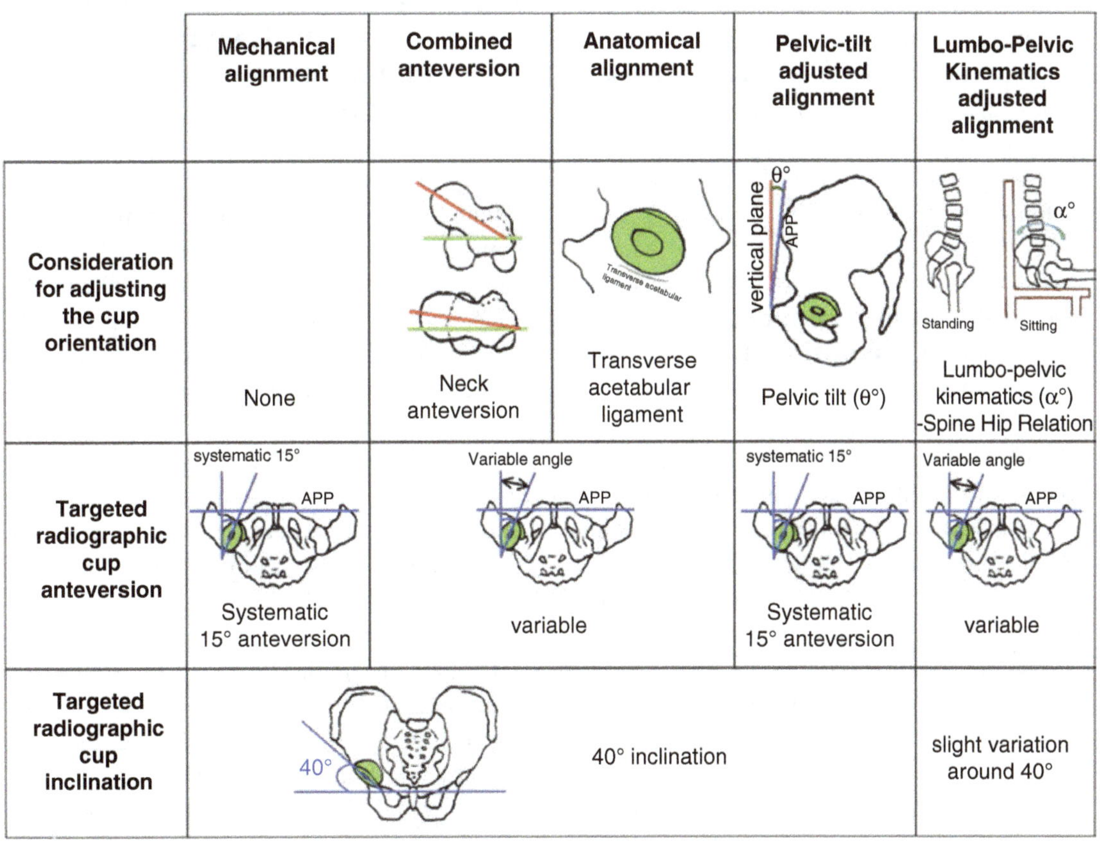

Fig. 3.7 This Figure illustrates the multiple techniques for aligning the acetabular component. *APP* Anterior pelvic plane

[34, 35] led to the development of the *combined anteversion technique* [24]: the femur is prepared first—with the final rasp left in place while preparing the acetabulum. The chosen cup anteversion angle depends on the observed stem anteversion, and the resulting combined anteversion is typically between 30° and 40°.

In contrast, the concept of *anatomic implantation* [25–30] of hip prostheses aims to restore the native hip anatomy with a focus on anatomical cup anteversion and restoration of hip center of rotation. The main rationale for an anatomical cup positioning is the limited ability to calculate an ideal cup orientation from preoperative images due to the multiple acetabular functional orientations and femoro-acetabular interplay combinations that an individual displays during ADLs [36–38]. It relies on intraoperative parameters such as the transverse acetabular ligament [25] and the use of calipers to precisely measure offset and neck length to define center of rotation. Anatomic implantation aims to restore native hip anatomy and improve prosthetic hip function and patient satisfaction by achieving physiological periprosthetic soft tissue balance and hip kinematics [29, 39]. The use of the neck-preserving femoral components (including resurfacing [27] or neck-sparing stem designs [16, 28]) facilitates anatomical restoration.

3.5 Residual Complications with Conventional Implantation

Although hip arthroplasty is considered a very successful procedure, and named the "operation of the century," there remain some residual complications [7, 31–33, 38]. Component loosening, late periprosthetic fracture, instability (0–10%) [6, 7], and residual pain in the absence of obvious complication (in 10–20%) [31] are reported, suggesting that there is still room for significant improvement in implant design, techniques, and implementation of technology. Failures leading to revision surgery remain excessive and vary from 3% to 8% at 14 years postoperatively [6, 7]. The main indications for revision surgery are aseptic loosening (48% of revisions), followed by dislocation (15%), periprosthetic fracture (10%), and then sepsis (9%) [6, 7]. The risk and indication for revision surgery dramatically vary with patient age at the time of primary surgery, with younger patients more likely to require revision surgery [6, 7]. Men implanted in their early 50s have a 30% lifetime revision risk compared to approximately 20% and 10% if the same primary replacement had occurred in their early 60s or 70s, respectively [7]. Many of these residual complications have been primarily related to poor component interaction, i.e., to the frequent occurrence of edge loading [33] and prosthetic impingement [32, 38, 39]. These may be mitigated by the use of more forgiving (tolerant to edge loading and prosthetic impingement) implants and/or more personalized surgical techniques for implanting hip components.

3.6 A Personalized Implantation May be the Next Step for Improvement of Clinical Outcomes

The risks of prosthetic edge loading, prosthetic impingement, dislocation, and suboptimal prosthetic hip function have been shown to be significantly influenced by the condition of the lumbar spine (individual spine–hip relationship) [14, 40–43]. In contrast, those risks remain poorly predicted by the radiographic orientation of conventionally aligned cup [10, 12, 14, 32, 35, 44, 45]. Despite our ability to precisely position implants using PSI, navigation, and robotic technology, there is limited evidence that they reduce dislocation or improve impingement-free range of motion [6, 46]. This may be a consequence of a consistent standard (excessively systematic) technique of implantation, with insufficient attention paid to the many unique aspects that characterize each patient including their hip anatomy and kinematics. The truly "safe" acetabular target for avoiding impingement and edge loading is much smaller than previously understood and varies considerably between patients [36, 37, 47, 48], thus supporting a personalized philosophy for the choice of implant and placement of the components.

To improve clinical outcomes of hip replacement for the next century, we advocate for a more personalized implantation that considers lumbar spine kinematics/spine-hip relationship [49–52] and hip constitutional anatomy [19, 51, 52] for a physiological and biomechanically sound hip arthroplasty. Surgical approach, implant design, and orientation should be dependent on a patient's unique anatomical and kinematic characteristics, and technological assistance can then be harnessed to precisely execute this patient-specific plan. By generating a physiological prosthetic hip (from anatomical restoration of the native) and by optimizing the components interaction during activities of daily living (from selecting a cup orientation that fits the spine flexibility), the kinematic alignment technique for hip replacement may perfect clinical outcomes of prosthetic hip. Precise kinematic alignment of forgiving, hard-wearing modern hip components may reach the ultimate goal of hip arthroplasty, which is generating a reproducible, durable, 'forgotten' prosthetic hip, and probably represents the future of hip arthroplasty.

References

1. Learmonth ID, Young C, Rorabeck C. The operation of the century: total hip replacement. Lancet. 2007;370(9597):1508–19.
2. Scheerlinck T, Casteleyn P-P. The design features of cemented femoral hip implants. J Bone Joint Surg Br. 2006;88-B(11):1409–18.
3. Langlais F, Kerboull M, Sedel L, Ling RSM. The 'French paradox'. J Bone Joint Surg Br. 2003;85-B(1):17–20.
4. Rivière C, Grappiolo G, Engh CA, Vidalain J-P, Chen A-F, Boehler N, et al. Long-term bone remodelling around 'legendary' cementless femoral stems. EFORT Open Rev. 2018;3(2):45–57.
5. Jaffe W, Scott D. Rationale and clinical application of hydroxyapatite coatings in pressfit total hip arthroplasty. Semin Arthroplast. 1993;4(3):159–66.
6. Ferguson RJ, Palmer AJ, Taylor A, Porter ML, Malchau H, Glyn-Jones S. Hip replacement. Lancet. 2018;392(10158):1662–71.
7. Commitee NS. National Joint Registry for England, Wales, Northern Ireland and the Isle of Man: 15th annual report, 2017. National Joint Registry Centre. 2018.
8. McCarthy TF, Nevelos J, Elmallah RK, Chughtai M, Khlopas A, Alipit V, et al. The effect of pelvic tilt and femoral head size on hip range-of-motion to impingement. J Arthroplast. 2017;32(11):3544–9.
9. Ezquerra L, Quilez MP, Pérez MÁ, Albareda J, Seral B. Range of movement for impingement and dislocation avoidance in total hip replacement predicted by finite element model. J Med Biol Eng. 2017;37(1):26–34.
10. Blakeney WG, Beaulieu Y, Puliero B, Lavigne M, Roy A, Massé V, et al. Excellent results of large-diameter ceramic-on-ceramic bearings in total hip arthroplasty. Bone Joint J. 2018;100(11):8.
11. McDonnell SM, Boyce G, Baré J, Young D, Shimmin AJ. The incidence of noise generation arising from the large-diameter Delta motion ceramic total hip bearing. Bone Jt J. 2013;95-B(2):160–5.
12. Tai SM, Munir S, Walter WL, Pearce SJ, Walter WK, Zicat BA. Squeaking in large diameter ceramic-on-ceramic bearings in total hip arthroplasty. J Arthroplast. 2015;30(2):282–5.
13. Heffernan C, Banerjee S, Nevelos J, Macintyre J, Issa K, Markel DC, et al. Does dual-mobility cup geometry affect posterior horizontal dislocation distance? Clin Orthop Relat Res. 2014;472(5):1535–44.
14. Dagneaux L, Marouby S, Maillot C, Canovas F, Rivière C. Dual mobility device reduces the risk of prosthetic hip instability for patients with degenerated spine: A case-control study. Orthop Traumatol Surg Res. 2019;105(3):461–6.
15. Darrith B, Courtney PM, Della Valle CJ. Outcomes of dual mobility components in total hip arthroplasty: a systematic review of the literature. Bone Jt J. 2018;100-B(1):11–9.
16. Khanuja HS, Banerjee S, Jain D, Pivec R, Mont MA. Short bone-conserving stems in cementless hip arthroplasty. J Bone Jt Surg Am. 2014;96(20):1742–52.
17. Mogliorini F, Biagini M, Rath B. Total hip arthroplasty: minimally invasive surgery or not? Meta-analysis of clinical trials. Int Orthop. 2018;43(7):1573–82.
18. Connolly KP, Kamath AF. Direct anterior total hip arthroplasty: comparative outcomes and contemporary results. World J Orthop. 2016;7(2):94.
19. Rivière C, Lazic S, Villet L, Wiart Y, Allwood SM, Cobb J. Kinematic alignment technique for total hip and knee arthroplasty: the personalized implant positioning surgery. EFORT Open Rev. 2018;3(3):98–105.
20. Bhaskar D, Rajpura A, Board T. Current concepts in acetabular positioning in total hip arthroplasty. Indian J Orthop. 2017;51(4):386.
21. Lazennec JY, Thauront F, Robbins CB, Pour AE. Acetabular and femoral anteversions in standing position are outside the proposed safe zone after total hip arthroplasty. J Arthroplast. 2017;32(11):3550–6.
22. Meftah M, Yadav A, Wong AC, Ranawat AS, Ranawat CS. A novel method for accurate and reproducible functional cup positioning in total hip arthroplasty. J Arthroplast. 2013;28(7):1200–5.

23. Maratt JD, Esposito CI, McLawhorn AS, Jerabek SA, Padgett DE, Mayman DJ. Pelvic tilt in patients undergoing total hip arthroplasty: when does it matter? J Arthroplast. 2015;30(3):387–91.
24. Dorr LD, Malik A, Dastane M, Wan Z. Combined anteversion technique for total hip arthroplasty. Clin Orthop Relat Res. 2009;467(1):119–27.
25. Archbold HAP, Mohammed M, O'Brien S, Molloy D, McCONWAY J, Beverland DE. Limb length restoration during total hip arthroplasty: use of a caliper to control femoral component insertion and accurate acetabular placement relative to the transverse acetabular ligament. Hip Int. 2006;16(1):33–8.
26. Hill JC, Archbold HAP, Diamond OJ, Orr JF, Jaramaz B, Beverland DE. Using a calliper to restore the Centre of the femoral head during total hip replacement. J Bone Joint Surg Br. 2012;94-B(11):1468–74.
27. Girard J, Lons A, Ramdane N, Putman S. Hip resurfacing before 50 years of age: a prospective study of 979 hips with a mean follow-up of 5.1 years. Orthop Traumatol Surg Res. 2018;104(3):295–9.
28. Shin Y-S, Suh D-H, Park J-H, Kim J-L, Han S-B. Comparison of specific femoral short stems and conventional-length stems in primary cementless total hip arthroplasty. Orthopedics. 2016;39(2):e311–7.
29. Patel AB, Wagle RR, Usrey MM, Thompson MT, Incavo SJ, Noble PC. Guidelines for implant placement to minimize impingement during activities of daily living after total hip arthroplasty. J Arthroplast. 2010;25(8):1275–1281.e1.
30. Meermans G, Van Doorn WJ, Koenraadt K, Kats J. The use of the transverse acetabular ligament for determining the orientation of the components in total hip replacement: a randomised controlled trial. Bone Jt J. 2014;96-B(3):312–8.
31. Beswick AD, Wylde V, Gooberman-Hill R, Blom A, Dieppe P. What proportion of patients report long-term pain after total hip or knee replacement for osteoarthritis? A systematic review of prospective studies in unselected patients. BMJ Open. 2012;2(1):e000435.
32. Marchetti E, Krantz N, Berton C, Bocquet D, Fouilleron N, Migaud H, et al. Component impingement in total hip arthroplasty: frequency and risk factors. A continuous retrieval analysis series of 416 cup. Orthop Traumatol Surg Res. 2011;97(2):127–33.
33. Hua X, Li J, Jin Z, Fisher J. The contact mechanics and occurrence of edge loading in modular metal-on-polyethylene total hip replacement during daily activities. Med Eng Phys. 2016;38(6):518–25.
34. Rivière C, Lazennec J-Y, Van Der Straeten C, Auvinet E, Cobb J, Muirhead-Allwood S. The influence of spine-hip relations on total hip replacement: a systematic review. Orthop Traumatol Surg Res. 2017;103(4):559–68.
35. Mayeda BF, Haw JG, Battenberg AK, Schmalzried TP. Femoral-acetabular mating: the effect of femoral and combined anteversion on cross-linked polyethylene wear. J Arthroplast. 2018;33(10):3320–4.
36. Nam D, Riegler V, Clohisy JC, Nunley RM, Barrack RL. The impact of total hip arthroplasty on pelvic motion and functional component position is highly variable. J Arthroplast. 2017;32(4):1200–5.
37. Mellon SJ, Grammatopoulos G, Andersen MS, Pandit HG, Gill HS, Murray DW. Optimal acetabular component orientation estimated using edge-loading and impingement risk in patients with metal-on-metal hip resurfacing arthroplasty. J Biomech. 2015;48(2):318–23.
38. McCarthy TF, Alipit V, Nevelos J, Elmallah RK, Mont MA. Acetabular cup anteversion and inclination in hip range of motion to impingement. J Arthroplast. 2016;31(9):264–8.
39. Shoji T, Yamasaki T, Izumi S, Kenji M, Sawa M, Yasunaga Y, et al. The effect of cup medialization and lateralization on hip range of motion in total hip arthroplasty. Clin Biomech. 2018;57:121–8.
40. Pierrepont JW, Feyen H, Miles BP, Young DA, Baré JV, Shimmin AJ. Functional orientation of the acetabular component in ceramic-on-ceramic total hip arthroplasty and its relevance to squeaking. Bone Jt J. 2016;98-B(7):910–6.
41. Heckmann N, McKnight B, Stefl M, Trasolini NA, Ike H, Dorr LD. Late dislocation following total hip arthroplasty: spinopelvic imbalance as a causative factor. J Bone Jt Surg. 2018;100(21):1845–53.
42. Grammatopoulos G, Dhaliwal K, Pradhan R, Parker SJM, Lynch K, Marshall R. Does lumbar arthrodesis compromise outcome of total hip arthroplasty? Hip Int. 2019;29(5):496–503.
43. Ochi H, Homma Y, Baba T, Nojiri H, Matsumoto M, Kaneko K. Sagittal spinopelvic alignment predicts hip function after total hip arthroplasty. Gait Posture. 2017;52:293–300.
44. Abdel MP, von Roth P, Jennings MT, Hanssen AD, Pagnano MW. What safe zone? The vast majority of dislocated THAs are within the Lewinnek safe zone for acetabular component position. Clin Orthop Relat Res. 2016;474(2):386–91.
45. Goyal P, Lau A, Naudie DD, Teeter MG, Lanting BA, Howard JL. Effect of acetabular component positioning on functional outcomes in primary total hip arthroplasty. J Arthroplast. 2017;32(3): 843–8.
46. Reininga IH, Zijlstra W, Wagenmakers R, Boerboom AL, Huijbers BP, Groothoff JW, et al. Minimally invasive and computer-navigated total hip arthroplasty: a qualitative and systematic review of the literature. BMC Musculoskelet Disord. 2010;11(1):92. http://bmcmusculoskeletdisord.biomedcentral.com/articles/10.1186/1471-2474-11-92
47. McCarthy TF, Alipit V, Nevelos J, Elmallah RK, Mont MA. Acetabular cup anteversion and inclination in hip range of motion to impingement. J arthroplast. 2016;31(9):264-8.
48. Pierrepont J, Hawdon G, Miles BP, Connor BO, Baré J, Walter LR, et al. Variation in functional pelvic tilt in patients undergoing total hip arthroplasty. Bone Jt J. 2017;99-B(2):184–91.
49. Stefl M, Lundergan W, Heckmann N, McKnight B, Ike H, Murgai R, et al. Spinopelvic mobility and

acetabular component position for total hip arthroplasty. Bone Jt J. 2017;99-B(1_Supple_A):37–45.
50. Phan D, Bederman SS, Schwarzkopf R. The influence of sagittal spinal deformity on anteversion of the acetabular component in total hip arthroplasty. Bone Jt J. 2015;97-B(8):1017–23.
51. Riviere C. Kinematic versus conventional alignment techniques for total hip arthroplasty: a retrospective case control study. Orthop Traumatol Surg Res. 2019;105(5):895–905.
52. Spencer-Gardner L, Pierrepont J, Topham M, Baré J, McMahon S, Shimmin AJ. Patient-specific instrumentation improves the accuracy of acetabular component placement in total hip arthroplasty. Bone Jt J. 2016;98-B(10):1342–6.

Part II

Application of Implants in Hip Arthroplasty

4

Hip Resurfacing Procedure and the Proximal Femur Anatomy

Julien Girard and Koen De Smet

Key Points

- Hip resurfacing (HR) is a personalized hip replacement procedure with restoration of biomechanical parameters with proximal femoral anatomy preservation.
- With HR, bone preservation is clearly an advantage on the femoral side.
- Hip joint stability allowing unrestricted range of motion with very low risk of dislocation.
- Possibility of returning to high-impact sports activities (running, football, judo, hockey, etc.).
- Better physiological restoration of spatial–temporal gait parameters versus standard head THA.
- Absence of thigh pain and optimal femoral loading.
- Preservation of hip joint proprioception.
- HR makes surgery easier in cases of femoral shaft deformity or when diaphysis implants are present.

J. Girard (✉)
Orthopedics C Unit, Hopital Roger Salengro, CHRU Lille, Lille Cedex, France

University of Lille, Lille, France
e-mail: julien.girard@chru-lille.fr

K. De Smet
Anca Medical Center, AMC, Xavier De Cocklaan 68.1, St Martens Latem Deurle, Belgium

4.1 Why Perform Hip Resurfacing (Pros and Cons)?

Today, we see younger patients with hip problems, so bone preservation and highly wear-resistant bearings are becoming more relevant. Metal-on-metal hip resurfacing (HR) has now been used for 20 years. To achieve bone preservation, less bearing wear, and higher patient activity, the trade-off has been a more technically difficult surgery and subsequent failures. The lack of knowledge about HR implant design, tribology, and mechanical properties has led to a general desire to try out this concept but also to this procedure being abandoned.

In this respect, the biggest downsides of this procedure are that it cannot be performed in all hip cases and cannot be performed by every orthopedic surgeon. A minimum number of surgeries a year are becoming necessary to be allowed to perform HR surgery. Other drawbacks of metal-on-metal HR is that high bearing wear debris can cause adverse local tissue reactions (ALTR) or pseudotumors, and high amounts of cobalt and chromium ions are released systemically. General health problems have been linked to high cobalt levels in these cases but not in the normal functioning HR case. Even if we have a perfect design and perfect technique, this complication is difficult to avoid, as no hip joint surgery has a 100% success rate. Besides the expected numbers of failures, there is an unforeseen allergy problem, which can develop in 1% of females and 0.1% of males.

The well-known bone stock preservation on the femoral side, now also holds for the pelvic side, where no more bone is removed than with a total hip arthroplasty (THA), if the technique is done correctly. This was not the case in the beginning of the HR practice because of the learning curve and lack of large-diameter implants or thin cups. In case of revision surgery, it has been shown that if the patient and implant are monitored closely, revision can be done at the correct time, and the outcomes should not differ greatly, relative to primary THA. The increase in cup size after revision surgery is negligible and does not reflect the concerns raised in many papers [1].

Where other failures can be attributed to HR such as femoral neck fracture and loosening of the femoral head, the frequency has become very low in modern practice. There are more benefits to doing HR if all the expert recommendations and current practices are followed. Bone preservation and easier revisions are obvious, but many other benefits of HR have emerged in the last decade. Bone mineral density studies have shown that the bone stock returns to normal after HR.

We believe HR allows younger and more active patients to resume physical and sports activities without restriction. This difference has been demonstrated in an increasing number of randomized studies [2]. The risks of wear in active patients with metal-on-metal HR have been shown to have no influence, whereas the wear products and metal ions decline over time in a normal functioning HR [3]. Biomechanics and muscular moment arms are more easily restored to the normal native hip anatomy. Risk of dislocation in HR has always been low relative to THA and has become extremely rare.

The revision rate of HR depends on type of implant and its size; however, it has become clear that surgeon's experience has a major impact. Some authors see this as a negative. But in the right patient, like a young male patient with osteoarthritis, there is only a revision burden of 9.5% at 16 years post HR versus 10.4% for THA in the same group based on registry data from the Australian Orthopedic Association National Joint Replacement Registry (AOANJRR 2017). Large volume/single surgeon groups improve the survivorship up to 98% in this cohort.

A more unexpected finding is that patients with hip osteoarthritis undergoing metal-on-metal HR have reduced mortality in the long term compared to those undergoing cemented or uncemented THA. This difference persisted after extensive adjustment for confounding factors available in the retrieved data. Although residual confounding is possible, the observed effect size is large [4] (Fig. 4.1). These findings require further validation but are starting to be reported in several national hip registries. At present, after 20 years of experience with the new generation of metal-on-metal HR, we have separated the wheat from the chaff, and must continue to use proven designs with the correct technique and experience, in the correct patient.

4.2 Clinical Evidence Supporting Hip Resurfacing

Registries data: Outcomes of THA in younger patients (≤50 years of age) are significantly worse compared to results in older patient groups. The 2016 Swedish Register found a cumulative survivorship in patients younger than 50 of 54.2% at 24 years' follow-up compared to 94.3% in patients older than 75 [5]. The 2016 AOANJRR indicated a cumulative percent revision of primary THA in patients aged less than 55 years of 8.5% and 12.7% at 10 and 15 years of follow-up, respectively [6]. On the other hand, HR in this specific population seems to work better. With the Birmingham Hip Resurfacing System (BHR), the 2016 National Joint Registry for England and Wales [7], the 2016 Australian Joint Registry [6], and the 2015 Swedish Registry [5] reported 90.1% survival at 12 years, 89.9% survival at 15 years, and 96.6% survival at 10 years, respectively.

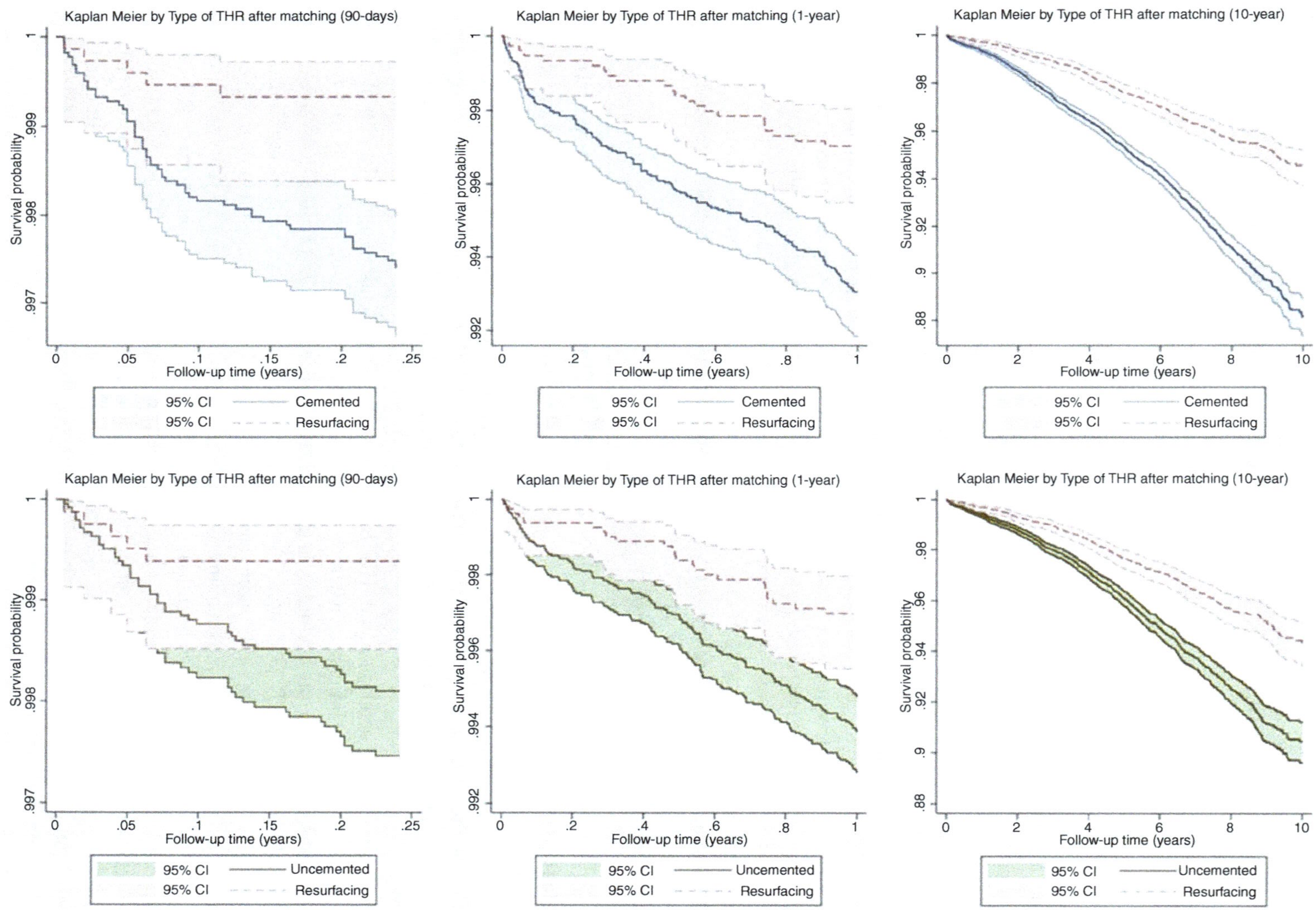

Fig. 4.1 Kaplan Meier survival curves by type of surgical procedure after matching. *THR* total hip replacement, *cemented* or *uncemented* type of total hip replacement, *resurfacing* metal-on-metal hip resurfacing

Recently, an international high-volume centers HR registry was created with patients ≤50 years at surgery with a minimum of 3 years' follow-up (11,386 cases with a mean age of 42.7 years) [8]. There were 8459 HR procedures in male patients (74.3%) and 2926 in female patients (25.7%) with a mean femoral head size of 49.7 mm and a mean follow-up time of 7.6 years (3 to 22). Overall survivorship was 89.1% at 22 years (95% CI: 88.5–89.7%). Survival was significantly superior in males—92.7% at 21 years—(95% CI: 92.1–93.3%) than in females—81.6% at 22 years (95% CI: 80.3–82.9%).

Return to sports activities: Return to sport after hip arthroplasty is an increasingly common functional demand. However, there are few published studies on this subject and returning to high-impact sports appears to be challenging. HR seems to fulfill this functional demand since the prosthetic femoral head diameter is close to the native diameter, and the bearing has high wear resistance (without the risk of head fracture). Several studies have reported a high rate of return to low-, medium-, and high-impact sports after HR. To date, no international consensus recommendations exist on the possibility of returning to sports after hip arthroplasty. Nevertheless, HR allows a patient to resume physical and sports activities without restriction. The rate of return to sports after HR appears to be excellent. It is important to point out that no long-term studies have analyzed the impact of these activities on aseptic loosening. The most iconic example is with patients who participate in triathlons. Girard et al. [9] found rates of return to swimming, cycling, and running of 38/48 (79%), 41/48 (85%), and 33/48 (69%), respectively, in 48 Ironman-distance triathletes. More interesting, during the preoperative period, all patients had taken part in at least one Ironman competition and at 4.7 years of follow-up, 28/48 (58.3%) had taken part in an Ironman competition with no decrease in their performance between the preoperative and postoperative periods.

Functional performance: The excellent hip function found after HR procedures is directly correlated with the conservative nature of the surgical procedure on the femoral head. With HR, the bone on the femoral bone side is preserved with two important effects: preservation of mechanoreceptors in the femoral neck and restoration of proximal femoral anatomy. Anatomical reconstruction after HR results in abductor and extensor moment arm preservation. In a prospective, randomized study comparing THA versus HR, biomechanical hip parameters were better restored with HR [10]. Leg length was restored to within±4 mm in 33 (60%) of THA and 42 (86%) of HR patients. Femoral offset was restored to within ±4 mm in 14 (25%) of THA and 29 (59%) of HR cases. Beyond biomechanical restoration, gait analysis showed that in all planes of motion, HR restored the patient's normal gait pattern while THA required an adaptation. At 6 months and 2 years post surgery, THA patients had a lower walking speed compared to normal subjects and HR patients [11]. It could enhance center of mass control and increase energy generation during the push off phase. The same conclusion was drawn based on static and dynamic stabilometric analysis and postural coordination studies [11, 12]. The advantage in terms of balance and postural control after HR results in better stability and motor patterns than observed after THA.

4.3 Optimal Positioning of Hip Resurfacing Implants (Tricks and Tips)

4.3.1 What Are the Keys to Successful Hip Resurfacing?

There are several keys to successful HR. The most important points are patient selection and appropriate surgical technique. Female patients have a greater risk of failure due to small femoral head size, high frequency of hip dysplasia, and potentially poor bone quality. Inflammatory disease, avascular necrosis, large femoral head cysts, and hip dysplasia appear to reduce survivorship. The best indication is primary osteoarthritis. Obesity is not a contraindication, but a minimum head diameter of 48 mm appears to be a prerequisite.

The posterolateral approach is the "Queen of surgical approaches" for HR. Detaching the gluteus maximus tendon is unnecessary. Preserving soft tissues is important for vascularization and gluteal function. The external rotators must be cut 5–8 mm from the bone, preserving a small cuff. The capsule is cut at the level at the piriformis and not at the head–neck junction. Coagulation should not be performed at the head–neck junction. Preserving the capsule is key; we do not recommend performing a full 360° capsulotomy.

Cup position is also crucial to the performance of metal-on-metal bearings. The cup should be positioned in 40° inclination with anatomical anteversion. A steep cup amplifies the risk of increased metal ion levels and higher failure rate. On the other hand, a cup implanted in less than 30° inclination can lead to impingement with the femoral neck in abduction and/or flexion. The transverse ligament is the key anatomical landmark. After impaction, the cup should be in line with the transverse ligament. This is the only prerequisite to impact the cup in an anatomical position and to avoid impingement. Preparing the femoral side first seems to be a smart option in order to optimize the acetabular exposure, to size the femoral neck perfectly and to achieve the optimal cup and femoral anteversion.

4.3.2 Femoral Component Position

It is very important to understand that the femoral neck is not circular in shape. Usually, it has more of an ovoid shape. The second important point is the definition of head–neck offset: distance between the head equator and femoral neck surface. Given that the femoral neck is not circular, this offset is not constant around the head/neck circumference. Third, HR has the worse head–neck offset of all the hip implant designs. After hip resurfacing, the femoral head–neck diameter offset is lower than conventional THA. In fact, the head–neck diameter ratio after conventional THA is close to 2 (assuming a 28-mm-diameter head and 12/14-mm-diameter neck), more than 3 for large-diameter heads, and around 1.2 for HR. This point is crucial. The risk of cam effect with impingement between the femoral neck and the cup or acetabular bone is one of the modes of failure of the HR. So correct component positioning is crucial and intraoperative testing is essential. The position of the cup and femoral components is interrelated, and excessive cup anteversion inexorably leads to a posterior cam effect. A retroverted cup leads to an anterior cam and an overly inclined cup to a superior cam.

In the same way, a low head–neck diameter offset may be detrimental to achieving better hip flexion. After conventional THA, range of motion is limited by "implant to implant" cam effect while with HR, it is limited by "cup component to femoral neck bone" contact. Hip flexion is the most important motion for daily activities. Maximum anterior head–neck offset is necessary to avoid cup–bone contact and increase the degree of flexion at which it occurs (Fig. 4.2). Anterior translation of the femoral component relative to the central femoral neck axis may improve anterior head–neck offset and hip flexion. Usually, the position of the femoral component is flush with the posterior cortex of the femoral neck. Considering that 1 mm of anterior offset increases hip flexion by 5°, anterior translation of the femoral component appears to be an attractive way to increase range of motion [13]. But anterior head–neck offset is very sensitive, and it is important to avoid drastically reducing the posterior offset.

HR is a surgical compromise. Each time the femoral position is optimized, the opposite position may be compromised. So, improving hip

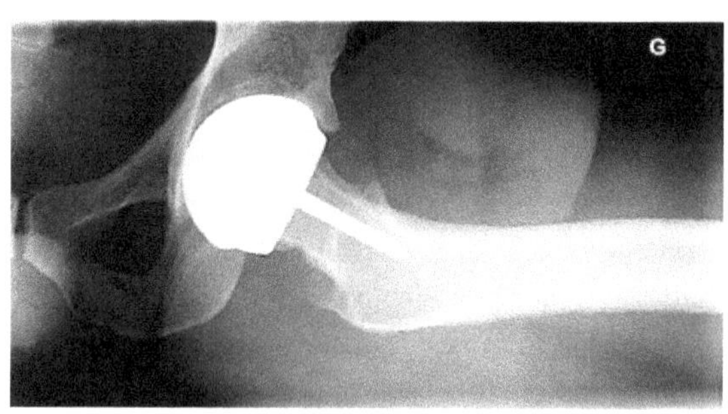

Fig. 4.2 Optimal femoral position. The femoral component is parallel to the neck with physiological anteversion. Notice the slight shift from posterior to anterior which led to better anterior head–neck offset

flexion by increasing anterior translation should be done carefully to avoid reducing the range of motion in the opposite direction. In fact, a completely symmetrical position of the femoral cup is not the rule. To summarize, more flexion than extension is required for daily activities. A posterior-to-anterior shift seems to be the most attractive option to improve range of motion. Removing osteophytes at head–neck junction can be done with caution after femoral impaction.

The last point in the offset femoral position is the femoral metallic offset of each implant. It reaches 3–4 mm and the cement mantle thickness adds 0–1.5 mm. Therefore, HR femoral head–neck offset varies from 3 to 5 mm. Other tricks can be used to increase range of motion:

- Careful anterior femoral osteoplasty can improve anterior offset and decrease the risk of a cam effect. But surgeons must be aware of the risk of neck fracture if the osteoplasty crosses the neck cortex.
- Acetabular rim osteophyte removal is essential. A 2–3 mm width of acetabular bone must be preserved on the anterior wall to avoid the risk of iliopsoas impingement. But if necessary, acetabular bone should be cleared around the cup.
- Modifying the femoral stem angle is not recommended. In fact, retroversion of the femoral component has little influence on the cam effect and leads to contact between the stem and neck.
- Increasing the implants' diameter could theoretically increase the femoral–head offset. But the risk of groin pain, acetabular bone fracture, and psoas irritation do not allow insertion of large cups. Moreover, the femoral component must be fitted on the bony femoral head without any defect.

A slight valgus placement of the femoral component leads to better biomechanical performance. A valgus of 5° to 10° compared to the native femoral neck is recommended [14]. A varus position exposes to neck a stress raiser while excessive valgus could produce a superior notch. Two useful intraoperative landmarks are the inferior part of the femoral neck and the femoral head fovea. The femoral K-wire should be placed in a slight valgus position relative to the inferior femoral neck line and about 1 cm higher than the fovea.

To achieve the optimal hip range of motion and avoid femoral neck impingement on the cup component, the goal is to reproduce the natural femoral head–neck offset around the entire femoral neck. That means the offset could be modified for each deformity (Legg–Calve–Perthes, post traumatic…). This is very different to conventional THA where the proximal femur is first resected and then reconstructed with a femoral stem. The stem should reproduce patient anatomy, biomechanical properties, and restore soft tissue tension. HR is an anatomy-preserving surgical procedure that keeps the proximal femur and minimizes anatomical distortion. With THA, surgeons have many implant options: multiple stem sizes, prosthetic head modularity, different stem neck–shaft angles, standard or high offset stems, different head diameters, anti-dislocation lips, etc. With HR, none of these possibilities exist and preserving the proximal femoral anatomy leads to exact biomechanical reconstruction of the joint (well described in randomized study). In fact, with THA, the biomechanical restoration is correlated with stem fixation. If stem stability is sub-optimal, it could lead to implant over-sizing and leg overlengthening and increase the femoral offset. With HR, the femoral component diameter is close to the native head diameter. The stability of the prosthetic head is immediate and optimal and under-sizing is impossible.

At the end of the procedure, the ability to view the position of both components is very valuable. In case of primary osteoarthritis without neck deformity and with a standard stem–shaft angle, the two components must be parallel to each other with the hip in neutral position (no rotation, no abduction, leg in line with trunk). This means the femoral component is in slight valgus (140°) and the cup is near 40° inclination. This point is crucial because it helps to avoid impingement between the neck and cup. The last check is performed to detect potential cam impingement (anterior or posterior). An acetabular rim osteoplasty or femoroplasty can be done at this point if needed.

4.3.3 Vascularization

Thorough knowledge of the vascular anatomy of the femoral head is necessary before starting a HR procedure. The retinacular vessels along the posterolateral and inferomedial femoral neck must be located. Throughout the procedure, the retinacular vessels should be preserved as well as all the soft tissues around the femoral head. Maintaining the blood supply to the femoral neck is vital. On the other hand, the posterior approach that inevitably disrupts the main blood supply is commonly used for HR. But the large majority of studies do not report head collapse or heat-induced bone necrosis. The blood supply of an arthritic femoral head can come from intraosseous vessels rather than from retinacular vessels. Moreover, some vascular anastomoses between the femoral epiphysis and metaphysis could increase the neck's blood supply. But the surgeon should be aware that these two possibilities do not mean the retinacular vessels do not need to be preserved.

Because of blood supply vulnerability during posterolateral approach, other approaches have been investigated. The main goal of each one is femoral head vascularization. These approaches are the direct lateral approach, anterior approach, and trochanteric flip approach. To date, none of these surgical approaches have been shown to lower the rate of head collapse. The most attractive surgical approach is still the posterolateral approach but with minimal soft tissue disruption: no release of the gluteus maximus extension, no circumferential capsulotomy, no release of the gluteus medius on the iliac bone and preservation of reticular vessels and soft tissues along the neck.

4.3.4 Femoral Cementing Technique

The femoral cementing technique is an important factor for long-term HR survival. Additional drill holes should be made in the prepared femoral head to increase the fixation area. A distance of at least 1 cm is required between cement holes to avoid thermal osteonecrosis. Five to ten anchoring holes 7 mm in depth and 4 mm in diameter are preferred. Some surgeons recommended placing a suction device into the lesser trochanter with femoral head pulse lavage in order to optimize cement penetration. However, this could lead to deep cement penetration and subsequently thermal necrosis. A dome hole seems sufficient before applying low viscosity cement. The merits of two cement application techniques—indirect filling with cement into the component or direct cement packing on the femoral head—continue to be debated. It is important to note that the cement mantle and penetration depth vary greatly depending on cement viscosity, head bone density, clearance between the reamed head and femoral component, and implant design.

4.4 Future Developments in Hip Resurfacing

There is an alternative type of surgery known as HR, which is carried out on younger patients. Unlike THA, the surgeon only removes the diseased cartilage from the hip joint and resurfaces it using a metal-on-metal implant. However, in some patients, the metal particles released by the implant cause tissue reactions with clinical implications. Because of the failures related to metallosis, the concern about metal ions and the risk of metal allergy has led to new developments, especially for female patients, who tend to have a smaller head size and higher percentage of allergy. While the need for surgeons to have substantial experience with the technique remains, some new developments are ready for the orthopedic joint market.

A new resurfacing implant with polyethylene cup is being tested, whereas ceramic-on-ceramic resurfacing looks to be a logical design for resurfacing implants. No matter what is produced or engineered, we should be aware there can be snags and unexpected problems can develop. Squeaking with ceramic-on-ceramic is a well-known problem in THA. The reported incidence of noisy ceramic-on-ceramic hips ranges from 1% to 29% depending on how the "noise" is defined [15]. Some acoustic studies have distinguished between squeaking and other types of noise such as clicking, clunking, popping, and grating in metal-on-metal resurfacing. The question remains whether these could appear in ceramic-on-ceramic resurfacing bearings. Squeaking in large-diameter metal-on-metal hip replacements has been associated with increased clearance and reduced lubrification [16]. In the newer ceramic-on-ceramic large-diameter total hips (head diameters up to 48 mm), the squeaking rate increases with head diameter (36 mm to 48 mm) [17]. These well-documented THA findings need to be addressed and documented during clinical trials of all new ceramic-on-ceramic resurfacing bearings coming on the market [18]. Ceramic fractures due to high impact should be a smaller concern based on stress tests done in the laboratory. Hopefully, resurfacing will not reproduce these complications, but we have to be aware that new problems can occur, like the trunnionosis problem with large metal heads on a stem in THA—a problem we never experienced in 60 years of joint surgery!

The custom polyethylene hip resurfacing was designed by pioneering orthopedic surgeon Derek McMinn. It is an alternative to patients with metal allergies. The cup is made from highly cross-linked polyethylene and has a layer of titanium porous coating on the outer surface, like the RM Pressfit cup (Matthys®) with a mean survival rate of 94.4% for aseptic loosening after 20 years. Dr. Pritchett (Seattle, USA) has produced Synovo Preserve implants made with cross-linked polyethylene which is stronger, lighter, and more wear resistant than conventional polyethylene. Both designs use a cobalt-chrome head, thus there still is a theoretical risk of allergy, just like in knee implants. But the fact these are hard-on-soft bearings that will not last a lifetime in younger active patients does not make them the ideal new HR development.

Ceramic-on-ceramic HR appears to be a better idea for reducing the risk of wear and allergy (Fig. 4.3). Justin Cobb at the Imperial College London was the first surgeon in the world to resurface patients' hips with ceramic-on-ceramic implants. A clinical trial has been designed to show ceramic implants are suitable for both men and women, as conventional HR techniques are currently less suitable for female patients. The new device, called "H1" (Fig. 4.3), has a contoured cup and BIOLOX® *delta* on BIOLOX® *delta* bearing. The contoured design is designed to better match the patient's anatomy and prevent impingement. The cup has a titanium porous coating, and the head is not cemented. It is important to realize that such designs are completely new; thus, unexpected problems may develop. They should be evaluated for a long time before they are made fully available to the orthopedic market. The same is true for the new ReCerf™ Hip Resurfacing Arthroplasty from MatOrtho® which uses ceramic monoblock components by Ceramtec®—femoral heads and acetabular cups—with no metal components.

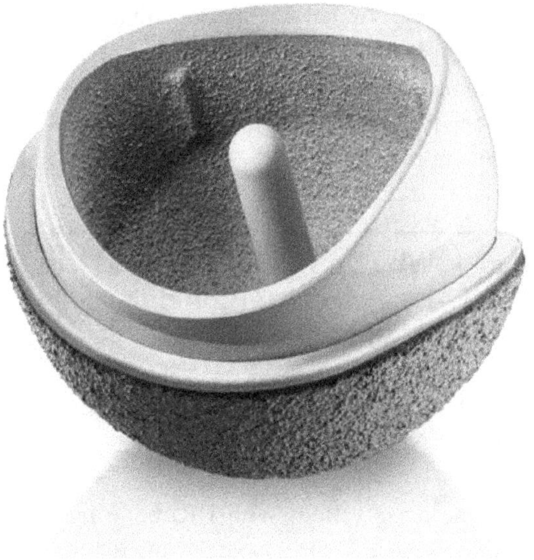

Fig. 4.3 Ceramic-on-ceramic H1® hip resurfacing components (Embody, London, UK) first implanted by Pr. Justin Cobb in 2017

Other companies are working on new HR designs with other bearing options. History always comes back to the resurfacing technique because it looks like a more anatomical, biomechanical, and logical treatment. From Charnley's soft Teflon bearing in the 1950s, to the Haboush (US) metal-on-metal bearing in 1953, to the 1970s with Gerard (France) and Muller (Switzerland) and the Wagner prosthesis in the 1980s, resurfacing will always remain an option. Today, there is extensive history with metal-on-metal resurfacing, with experimental work done than in typical THA implants. It is vital that we do not make the same mistakes twice, and we should be wary of any newly introduced solution that is inadequate at this moment.

4.5 Why Do We Recommend Hip Resurfacing? (Convincing Arguments)

The main reasons I recommend HR rather than THA for younger patients are:

- Bone preservation: With HR, bone preservation is clearly an advantage on the femoral side. Moreover, femoral neck bone density increases postoperatively due to physiological loading.
- No dislocation: In a randomized controlled trial, Vendittoli and al. [10] reported a 0% dislocation rate in the HR group compared to 3% in the THA group. Pollard et al. [19] reported a dislocation rate of 7.4% among 54 THA patients while none occurred in a group of 54 HR patients.
- Possibility of returning to high-impact sports activities (running, football, judo, hockey, etc.).
- Physiological restoration of spatial–temporal gait parameters.
- Restoration of biomechanical parameters: No leg length discrepancy and normal femoral offset are possible after HR.
- Absence of thigh pain.
- Optimal femoral loading.
- Preservation of hip joint proprioception.
- Possibility of performing HR even in cases of femoral shaft deformity or when existing implants cannot be removed.

References

1. De Smet K, Van Der Straeten C, Van Orsouw M, Doubi R, Backers K, Grammatopoulos G. Revisions of metal-on-metal hip resurfacing: lessons learned and improved outcome. Orthop Clin N Am. 2011;42(2):259–69.
2. Lavigne M, Masse V, Girard J, Roy AG, Vendittoli PA. Return to sport after hip resurfacing or total hip arthroplasty: a randomized study. Rev Chir Orthop Reparatrice Appar Mot. 2008;94(4): 361–7.
3. Van Der Straeten C, Van Quickenborne D, De Roest B, Calistri A, Victor J, De Smet K. Metal ion levels from well-functioning Birmingham hip resurfacings decline significantly at ten years. Bone Joint J. 2013;95-B(10):1332–8.
4. Kendal AR, Prieto-Alhambra D, Arden NK, Carr A, Judge A. Mortality rates at 10 years after metal-on-metal hip resurfacing compared with total hip replacement in England: retrospective cohort analysis of hospital episode statistics. BMJ. 2013;347:f6549. https://doi.org/10.1136/bmj.f6549.
5. Swedish Register. https://registercentrum.blob.core.windows.net/shpr/r/Annual-Report-2015-H19dFINOW.pdf20.
6. Australian Orthopedic Association National Joint Replacement Registry. https://aoanjrr.sahmri.com/fr/annual-reports-2016.
7. 2016 National Joint Register of England and Wales. http://www.njrcentre.org.uk/njrcentre/NewsandEvents/NJR14thAnnualReportrecordnumberofproceduresduring201617/tabid/1453/Default.aspx.
8. Van Der Straeten C. Results from a worldwide HR data base. Seoul: International Society for Technology in Arthroplasty; 2017.
9. Girard J, Lons A, Pommepuy T, Isida R, Benad K, Putman S. High-impact sport after hip resurfacing: The Ironman triathlon. Orthop Traumatol Surg Res. 2017;103(5):675–8.
10. Vendittoli PA, Ganapathi M, Roy AG, Lusignan D, Lavigne M. A comparison of clinical results of hip resurfacing arthroplasty and 28 mm metal on metal total hip arthroplasty: a randomised trial with 3-6 years follow-up. Hip Int. 2010;20(1):1–13.
11. Szymanski C, Thouvarecq R, Dujardin F, Migaud H, Maynou C, Girard J. Functional performance after hip resurfacing or total hip replacement: a comparative assessment with non-operated subjects. Orthop Traumatol Surg Res. 2012;98(1):1–7.
12. Bouffard V, Nantel J, Therrien M, Vendittoli PA, Lavigne M, Prince F. Center of mass compensation during gait in hip arthroplasty patients: comparison between large diameter head total hip arthroplasty and hip resurfacing. Rehabil Res Pract. 2011;2011:586412.
13. Girard J, Krantz N, Bocquet D, Wavreille G, Migaud H. Femoral head to neck offset after hip resurfacing is critical for range of motion. Clin Biomech (Bristol, Avon). 2012;27(2):165–9.
14. Beaulé PE, Harvey N, Zaragoza E, Le Duff MJ, Dorey FJ. The femoral head/neck offset and hip resurfacing. J Bone Joint Surg Br. 2007;89(1):9–15.
15. Keurentjes, et al. High incidence of squeaking in THAs with alumina ceramic-on-ceramic bearings. Clin Orthop Relat Res. 2008;466(6): 1438–43.

16. Brocket, et al. The influence of clearance on friction, lubrication and squeaking in large diameter metal-on-metal hip replacements. J Mater Sci Mater Med. 2008;19(4):1575–9.
17. Blakeney WG, Beaulieu Y, Puliero B, Lavigne M, Roy A, Massé V, Vendittoli PA. Excellent results of large-diameter ceramic-on-ceramic bearings in total hip arthroplasty. Bone Joint J. 2018;100-B(11): 1434–41.
18. Tai S, et al. Squeaking in large diameter ceramic-on-ceramic bearings in total hip arthroplasty. J Arthroplast. 2014;30(2) https://doi.org/10.1016/j.arth.2014.09.010.
19. Pollard TC, Baker RP, Eastaugh-Waring SJ, Bannister GC. Treatment of the young active patient with osteoarthritis of the hip. A five- to seven-year comparison of hybrid total hip arthroplasty and metal-on-metal resurfacing. J Bone Joint Surg Br. 2006;88(5):592–600.

5

Neck Anchorage Stem Design for Reconstructing Proximal Femur Anatomy

Philippe Piriou and James Sullivan

5.1 Introduction

Neck-sparing stem designs enable a personalized (patient-specific) surgery by reproducing the native proximal femur anatomy. This facilitates physiological soft-tissue tension and hip kinematics, hopefully responsible for higher prosthetic hip function and patient satisfaction, as well as reduced risk of dislocation. Moreover, the bone economy achieved by this implant design is an obvious advantage in terms of easing revision surgery and decreasing stress-shielding-induced bone loss. The authors present their experience of using a neck-only tapered prosthesis with hydroxyapatite (HA) and porous coating: the Silent™ Hip system. The concept of the silent hip (Fig. 5.1) was first considered by Dr. Allan Ritchie in the mid-1990s when the need for a better solution for younger, more active and demanding patients was first recognised. Following this, a group of engineers and surgeons took this concept to development in conjunction with the University of Hamburg [1]. The implant went on to satisfy pre-clinical in vitro evaluation, and in 2003, the clinical study began to assess the stability of the implant, using two surgeons (Dr. Honl and Sullivan) to assist DePuy with the findings. Between January and November of 2003, 41 implantations were performed. Following this, a wider study began to test the validity of the technique with a wider range of surgeons, with encouraging results.

The reader might be surprised to read an article about an implant that is no longer marketed. The authors' experience with this implant was entirely satisfactory. It was unfortunately marketed in association with the large-diameter metal-on-metal bearings found to have high failure rates. The company, under the pressure of lawyers and regulators, decided to suddenly withdraw it when it had given excellent results. This innovation, for us, deserves to be reported until the concept is reborn in the future.

Healthy bone stock preservation at the time of primary total hip arthroplasty remains a goal for surgeons performing surgery on younger patients. The advent of short-stemmed femoral prostheses designed to conserve bone and load the femoral neck in a physiological way has enabled use in the general patient population requiring total hip arthroplasty. Indeed, the preservation of the elasticity of the proximal femur eliminates the proximal femoral stress shielding of conventional stems. Of principal benefit to the patient is that a subsequent revision of the prosthesis can potentially be made to a standard primary stem. Patients are often younger, more active and have

P. Piriou (✉)
Clinique Ambroise Paré, Neuilly sur Seine, France

J. Sullivan
The Australian School of Advanced Medicine, Macquarie University Hospital, Sydney, NSW, Australia

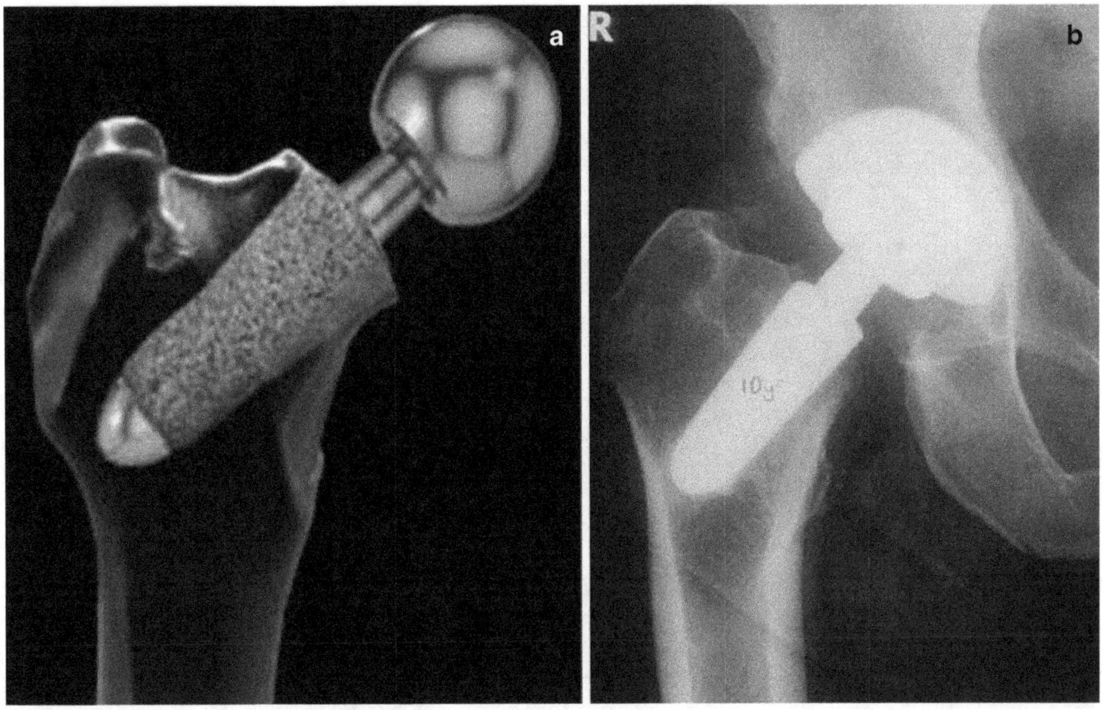

Fig. 5.1 The Silent™ stem is a neck-only tapered prosthesis with HA and porous coating (**a**). This stem is designed to load the calcar. (**b**) Illustrates a well-fixed silent™ stem at 10 years follow-up

increased expectations regarding function. As such, these patients are more likely to require a revision procedure.

5.2 Design Rationale and Development of the Silent™ Stem

In the years 2000–2010, there existed on the market several types of femoral bone-conserving THA (Fig. 5.2) [2]: short-stemmed prostheses, neck-plate devices, neck-only stems and resurfacing. The thrust plate prosthesis (TPP) has been available since 1978. Now in its third generation of design, which has been in clinical use since 1992, it is made of titanium and has a coarse blasted surface to allow bony ongrowth. This third-generation TPP is reported to have improved survival and better functional outcomes than the second-generation TPP design. The Silent™ stem was born from the observation that sometimes, because of lateral thigh pain in the TPP, it was necessary to remove the side plate. In these cases, the implant in the centre of the neck continued to give good results.

Michael M Morlock and Matthias Honl in collaboration with Depuy's teams developed the Silent™ rod in its final version. First, there was a preclinical test phase to understand the biomechanics of the implant and to specify its conditions of use (Figs. 5.3 and 5.4). A press-fit implantation in good quality bone is essential to resist the varus forces and obtain sufficient stability to ensure that bony ongrowth is achieved. Regarding the surgical technique, the placement of the stem required an initial femoral head resection followed by neck cavity preparation with reaming. The final component is then implanted with a press fit.

5.3 Clinical Data

We report here the results of the first clinical study of the Silent™ implant. A cohort study was prospectively designed and carried out in two centres (M Honl—Germany, J Sullivan—Australia). The

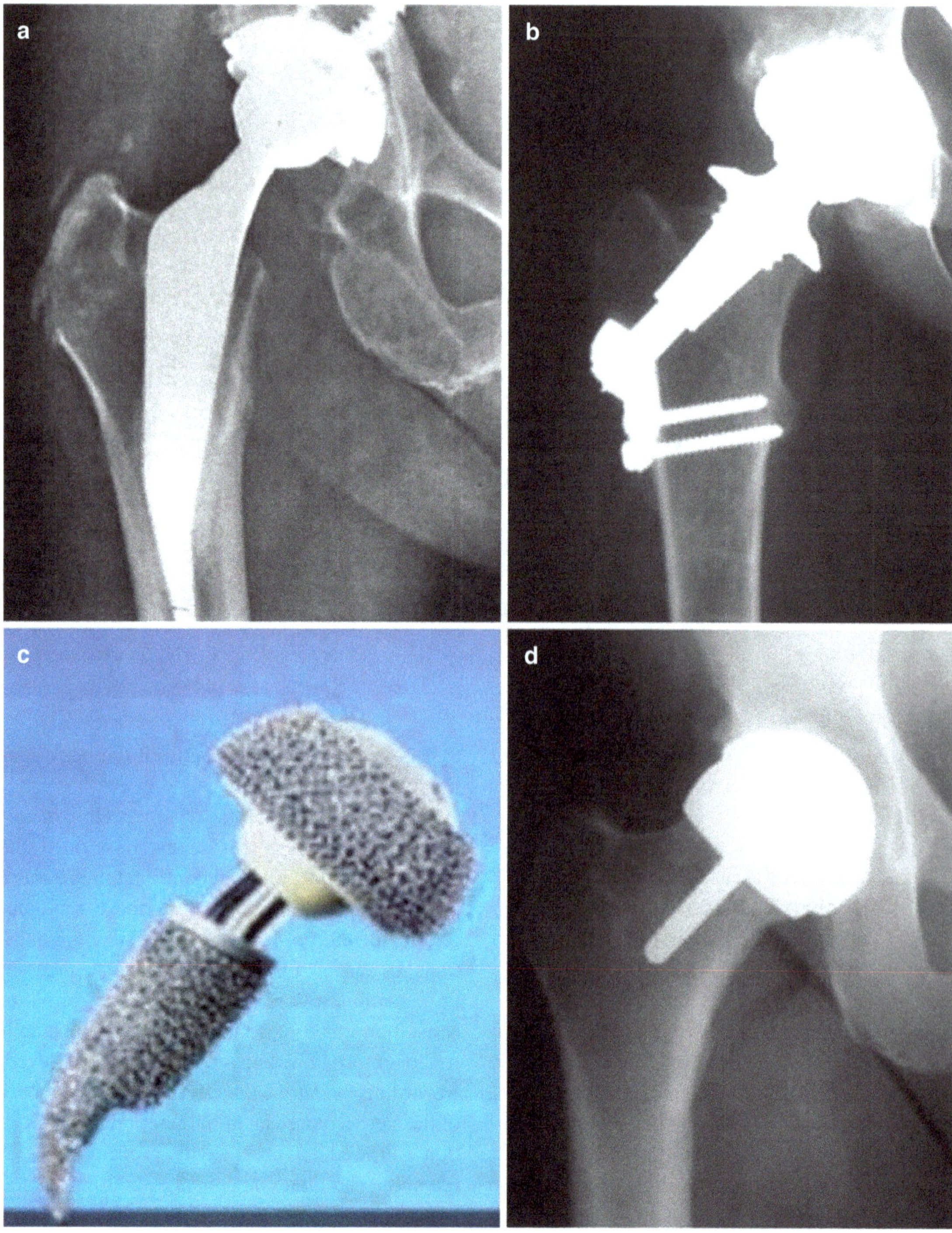

Fig. 5.2 Illustration of short stem (**a**), thrust plate (**b**), neck anchorage stem (**c**), and resurfacing (**d**) femoral component designs

outcomes of interest were a combination of clinical (occurrence of complications and functional assessment with Harris Hip and Oxford Hip scores) and radiographic (standard and RSA X-rays at post-op, 3, 6, 12, 18, 24 and 60 months) measures. The Harris and Oxford Hip Scores were gathered pre-operatively and then at regular intervals over a 5-year period. The local research

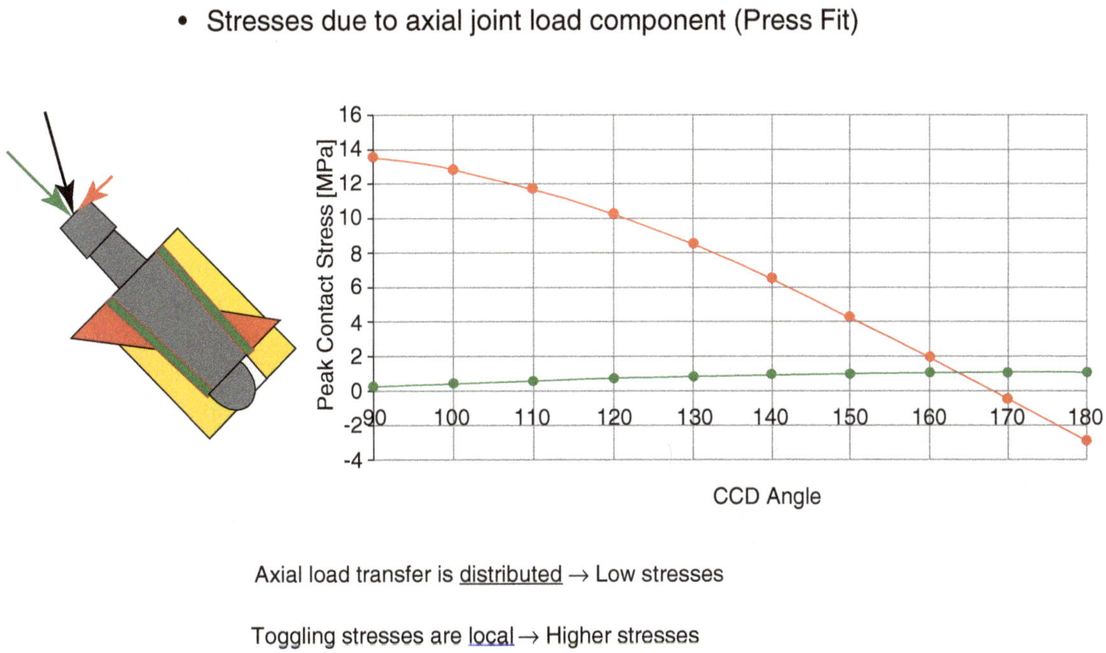

Fig. 5.3 This figure shows the stress distribution on the femoral neck (left image) and the influence of the neck-shaft angle (CCD angle) on the axial (green) and toggling (red) peak contact stress when the Silent™ stem is physiologically loaded (black arrow on left image)

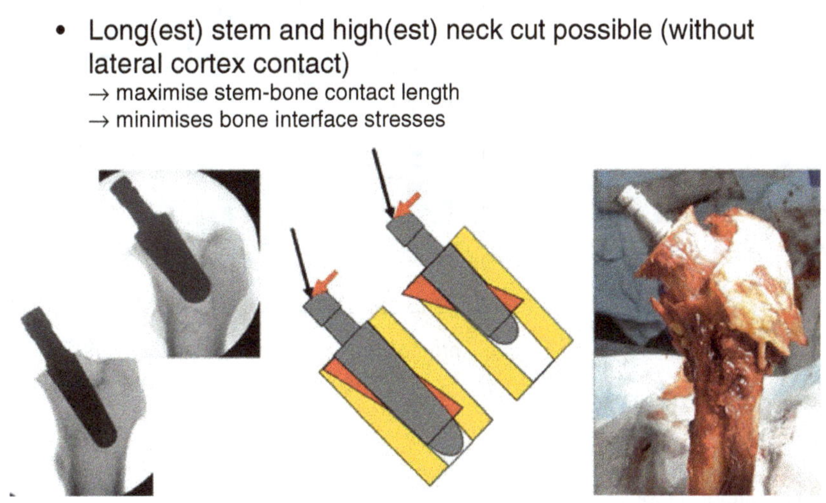

Fig. 5.4 The recommendations for implanting the Silent™ stem were to use the longest stem possible without lateral cortex contact in order to not reduce its press fit. This would maximise the stem–bone contact length and minimise stress on the calcar, therefore optimising stem osteointegration and reducing risk of peri-prosthetic fracture

ethics committees and the regulatory authorities in both countries approved this study.

Patients with hip osteoarthritis (OA) between 25 and 65 years old and weighing less than 90 kg were included in this study. Significant bone loss or gross deformity of the femoral neck, osteonecrosis extending into the femoral neck, coxa vara (anatomical CCD angle of less than 125°), being C on the Charnley classification and subjects with inflammatory or Paget hip disease were criteria for exclusion.

Forty-one patients received a Silent™ Hip between January and November 2003, with additional tantalum beads inserted in the femur and attached to the stem for radio stereometric analysis (RSA). The characteristics of the cohort were as follows: mean age of 50.4 years (range 26–65), mean BMI of 26.6 (range 19–37) and 18 females/23 males. The cause of the hip degeneration was primary OA in 28 cases, dysplasia in 3, avascular head necrosis in 6, postinfection in 2 and 'other' in 2 cases. All patients received a ceramic-on-ceramic bearing except one with ceramic-on-polyethylene. The German group favoured the anterolateral approach with a 28-mm femoral head, while the Australian group used a posterior approach with a 32-mm head.

Five-year review was achieved with only one patient lost to follow-up. Good Harris and Oxford Hip Scores were obtained as illustrated on Figs. 5.5 and 5.6, respectively. Regarding the radiographic performance, no progressive femoral radiolucencies were observed; there was an increase of bone density in the calcar region (Fig. 5.7). The RSA showed satisfactory stem migration over a period of 18 months (Fig. 5.8) demonstrating good primary stability and secondary fixation (osteointegration) of the Silent™ stem.

There were five reoperations involving the acetabulum but no revisions of the Silent stem; three cups were revised: one for recurrent dislocation, one following an early acetabular fracture and one for psoas impingement. One acetabular liner was exchanged as the ceramic liner fractured after the patient had a fall. Finally, one acetabular liner and femoral head were exchanged during washout procedure for an acute haematogenous periprosthetic infection occurring at 18 months post-op.

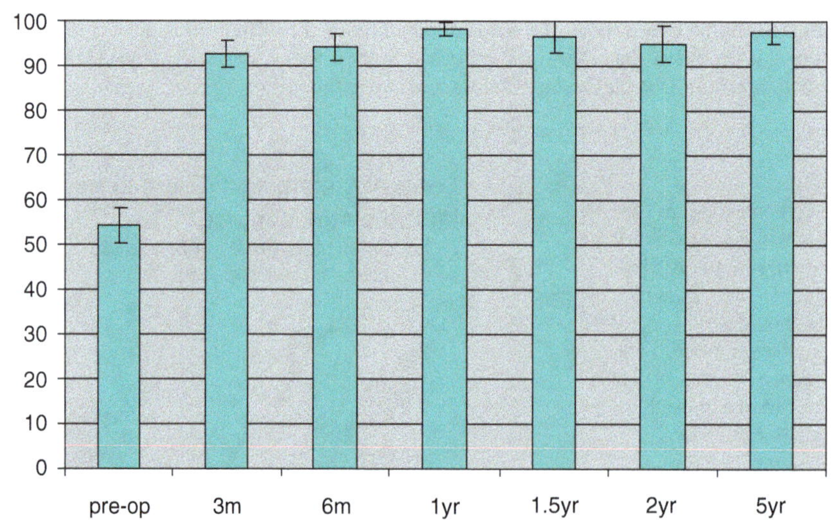

Fig. 5.5 Harris Hip Score pre-operatively and during 5-year follow-up

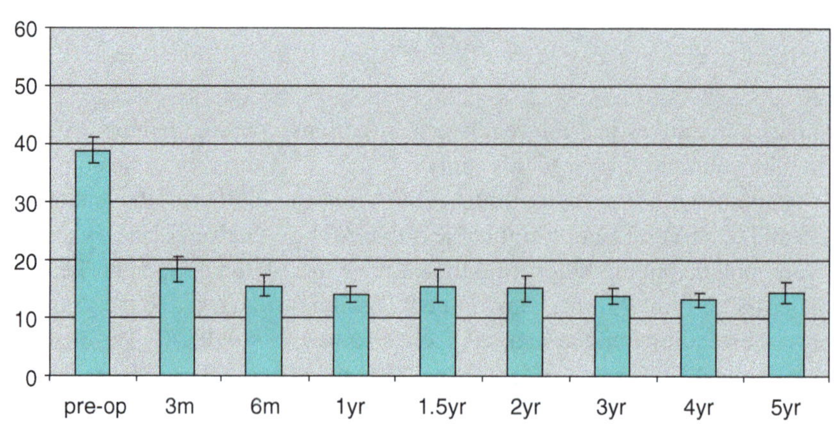

Fig. 5.6 Oxford Hip Score pre-operatively and during 5-year follow-up (0 best, 60 worst)

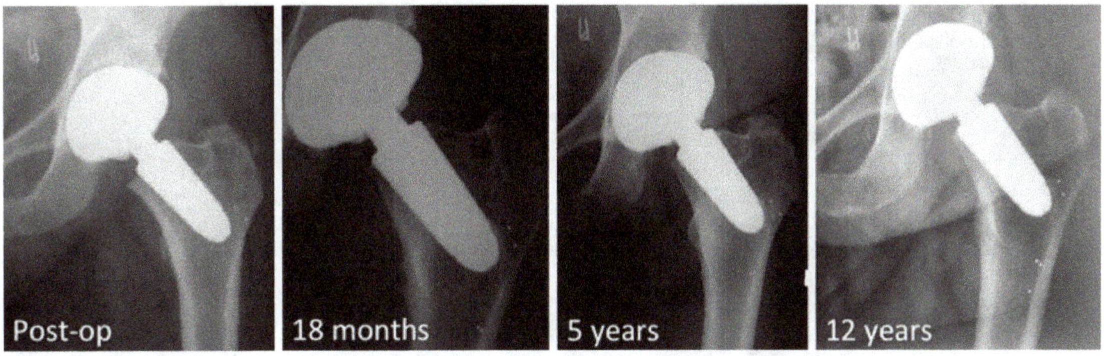

Fig. 5.7 Radiographic appearance of the bone remodelling around the Silent™ stem over a 12-year period

Fig. 5.8 This graphs shows the negligible migration of the Silent™ stems at 3, 6, 12 and 18 months after implantation, as measured via RadioStereometric Analysis

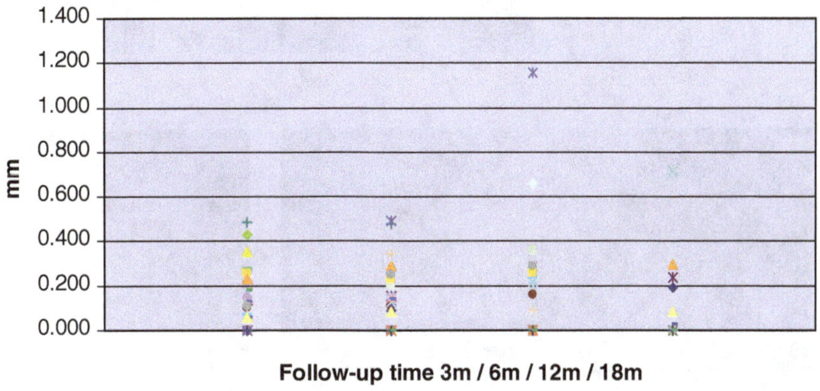

5.4 Discussion

The silent stem is a bone-preserving implant that gets its anchorage in the femoral neck and so loads the proximal femur more physiologically than stemmed or short-curved implants. This is reflected by the bone remodelling [3] and preservation of the calcar as seen on radiographs [4]. Unlike the resurfacing procedure, the Silent™ stem can be used with destruction or deformity of the femoral head as it relies on fixation in the neck (Fig. 5.9). In addition, the resection of the femoral head enables easier access to the acetabulum for reaming and implantation of the acetabular component.

Previous RSA studies have suggested that distal intramedullary migration should be less than 1–1.5 mm in the first 2 years after implantation. The data for the Silent™ stem fell well within this limit, suggesting excellent stability of the stem. Preparation of the femur is performed by reaming. This creates an accurate bone defect for the tapered implant and would explain the excellent initial stability achieved.

The neck-sparing stem was a real innovation for young patients. It has proven its effectiveness in several clinical studies [5, 6]. It is unfortunate that the economic, political and regulatory climate has not given this stem an opportunity to demonstrate success on a wider platform. In any case, both authors regret it [7].

Case Report

The concept of using a short stem, anchored only in the femoral neck, was not exclusively developed by Depuy. This is evidenced by the following case of a 42-year-old man who was implanted by one of the authors with a Primoris stem. This stem was developed by Biomet and, similar to the Silent stem, fell into oblivion despite excellent preliminary results. The patient enjoyed running but had to stop due to right hip osteoarthritis

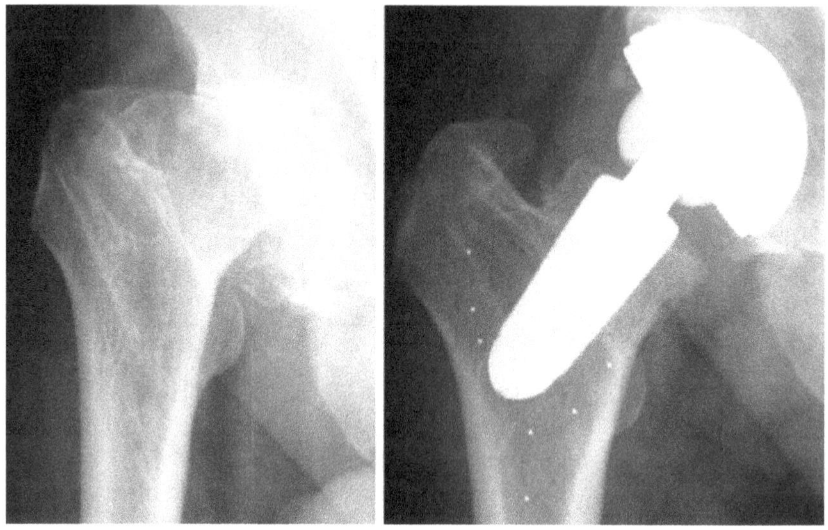

Fig. 5.9 Leg Calve Perthes hip implanted with a Silent™ stem

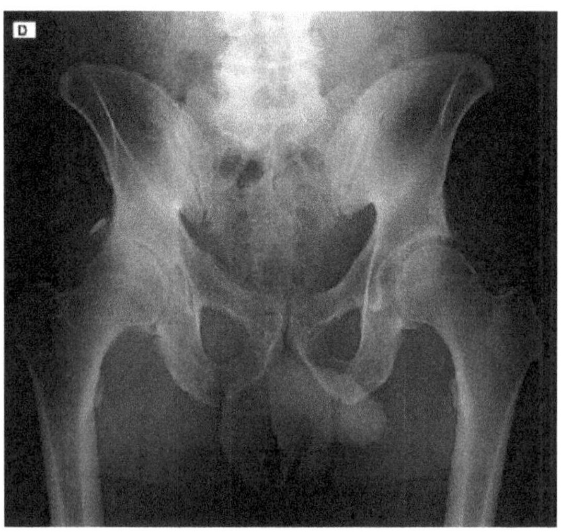

Fig. 5.10 Antero-posterior pelvic radiograph of a 42-year-old man showing right hip osteoarthritis

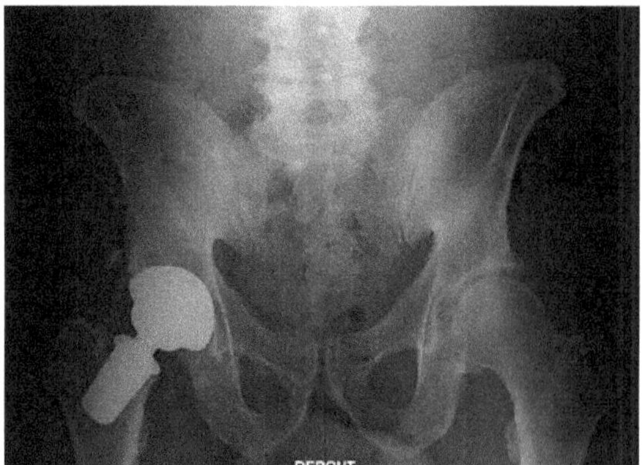

Fig. 5.11 Post-operative pelvic radiograph at 6 weeks

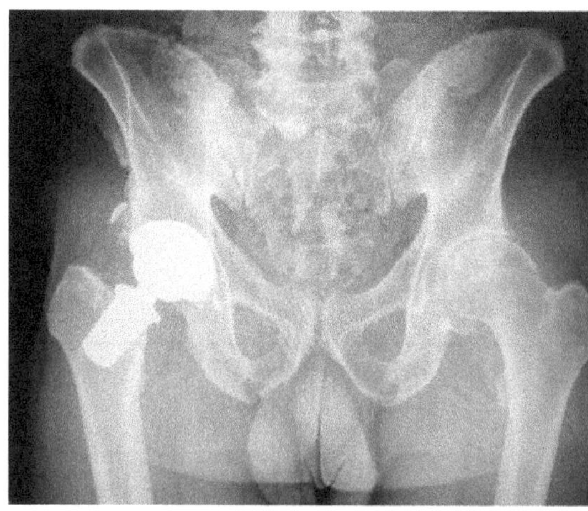

Fig. 5.12 Post-operative pelvic radiograph at 4 years, showing well-fixed components and no significant stress-shielding

(Fig. 5.10). After having undergone a total hip replacement through a direct anterior approach, the patient resumed his running activities as early as the sixth post-operative week (Fig. 5.11). At 4 years post-op, the patient continues to run with no detrimental effect on implant fixation (Fig. 5.12).

References

1. Falez F, Casella F, Papalia M. Current concepts, classification, and results in short stem hip arthroplasty. Orthopedics. 2015;38(3 Suppl):S6–13.

2. Rajakulendran K, Field RE. Neck-preserving femoral stems. HSS J. 2012;8(3):295–303.
3. Tran P, Zhang BX, Lade JA, Pianta RM, Unni RP, Haw CS. Periprosthetic bone remodeling after novel short-stem neck-sparing total hip arthroplasty. J Arthroplast. 2016;31(11):2530–5.
4. Burchard R, Braas S, Soost C, Graw JA, Schmitt J. Bone preserving level of osteotomy in short-stem total hip arthroplasty does not influence stress shielding dimensions - a comparing finite elements analysis. BMC Musculoskelet Disord. 2017;18(1):343.
5. Hauer G, Vielgut I, Amerstorfer F, Maurer-Ertl W, Leithner A, Sadoghi P. Survival rate of short-stem hip prostheses: a comparative analysis of clinical studies and national arthroplasty registers. J Arthroplast. 2018;33(6):1800–5.
6. Molfetta L, Capozzi M, Caldo D. Medium term follow up of the biodynamic neck sparing prosthesis. Hip Int. 2011;21(1):76–80.
7. Giardina F, Castagnini F, Stea S, Bordini B, Montalti M, Toni A. Short stems versus conventional stems in cementless Total hip arthroplasty: a long-term registry study. J Arthroplast. 2018;33(6):1794–9.

6

Custom Stems and the Reconstruction of the Proximal Femur Anatomy

Elhadi Sariali, Alexandre Mouttet, Xavier Flecher, and Jean Noel Argenson

6.1 Introduction

The proximal femur anatomy is highly variable between hip osteoarthritic patients [1–4]. This variability may render reliable restoration of the native hip anatomy and biomechanics difficult when performing total hip arthroplasty (THA) with conventional off-the-shelf stemmed femoral components. Poor restoration of biomechanical hip parameters such as femoral offset (FO), leg length (LL), and the femoral anteversion (FA) may compromise clinical outcome due to the resultant limp [5], edge loading [6], prosthetic impingement, and dislocation [5]. For instance, as little as a 15% decrease in FO reduces the abductor moment arm and hampers gait [7], suggesting that accurately restoring the FO is important, especially for younger patients with high functional demands.

E. Sariali (✉)
Hôpitaux Universitaires La Pitié Salpêtrière-Charles Foix, AP-HP, Paris, France

A. Mouttet
Polyclinique Médipôle Saint-Roch, Perpignan, France

X. Flecher · J. N. Argenson
Department of Orthopaedics and Traumatology, Aix Marseille Univ, APHM, CNRS, ISM, Sainte-Marguerite Hospital, Institute for Locomotion, Marseille, France
e-mail: Jean-noel.ARGENSON@ap-hm.fr

To assist surgeons in reproducing proximal femur anatomy in THA, conventional stems are typically available in two neck-shaft angles and two femoral offsets. Nevertheless, restoration of patient-specific femoral anteversion remains technically challenging—particularly for uncemented stems. Femoral stems with modular necks have therefore been developed to assist in the restoration of hip biomechanics (FO, LL, and FA) and to reduce the risk of prosthetic impingement. However, this results in excessive corrosion at the modular junction and leads to unacceptable rates of prosthetic neck fracture and adverse local tissue reaction to metal debris [8]; this has stymied their widespread adoption. The use of proximally loaded (metaphyseal fixation) custom stems has been proposed to precisely restore patient-specific proximal femur biomechanical parameters [9]. Their long-term clinical outcomes are excellent, with a survival rate of 97% at 20-year follow-up, including in very active below 50-year-old patients [10].

However, custom stems require three-dimensional (3D) imaging and planning, a longer lead time before surgery to allow for manufacture, and are typically more expensive than conventional stems. Therefore, it remained unclear what proportion of THA patients requires a custom stem to achieve an accurate 3D restoration of proximal femur anatomy. To address this question, we conducted a prospective observational study between January 2009 and November

2014, including all patients who underwent a 3D-planned primary THA using either an anatomic proximally hydroxyapatite (HA)-coated cementless modular-neck stem (off the shelf SPS® stem, Symbios, Switzerland) or a custom stem (Symbios, Switzerland).

6.2 Methods

Cohort description. Between 2009 and 2014, 578 consecutive patients underwent 3D-planning guided THA through a minimal invasive direct anterior approach. They were composed of 284 women and 294 men, aged 61 years (±SD 13) with a mean BMI of 26.5 ± 5. To restore hip biomechanics using 3D reconstruction, our prespecified guidelines determined that a custom stem was required in 72 (12%) patients composed of 40 women and 32 men aged 48 years (SD 15.4) with a mean BMI of 26.7 ± 5 kg/m^2, amongst whom 12 patients had previous hip surgery. In the custom group, the most frequent etiologies were DDH in 33 (46%) patients, primary osteoarthritis in 27 (38%) patients, AVN in 6 (8%) cases, and Legg–Perthes–Calve disease in 6 (8%) cases. In the SPS® group, the most frequent etiologies were primary osteoarthritis in 456 (80%) patients, DDH in 18 (3.5%) patients, AVN in 65 (13%) cases, and Legg–Perthes–Calve disease in 6 cases (1%). Patients in the custom group were significantly younger ($p < 0.001$) and more frequently suffered DDH ($p < 0.001$). All patients had an HA-coated acetabular component (APRIL®, Symbios, Switzerland) with a Biolox delta ceramic head and liner (CeramTec, Germany). A 28 mm head was used for cup diameters under 44 mm, a 32 mm head for cup diameters under 50 mm, and a 36 mm for larger cups. All the surgical procedures were performed by one surgeon (E. Sariali) who used a minimally invasive direct anterior approach (DAA), with patients positioning supine on a traction table [11]. Prior to surgery, patients had a low-dose CT scan [12] and 3D planning using the HIP-PLAN® software [13] to determine the prosthetic components size and position and to anticipate any surgical difficulties. The study was conducted according to the French bioethics law (Article L. 1121-1 of law no 2004-806, August 9, 2004), and an approbation was accorded by the patient protection committee responsible for this hospital.

Surgical planning. Cup implantation was simulated. The 3D-cup template was positioned relative to the medial acetabular wall, which was not breached. The cup was completely covered by the acetabular bone in order to avoid any impingement with surrounding soft tissues, especially the psoas tendon. The goal was to restore the native acetabular anteversion and to achieve a cup inclination of 40° (Fig. 6.1). In patients with developmental dysplasia of the hip (DDH), a standard 20° acetabular anteversion was planned. The stem size was chosen to maximize both the fit and fill in the metaphysis. To determine the cranio-caudal stem positioning, a colored image mode reflecting the density of the bone (based on Hounsfield units) in contact with the stem was used. To achieve good primary mechanical stability, the surgeon assumed that the stem should be in contact with highly dense (i.e., cortical) bone at least on the stem's lateral flare and the calcar (Fig. 6.2). The goal was also to restore the global hip offset corresponding to the sum of the acetabular offset and the femoral offset. Indeed, if a medial translation of the cup was required in order to achieve a good bony coverage of the cup, the femoral offset was increased by the same amount in order to restore the native global offset. Once the cup and the stem implantation were simulated, four points were determined during the preoperative planning in order to simulate the alteration of the hip anatomy induced by the arthroplasty (Fig. 6.3): (1) the centers of the acetabulum (Ac) and the cup (Cc)—the vector between these two points Ac and Cc was labeled acetabular displacement (AD); (2) the centers of the femoral head (FHc) and the femoral ball (FBc)—the vector between these two points FHc and FBc was labeled femoral head displacement (FHD). The global femoral displacement (FD) was measured as the sum of these two vectors AD and FHD. The goal was to achieve FD = 0, which means that the relative positions of the two native centers Ac and FHc were not altered by THA. A rotational analysis of the entire lower limb was

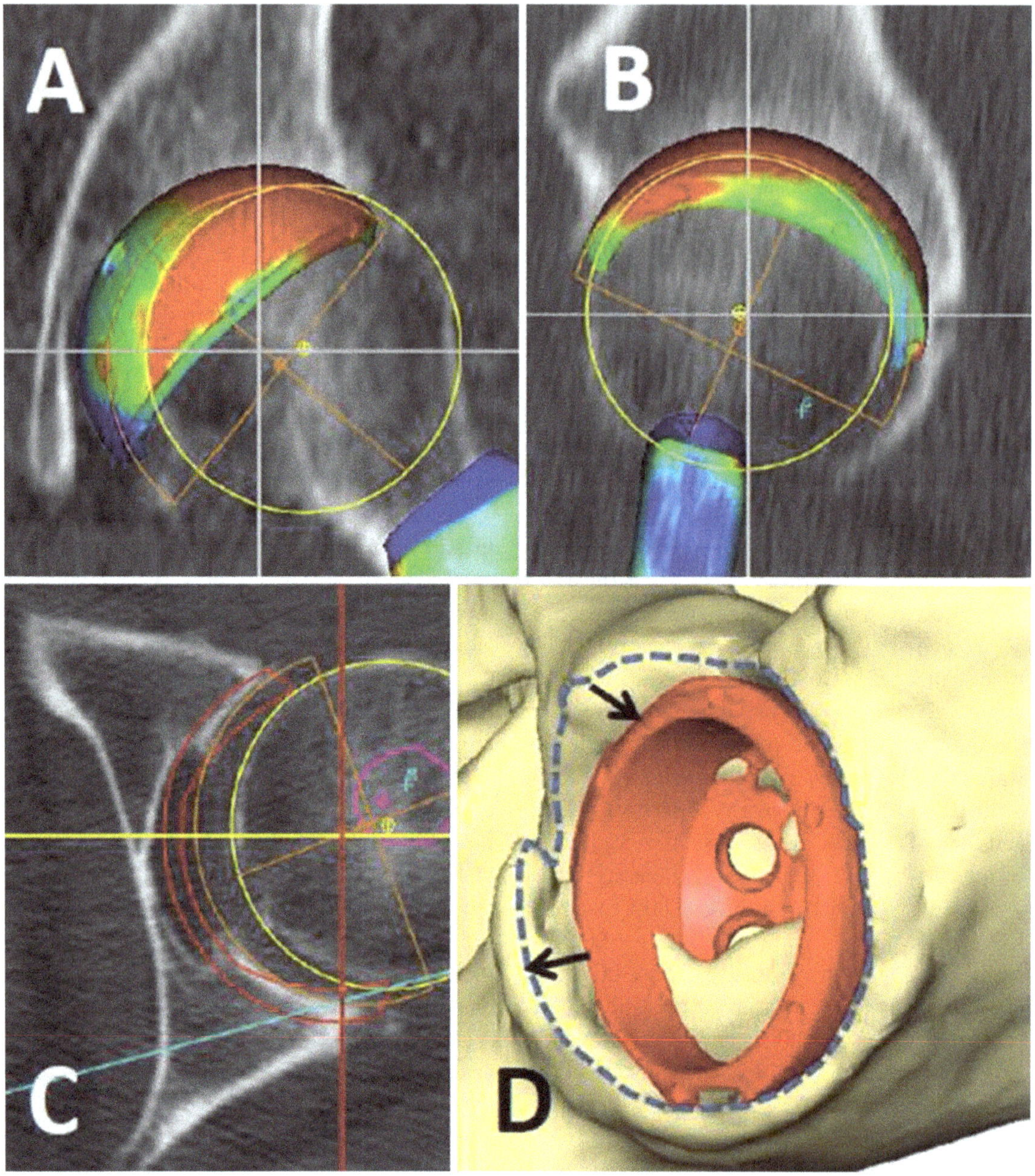

Fig. 6.1 Simulated 3D cup position (Coronal view (**a**), sagittal view (**b**), axial view (**c**) and 3D view (**d**)). To achieve primary stability, we assumed that the cup had to be in contact with highly dense bone on at least three points: the two walls and the roof. The 3D position of the cup was determined by measuring the distance from the edge of the cup to the edge of the bony acetabulum, especially relatively to the two walls (*black arrows*) and the lateral part of the roof

also performed, which included measuring the acetabular anteversion, the femoral neck anteversion, and the foot orientation angle—defined as the angle between the bi-malleolar axis and the posterior knee bicondylar plane line (Fig. 6.4). Based on previously reported results regarding the dislocation risk of DAA-THA [14], the goal was to restore the native femoral anteversion unless the femoral displacement (FD) in the anteroposterior direction was above 8 mm. This situation is typically observed when a posterior shift in the hip's center of rotation (COR) is combined with an increase in the femoral anteversion. In this case, a custom stem with a retroverted

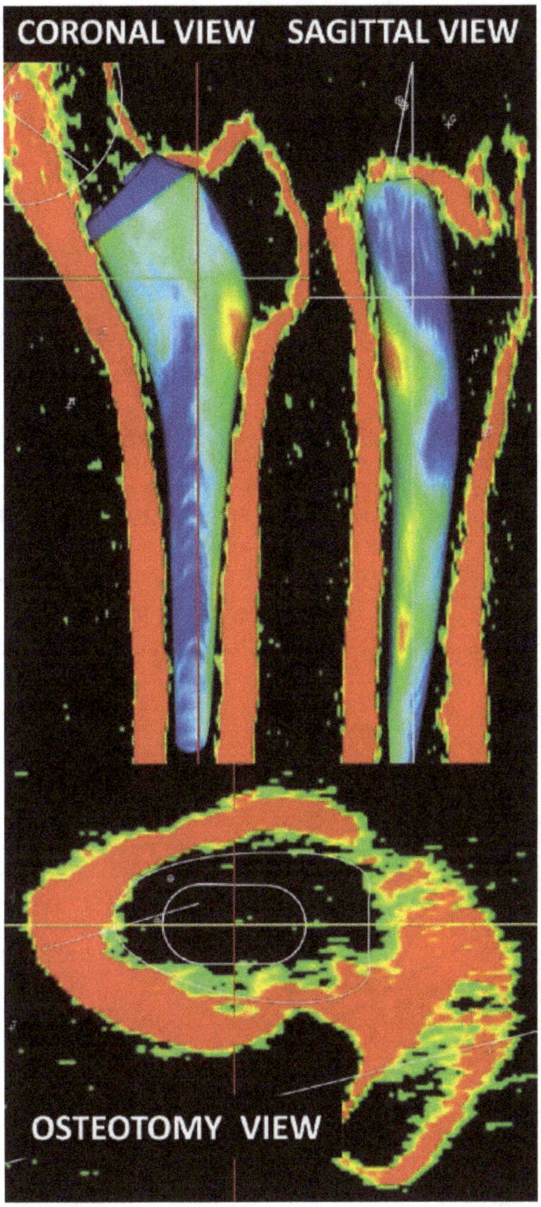

Fig. 6.2 3D planning of the stem including a coronal and sagittal analysis. A view of the osteotomy plane was available at the time of surgery to assist in controlling stem torsion

neck was used to make the femoral ball center coincide with the cup center (Fig. 6.5). When a decreased foot angle was observed, the femoral anteversion was slightly decreased in order to achieve a 15° foot orientation. For the femoral ball, four lengths could be used to alter neck length: −4 mm, 0, +4 mm, and + 8 mm. A custom femoral stem was used if the 3D reconstruction was not achievable with our standard stem (SPS®, Symbios SA). In this purpose, we used a tolerance of 15% for the offset and length and a tolerance of 6 mm for the anteroposterior position of the hip rotation center. The stem was designed to maximize the fit and fill in the metaphyseal zone (20 mm on each side of the middle of the lesser trochanter). The minimum stem length was calculated to withstand the fatigue tests.

Surgical technique. Minimally invasive DAA was used for all the patients. The cup was leveled with the tear drop and placed relative to the medial acetabular wall. The surgeon visually reproduced the preoperative planned position of the cup relatively to the acetabular rim by checking the distances from the edge of the cup to the acetabular roof and to the anterior and the posterior walls, using a 3D view of the simulated cup as a guide. The surgeon checked the final stem position with two parameters measured during the 3D planning. Firstly, he measured the distance from the top of the lesser trochanter to the top of the stem. Secondly, in order to control the stem anteversion, the surgeon performed a visual check of the position of the stem relative to the femur cross section corresponding to the neck osteotomy; this view was planned preoperatively. For the custom stems, only one custom rasp was used for the femur preparation. The postoperative protocol included full immediate weight-bearing for all patients.

Quality control of the implantation. In order to assess the accuracy of anatomically reconstructing the hip when using custom stem, we compared the native and prosthetic anatomical parameters in 30 consecutive patients who underwent a custom THA. For this, a pre- and postoperative CT scans were matched with the HIP-PLAN® software by independently aligning pelvic and then femoral bony landmarks (Fig. 6.6). We measured limb length discrepancy and changes to femoral offset and femoral anteversion.

Anticipation of surgical difficulties. The surgeon tried to forecast the following difficulties: (1) femoral perforation or femoral fracture which, in our experience, are more likely to occur if three conditions are combined: (a) a

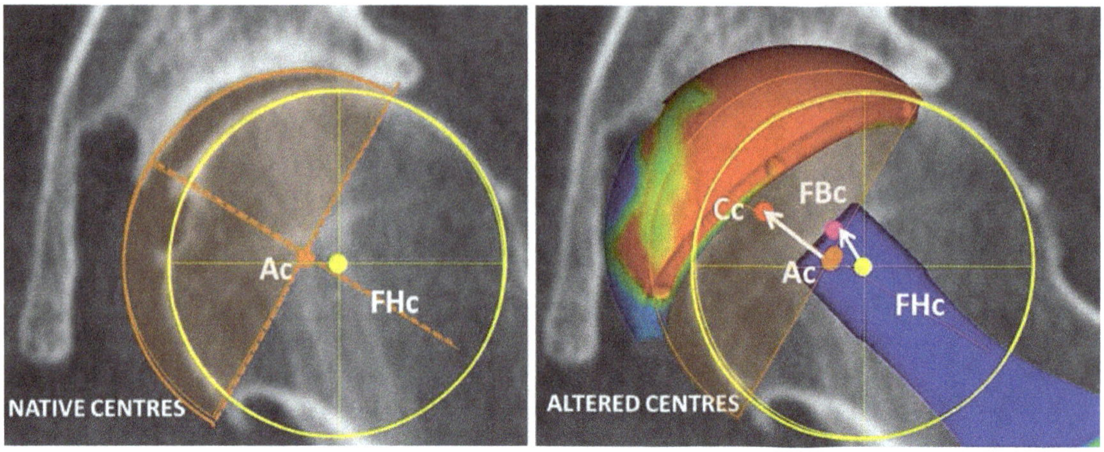

Fig. 6.3 The centers of the native acetabular (Ac) and femoral head (FHc) were determined. The distance between these two points was labeled initial displacement (ID) which corresponds to the articular surfaces wear. The centers of the final cup (Cc) and femoral prosthetic ball (FBc) were determined. The vector AcCc was labeled acetabular displacement (AD). The vector FHcFBc was labeled femoral head displacement (FHD). The global femoral displacement FD was measured as the sum of AD and FHD. We aimed for FD = 0. A XL head (long neck) is simulated

Fig. 6.4 Lower limb torsion was analyzed including the acetabular anteversion, the femoral anteversion, and the foot orientation

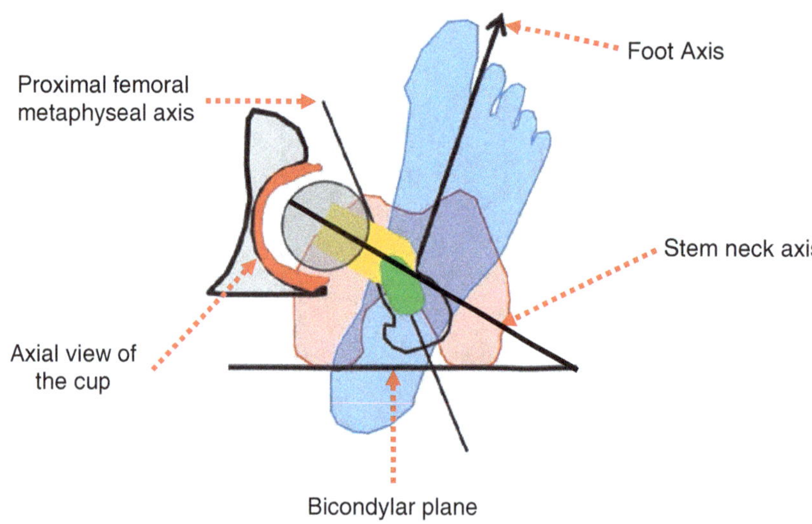

high anterior curvature of the femur, (b) a high density of cancellous bone at the upper part of the femur, and (c) and a narrow femoral isthmus. In these cases, before starting the rasping procedure, the femoral canal was reamed using a power tool and flexible reamers. (2) Any difficulties in simultaneously restoring femoral offset and length, especially in patients who have a femoral canal size incongruent with femoral offset (i.e., large femoral canal and low offset and vice versa). (3) Inappropriate final femoral anteversion (±10° compared to the native femoral anteversion) as a result of abnormal femoral torsion. For these cases, a suitably retroverted or anteverted neck was proposed to reduce the risk of prosthetic impingement and therefore increase stability.

Clinical assessment. Patients were assessed at the last follow-up with two self-completed questionnaires: the Harris Hip Score (0 worst and 100 best) and the Oxford Hip Score (0 worst and 60 best).

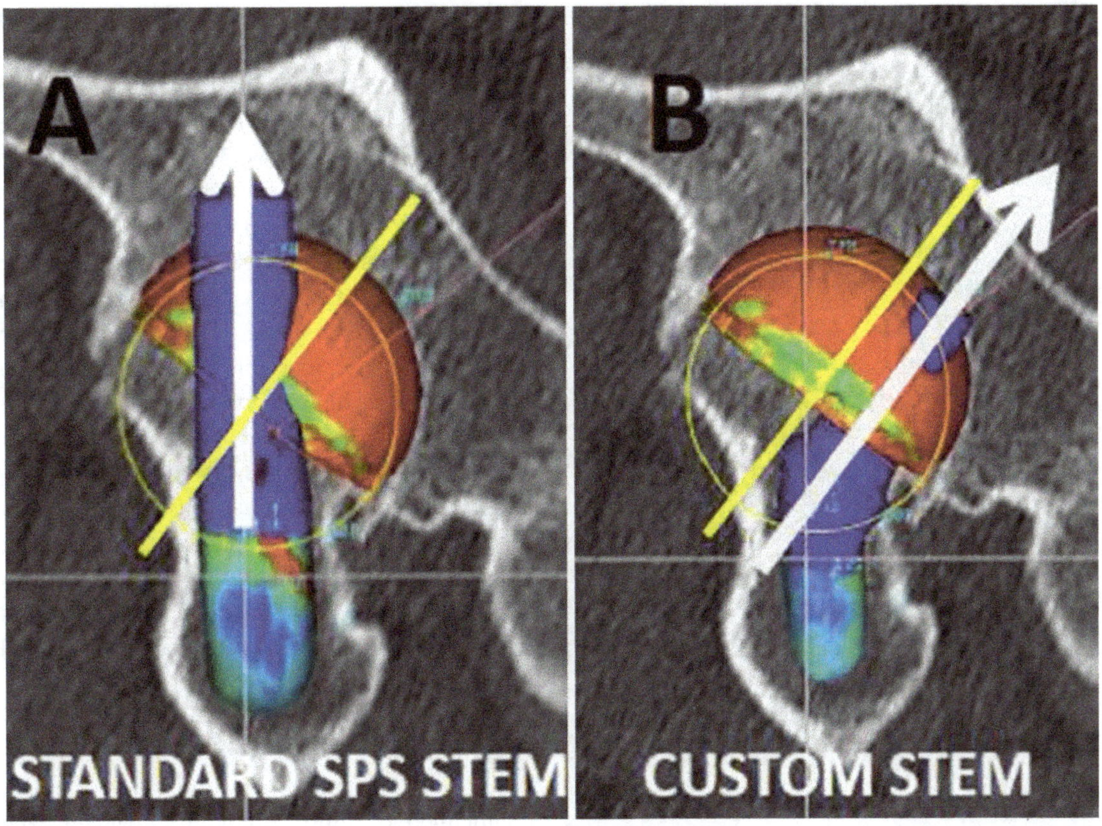

Fig. 6.5 This case shows a dysplastic hip with a mismatch between the femoral ball center and the cup center due to excessive antetorsion of the proximal metaphyseal part of the femur. The acetabular reaming procedure generates a posterior translation of the center of rotation and consequently an anterior hip instability. A custom stem with a retroverted neck (**b**) was used to make the femoral ball center coincide with the cup center at contrary to a standard straight-neck stem (**a**)

Statistical analysis method. Pearson correlation coefficient was used to study the relationship between two variables (preoperative and postoperative anteversion values). Surgical precision was defined by assessing the difference in matched anatomical parameters between the planned and the postoperative values (mean ± SD). Data were assessed for normality using the Ryan–Joiner and Shapiro–Wilk tests. For normally distributed variables, when two groups had the same variances, differences between them were analyzed using Student's *t*-test. For abnormally distributed variables or normally distributed variables with different variances, the Mann and Whitney test was used. A *p*-value of less than 0.05 was considered significant. Statistical analysis was performed with JMP software (version-11; SAS Institute).

6.3 Results

Implantation accuracy. There was excellent agreement between the planned and the performed femoral stem anteversions with an implantation accuracy of 1° (±4°). The difference between the planned (20° ± 8°) and the postoperatively measured femoral anteversion (21° ± 8°) was not statistically significant ($p = 0.3$), and their correlation was very strong

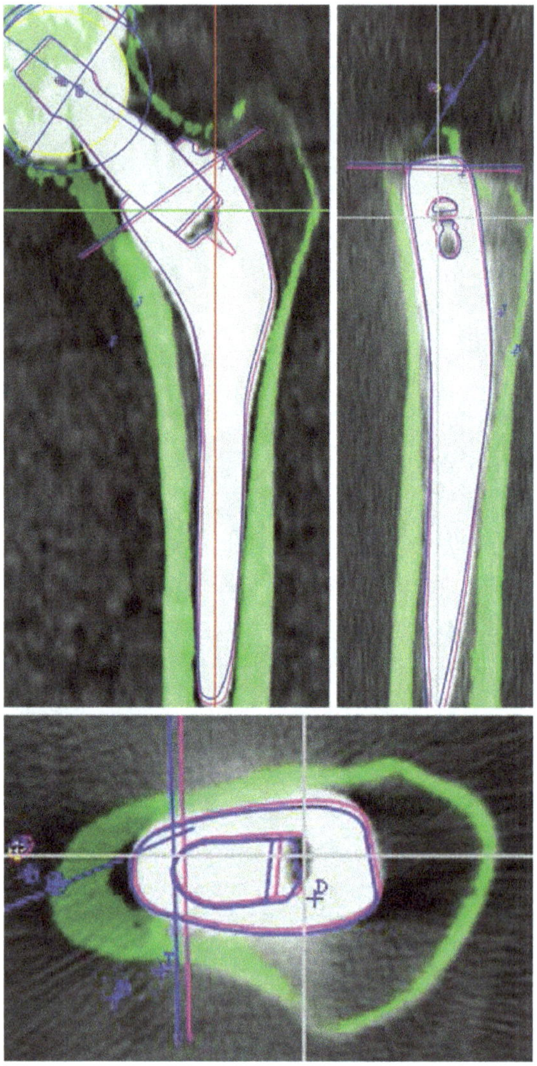

Fig. 6.6 Matching of preoperative and postoperative CT scans was performed with the HIP-PLAN® software in a group of 30 patients in order to compare the planned and performed positioning of components

($r = 0.9$, $p < 0.001$) (Fig. 6.7a). There was excellent agreement between the planned and performed lower limb length (LL) with an implantation accuracy of −0.6 ± 2.5 mm. There was no significant difference between the planned (5 ± 4.6 mm) and the executed (4.4 ± 5.5 mm) LL ($p = 0.3$), and the correlation between them was found very strong ($r = 0.9$, $p < 0.001$) (Fig. 6.7b). Last, there was excellent agreement between the planned and performed femoral offset with an implantation accuracy of −1.2 ± 2.4 mm. There was no significant difference between the planned FO value (43.3 ± 6.8 mm) and the postoperative one (42.1 ± 7.0 mm) ($p = 0.3$), and furthermore, a very strong correlation between these two values was found ($r = 0.95$, $p < 0.001$) (Fig. 6.7c).

Anticipation of surgical difficulties. The main anatomic reasons that led to use a custom stem were: (1) torsional abnormalities of the proximal femur that prevented restoring a planned femoral anteversion (Fig. 6.8) and potentially made the patient prone to dislocation or foot malorientation, (2) severe coxa vara or coxa valga making the simultaneous restoration of femoral offset and length challenging when using conventional stems (Fig. 6.9), and (3) severe outlier morphotypes such as dwarf and giant patients where off-the-shelf stems are inappropriate and either too big or too small, respectively.

Clinical outcomes. At 5 years ±2 mean follow-up, no stem was revised for an aseptic reason, no dislocation occurred, no patient complained of limb length discrepancies, and excellent clinical results were achieved. The mean HHS improved from 30 to 93 (±16) and the Oxford score improved from 23 to 56 (±9).

6.4 Discussion

The main results from our study were that (1) 12% of patients required a custom stem to reconstruct their native femoral anatomy, the main reasons being torsional abnormalities and severe coxa vara or coxa valga; (2) the manual implantation (technology free) of custom stem was precise; and (3) performing anatomic restoration of hip biomechanics using 3D planning, intraoperative checks, and custom implants resulted in excellent functional outcome for patients with atypical proximal femoral anatomy.

The main limitation of this study is that our results are implant and patient specific. Our

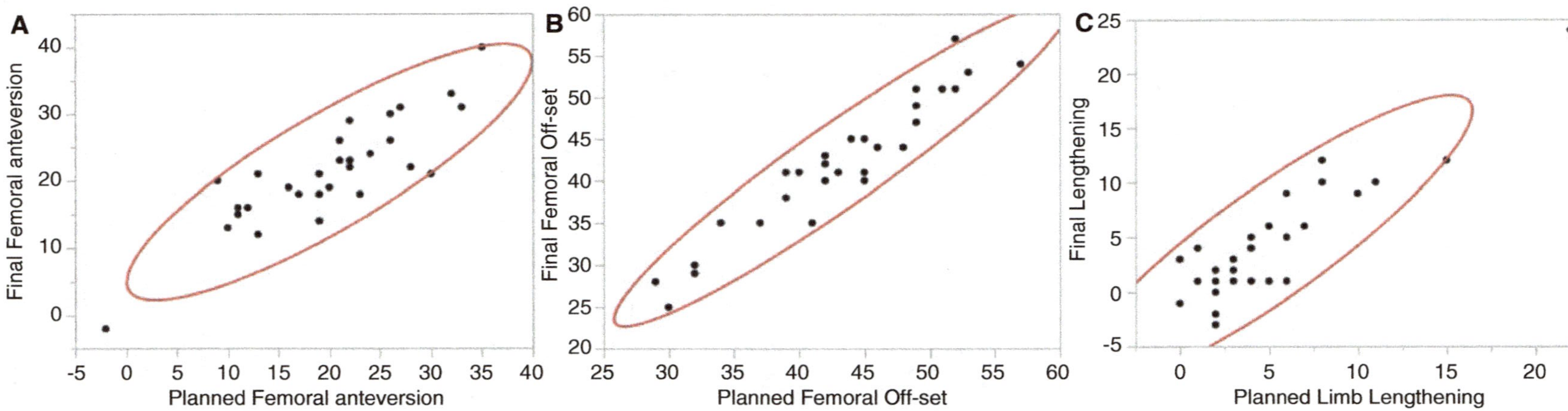

Fig. 6.7 Very high precision was achieved when manually implanting the cementless custom stems. Those charts illustrate the strong relationship between planned and performed femoral anteversion (**a**, $r = 0.90$), femoral offset (**b**, $r = 0.95$), and limb lengthening (**c**, $r = 0.90$)

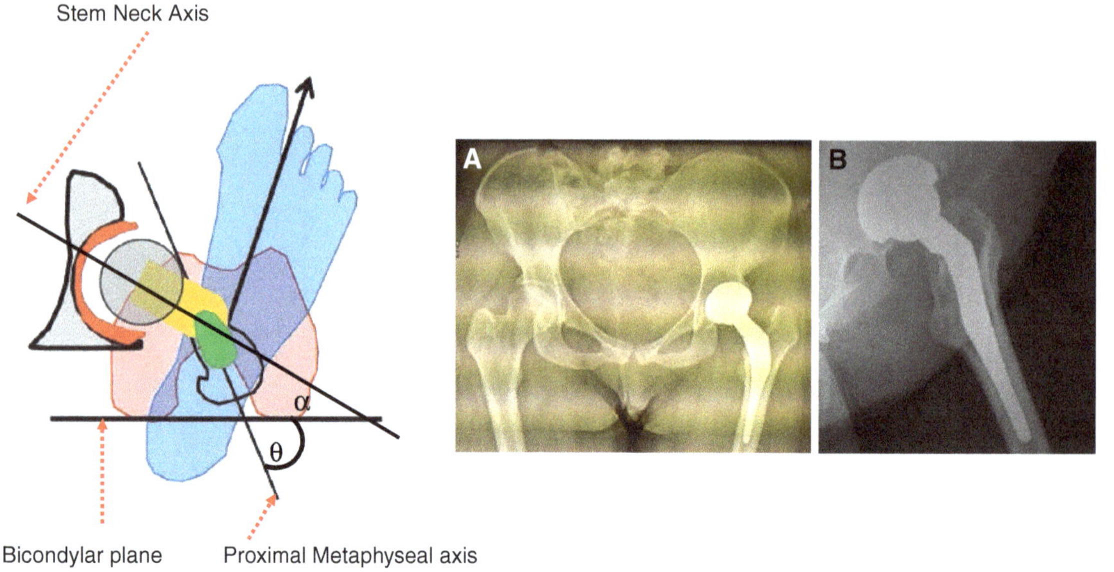

Fig. 6.8 The post operative radiographies are presented: (**a**) Antero-posterior view (**b**) lateral view. Illustration of a 3D plan for a patient with a severe torsional disorder with a proximal femoral metaphyseal version of 63°—increased by 40° compared to native femoral anteversion. A 40° retroversion of the neck relatively to the shaft was required to stabilize the hip. The use of standard straight-neck SPS Stem would have led to a 40° excess in stem anteversion. A 40° retroversion of the neck relatively to the shaft was required to stabilize the hip

results regarding the proportion of patients needing a custom stem, and the reasons for this, only apply to the SPS stem design. Different results would probably be found with other stem designs.

The accuracy for anatomically reconstructing the hip with custom stem technology was judged to be excellent. This accuracy compares well with previously reported results for 3D planning-based off-the-shelf THA [4, 11]. However, patients in the custom group had complex hip anatomy, primarily regarding their proximal femoral morphology, and restoration of normal biomechanics would not be achievable with conventional implant designs such as the SPS® stem (anatomic design).

Few studies have assessed the accuracy of postoperative hip anatomical restoration using a CT scan, as it requires careful 3D analysis of preoperative anatomy and accurate matching. Contrary to literature on optimal acetabular cup positioning, there is no "safe zone" recommended for femoral anteversion. In this study, we propose a new method for defining the target femoral anteversion. Surgeons should compensate for changes in the acetabular center induced by reaming. Typically, acetabular preparation induces a posterior, medial, and cranial shift of the hip center of rotation. In response, we advise that femoral offset and anteversion/retroversion are adapted accordingly during 3D planning. In the case of a high-grade dysplastic hip (dislocated), a 15–20° anteversion was aimed for.

Kirshnan et al. [15] reported that the intracanalar (femur flares and volume) and the extracanalar proximal femur anatomy (femoral offset, neck length, and femoral anteversion) are not correlated, suggesting that the same proximal femur volume may correspond to a highly variable femoral offset. Interestingly, Sariali et al. [13] showed that for a given stem size, the required range for stem FO was 22 mm in order to restore accurately the patient native FO. Hence, for outlier patients, custom stems are the favored solution. They allow the surgeon to accurately address the extramedullary anatomy independent of the intracanalar anatomy, while avoiding the complications related to the use of modular necks such as modular neck fractures and adverse local tissue reaction to metal debris.

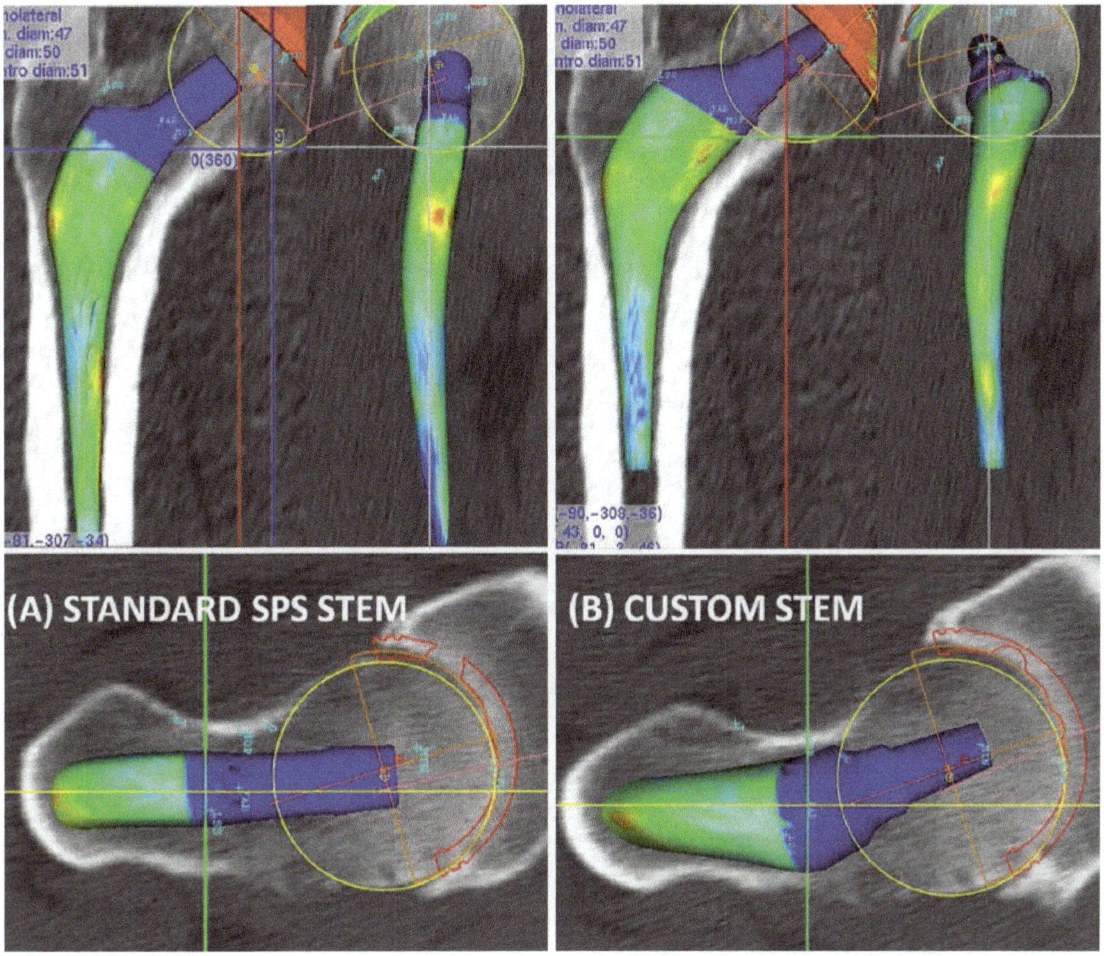

Fig. 6.9 The 3D plan in this case shows a hip with severe coxa vara and a high femoral offset. The standard 129° CCD angle stem (**a**) would not allow the restoration of proximal femur anatomy. The custom stem (**b**) included a higher offset and a 15° retroversion of the neck relative to the shaft

6.5 Conclusion

Custom stem technology is a reliable solution to treat degenerated hip patients having an atypical hip anatomy. Approximately, 12% of patients require a custom stem to achieve an accurate reconstruction of their proximal femur anatomy. Performing 3D planning for all osteoarthritic hip patients and checking intraoperative anatomical parameters are key steps to anticipate the surgical difficulties, select the appropriate implants, and restore normal hip biomechanics.

References

1. Argenson J, Ryembault E, Flecher X, Brassart N, Parratte S, Aubaniac J. Three-dimensional anatomy of the hip in osteoarthritis after developmental dysplasia. J Bone Joint Surg Br. 2005;87(9):1192–6.
2. Husmann O, Rubin P, Leyvraz P, de Roguin B, Argenson J. Three-dimensional morphology of the proximal femur. J Arthroplast. 1997;12:444–50.
3. Schmidutz F, Graf T, Mazoochian F, Fottner A, Bauer-Melnyk A, Jansson V. Migration analysis of a metaphyseal anchored short-stem hip prosthesis. Acta Orthop. 2012;83(4):360–5.
4. Sariali E, Mouttet A, Pasquier G, Durante E. Three dimensionnal hip anatomy in osteoarthritis. Analysis of the femoral off-set. J Arthroplast. 2009;24(6):990–7.

5. Asayama I, Chamnongkich S, Simpson K, Kinsey T, Mahoney O. Reconstructed hip joint position and abductor muscle strength after total hip arthroplasty. J Arthroplast. 2005;20:414–20.
6. Sariali E, Klouche S, Mamoudy P. Ceramic-on-ceramic total hip arthroplasty: is squeaking related to an inaccurate three-dimensional hip anatomy reconstruction? Orthop Traumatol Surg Res. 2012;100(4):437–40.
7. Sariali E, Klouche S, Mouttet A, Pascal-Moussellard H. The effect of femoral offset modification on gait after total hip arthroplasty. Acta Orthop. 2014;85(2):123–7. Epub 2014/02/26.
8. Kwon YM, Khormaee S, Liow MH, Tsai TY, Freiberg AA, Rubash HE. Asymptomatic pseudotumors in patients with taper corrosion of a dual-taper modular femoral stem: MARS-MRI and metal ion study. J Bone Joint Surg Am. 2016;98(20):1735–40. Epub 2016/11/22.
9. Flecher X, Pearce O, Parratte S, Aubaniac J, Argenson J. Custom cementless stem improves hip function in young patients at 15-year followup. Clin Orthop Relat Res. 2010;468(3):747–55.
10. Dessyn E, Flecher X, Parratte S, Ollivier M, Argenson JN. A 20-year follow-up evaluation of total hip arthroplasty in patients younger than 50 using a custom cementless stem. Hip Int. 2018;23:1120700018803290. Epub 2018/10/24.
11. Sariali E, Catonne Y, Pascal-Moussellard H. Three-dimensional planning-guided total hip arthroplasty through a minimally invasive direct anterior approach. Clinical outcomes at five years' follow-up. Int Orthop. 2017;41(4):699–705. Epub 2016/06/18.
12. Huppertz A, Lembcke A, Sariali E, Durmus T, Schwenke C, Hamm B, et al. Low dose computed tomography for 3D planning of total hip arthroplasty: evaluation of radiation exposure and image quality. J Comput Assist Tomogr. 2015;39(5):649–56.
13. Sariali E, Mouttet A, Pasquier G, Durante E, Catonne Y. Accuracy of reconstruction of the hip using computerised three-dimensional pre-operative planning and a cementless modular-neck stem. J Bone Joint Surg Br. 2009;91(3):333–40.
14. Sariali E, Klouche S, Mamoudy P. Investigation into three dimensional hip anatomy in anterior dislocation after THA. Influence of the position of the hip rotation centre. Clin Biomech. 2012;27(6):562–7.
15. Krishnan S, Carrington R, Mohiyaddin S, Garlick N. Common misconceptions of normal hip joint relations on pelvic radiographs. J Arthroplast. 2006;21:409–12.

7

Large-Diameter Head THA and the Reconstruction of the Proximal Femur Anatomy

William G. Blakeney, Jean-Alain Epinette, and Pascal-André Vendittoli

Key Points

Large Diameter Head THA

- Is defined as a bearing diameter >36 mm and includes monobloc or dual-mobility femoral head designs.
- Allows supraphysiologic postoperative hip range of motion and return to unrestricted activities.
- Is a forgiving procedure, minimizing the risk of femoral neck impingement on the acetabular component rim.
- Dislocation rate is extremely low whatever the surgical approach.
- Helps restore hip biomechanics, minimizing the requirement for surgical modifications linked to intraoperative stability.
- CoC THA has the potential to provide long-term implant survivorship with unrestricted activity, while avoiding implant impingement, liner fracture at insertion, and hip instability.
- With the recently reported low wear rate, Dual Mobility THA could be considered for a larger proportion of THA patients.

W. G. Blakeney
Department of Surgery, CIUSSS-de-L'Est-de-L'Ile-de-Montréal, Hôpital Maisonneuve Rosemont. 5415, Montréal, QC, Canada

Department of Surgery, Albany Health Campus, Albany, WA, Australia

J.-A. Epinette
Clinique Médico-chirurgicale, Bruay la Buissière, France
e-mail: jae@orthowave.net

P.-A. Vendittoli (✉)
Department of Surgery, CIUSSS-de-L'Est-de-L'Ile-de-Montréal, Hôpital Maisonneuve Rosemont. 5415, Montréal, QC, Canada

Department of Surgery, Université de Montréal, Montréal, QC, Canada

7.1 Introduction

There are many potential benefits to using large-diameter femoral heads (LDHs, >36 mm) in total hip arthroplasty (THA). They provide a supraphysiologic range of motion (ROM), which makes them more forgiving with regard to component positioning. This is of particular benefit to high-demand patients involved in manual work or with an active lifestyle. These are frequently young patients, in which the use of a hard-on-hard bearing also offers the promise of prosthetic longevity. The move toward large head ceramic-on-ceramic (CoC) bearings ought to diminish the incidence of local adverse reaction to metal debris (ARMD) experienced with some LDH metal-on-metal (MoM) bearings.

7.2 Hip Stability and Range of Motion

Throughout the world, LDH has been increasingly used in THA mainly because of the perceived benefits of reduced dislocation risk. This has been demonstrated in a number of trials. A series of 1748 patients operated on with LDH THAs reported a dislocation rate as low as 0.05% at a mean follow-up of 31 months [1]. A retrospective review of all primary THAs performed by two experienced arthroplasty surgeons reported a significantly higher rate of dislocation in small-diameter head THAs (1.8%, 10 of 559) compared to the LDH group (0%, 0 of 248) at a mean follow-up of 5 years [2]. Improved outcomes have also been seen in patients undergoing revision THA. A randomized trial demonstrated a significantly lower instability with only 1.1% dislocation risk in patients with larger heads (36 or 40 mm) compared to 8.7% in those with small heads (32 mm) at a mean of 5 years post-surgery [3]. These results have been replicated in national joint registries [4, 5].

The reduced dislocation rate seen in LDH THAs is a result of many possible factors. Primarily, it is a result of the greater head-to-neck ratio and increased jump distance (Fig. 7.1). It has also been proposed that large heads may provide passive resistance to dislocation through a suction effect, preventing microseparation [6]. A large head fills the capsular void left by resection of the native femoral head and has an increased volume to displace, which may further resist dislocation. They may also be favorable for joint perception and proprioception.

LDHs increase the ROM of the hip before prosthetic impingement. Burroughs et al., in a biomechanical study, found that the effect of increasing the head–neck ratio on range of motion plateaued at 38 mm. This was because the impingement was no longer on the prosthesis but extra-articular (soft

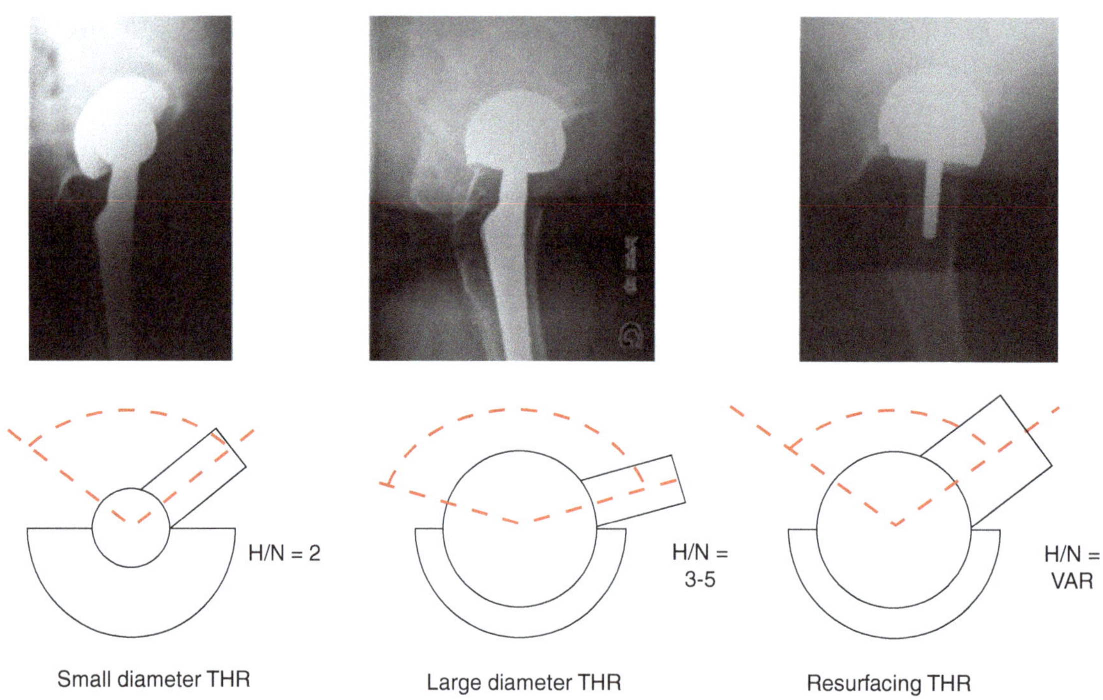

Fig. 7.1 Different head–neck ratios and related arc of motion before component–component impingement for small diameter THA, LDH THA, and hip resurfacing

tissue or bony) impingement, which was independent of head size [7]. Avoiding component impingement may be a significant advantage for hard bearings like ceramic. Contact between the metallic femoral neck and the ceramic liner has been associated with liner chipping, neck wear (metallosis), pain, and noise generation (squeaking) [8]. Moreover, Scifert et al. reported that with extra-articular contact, rather than impingement of the prosthetic neck on the liner, the moment resisting dislocation increased substantially (about fourfold larger) [9]. Cinotti et al. similarly found increased range of motion with larger head sizes and reported that the benefit of larger heads on ROM was even greater in mal-positioned acetabular components; thus, it is a more forgiving implant [10]. This is of importance, given the high number of patients with lumbosacral degeneration undergoing THA, and the known difficulties faced by the surgeon in optimally placing the acetabular component in this subset of patients at high risk of impingement and dislocation [11, 12].

Young and active patients frequently suffer from secondary OA associated with anatomical challenges, such as acetabular retroversion, hip dysplasia, femoral retroversion, Perthes deformity, and pistol-grip femur. These extreme anatomies may not be ideal for hip resurfacing procedures where anatomy correction is limited. In THAs, ideal component positioning for most advantageous ROM and wear may be limited by suboptimal primary fixation. Using LDH THAs helps the surgeon to manage these challenges.

Although the range of motion may plateau with increasing head size, the jump distance required for dislocations to occur will continue to increase. The jump distance is the amount of lateral translation of the femoral head center required for dislocation. The greater the head size, the greater is the jump distance required for dislocation. The jump distance, however, decreases with increasing offset of the center of rotation of the femoral head. This is of importance as the current designs of cups for LDH articulations are often truncated hemispheres of ~160° with offset of 3–4 mm. Increasing cup abduction and to a lesser degree anteversion also affect the jump distance, so an LDH will offset the risk of dislocation due to component malpositioning [13].

Micro-separation has been reported in vivo by many authors, who demonstrated that during the swing phase, the femoral head may not stay centered inside the cup. A metal-on-polyethylene (MoP) THA has a larger clearance between the femoral head and the polyethylene liner. Furthermore, polyethylene has reduced wettability that may result in less cohesiveness of the lubricating film, allowing hip separation to occur. A video fluoroscopy study has shown absence of micro-separation in large-head metal-on-metal (MoM) THAs compared to frequent micro-separations in small-head MoP THAs [14]. Potential detrimental effects resulting from this micro-separation include premature wear and component loosening. It has also been linked to clicking and squeaking sounds coming from the hip. In a trial of 24 patients with a variety of tribological combinations, the only patient who did not generate sound was the only one not to experience femoral head micro-separation during gait [15]. CoC LDH THA with small clearance and broad contact surface may help to reduce or avoid bearing micro-separation during gait and improve muscle function and joint kinematics.

7.3 Anatomical Reconstruction

The other benefit to an LDH is in providing a more anatomical joint. By maintaining similar biomechanics as the native hip joint with regard to restoration of hip offset, leg length, and femoral head diameter on an individual case-by-case basis, it is thought the patient will have a more natural-feeling hip. Because of its intrinsic stability and low dislocation risk, surgeons performing LDH THA can tailor the patient's leg length and femoral offset to their individual anatomy without having to make adjustments or compromises to ensure hip stability. In the gait lab, it has been demonstrated that LDH THA restores the center of gravity and gait pattern to normal [16]. A number of studies have demonstrated that restoration of the femoral head diameter better restores normal gait parameters in comparison to conventional small head

THAs [17, 18]. LDH THA has been demonstrated to better restore hip ROM, compared to 28-mm head THA and hip resurfacing [19]. In our experience, patients who have had a hip resurfacing and an LDH THA on the contralateral side, often prefer the more supple joint offered by the LDH THA.

As femoral head sizes have increased with a concomitant decrease in dislocations, surgeons have been removing more and more patient restrictions. A study of the Danish registry showed no increased risk of dislocation in a cohort of patients with 32 mm and 36 mm heads when immediately mobilized without restrictions following THA, compared to a historic cohort with 28 mm heads that had standard restrictions [20]. In our institution, using a posterior approach with LDH THAs, we have removed all postoperative restrictions, and review of our first 276 hips at a mean of 66.5 months (range 48.0–78.5) post surgery demonstrated a dislocation rate of 0% [21]. It also significantly simplifies the postoperative management of patients undergoing bilateral procedures or outpatient THA surgery. The need for patient education is considerably reduced and confidence in the hip is much higher.

Once the hip capsule is healed (2–3 months), we allow LDH THA patients to go back to unrestricted activities. At-risk activities, like kayaking, rock climbing, and skiing, are performed as with a natural hip. Professional activities are also resumed without limitations. Roof workers, plumbers, firemen, or policemen are allowed to go back to their original occupation. This lack of restrictions was not accepted by employers with the previously used smaller head diameter (28–32 mm) MoP bearings. Furthermore, with the low wear rates of a CoC bearing, no limitation on the activity volume is imposed.

7.4 Potential Concerns: Trunnionosis, ARMD, and Noise

There are some potential disadvantages to using LDH THA. With the introduction of highly cross-linked polyethylene, concerns about volumetric wear in a polyethylene liner have proven unfounded on results to date. Clinically deleterious taper corrosion (or trunnionosis) has gained a lot of media attention with the well-documented problems, following the widespread introduction of LDH MoM THAs. A randomized trial reported higher serum metal ion levels in LDH MoM THAs compared to MoM hip resurfacings, suggesting that the problem is greater at the trunnion than at the articulation [22]. Though taper corrosion has been documented to occur with most head–neck material combinations and tribological combinations, reports of clinical sequelae were rare until the era of LDH MoM THAs. It is now understood to be associated with adverse local tissue reactions (ALTR), which may lead to clinical failure. It has been hypothesized that the small diameter of the trunnion in THAs, which was initially designed for a 28 mm head, may be more prone to corrosion due to increased frictional torque at the head–neck junction with a larger head. A conceivable solution is to increase the taper size for LDH. However, the degree to which LDH size is the cause of this problem is currently unknown. Implant retrieval as well as finite element analysis studies have identified multiple mechanical factors associated with the risk of trunnionism, including taper length, taper angle, surface finish, rigidity, and mixed alloys, which may result in corrosion. We compared whole blood titanium (Ti) ion levels at a minimum 1-year follow-up in 27 patients with unilateral primary LDH CoC THA with head sizes ranging from 36 to 48 mm using a Ti stem and acetabular component [23]. Mean Ti ion levels in patients with 36- to 40-mm head diameters (without Ti sleeve) was 2.3 µg/L and 1.9 µg/L for the 44- and 48-mm femoral head (with Ti sleeve). These Ti levels are low and probably related to unavoidable passive corrosion of implant surfaces. No patients presented clinical signs of ALTR.

LDH CoC bearings were introduced to reduce component impingement, increase stability, and optimize tribology without the associated problems seen in metal-on-metal bearings. With ceramic heads, metal ion release from the head–neck junction is substantially lower than with metallic heads [23, 24]. The Australian joint registry has reported a decreasing rate of revision at 5 years for increasing head size of a ceramic-on-ceramic bearing. A high revision rate of 4.7% is seen with heads of less than 28 mm compared to 3.3% for 32 mm, 2.8% for 36–38 mm, and 2.6% for head size of 40 mm or greater [4]. This reduced revision rate is mainly a result of a reduced dislocation rate. At 1 year, the cumulative incidence of revision for dislocation is 2.0% for head sizes 28 mm or smaller compared to 0.4% for 32 mm, 0.3% for 36–38 mm, and 0.1% for head sizes 40 mm or larger.

One problem that has been noted, specific to hard-on-hard bearings, is squeaking. McDonnell et al. reported on the Delta Motion Hip System (DePuy Synthes, Warsaw, IN, USA), the first LDH monoblock delta ceramic acetabular system (since withdrawn from production) [25]. They reported an overall squeaking incidence of 21% in 208 hips at a mean follow-up of 21 months. Goldhofer et al. reported an incidence of squeaking of 17% at 5-year follow-up [26], increased from 7% at 2 years [27]. There were, however, no significant differences with regard to patient satisfaction or clinical outcomes (Oxford Hip Score and Harris Hip Score) between the patients with squeaking and silent hips. In our institution, review of the first 276 hips using the Maxera (Zimmer, Warsaw, IN, USA; Fig. 7.2) LDH CoC hip system revealed a similar squeaking rate (22.7%) [21]. Squeaking was significantly associated with younger age and more active patients (higher SF-12 PCS and UCLA scores). Greater femoral head size was also associated with increased squeaking. Despite the squeaking, functional scores and patient satisfaction were high. After 9 years of clinical use, we have replaced more than 2700 hips with CoC LDH THA. No revisions were performed for component loosening, osteolysis, adverse reaction to metal debris (trunnionosis), implant fracture, or squeaking. There were five cases of early implant mobilization secondary to insufficient primary press fit fixation and four early postoperative dislocations treated with closed reduction without recurrence.

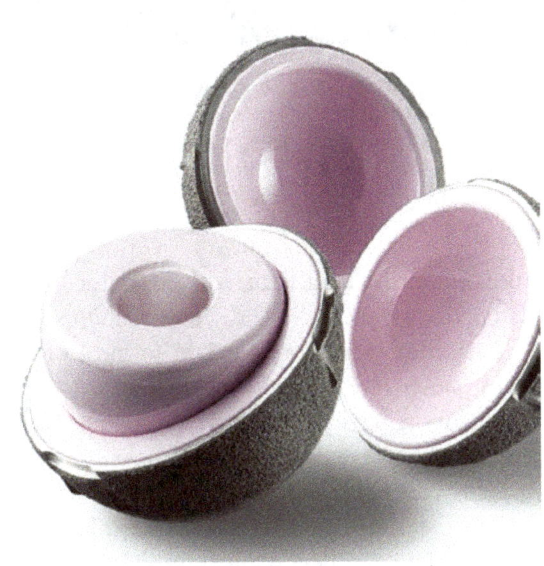

Fig. 7.2 LDH delta ceramic with the monoblock Maxera acetabular component

7.5 LDH with Dual-Mobility Femoral Head

Another hip component design that could be incorporated into an LDH option is the dual mobility (DM) articulation. This "old French invention," used since 1974 by Gilles Bousquet in Saint-Etienne (France), takes the double principle of a small articulation to minimize the problems of wear, coupled with a "big articulation" to stabilize the hip and prevent instability (Fig. 7.3) [28–30]. We know that DM implants are performing well for cases of primary THA with a high risk of dislocation (neurological patient, major muscle deficit, etc.) and complex prosthetic revisions. In comparison with conventional implants, DM cups can add an extra arc of movement before impingement of 30.5° in flexion, 15.4° in abduction, and 22.4° in external rotation [31]. This high prosthetic stability is supported by the conclusions of a literature review done by Stroh et al. [32] that showed DM devices significantly reduce the risk of dislocation, both in primary arthroplasty (0.1% for DM vs. 2–7% for fixed inserts) and in revision surgery (3.5% for DM vs. 10–16% for fixed inserts). Since the early 2000s, improved DM implant designs have allowed a different assessment of the risk–benefit ratio, therefore creating potential new indications

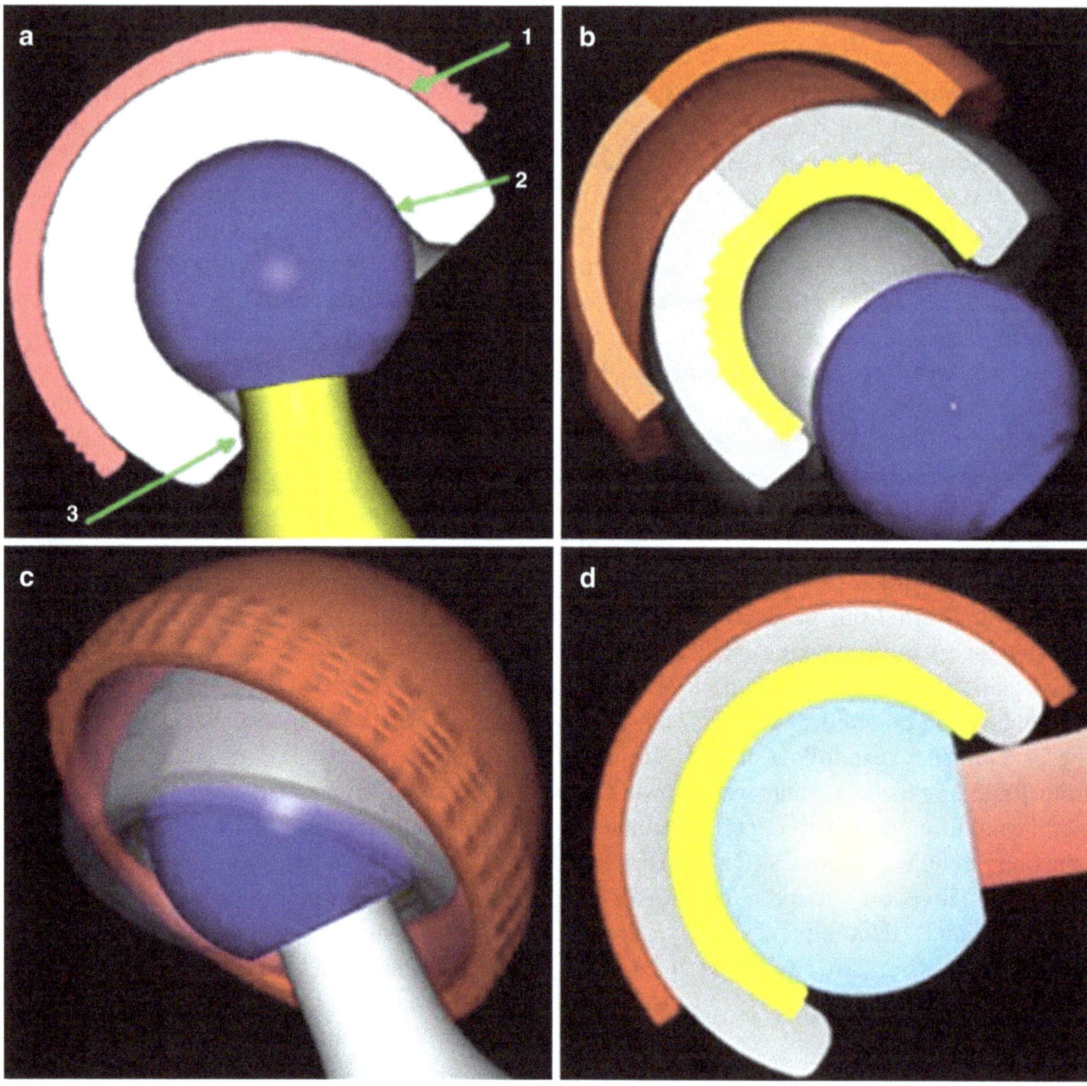

Fig. 7.3 The three articulating surfaces in DM cups: (**a**, **b**) demonstrate these three bearings as the large one (**a**.**1**) between the PE liner and metallic shell, the small one (**a**.**2**) between the femoral head and liner, and the so-called third articulation (**a**.**3**) between the femoral neck and the PE liner. (**c**) Illustrates the rotation of the PE liner upon contact with the femoral neck, while (**d**) shows the relationship during movements between the femoral neck, on the one hand, and first the liner, and second the rim of the metallic shell, on the other

for this DM solution [33]. The current implants' outer shell coatings now have optimized surfaces for bone fixation, resulting in comparable loosening rate to their fixed insert counterparts [34]. Second, better cup designs, smooth and round femoral necks, improved mechanisms for retention of the head in the mobile polyethylene liner, and new-generation polyethylene have almost eliminated the complication of intra-prosthetic dislocation (seen with early implants) and minimized wear. These improvements are expected to continue in the long term, as well as for young and active subjects. Should we then endorse the extension of indications for DM to most of our THA patients? [35]

Encouraging early results, given this background of expanded indications, was presented at the 2015 EFORT congress (Prague). A total of 747 primary hips in 661 patients aged less than 55 years had excellent clinical results with mean Harris Hip Score scores of 93.4 points and a survivorship at 12.7 years with all-cause revision at

98.9% (0.976–1), with only three revisions (one early cup migration at 10 days, one neurotrophic pain at 2 years, and one anterior soft tissue impingement at 3 years). There was no dislocation, no instability, no loosening, no osteolysis or noticeable wear, and especially no intra-prosthetic dislocation. A final element in the assessment of DM versus fixed insert bearings concerns the medico-economic aspect of this prosthetic option. Rehospitalizations for hip dislocations (even closed reduction), or for revisions in case of recurrent instability, have a significant overall cost in the national health budget. A recent French, national-level socioeconomic modeling (sample of 80,405 patients) looking at the comparative costs of these instability episodes, compared DM with fixed insert cups. They concluded that 3283 dislocations would be avoided per 100,000 patients if DM components were systematically used, with a potential annual gain for 140,000 prostheses of 39.6 million Euros [36]. What was demonstrated in France would probably be similarly observed on an international scale.

7.6 LDH THA Summary

LDH THAs either with monobloc or dual-mobility femoral head have proven highly valuable in reducing the risk of dislocation. The supraphysiologic arc of motion provided by the large head–neck ratio makes it a forgiving procedure, leaving some room for imprecision by the surgeon and for suboptimal functional acetabular orientation, resulting from abnormal lumbo-pelvic kinematics. It may also permit a better reproduction of individual hip anatomy (femoral offset and leg length) for more physiological peri-prosthetic soft tissue tension that would likely favor more natural joint kinematics and optimize functional outcomes and patient satisfaction. Bilateral and outpatient procedures are simplified. It allows unrestricted ROM and return to usual activities and vocation. There is evidence that patients return to a more normal gait and have a greater ROM than conventional THAs. Patients often experience a much suppler hip, especially when preoperative contractures are present, with increased likelihood of having a forgotten hip. LDH THAs aim to better replicate normal human anatomy, which should lead to greater function and a more natural hip. Early results of LDH CoC bearings have been promising. Although there is a significant incidence of occasional squeaking, it does not appear to be bothersome to the patient. CoC LDH has a reduced risk of early and late instability due to bearing wear. LDH with dual-mobility femoral head is also very attractive because it has a lower cost, it does not produce noise and it is not linked with fracture. With the recently reported low wear rate, DM could be considered for a larger proportion of our THA patients, keeping LDH CoC bearings for a selected group of young and active subjects.

Case Example

A 40-year-old man, who had bilateral Perthes disease of the hips at a young age (Fig. 7.4), presents because of bilateral severe hip pain resistant to conservative treatment. He has worked as a fireman for the last 17 years and enjoys sporting activities like kayaking, cycling, and rock climbing. He has had to stop all leisure activities a year ago and has been off work for the last 3 months.

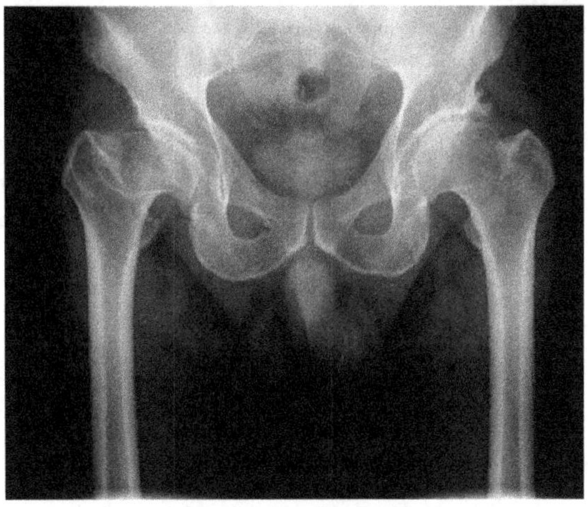

Fig. 7.4 Anteroposterior radiograph of the pelvis of a patient who had bilateral Perthes disease of the hips at a young age and secondary hip joint degeneration

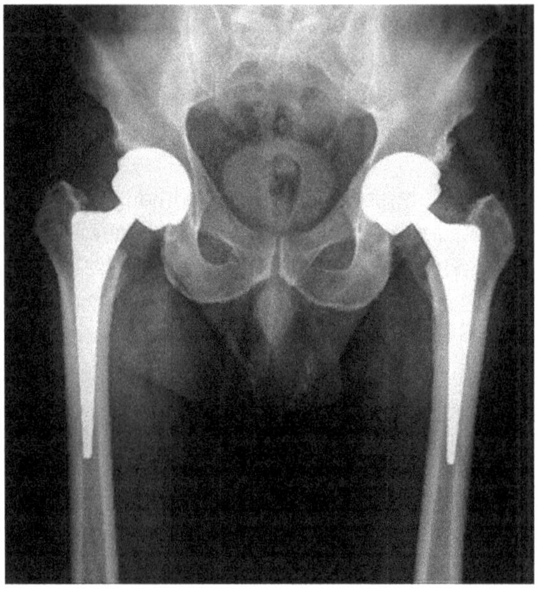

Fig. 7.5 Postoperative AP pelvis radiograph after bilateral CoC LDH THAs

He would like to resume his normal life as soon as possible.

We offered him bilateral CoC LDH THAs, performed in one stage through our standard posterior approach. Surgery was uneventful and took a total of 1 h 45 min including time to switch sides, with total blood loss of 450 cc (Fig. 7.5). The patient stayed in hospital for 2 days. No range of motion restrictions were imposed. He was full weight-bearing without walking aids by 4 weeks and started stationary bike exercising. He resumed his work and leisure activities without restriction after 4.5 months. At 5-years follow-up, he is still very satisfied with his clinical results. He has heard some squeaking noise in his left hip on a few occasions but describes it as "not annoying." He considers his right hip as a natural or forgotten hip and the left one as an artificial hip without limitations.

References

1. Lombardi AV Jr, Skeels MD, Berend KR, Adams JB, Franchi OJ. Do large heads enhance stability and restore native anatomy in primary total hip arthroplasty? Clin Orthop Relat Res. 2011;469:1547–53.
2. Stroh DA, Issa K, Johnson AJ, Delanois RE, Mont MA. Reduced dislocation rates and excellent functional outcomes with large-diameter femoral heads. J Arthroplast. 2013;28:1415–20.
3. Garbuz DS, Masri BA, Duncan CP, et al. The frank Stinchfield award: dislocation in revision THA: do large heads (36 and 40 mm) result in reduced dislocation rates in a randomized clinical trial? Clin Orthop Relat Res. 2012;470:351–6.
4. Author N. Australian Orthopaedic Association National Joint Replacement Registry. Annual report. Adelaide: AOA; 2017. https://aoanjrr.sahmri.com/annual-reports-2017. Accessed 10 Oct 2017.
5. Malkani AL, Ong KL, Lau E, Kurtz SM, Justice BJ, Manley MT. Early- and late-term dislocation risk after primary hip arthroplasty in the Medicare population. J Arthroplast. 2010;25:21–5.
6. Peters CL, McPherson E, Jackson JD, Erickson JA. Reduction in early dislocation rate with large-diameter femoral heads in primary total hip arthroplasty. J Arthroplast. 2007;22:140–4.
7. Burroughs BR, Hallstrom B, Golladay GJ, Hoeffel D, Harris WH. Range of motion and stability in total hip arthroplasty with 28-, 32-, 38-, and 44-mm femoral head sizes. J Arthroplast. 2005;20:11–9.
8. Elkins JM, O'Brien MK, Stroud NJ, Pedersen DR, Callaghan JJ, Brown TD. Hard-on-hard total hip impingement causes extreme contact stress concentrations. Clin Orthop Relat Res. 2011;469:454–63.
9. Scifert CF, Noble PC, Brown TD, et al. Experimental and computational simulation of total hip arthroplasty dislocation. Orthop Clin North Am. 2001;32:553–67, vii.
10. Cinotti G, Lucioli N, Malagoli A, Calderoli C, Cassese F. Do large femoral heads reduce the risks of impingement in total hip arthroplasty with optimal and non-optimal cup positioning? Int Orthop. 2011;35:317–23.
11. Malkani AL, Garber AT, Ong KL, et al. Total hip arthroplasty in patients with previous lumbar fusion surgery: are there more dislocations and revisions? J Arthroplast. 2018;33(4):1189–93.
12. Sing DC, Barry JJ, Aguilar TU, et al. Prior lumbar spinal arthrodesis increases risk of prosthetic-related complication in total hip arthroplasty. J Arthroplast. 2016;31:227–32 e1.
13. Sariali E, Lazennec JY, Khiami F, Catonne Y. Mathematical evaluation of jumping distance in total hip arthroplasty: influence of abduction angle, femoral head offset, and head diameter. Acta Orthop. 2009;80:277–82.
14. Komistek RD, Dennis DA, Ochoa JA, Haas BD, Hammill C. In vivo comparison of hip separation after metal-on-metal or metal-on-polyethylene total hip arthroplasty. J Bone Joint Surg Am. 2002;84-A:1836–41.
15. Glaser D, Komistek RD, Cates HE, Mahfouz MR. Clicking and squeaking: in vivo correlation of sound and separation for different bearing surfaces. J Bone Joint Surg Am. 2008;90(Suppl 4):112–20.

16. Bouffard V, Nantel J, Therrien M, Vendittoli PA, Lavigne M, Prince F. Center of mass compensation during gait in hip arthroplasty patients: comparison between large diameter head total hip arthroplasty and hip resurfacing. Rehabil Res Pract. 2011;2011:586412.
17. Nantel J, Termoz N, Ganapathi M, Vendittoli PA, Lavigne M, Prince F. Postural balance during quiet standing in patients with total hip arthroplasty with large diameter femoral head and surface replacement arthroplasty. Arch Phys Med Rehabil. 2009;90:1607–12.
18. Nantel J, Termoz N, Vendittoli PA, Lavigne M, Prince F. Gait patterns after total hip arthroplasty and surface replacement arthroplasty. Arch Phys Med Rehabil. 2009;90:463–9.
19. Lavigne M, Ganapathi M, Mottard S, Girard J, Vendittoli PA. Range of motion of large head total hip arthroplasty is greater than 28 mm total hip arthroplasty or hip resurfacing. Clin Biomech (Bristol, Avon). 2011;26:267–73.
20. Gromov K, Troelsen A, Otte KS, Orsnes T, Ladelund S, Husted H. Removal of restrictions following primary THA with posterolateral approach does not increase the risk of early dislocation. Acta Orthop. 2015;86:463–8.
21. Blakeney WG, Beaulieu Y, Puliero B, et al. Excellent results of large-diameter ceramic-on-ceramic bearings in total hip arthroplasty. Bone Joint J. 2018;100-B:1434–41.
22. Garbuz DS, Tanzer M, Greidanus NV, Masri BA, Duncan CP. The John Charnley award: metal-on-metal hip resurfacing versus large-diameter head metal-on-metal total hip arthroplasty: a randomized clinical trial. Clin Orthop Relat Res. 2010;468:318–25.
23. Deny A, Barry J, Hutt JRB, Lavigne M, Masse V, Vendittoli PA. Effect of sleeved ceramic femoral heads on titanium ion release. Hip Int. 2018;28(2):139–44.
24. Hallab NJ, Messina C, Skipor A, Jacobs JJ. Differences in the fretting corrosion of metal-metal and ceramic-metal modular junctions of total hip replacements. J Orthop Res. 2004;22:250–9.
25. McDonnell SM, Boyce G, Bare J, Young D, Shimmin AJ. The incidence of noise generation arising from the large-diameter Delta motion ceramic total hip bearing. Bone Joint J. 2013;95-B:160–5.
26. Goldhofer MI, Munir S, Levy YD, Walter WK, Zicat B, Walter WL. Increase in benign squeaking rate at five-year follow-up: results of a large diameter ceramic-on-ceramic bearing in total hip arthroplasty. J Arthroplast. 2018;33(4):1210–4.
27. Tai SM, Munir S, Walter WL, Pearce SJ, Walter WK, Zicat BA. Squeaking in large diameter ceramic-on-ceramic bearings in total hip arthroplasty. J Arthroplast. 2015;30:282–5.
28. Fessy M. La double mobilité ; Maîtrise Orthopédique (152) 2006; http://www.maitrise-orthopedique.com/articles/la-double-mobilite-86.
29. Guyen O, Pibarot V, Vaz G, Chevillotte C, Bejui-Hugues J. Use of a dual mobility socket to manage total hip arthroplasty instability. Clin Orthop Relat Res. 2009;467:465–72.
30. Grazioli A, Ek ET, Rudiger HA. Biomechanical concept and clinical outcome of dual mobility cups. Int Orthop. 2012;36:2411–8.
31. Guyen O, Chen QS, Bejui-Hugues J, Berry DJ, An KN. Unconstrained tripolar hip implants: effect on hip stability. Clin Orthop Relat Res. 2007;455:202–8.
32. Stroh A, Naziri Q, Johnson AJ, Mont MA. Dual-mobility bearings: a review of the literature. Expert Rev Med Devices. 2012;9:23–31.
33. Epinette JA. Clinical outcomes, survivorship and adverse events with mobile-bearings versus fixed-bearings in hip arthroplasty-a prospective comparative cohort study of 143 ADM versus 130 trident cups at 2 to 6-year follow-up. J Arthroplast. 2015;30:241–8.
34. Epinette JA, Beracassat R, Tracol P, Pagazani G, Vandenbussche E. Are modern dual mobility cups a valuable option in reducing instability after primary hip arthroplasty, even in younger patients? J Arthroplast. 2014;29:1323–8.
35. Blakeney WG, Epinette JA, Vendittoli PA. Dual mobility total hip arthroplasty: should everyone get one? EFORT Open Rev. 2019;4(9):541–7.
36. Epinette JA, Lafuma A, Robert J, Doz M. Cost-effectiveness model comparing dual-mobility to fixed-bearing designs for total hip replacement in France. Orthop Traumatol Surg Res. 2016;102:143–8.

8

Modular Femoral Component: Reconstruction of the Proximal Femur Anatomy

Aldo Toni, Francesco Castagnini, and Susanna Stea

8.1 Neck Modularity

Stem modularity can be classified according to the coupling location: distal, mid-stem, and proximal [1]. Mid-stem and proximal modularity have been more frequently used. Either the junction is located proximal or distal (mid-stem) to the neck osteotomy (Fig. 8.1). Proximal modularity with modular necks was introduced in 1987 by Cremascoli Ortho (Milan, Italy), in order to provide independent combinations of version, offset, and length [1].

Rationale of modular necks. The rationale for proximal modularity with modular necks was the achievement of a better soft tissue balancing and was to reduce the occurrence of prosthetic impingement [1, 2]. The best candidates for neck modularity, where the most remarkable benefits are obtained, are subjects with unconventional hip anatomies and biomechanics [1, 2]. In these cases, standard acetabular and femoral component orientation adjustment to achieve adequate reciprocal positioning may be ineffective due to the limited bone fit and coverage. Such suboptimal implant orientation may result in restricted range of motion, abductor dysfunction, and increased risks of dislocations and other impingement-related events [1, 3]. The bony and soft tissue alterations in hip dysplasia are a clear example (Fig. 8.2) [1, 2]. The short anteverted neck and the inadequate abductor muscles may be correctly reconstructed using modular components, independently tuning the soft tissue tension and the leg length. Moreover, modularity may provide adequate correction of the combined version. Similar considerations can be made for coxa vara: a conventional implant, with progressive neck lengths according to implant size, may restore the offset using a larger size, but sometimes at the cost of an unacceptable leg length discrepancy (Fig. 8.3) [1–3]. Modularity may also be beneficial in post-traumatic cases, where the abnormal acetabular or femoral morphologies may influence the component position. In revision cases, when the acetabular bone loss may compromise the socket positioning, modularity may improve joint stability and reduce impingement, compensating imperfect acetabular implant orientation and/or soft tissue tension [1]. Even in case of standard primary arthroplasties looking relatively simple, as the proximal femoral anatomy significantly varies between patients and is not that predictable [2], proximal modularity

A. Toni (✉)
Casa di Cura Madre Fortunata Toniolo, Bologna, Italy

F. Castagnini
Ortopedia-Traumatologia e Chirurgia protesica e dei reimpianti d'anca e di ginocchio, IRCCS Istituto Ortopedico Rizzoli, Bologna, Italy

S. Stea
Laboratorio di Tecnologia Medica, IRCCS Istituto Ortopedico Rizzoli, Bologna, Italy
e-mail: stea@tecno.ior.it

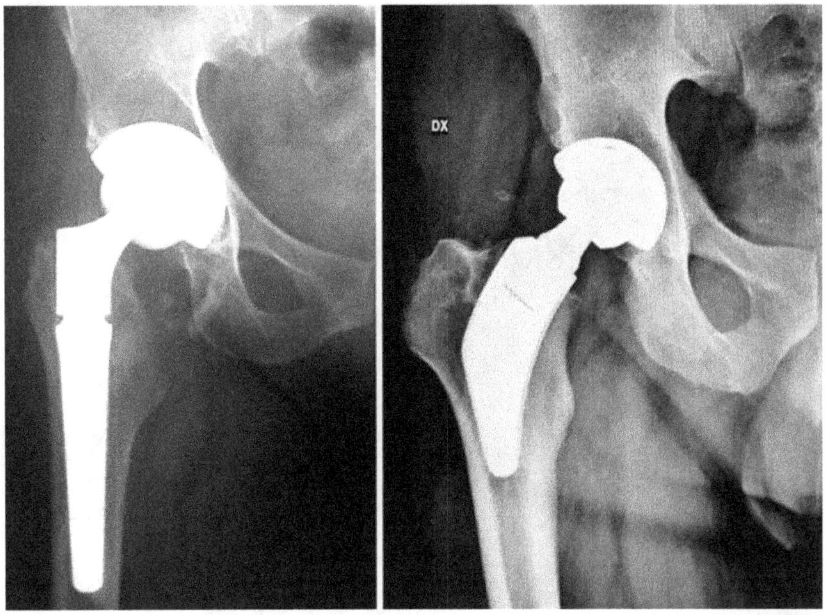

Fig. 8.1 Stem modularity can be classified according to the junction location: on the left mid-stem modularity (junction distal to the neck osteotomy) and on the right proximal femoral modularity (junction proximal to the neck osteotomy)

with modular necks may be of clinical interest. Males usually have long necks with higher neck-shaft angles and low anteversion; on the contrary, females show short, varus, and anteverted necks [2]. Most stem designs have size-proportional neck lengths, affecting leg length and offset, which may address partially this wide variability [2]. It was estimated that tapered stems with metaphyseal fit designs require at least 15 sizes distributed in three metaphyseal configurations, and two different neck-shaft angles to match the frontal anatomy of 85% of the femurs [4]. Moreover, uncemented stems often have limited version freedom during implantation. Thus, proximal modularity with modular necks has theoretical advantages in outlier anatomies as well as in standard cases, more closely matching the native proximal femur anatomy than conventional stems. Due to these reasons, we frequently used in our institution the modular neck implants in cases of conventional and, mostly, unconventional hip anatomies.

Clinical results of modular necks. There is solid evidence that shows the reliability of well-designed modular neck implants regarding their capacity to restore the native proximal femoral anatomy and to provide good long-term clinical outcomes. Montalti et al. [5] reported good anatomical reconstructions in severe dysplastic hips using modular necks (AncaFit® stem, Cremascoli Ortho, Milan, Italy). In particular, the use of a high prosthetic hip center reconstruction, combined with modular necks, improved the biomechanics and the offset restoration, with good to excellent clinical results and only a case of cup aseptic loosening after a minimum follow-up of 10 years. Archibeck et al. [6] reported a comparison between 100 primary total hip arthroplasties (THAs) with modular neck stem design and 100 primary THAs without (respectively Kinectiv® and M/L Taper® stems, Zimmer-Biomet, Warsaw, USA). The offset and leg length were restored to within 1 mm in 85% of the modular hips and in 60% of the monoblock stems. On the contrary, Duwelius et al. [7] failed to demonstrate superior clinical outcomes at 2-years follow-up in a similar comparison involving the same implants. Nevertheless, a better reconstruction of leg length and offset characterized the modular neck cohort.

Our experience: The regional arthroplasty registry of Emilia Romagna. In the regional arthroplasty registry of Emilia Romagna, the 15-year cumulative implant survival rates were found to be similar between 16,575 modular implants (557 being exposed to risk at 15 years) and 35,620 monoblock implants (1781 being exposed to risk at 15 years) performed for primary osteoarthritis, at 90.8% and 91%, respectively [8]. The rates of aseptic loosening were

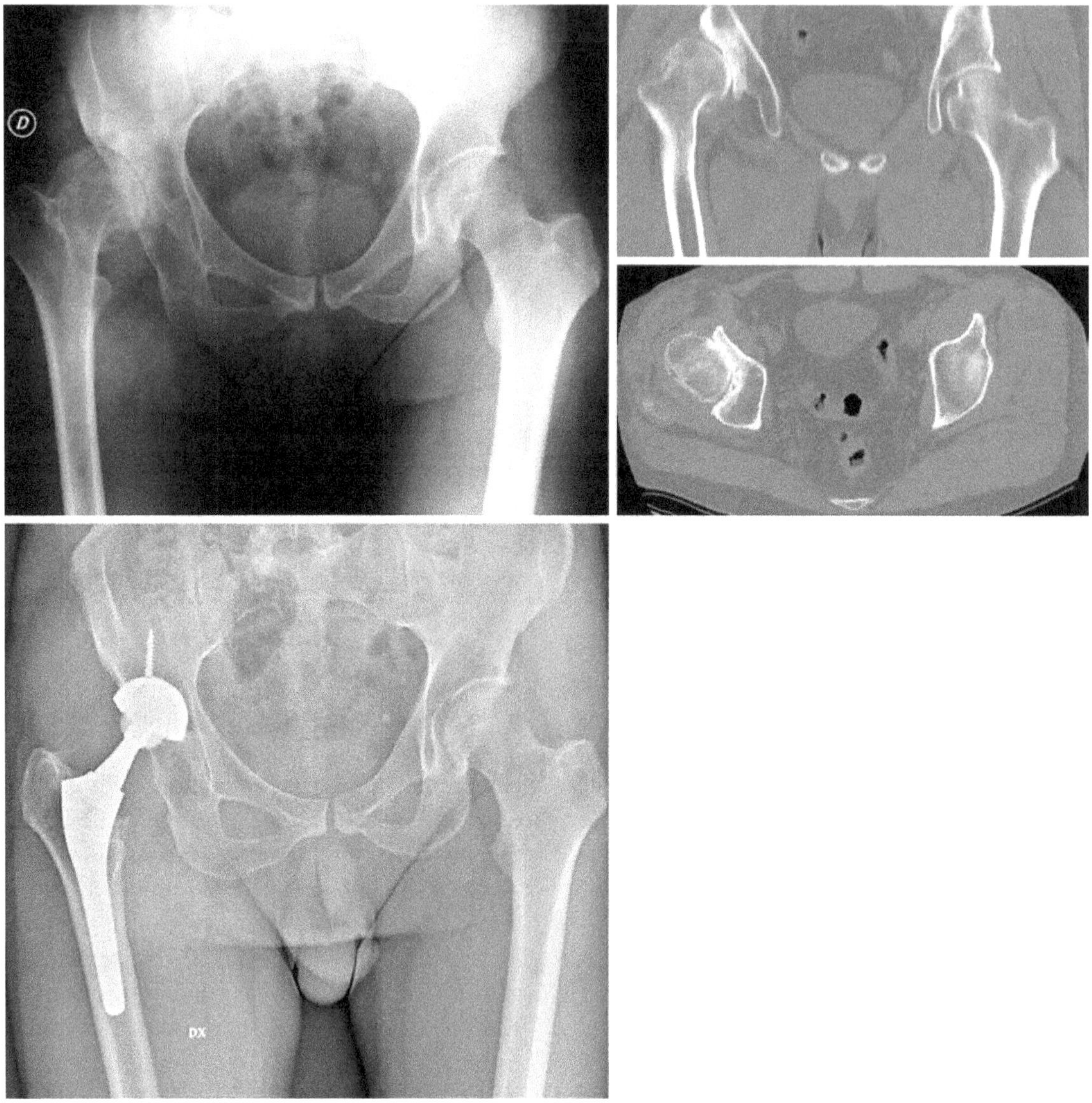

Fig. 8.2 A Crowe III dysplasia in a 45-year-old male was treated with a Ti modular neck implant (Ancafit, Cremascoli Ortho, Milan, Italy): the use of a long neck allowed for the proper restoration of leg length and offset, achieving an excellent result at 13 years

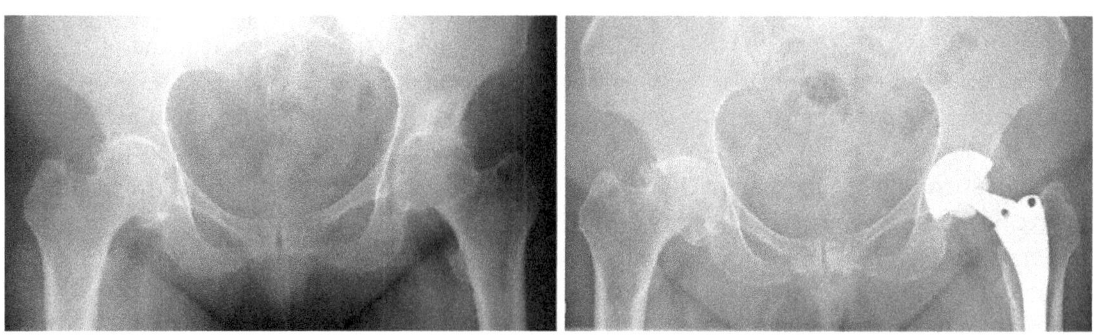

Fig. 8.3 Modular implants are particularly useful in outlier anatomies, like coxa vara. A varus, retroverted neck (Apta, Adler Ortho, Milan, Italy) was used to restore the proper neck-shaft angle, offset, and leg length, achieving a satisfying result at 8 years

inferior in the modular group (0.4% vs. 0.7% for isolated acetabular implant loosening; 0.6% vs. 0.8% for isolated femoral stem loosening; and 0.1% vs. 0.4% for loosening of both the components), as well as the rate of revision due to polyethylene wear (0.04%, 7 implants out of 16,575 THAs), but none of those differences reached statistical significance. In terms of revisions due to prosthetic instability, no differences could be detected between the two groups. These data may suggest that modular necks allow for a better component interaction, enabling to reduce the mechanical stresses on component fixation and preserving them from aseptic loosening. Considering only the THAs performed due to congenital pathologies (e.g., developmental hip dysplasia), the results between the two groups were more striking. The modular neck implants (2805 cases with 238 being exposed to risk at 15 years) achieved a survival rate of 93.3% at 15 years, whereas conventional implants (3707 cases with 389 being exposed to risk at 15 years) had a lower performance with 89.6% of survivorship. Regarding the reasons for revision, the two groups had similar revision rates for early prosthetic instability (within the first 3 months), but modular neck THAs had an inferior revision rate for recurrent dislocations (0.5% vs. 0.8%). Revisions for aseptic cup loosening were significantly lower with modular necks (0.5% vs. 1.9%). This finding showed that, in the modular neck cohort, the revision rate for aseptic cup loosening was comparable to THAs implanted for primary osteoarthritis and was four times lower than conventional implants used for congenital pathologies. On the other hand, in the cohort of congenital pathologies, a rate of 0.5% of neck fractures was reported for the modular neck implants.

Insight into modular neck failure. Due to the frequent excessive corrosion at the modular neck-stem junction and the related clinical complications (e.g., neck breakage, adverse local tissue reaction to metal debris), the routine use of modular neck implants has been frequently questioned [1, 9]. In a recent study by Graves et al. [9] that describes the outcomes of the Australian registry, the revision rate for all reasons at 10 years was 9.7% in modular necks, whereas 5.1% for the conventional stem. However, when the modular neck cohort was split into chromium–cobalt (Cr–Co) necks and Titanium (Ti) necks, the latter performed better: at 10 years, 7.4% of the Ti implants were revised, suggesting that the neck alloy is an important predictive factor. The first modular necks were fabricated in Ti alloy, with a taper connection mated to a Ti alloy stem [1]. Of the reported breakage and dissociation of the components, neck failures were mostly due to insufficient fatigue strength (Fig. 8.4) [1, 9]. Thus, Cr–Co alloy necks were proposed as a stronger alloy alternative and implanted on Ti

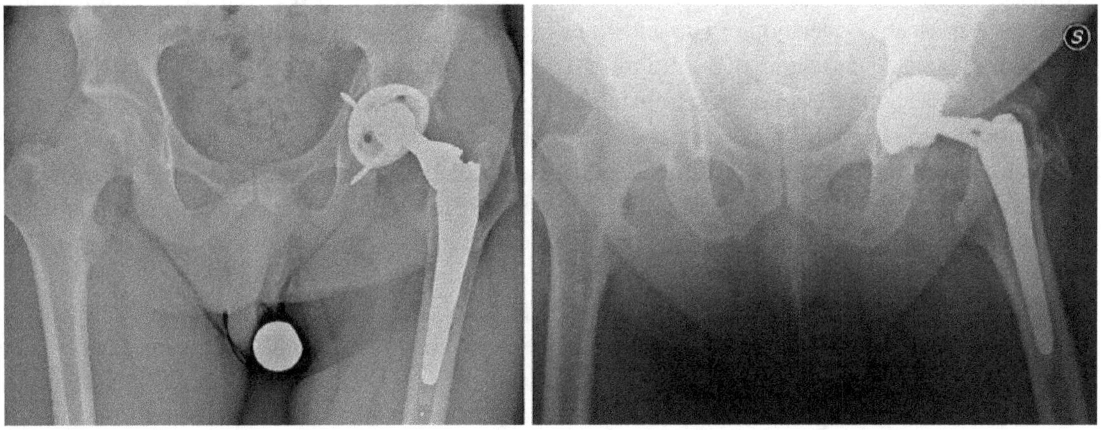

Fig. 8.4 Ti proximal modularity may face disassembling (left image) and neck failure (right image): disassembling occurred after a trauma 20 years after the implantation. The fracture occurred in severe obesity (150 kg, 65-year-old male)

alloy stems in order to prevent fractures [1, 10, 11]. The new Cr–Co necks experienced lower rates of fractures (to date, no implant breakage in the Australian registry) [9]. However, excessive corrosion at the taper junction, primarily related to abnormal micromotions at its site (mechanically assisted crevice corrosion), emerged as a devastating complication [1, 10–15]. A famous example may be given by the 2012 recall of the Rejuvenate devices (Stryker, Mahwah, USA) where Cr–Co necks were mated to Ti alloy stems. De Martino et al. [10] analyzed 60 Rejuvenate stems that were removed for multiple reasons; the totality of the retrievals showed severe signs of fretting corrosion at the neck-stem modular taper junction, starting soon after the implantation (less than 4 weeks) and increasing over the time. In contrast, the head–neck tapers only showed negligible corrosion signs. The authors suggested that the neck–stem junction was subject to a cantilever bending: the medial and lateral sides of the neck were cyclically compressed against the correspondent part of the stem, describing a small amplitude oscillatory motion [10]. Nawabi et al. [11] described the results of 216 Rejuvenate THAs, highlighting necrosis and adverse local tissue reactions similar to metal-on-metal bearing prostheses as a consequence of the cantilever bending. The source of metal ions was the mechanically assisted crevice corrosion: the fluid entering the modular junction repassivated the titanium alloy, causing acid release and Ti or Co dissolution [10–15]. Due to these severe problems, the American Association of Hip and Knee Surgeons elaborated a specific algorithm for risk stratification, designing Cr–Co neck implants at moderate or severe risk [12]. A strict follow-up including standard radiographs, periodical metal ion level tests, and cross-sectional images (MARS-MRI or CT scan) was suggested, in order to establish if a revision surgery was recommended. On the other hand, when Ti necks were compared to Cr–Co necks, less degradation was evident and ion release was modest and within a noncritical range [13–15]. A study by Kop et al. [13] suggested that Ti necks are more corrosion resistant and frequently subject to cold welding. The cold welding at the neck–stem modular junction was probably beneficial in terms of reducing fretting corrosion but rendered disassembling a troublesome (impossible) procedure in 22% of the cases. Despite the safer Ti neck profile, a few catastrophic events related to neck breakage should not be forgotten (0.2% in the Australian registry) [9]. It is not easy to delineate the reasons for Ti neck breakage: the implant design plays a capital role, as few models have been frequently involved [13–15]. Moreover, retrieval studies on Ti neck breakage found that varus high-offset modular necks were at higher risk of fracture when implanted in young, active, overweight patients [1, 13–15].

8.2 Head Modularity

Similarly to modular necks, modular heads were introduced in the 1980s, aiming to restore better prosthetic hip biomechanics [16]. The success was outstanding and, in the 1990s, 90% of the implants had a head–neck modularity [16]. Nowadays, head modularity is a capital element in THA as it allows the surgeon to use different bearing surfaces, to more accurately restore offset and leg length, to improve stability, and to facilitate revision procedures [16–18]. Usually, head modularity occurs at a Morse taper, resulting in a force-fit connection (taper locking) that resists the axial and torsional forces [16]. Unfortunately, there is no standard taper. Tapers are fabricated with different configurations and angles, with several variations among manufacturers and hip devices [16–18]. Thus, the surgeons must carefully assess the compatibility between the new head and the well-fixed stem in case of partial revisions [16–18]. Although the benefits related to head modularity remarkably outweigh the cons, few drawbacks should be noticed: disassembling and excessive corrosion [17]. Dissociation of the head is anecdotic in the modern implants, usually occurring after trauma and secondary to mismatches [17]. Severe and clinically troublesome corrosion almost uniquely occurs with large metal heads, being ceramic balls involved in very few cases. The taper is subjected to mechanically assisted crevice corrosion due to oxidation and micromotion, similarly to the neck-stem junctions that are usually Morse tapers too [17]. The main factors increasing corrosion at the head–neck interface occur with different metal combinations, larger heads (>32 mm), shorter tapers, high head offset (e.g., XL head), and active and/or obese patients [17]. Despite those few concerns, the routine use of head–neck modularity in primary THAs is not challenged. Furthermore, the use of modular head–neck adapter systems seems particularly important in revision settings [18]. Such systems allow the reduction of leg length discrepancy and the loss of offset, improving the biomechanics and the stability of the revised prosthetic hip. In a retrospective series including 95 patients, Hoberg et al. [18] described 95 revisions requiring the use of BioBall® system (Merete, Berlin, Germany). The survival rate was 92.8% at 8 years, two patients requiring a further procedure due to recurrent dislocations. No corrosion was noticed in the revised cases.

8.3 Femoral Component Modularity Contributes to Personalizing the Hip Reconstruction

Proximal femoral modularity is a useful tool to optimize prosthetic hip biomechanics and to potentially reduce complications related to poor component interaction (edge loading, prosthetic impingement, and related complications such as instability). Each patient has a unique hip biomechanics that may even vary with age. Three capital parameters of hip biomechanics, femoral offset and hip rotation center and combined anteversion of femur and acetabulum, are randomly and independently located even in conventional hip morphologies [1–4]. Restoring the native hip anatomy when performing hip replacement is a sound option for optimizing prosthetic function and biomechanics, and overall clinical outcomes and patients' satisfaction. However, as conventional implants, even with modular heads, may only address a few hip anatomies, most of the patients have their native hip anatomy altered after reconstruction. Thanks to the independent tuning of lengths and angles in the three planes, regardless the stem size, proximal modularity (head and neck) may effectively reproduce the constitutional hip biomechanics within millimeters [1, 2]. Thus, the muscle lever arms can be finely reconstructed and the combined anteversion optimized. A wider articular excursion, a more uniform distribution of joint forces, and an improved component interaction consequently result, highlighting that personalizing hip replacement using modularity is not without tangible outcomes [4]. Proximal femoral modularity is even more desirable in case of outlier anatomies, when conventional implants with minimal modularity (head) grossly fail to reconstruct the hip biomechanics [1, 2, 5].

8.4 Modularity: Guidelines for Users

Complex cases with unusual anatomies and biomechanics, like dysplastic hips, may be the best candidates for modular implants [2, 5]. Up to now, well-designed femoral head/neck modularity has proven to be reliable, achieving positive long-term results in such cases (Fig. 8.5) [1, 5]. On the contrary, a regular use of modular neck implants has been universally discouraged [9]. Excluding its costs (15–25% more expensive than conventional implants), adding a modular junction carries some additional risks related to corrosion, disassembling, and modular implant failure [1]. Lessons learned with modular implant failures helped us to draw important recommendations and restrictions [16]. Mixing alloys should be avoided due to corrosion and ion release. Cr–Co heads on Ti necks can be admitted; on the contrary, Cr–Co necks in Ti stem junctions should be avoided [1, 9–13]. Every taper is designed to better resist torsional loading rather than bending one [16]. Thus, in young, active, and overweight patients, modular head and neck options that provide high femoral offset should be adopted with care, or better, discouraged [13–15]. In these cases, modular junction corrosion and Ti neck fatigue fractures are more likely to occur [13–15].

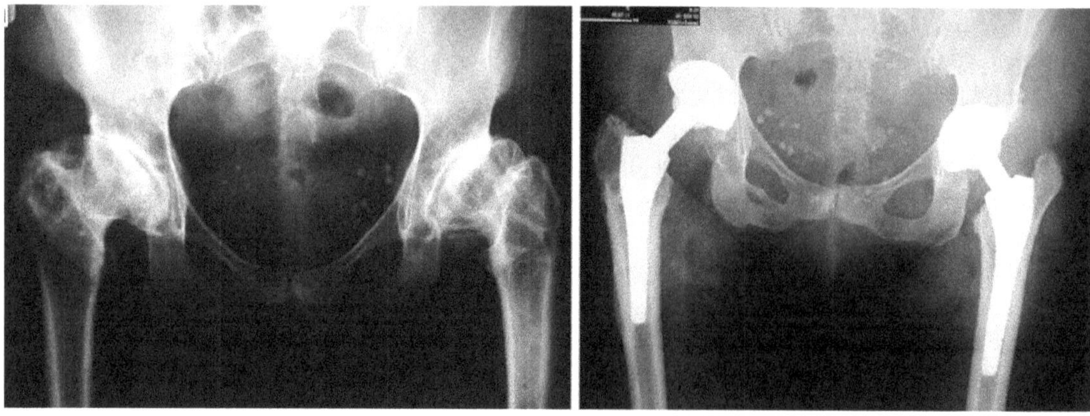

Fig. 8.5 Modular necks are useful implants in case of difficult anatomies. A case of dysplasia was treated with modular THAs (Ancafit, Cremascoli Ortho, Milan, Italy), achieving a good radiographic result after 15 years

Thus, problems with taper can be avoided reducing the bending load at taper interface and, in case of modular heads, increasing the taper strength acting on diameter and length [13–15]. It is important to highlight that a proper assembly is capital: no third body should be entrapped in the taper connections [9–17]. A careful surgical technique is universally recommended to avoid taper failures [9–17]. Although modularity was proven reliable when handled with the abovementioned recommendations, new developments should be welcomed, aiming to produce safer modular junctions. The microstructure and the grain size of the Ti alloy were advocated as important factors: in particular, as most of the cracks initiated and propagated between two alfa-lamellae, avoiding or reducing such elements might be beneficial [14]. Such a development should be accompanied by a proper implant design, a factor significantly affecting the long-term results [13–15]. Up to now, a 100% safe design has not been found. The modular junction design of Ancafit® implants proved good [8]: only 2 neck breakages out of 3148 cases occurred at a minimum follow-up of 5 years. The modest offset range (13.5 mm) may have probably played an important role in such a success. Another positive experience was the Modula® system (Adler Ortho, Milan, Italy), which is available for different stem designs. This modular Ti neck system provides independent tridimensional tuning of three parameters (length, offset, version) achieving 27 combinations per side and an offset range of 26 mm [19]. Although initial data showed an excessive rate of neck fractures, in particular in young patients and high-offset implants (unpublished results), the more recent use of a second generation "reinforced" neck system has generated a significant improvement in the fracture rate. To date, at the last follow-up (December 2015), no fracture occurred with the second-generation system in 1689 implants at a mean follow-up of 1.8 years (range: 0–3.7) [8].

Clinical Case

A 64-year-old female patient came presented to our clinic after a long history of right groin pain. When she was a child, the patient was conservatively treated for congenital hip dysplasia, achieving modest results. The patient had a residual limping, requiring the regular use of a walking cane and a severe lower limb discrepancy (Harris hip score: 23.8 points).

The anteroposterior X-rays demonstrated a bilateral Crowe III dysplasia (Fig. 8.6). In both hips, the articular degeneration was severe and the greater trochanters were very deformed. The right lower limb was 2 cm shorter. The computed tomography (CT) scan showed a dysplastic, small and shallow acetabulum, and a remarkable neck antetorsion (27°). The gluteal muscles were short and hypotrophic.

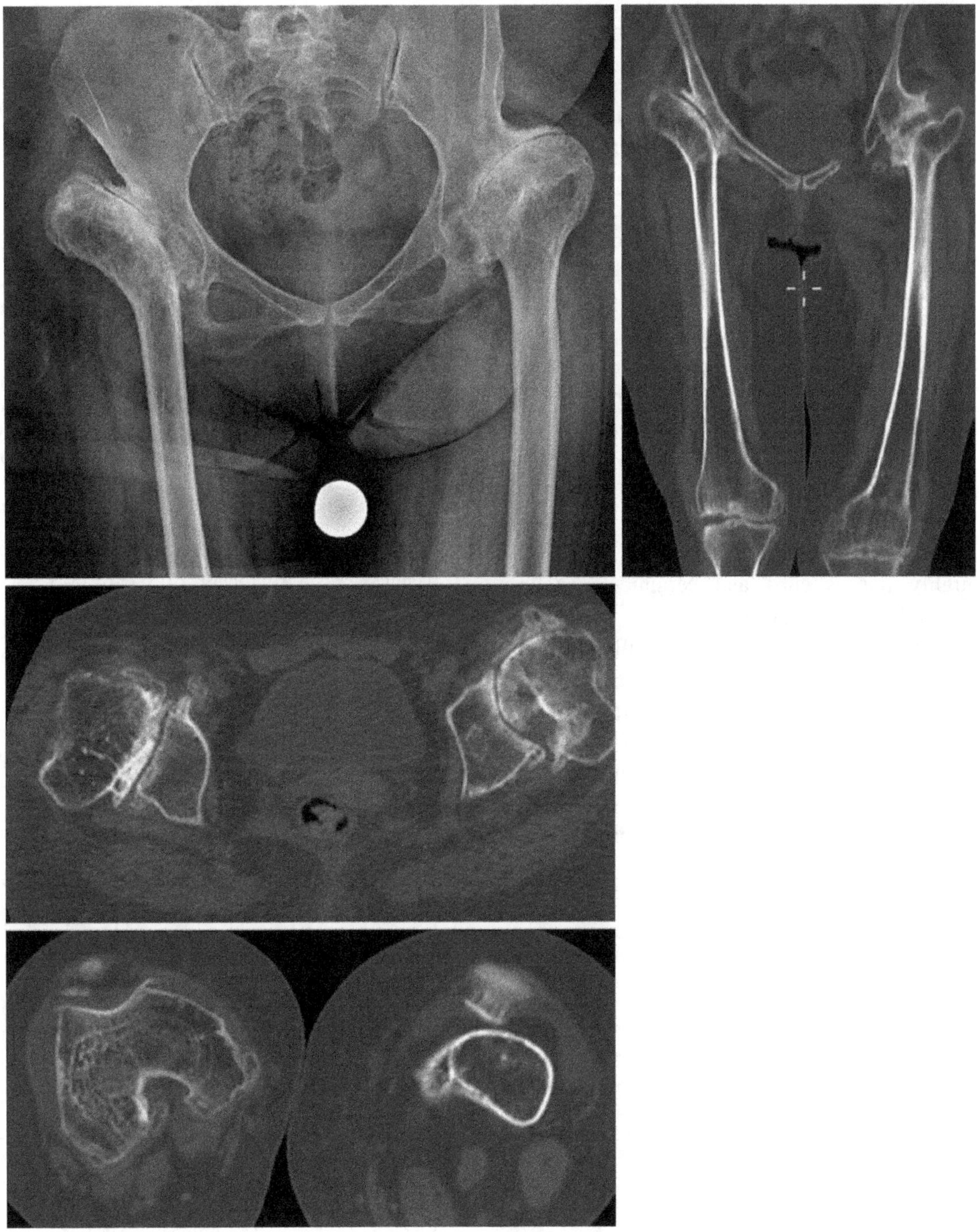

Fig. 8.6 (clinical case) The anteroposterior radiograph and CT scan showed bilateral dysplastic hips, severely deformed trochanters, leg length discrepancy, small and shallow acetabula, and marked femoral antetorsion, with minimum femoral offsets and abductor deficiencies

A right cementless total hip arthroplasty was performed, using an anterolateral approach. The cup was a highly porous titanium socket (TiPor, Adler Ortho, Milan, Italy), positioned in a high hip center. A modular tapered stem was implanted (Acuta, Adler Ortho, Milan, Italy). The shortest varus titanium (Ti) neck was positioned in order to restore the offset without damaging the weak abductors. The stem antetorsion was controlled, using the tapered stem—retroverted modular necks were not necessary. Delta ceramic bearing surfaces were chosen with a 32 mm ball (CeramTec, Plochingen, Germany). The greater trochanter was modeled and the abductors were sutured and re-tensioned. The implant proved stable and a good range of motion was achieved, with a residual 0.8-cm lower limb discrepancy to avoid excessive stresses on the gluteal muscles.

After 5 years, the patient was satisfied with the final result: the Harris hip score was 85.8 points. The gluteal muscles were still hypotrophic and a slight limping was evident: a walking cane was required only for long distances. On the radiographs, the implant showed good osseointegration (Fig. 8.7).

Severe dysplastic cases should be treated with specific modular implants. The use of highly porous cups and ceramic-on-ceramic couplings reduce the rate of wear and aseptic loosening, even in case of abnormally high joint reaction forces. Tapered stems may efficaciously control the combined anteversion, mostly when the stem antetorsion is higher than 25°. Modular necks are useful to independently fine-tune the offset, the length, and the version, restoring a good abductor lever arm and physiological soft-tissue tension.

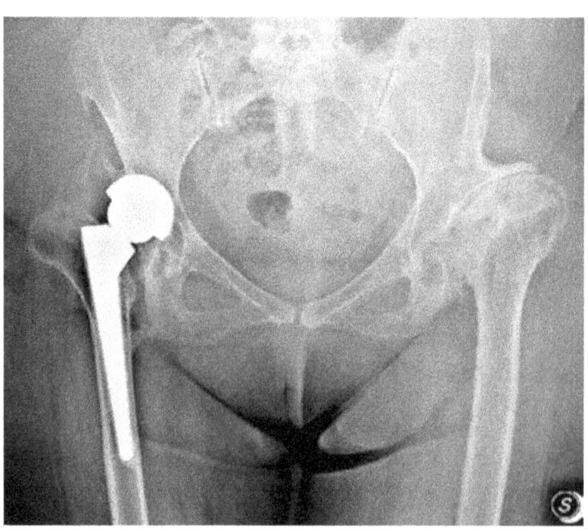

Fig. 8.7 (clinical case) After 5 years, the anteroposterior radiograph showed a very good osseointegration of the components and the restoration of a proper offset, avoiding excessive elongation of the gluteal muscles. In this case, proximal modularity was necessary to manage a very complex hip anatomy

References

1. Srinivasan A, Jung E, Levine BR. Modularity of the femoral component in total hip arthroplasty. J Am Acad Orthop Surg. 2012;20(4):214–22.
2. Traina F, De Clerico M, Biondi F, Pilla F, Tassinari E, Toni A. Sex differences in hip morphology: is stem modularity effective for total hip replacement? J Bone Joint Surg Am. 2009;91(Suppl 6):121–8.
3. Matsushita A, Nakashima Y, Fujii M, Sato T, Iwamoto Y. Modular necks improve the range of hip motion in cases with excessively anteverted or retroverted femurs in THA. Clin Orthop Relat Res. 2010;468(12):3342–7.
4. Massin P, Geais L, Astoin E, Simondi M, Lavaste F. The anatomic basis for the concept of lateralized femoral stems: a frontal plane radiographic study of the proximal femur. J Arthroplast. 2000;15(1): 93–101.
5. Montalti M, Castagnini F, Giardina F, Tassinari E, Biondi F, Toni A. Cementless total hip arthroplasty in Crowe III and IV dysplasia: high hip center and modular necks. J Arthroplast. 2018;33(6):1813–9.
6. Archibeck MJ, Cummins T, Carothers J, Junick DW, White RE Jr. A comparison of two implant systems in restoration of hip geometry in arthroplasty. Clin Orthop Relat Res. 2011;469(2):443–6.
7. Duwelius PJ, Burkhart B, Carnahan C, Branam G, Ko LM, Wu Y, Froemke C, Wang L, Grunkemeier G. Modular versus nonmodular neck femoral implants in primary total hip arthroplasty: which is better? Clin Orthop Relat Res. 2014;472(4):1240–5.
8. Registro dell'implantologia protesica ortopedica RIPO. https://ripo.cineca.it/. Accessed 25 May 2018.
9. Graves SE, de Steiger R, Davidson D, Donnelly W, Rainbird S, Lorimer MF, Cashman KS, Vial RJ. The use of femoral stems with exchangeable necks in primary total hip arthroplasty increases the rate of revision. Bone Joint J. 2017;99-B(6):766–73.
10. De Martino I, Assini JB, Elpers ME, Wright TM, Westrich GH. Corrosion and fretting of a modular hip system: a retrieval analysis of 60 rejuvenate stems. J Arthroplast. 2015;30(8):1470–5.
11. Nawabi DH, Do HT, Ruel A, Lurie B, Elpers ME, Wright T, Potter HG, Westrich GH. Comprehensive analysis of a recalled modular total hip system and recommendations for management. J Bone Joint Surg Am. 2016;98(1):40–7.
12. Kwon YM, Fehring TK, Lombardi AV, Barnes CL, Cabanela ME, Jacobs JJ. Risk stratification algorithm for management of patients with dual modular taper total hip arthroplasty: consensus statement of the American Association of hip and knee surgeons, the American Academy of orthopaedic surgeons and the hip society. J Arthroplast. 2014;29(11):2060–4.
13. Kop AM, Keogh C, Swarts E. Proximal component modularity in THA--at what cost? An implant retrieval study. Clin Orthop Relat Res. 2012;470(7): 1885–94.

14. Fokter SK, Rudolf R, Moličnik A. Titanium alloy femoral neck fracture--clinical and metallurgical analysis in 6 cases. Acta Orthop. 2016;87(2):197–202.
15. Kretzer JP, Jakubowitz E, Krachler M, Thomsen M, Heisel C. Metal release and corrosion effects of modular neck total hip arthroplasty. Int Orthop. 2009;33(6):1531–6.
16. Morlock M. Modularity in orthopaedics. J Traum Orthopae. 2017;5(3):60–3.
17. Wight CM, Lanting B, Schemitsch EH. Evidence based recommendations for reducing head-neck taper connection fretting corrosion in hip replacement prostheses. Hip Int. 2017;27(6):523–31.
18. Hoberg M, Konrads C, Huber S, Reppenhagen S, Walcher M, Steinert A, Barthel T, Rudert M. Outcome of a modular head-neck adapter system in revision hip arthroplasty. Arch Orthop Trauma Surg. 2015;135(10):1469–74.
19. Ollivier M, Parratte S, Galland A, Lunebourg A, Flecher X, Argenson JN. Titanium-titanium modular neck for primary THA. Result of a prospective series of 170 cemented THA with a minimum follow-up of 5 years. Orthop Traumatol Surg Res. 2015;101(2):137–42.

Part III

Patient Specific Hip Arthroplasty: Technological Tools and Implants Position

9

Reconstructing the Proximal Femur Anatomy

Tyler A. Luthringer and Jonathan M. Vigdorchik

Key Points

- Custom femoral cutting guides may increase the accuracy and precision of the femoral neck osteotomy based on patient-specific targets from 3D preoperative planning.
- The level and angle of the neck cut affects final stem height and coronal alignment, while proximal femur anatomy and canal morphology influence femoral stem version in uncemented designs.
- Available femoral PSI systems only control the level and angle of the osteotomy and do not yet guide stem version, although they provide a useful preoperative reference to help decision making.
- Additional research is necessary to confirm the efficacy of femoral guidance PSI in achieving targeted stem height, position, and version, as well as reveal the effect on clinical outcomes compared to traditional techniques.

T. A. Luthringer
NYU Langone Orthopedic Hospital,
NYU Langone Health, New York, NY, USA
e-mail: Tyler.Luthringer@nyulangone.org

J. M. Vigdorchik (✉)
Hospital for Special Surgery, New York, NY, USA
e-mail: VigdorchikJ@HSS.edu

9.1 What Is the Rationale?

Successful outcomes of total hip arthroplasty (THA) depend upon patient-specific factors, surgical technique, and appropriate implant selection. Proper surgical technique requires meticulous preoperative templating, followed by accurate and precise component positioning, a modifiable risk factor which may prevent poor clinical function following THA. Restoration of native hip biomechanics serves to optimize implant wear and THA stability. Closely approximating native hip biomechanics also avoids abductor insufficiency, limb-length inequality, and early construct failure. A key challenge to accurate component placement includes accommodating for variations in individual patient anatomy, functional spinopelvic mobility, and intraoperative positioning. Three-dimensional (3D) preoperative templating and patient-specific instrumentation (PSI) have emerged to enhance the surgical precision of bone resection and individualize component placement in THA.

Ideal femoral component position restores leg length, femoral offset, and femoral version. Conventional templating on two-dimensional (2D) anteroposterior (AP) pelvic radiographs is often limited by inaccurate magnification and variable rotational alignment of the proximal femur. Femoral offset may be underestimated on AP pelvis radiographs due to the projectional effects of femoral anteversion and external rotation contractures that may be present in late-stage osteoarthritis [1]. Uncemented stem designs follow the medullary canal from the aperture of the neck cut to achieve mediolateral metaphyseal and distal diaphyseal fixation [2]. The shape of the proximal femur thereby influences the final stem anteversion and coronal alignment [3]. Additionally, femoral canal morphology varies significantly at different planes of axial resection due to the complex anatomy of the proximal metaphyseal bone [4]. As a result, the angle and level of the osteotomy respectively influence the anteversion and varus/valgus alignment of the femoral component [4]. Freehand femoral osteotomy is accurate to within 4 mm of conventionally templated targets in only 87% of cases, which may introduce significant variability in final stem height and position and ultimately result in alterations in limb length [4].

Three-dimensional templating optimizes stem size and position to achieve optimal metaphyseal loading for fixation and anatomical restoration. The addition of axial imaging mitigates the shortcomings of 2D coronal templating while the use of custom femoral cutting guides helps to limit variability in surgical technique and minimize outliers of leg length, offset, and version. Femoral guidance PSI systems additionally incorporate kinematic simulation of the hip, pelvis, and lumbar spine in preoperative planning to assess impingement-free range of motion throughout functional extremes of posture [5]. Currently, there are four commercially available PSI hip systems, two of which include femoral guides (MyHip from Medacta and OPS™ from Corin). As of early 2019, the OPS™ is the only femoral PSI system approved by the Food and Drug Administration (FDA) for use in the United States. While the OPS™ will serve as the primary example system for the purposes of this chapter, the methodology and implementation of each system is generally the same. As the roles of 3D preoperative planning and the intraoperative use of femoral PSI guides are intimately intertwined, the indication for and potential benefit of their utilization is mutually considered.

9.2 What Are the Best Indications?

Relatively healthy bone stock is required for rigid fixation of PSI guides intraoperatively [5]. Femoral guides are fixed into place via two interosseous pins prior to performing the osteotomy. If the integrity of pin fixation is compromised by poor bone quality, or if the guide cannot be reliably secured in the intended position, the accuracy of the neck cut will be affected. The adjunct of 3D preoperative templating and femoral guidance PSI may be particularly valuable in young, active patients, in patients prone to postoperative instability, in patients suspected to have excessive native femoral ante- or retroversion or extreme neck-shaft angles, and for surgeons who employ minimally invasive approaches to the hip.

Young, active patients: In young, active THA patients, restoration of native hip biomechanics is not only important to increase construct longevity but also for the maintenance of physiological hip soft-tissue balance and native hip joint kinematics. Patients with high levels of activity are more likely to notice small inconsistencies between their native and artificial hips as well as overall limb lengths, placing them at greater risk for postoperative dissatisfaction. Femoral guidance PSI can help to limit postoperative limb-length outliers in younger patients who may be sensitive to such minimal discrepancies. Younger, active patients also more regularly assume positions of extreme hip flexion and extension compared to their older counterparts. Femoral PSI systems combine 3D anatomic model reconstruction with dynamic spinopelvic imaging to plan for optimal component position in a variety of functional positions. This kinematic simulation estimates the magnitude and direction of hip joint reaction forces across extreme ranges of motion. Imparting this knowledge to surgeons preoperatively allows for consideration of potential wear rates in young patients and impingement risk in more active candidates (such as those who wish to return to yoga or extreme sports).

Instability-prone patients: A growing body of evidence has questioned the universal application of traditional acetabular "safe zones" in all patients undergoing THA. Certain populations have been identified to be at increased risk for dislocation secondary to "functionally" malpositioned acetabular components. Arthroplasty surgeons have begun to mitigate this risk by tailoring traditional cup position to individual spinopelvic kinematics. While evidence supports that candidates with limited spinopelvic mobility may particularly benefit from patient-specific cup placement, the implications of femoral component position on THA stability are relatively less well understood. Nonetheless, due to the known effect of the combined anteversion of the cup and stem in conferring impingement-free range of motion [3], complementary use of acetabular and femoral PSI may be considered in patients with stiff spines or prior lumbar fusions who are at higher risk for dislocation. Similar to that in young, active patients, the preoperative aspect of dynamic spinopelvic imaging and kinematic simulation is of equal importance to the intraoperative implementation of planned component positioning with PSI in this population.

Femoral neck variants: Variation in femoral canal morphology in the periaxial plane of resection and overall proximal femur anatomy influences the final version and coronal alignment of the femoral stem with uncemented implant designs [3, 4]. Aberrant femoral neck version or neck-shaft angle alters the habitual anatomic orientation of the osteotomy relative to the surgeon and patient. This may introduce significant variability in the angle and level of a freehand neck cut relative to templated targets. Provided the extent of the anatomy does not preclude adequate guide fixation, there is a theoretical advantage to femoral guidance PSI in patients with significant femoral neck ante- or retroversion, as well as coxa valga or vara. Custom femoral cutting guides may help to reproduce the height and plane of the intended osteotomy and more reliably achieve targeted femoral stem level and position in these challenging cases.

Minimally invasive approaches: Patient-specific instrumentation may be a particularly valuable tool in improving the precision of femoral neck osteotomies for surgeons who employ minimally invasive approaches in THA. In minimally invasive hip surgery, limited exposure of the operative field leaves bony landmarks less accessible. As the femoral neck osteotomy is typically referenced from the lesser trochanter, use of femoral guidance PSI may reduce the margin of error and obviate the need for intraoperative imaging when performing the femoral neck cut with limited exposure.

9.3 What Is the Process?

3D preoperative planning: PSI systems require preoperative imaging with computed tomography (CT) or magnetic resonance imaging (MRI) to create the patient-specific joint model as well as make a template of the custom cutting guides and implants. A 3D computer model is generated and utilized to virtually plan the position and size of the prosthesis. In addition, functional spinopelvic imaging in sitting/standing positions may be used in some systems to define the limits of hip extension and flexion and assess the effect of chosen component position on implant and bony impingement in those functional positions. Inputs from these functional radiographs are also used for a kinematic simulation that shows the direction and magnitude of hip joint reactive forces throughout range of motion [6]. Preoperatively, surgeons may view the expected alterations in bearing contact mechanics at different component positions. Final planned implant positions may ultimately be tailored to the surgeon's preference for each patient prior to instrumentation manufacturing.

Manufacturing: Custom cutting guides are designed to fit and complement the native anatomy using bony or cartilage landmarks on CT or MRI, respectively. The guides are produced by either selective laser sintering or 3D printing and sterilized for delivery to the surgeon's center. Both posterior and anterior femoral cutting guides are offered to the surgeon to best suit the preferred surgical approach (dislocating versus in situ neck cut, respectively) (Fig. 9.1). The whole process from preoperative imaging to guide acquisition generally takes between 3 and 8 weeks [5].

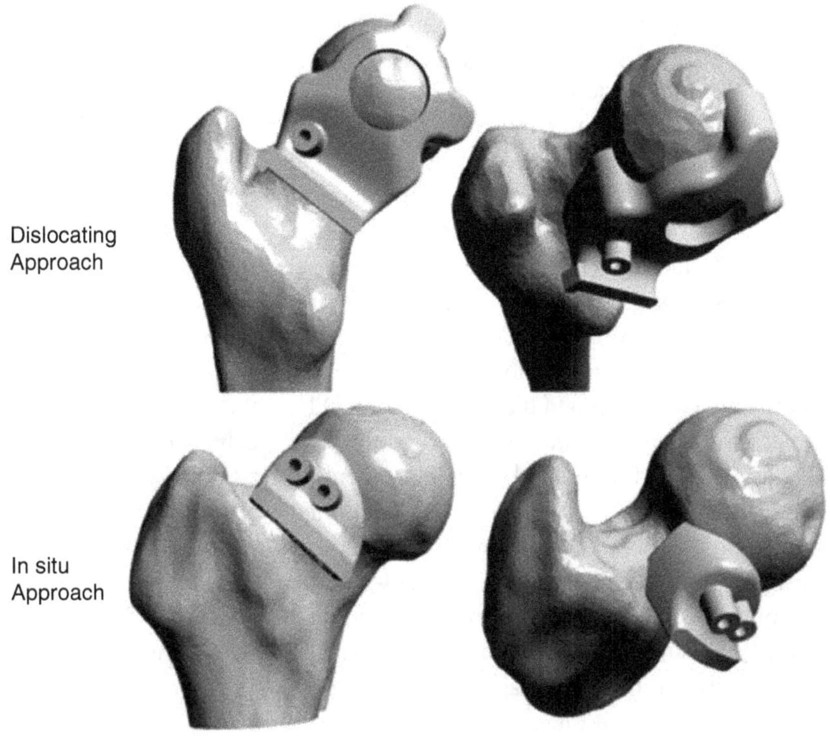

Fig. 9.1 Custom cutting guides for femoral neck osteotomy

Intraoperative implementation: Following routine exposure intraoperatively, the femoral guide is positioned on the head–neck junction and secured in place with a pin. The osteotomy is done with a standard oscillating saw along an open capture feature of the guide, which controls the level and angle of the neck cut but does not directly guide stem version.

9.4 What Are the Specific Related Complications?

There have been no reports of specific complications related to the use of femoral PSI in THA in the literature; however, most published series have been limited to approximately 30 patients or less [5, 7, 8]. No significant differences in blood loss or operative time have been shown to exist between patient-specific and conventional instrumentation. Comparisons to date have been limited to acetabular PSI and are undoubtedly influenced by surgeon experience [5]. Theoretical complications of currently available femoral guidance PSI include improper guide-anatomy fit, inadequate or loss of guide fixation, and iatrogenic fracture caused by pin fixation or guide misuse.

Use of PSI and 3D custom cutting guides requires the patient to undergo a CT scan in the preoperative period, and thus, it is associated with additional time, cost, and radiation exposure (unless using an MRI-based PSI system). The effective dose of radiation associated with the CT scan has been determined to be 2.8 mSv, which is similar to average annual background radiation exposure [9, 10]. There is currently no evidence to support the superiority of either CT or MRI for the creation of PSI in THA. The preferred PSI system determines which imaging modality is employed.

9.5 What Is the Supporting Clinical Evidence?

Due to the recent advent of femoral guidance PSI in THA, there are limited published reports on its clinical use yet available in the literature. Generic osteotomy guides have been shown to improve the accuracy of femoral neck resection height and limit postoperative limb length discrepancy (LLD). Yang et al. developed a set of six osteotomy guides with 1-mm interval height differences suitable for use on a variety of femoral neck configurations [11]. In 48 patients randomized to undergo THA with and without use of the guides, the mean average differences in femoral neck resection height were 0.84 mm and 1.69 mm, respectively [11]. The mean postoperative LLD was 5.45 mm among the guide group compared to 13.37 mm in the control group [11]. Ito et al. conducted an initial feasibility study on the use of PSI for femoral stem placement in THA. Using CT scan data for 3D planning and computer modeling software, the authors designed and manufactured 10 patient-specific femoral osteotomy guides for individual clinical use [7]. Compared to their preoperative targets, postoperative CT demonstrated the mean accuracy of femoral stem tilt, varus/valgus, and anteversion to be 2.1° ± 4.1°, 1.0° ± 0.7°, and 4.7° ± 1.2° with use of their PSI guides, respectively [7].

Early clinical data have supported the efficacy of the commercially available OPS proximal femoral cutting guide in achieving accurate osteotomies [8, 12, 13]. In an analysis of 33 patients, early use of the OPS femoral cutting guide by two surgeons was found to be clinically accurate within 1 mm of the planned osteotomy level in 85% of cases, with a mean difference of 0.7 mm between achieved osteotomy levels and templated targets [12]. In a subsequent series, 100 patients underwent posterior THA by one of three surgeons; use of PSI yielded femoral neck osteotomies within 1 mm and 2 mm of the preoperative plan in 83% and 96% of cases, respectively [13]. The mean difference between the planned and achieved osteotomy level was 0.3 mm, with a maximum reported error of 4 mm [13]. Schneider et al. subsequently analyzed the radiographic outcomes of 30 patients who underwent uncemented PSI–THA via the minimally invasive direct superior approach [8]. A total of 29 of 30 osteotomies were found to be within 3 mm of planned height [8]. In each of these studies, the achieved level of the femoral neck osteotomy at the medial calcar was compared to the planned level of resection using a 3D/2D matching analysis (Mimics X-ray module, Materialise, Belgium), and all patients received a Trinity/TriFit TS uncemented THA (Corin, Cirencester, UK) [8, 12, 13].

A single-center pilot study of 100 patients analyzed restoration of femoral head center of rotation using the OPS 3D femoral planning. In this series, the mean differences in planned and achieved head height, medial offset, and anterior offset were 0.9 mm, −0.9 mm, and 3.2 mm, respectively [14]. The resulting 3D change in planned and achieved head center was 4.4 mm; changes in anterior offset were strongly correlated to differences in achieved stem anteversion compared to planned targets (16.3° vs. 10.5°, respectively) [14]. While there was no comparison group, the authors conclude that use of 3D templating and PSI femoral guides accurately reproduce femoral center of rotation.

The OPS 3D planning software has also been evaluated for the sizing accuracy of the Trinity/TriFit TS components. In a consecutive series of 49 THAs, 92% of implanted TriFit TS femoral stems were within one size of that predicted, and use of standard or high-offset stems was predicted correctly in 80% of cases [15]. Variability in final stem offset chosen was largely attributed to the extent of medialization of the acetabular component.

Despite reports of the operative reproducibility of PSI femoral guidance, there have been no published studies on the clinical or functional outcomes following use of the technology in THA. Commercially available instrumentation has been validated in its ability to aid surgeon execution of femoral neck osteotomies at the desired (templated) level based on radiographic outcomes. However, data that directly compares the accuracy of femoral guidance PSI to conventional techniques have not yet been reported. Further study needs to address whether these radiographic outcomes correlate with functional and clinical outcomes in patients undergoing THA with femoral PSI. The body of literature on femoral guidance PSI in THA will undoubtedly grow with the continued use of this technology and appropriate patient follow-up.

9.6 Convincing Arguments: Why Recommend?

Variable magnification and out-of-plane rotations limit the reliability of 2D X-rays for accurate templating. Native proximal femur anatomy tends to guide femoral component alignment with use of uncemented stem designs [2, 3], while the level and angle of the femoral neck cut has been shown to influence final stem height and position [4]. Undersized femoral components can lead to a limb shortening, stem subsidence, and instability secondary to insufficient offset. Oversizing the femoral component may restrict hip motion, cause excessive limb lengthening, and increase the risk of intraoperative fracture. Three-dimensional preoperative planning includes assessment of femoral version and proximal canal morphology to more reliably measure true native offset and predict implant size. Patient-specific instrumentation may enhance the precision and accuracy of the osteotomy technique to increase consistency between final stem position and templated targets. Together, use of patient-specific 3D preoperative templating and custom femoral guides can help minimize outliers of limb length, offset, and stem version, and ultimately benefit clinical outcomes.

Limb length discrepancy (LLD) is the most common reason for patient dissatisfaction and litigation following THA [16, 17]. Errors in limb length are due to improper femoral stem positioning in 98% of cases [18]. Although conventional templating and techniques may effectively keep LLD to <10 mm in 97% of cases [19], evidence has shown that discrepancies >5 mm are likely to be perceived by patients [20, 21]. Greater discrepancies may result in the need for a shoe lift, potentiate back and radicular pain, increase pelvic obliquity, and cause implant failures such as instability, accelerated wear, and early loosening [16]. Residual LLD after THA has been associated with abnormal hip biomechanics, alterations in gait, and worse functional outcome scores [18, 20, 22, 23]. The extent of these adverse clinical effects is relative to the magnitude of the LLD, tends to be patient-specific, and may or may not improve with time elapsed from surgery. Younger, more active patients are far less likely to tolerate any significant alterations in limb length following THA; they may particularly benefit from PSI.

Femoral offset is the horizontal distance from the center of rotation of the femoral head to a line bisecting the anatomic axis of the femur. This length is underestimated by up to 20% on 2D radiographs [24]. In THA, femoral offset is influenced by the coronal (varus/valgus) alignment and anteversion of the stem, as well as the neck-shaft angle of the implant design. Global offset, defined as the sum of acetabular offset and femoral offset, should invariably be restored in THA [25]. Reductions in global offset result from imbalanced positioning of both the acetabular cup and femoral stem [18, 26]. While medialization of the acetabular cup (a decrease in acetabular offset) serves to reduce joint reactive forces and optimize bearing surface wear, a compensatory increase in femoral offset is required to maintain soft-tissue tension and avoid impingement. Decreasing offset in THA may result in abductor weakness, altered gait, and instability [16, 24, 27]. A significant increase in offset may contribute to lateral-sided hip pain and greater trochanteric bursitis. Accordingly, failure to restore offset has been shown to decrease patient satisfaction, quality of life, and yield worse functional outcomes [16, 25].

Acetabular and femoral component positions are mutually important for THA stability. Dorr et al. have suggested that the combined anteversion of the cup and stem (optimal range 25–50°) is more important in conferring impingement-free motion and constructing stability than acetabular "safe zone" position alone [3]. As our appreciation of the importance of combined anteversion continues to grow, the demand for accurate femoral component delivery systems such as PSI is likely to rise. Presently, femoral PSI guides control only the level and angle of the neck cut and do not yet control stem version. Nonetheless, accurate cup positioning and assessment of femoral version and canal morphology with available PSI–THA systems is beneficial for the surgeon in achieving combined anteversion targets.

Patient-specific instrumentation is a novel modality designed to enhance surgical technique and improve the accuracy of component positioning in THA. Currently available systems offer an alternative approach to patient-specific THA for surgeons without access to computer navigation or robotic-assisted platforms. Ongoing research will determine the efficacy of custom femoral cutting guides in reproducing desired femoral component position, as well as the effect on patient-reported and functional outcomes.

9.7 Case Example

The following section offers a generic visual guide to further explain the 3D preoperative templating for femoral component position using the OPS™, Corin Group. An example of a final OPS Plan for PSI-THA is shown in conclusion.

9.7.1 Length Planning

- The planned position of the entire femoral component (stem/head) is measured relative to the tip of the greater trochanter to reproduce the native femoral head center (Fig. 9.2). In patients who have undergone a contralateral THA, the stem/head combination is planned to match the head center of the contralateral prosthesis (Fig. 9.2).
- Postoperative length change is measured in the superior–inferior direction from the templated center of rotation of the liner (green) to the templated prosthetic head center (pink), and is compared to the preoperative state. The stem height is planned such that the osteotomy level is at least 5 mm superior to the lesser trochanter (unless otherwise specified) (Fig. 9.3).

9.7.2 Offset Planning

- As the acetabular component is often medialized, planned femoral offset of the stem/head combination is generally increased to maintain global offset.
- Center of rotation medialization is measured from the native femoral head center to the templated center of rotation of the liner. Femoral offset is measured from the native femoral head center to the templated prosthetic head center (Fig. 9.4). Offset is the planned overall change in hip offset when the femoral prosthesis is concentrically reduced into the acetabular component (Offset = femoral offset − Center of rotation medialization) (Fig. 9.4).

9.7.3 Stem Version Planning

- The femoral stem position is templated to reproduce the native femoral head center in the axial or transverse plane.
- Native femoral version is measured as the angle subtended by axis of the native femoral neck and the line tangent to the posterior condyles of the knee viewed down the long axis of the femur (Fig. 9.5).

Stem version is the angle between the axis of the neck of the femoral stem and the line tangent to the posterior condyles of the knee, again viewed down the long axis of the femur (Fig. 9.6).

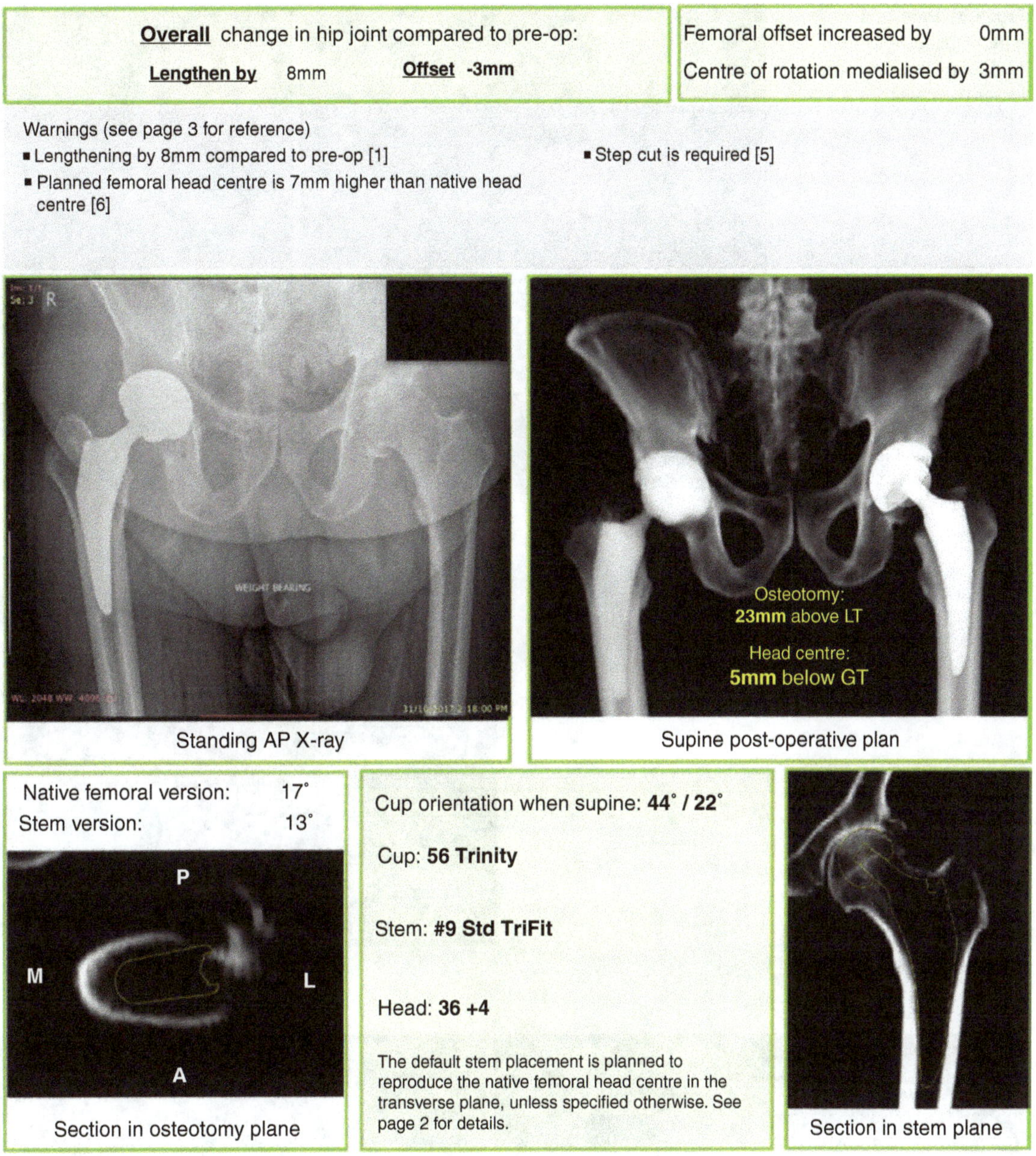

Fig. 9.2 Example of OPS plan targeted to contralateral implant head height

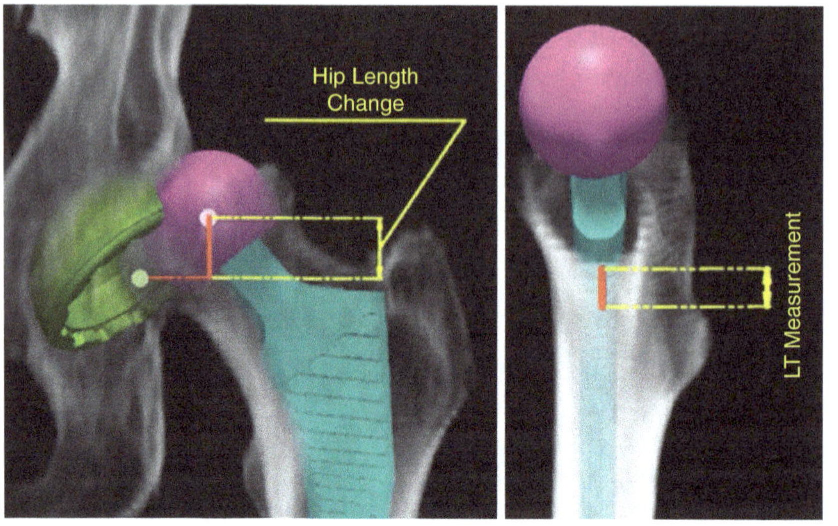

Fig. 9.3 Predicted length change and osteotomy relative to the lesser trochanter

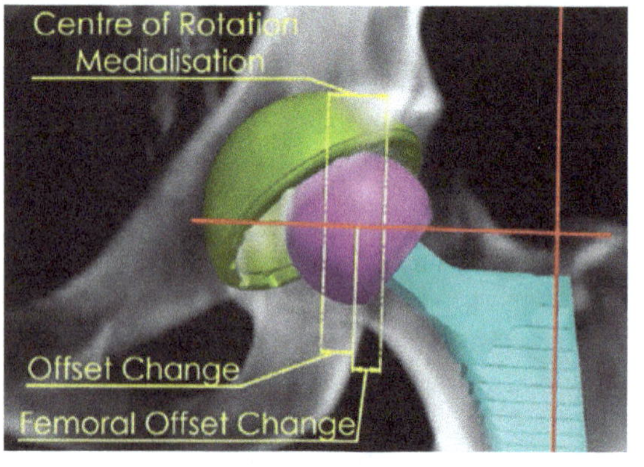

Fig. 9.4 Predicted change in global offset

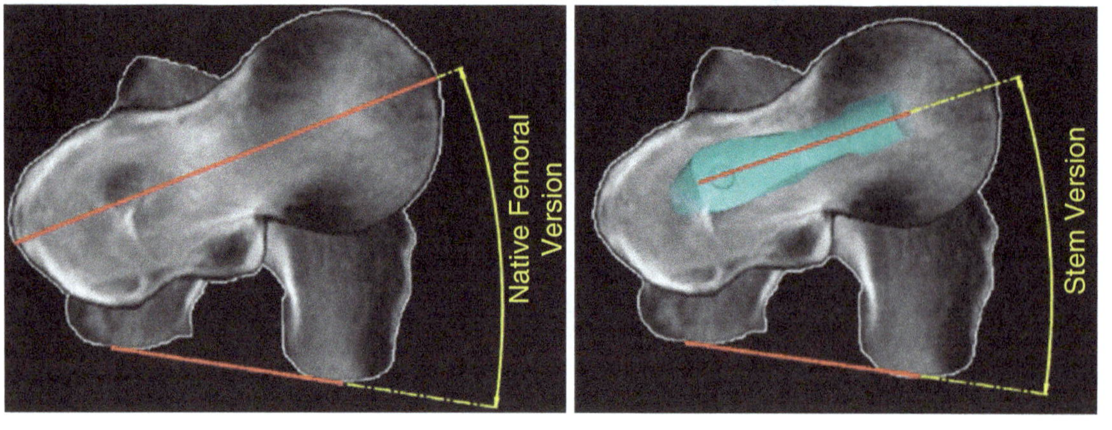

Fig. 9.5 Planned femoral stem version based on native femoral version

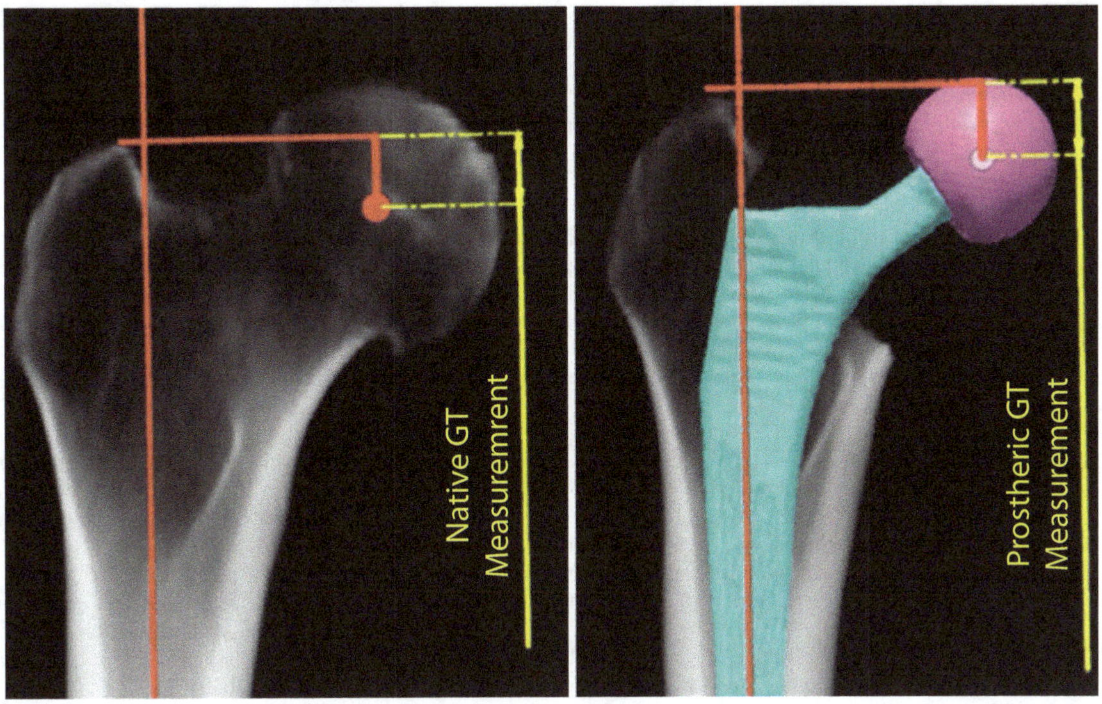

Fig. 9.6 Native and prosthetic greater trochanter measurement

References

1. Merle C, Waldstein W, Pegg E, Streit MR, Gotterbarm T, Aldinger PR, et al. Femoral offset is underestimated on anteroposterior radiographs of the pelvis but accurately assessed on anteroposterior radiographs of the hip. J Bone Joint Surg Br. 2012;94:477–82. https://doi.org/10.1302/0301-620X.94B4.28067.
2. Khanuja HS, Vakil JJ, Goddard MS, Mont MA. Cementless femoral fixation in total hip arthroplasty. J Bone Joint Surg Am. 2011;93:500–9. https://doi.org/10.2106/JBJS.J.00774.
3. Dorr LD, Malik A, Dastane M, Wan Z. Combined Anteversion technique for Total hip Arthroplasty. Clin Orthop Relat Res. 2009;467:119–27. https://doi.org/10.1007/s11999-008-0598-4.
4. Dimitriou D, Tsai T-Y, Kwon Y-M. The effect of femoral neck osteotomy on femoral component position of a primary cementless total hip arthroplasty. Int Orthop. 2015;39:2315–21. https://doi.org/10.1007/s00264-015-2739-1.
5. Henckel J, Holme TJ, Skinner JA, Hart AJ. 3D-printed patient-specific guides for hip Arthroplasty. J Am Acad Orthop Surg. 2018;26:e342–8. https://doi.org/10.5435/JAAOS-D-16-00719.
6. Pierrepont J, Stambouzou C, Miles B, O'Connor P, Ellis A, Molnar R, et al. Patient-specific component alignment in total hip arthroplasty. Reconstr Rev. 2016;6:27–33. https://doi.org/10.15438/rr.6.4.148.
7. Ito H, Tanaka S, Tanaka T, Oshima H, Tanaka S. A patient-specific instrument for femoral stem placement during total hip arthroplasty. Orthopedics. 2017;40:e374–7. https://doi.org/10.3928/01477447-20161108-06.
8. Schneider AK, Pierrepont JW, Hawdon G, McMahon S. Clinical accuracy of a patient-specific femoral osteotomy guide in minimally-invasive posterior hip arthroplasty. Hip Int. 2018;28:636–41. https://doi.org/10.1177/1120700018755691.
9. Huppertz A, Lembcke A, Sariali EH, Durmus T, Schwenke C, Hamm B, et al. Low dose computed tomography for 3D planning of total hip arthroplasty: evaluation of radiation exposure and image quality. J Comput Assist Tomogr. 2015;39:649–56. https://doi.org/10.1097/RCT.0000000000000271.
10. Schauer DA, Linton OW. Ionizing radiation exposure oh the population of the United States. Med Phys. 2009;36:5375. https://doi.org/10.1118/1.3245881.
11. Yang L, Zheng Z, Chen W, Wang J, Zhang Y. Femoral neck osteotomy guide for total hip arthroplasty. BMC Surg. 2015;15:1–6. https://doi.org/10.1186/s12893-015-0015-3.
12. Pierrepont J, Riddell W, Miles B, Baré J, Shimmin A. Clinical accuracy of a patient-specific guide for delivering a planned femoral neck osteotomy. Orthop Proc. 2016;98–B:131.
13. Bare J, Selim J, Stambouzou C, Pierrepont J, McMahon S, Shimmin A. Clinical accuracy of a patient specific femoral neck osteotomy guide. Liverpool: Br Orthop Assoc Ann Congr; 2016.

14. Reitman R, Pierrepont J, Shimmin A, McMahon S, Kerzhner E. Accurate reproduction of femoral Centre of rotation using 3d templating and a PSI guide. Orthop Proc. 2017;99:109.
15. Pierrepont J, Miles B, Walter L, Marel E, McMahon S, Solomon M, et al. Sizing accuracy of the trinity 3D planning software for total hip replacement conclusions. In: Paris: Int Congr Jt Reconstr; 2015.
16. Flecher X, Ollivier M, Argenson JN. Lower limb length and offset in total hip arthroplasty. Orthop Traumatol Surg Res. 2016;102:S9–20. https://doi.org/10.1016/j.otsr.2015.11.001.
17. Hofmann AA, Skrzynski MC. Leg-length inequality and nerve palsy in total hip arthroplasty: a lawyer awaits. Orthopedics. 2000;23:943–4.
18. Konyves A, Bannister GC. The importance of leg length discrepancy after total hip arthroplasty. J Bone Joint Surg Br. 2005;87:155–7. https://doi.org/10.1302/0301-620X.87B2.14878.
19. Woolson ST, Hartford JM, Sawyer A. Results of a method of leg-length equalization for patients undergoing primary total hip replacement. J Arthroplast. 1999;14:159–64.
20. Renkawitz T, Weber T, Dullien S, Woerner M, Dendorfer S, Grifka J, et al. Gait & posture leg length and offset differences above 5 mm after total hip arthroplasty are associated with altered gait kinematics. Gait Posture. 2016;49:196–201. https://doi.org/10.1016/j.gaitpost.2016.07.011.
21. Sykes A, Hill J, Orr J, Humphreys P, Rooney A, Morrow E, et al. Patients' perception of leg length discrepancy post total hip arthroplasty. Hip Int. 2015;25:452–6. https://doi.org/10.5301/hipint.5000276.
22. Mahmood SS, Mukka SS, Crnalic S, Sayed-Noor AS. The influence of leg length discrepancy after total hip arthroplasty on function and quality of life: a prospective cohort study. J Arthroplast. 2015;30:1638–42. https://doi.org/10.1016/j.arth.2015.04.012.
23. Li J, McWilliams AB, Jin Z, Fisher J, Stone MH, Redmond AC, et al. Unilateral total hip replacement patients with symptomatic leg length inequality have abnormal hip biomechanics during walking. Clin Biomech (Bristol, Avon). 2015;30:513–9. https://doi.org/10.1016/j.clinbiomech.2015.02.014.
24. Sariali E, Klouche S, Mouttet A, Pascal-Moussellard H. The effect of femoral offset modification on gait after total hip arthroplasty. Acta Orthop. 2014;85:123–7. https://doi.org/10.3109/17453674.2014.889980.
25. Clement ND, S Patrick-Patel R, MacDonald D, Breusch SJ. Total hip replacement: increasing femoral offset improves functional outcome. Arch Orthop Trauma Surg. 2016;136:1317–23. https://doi.org/10.1007/s00402-016-2527-4.
26. Al-amiry B, Mahmood S, Krupic F. Leg lengthening and femoral-offset reduction after total hip arthroplasty: where is the problem – stem or cup positioning? Acta Radiol. 2017;58:1125–31. https://doi.org/10.1177/0284185116684676.
27. Mahmood SS, Mukka SS, Crnalic S, Sayed-Noor AS. Association between changes in global femoral offset after total hip arthroplasty and function, quality of life, and abductor muscle strength a prospective cohort study of 222 patients. Acta Orthop. 2016;87:36–41. https://doi.org/10.3109/17453674.2015.1091955.

10

Computer-Assisted Surgery and Reconstructing the Hip Anatomy

Marius Dettmer, Stefan W. Kreuzer, and Stefany Malanka

10.1 What Is the Rationale for Computer-Assisted Hip Arthroplasty?

Total hip arthroplasty (THA) is a very successful procedure with 95% survivorship after 10 years and 80% survivorship at 25 years [1]. Despite this success, there are also reports about patient dissatisfaction, (early) revisions, and other issues.

Research has shown that appropriate femoral and acetabular component positioning and placement is crucial for prevention of hip dislocations, accelerated wear, leg length inequality, unfavorable biomechanics, and suboptimal function. One of the persisting challenges of appropriate acetabular component placement is its dependence on correct evaluation of the individual lumbopelvic kinematics and spine–hip relation.

Over the past decades, there have been multiple innovative approaches to improve positioning and placement of components to enhance alignment or to recreate native characteristics of the hip and femur, such as intraoperative fluoroscopy and mechanical navigation [2] technology. Potentially, the most influential innovation related to efforts in improving implant positioning was the introduction of computer-assisted surgery (CAS), built on the technological foundations and innovation and advances in major fields such as computing and optics.

When defining CAS, often computer technology for planning, navigating, and guiding surgery and the use of robotic assistance in surgery are used interchangeably to describe the term. While the fields of robotic assistance and computer-assisted navigation are heavily intertwined and most robotics currently rely on computers and image-based preplanning for navigation (an exemption being the imageless NAVIO robotic system for knee arthroplasty by Smith & Nephew, LPC), the underlying methods and techniques are distinct.

CAS systems comprise of a number of different technologies and methods to overcome challenges posed by arthroplasty. In total hip arthroplasty, CAS tracks the intraoperative position and alignment of the pelvis, femur, and surgical instruments. Orthopedic surgery may specifically benefit from this development, since bone matter is a great candidate for such measures due to its relative rigidity and its distinction from soft tissue in the body. For THA, CAS allows for accurate and appropriate placement of the acetabular component within the "safe zone" [3] and for recreation of the native femoral offset and leg

M. Dettmer · S. Malanka
Memorial Bone & Joint Research Foundation, Houston, TX, USA
e-mail: mdettmer@mbjc.net; SMalanka@mbjc.net

S. W. Kreuzer (✉)
Memorial Bone & Joint Research Foundation, Houston, TX, USA

Inov8 Orthopedics, Houston, TX, USA
e-mail: stefan@inov8hc.com, fcheney@inov8hc.com

length. Some devices further provide information about joint biomechanics, surgery progress, joint irregularities, and cutting accuracy [4].

10.2 Imageless and Image-Based CAS

A number of established navigation systems rely either on accelerometer-based tools or position/motion capture technology that combines infrared cameras and reflective (passive) or light-emitting (active) markers or diodes attached to arrays/platforms, bony landmarks, and surgical tools. Software is then used to determine the position and orientation of the bone structures and instruments in 3D space for monitoring and provision of feedback. Imageless CAS includes an intraoperative bone registration process, where the identification and digitization of bony landmarks are crucial for developing a 3D model of the hip and to establish femoral position and orientation.

After registration and definition of planes, e.g., anterior pelvic plane, reaming depth/direction, and implant placement can be intraoperatively planned and modified. For image-based CAS, CTs or MRI is used for 3D modeling and subsequent preoperative planning, with intraoperative flexibility to modify the plan.

10.3 Benefits, Complications, and Specific Risks of CAS

Overall, both imageless and image-based computer navigation systems in THA are considered reliable and accurate. For imageless navigation, one study showed about 97% of acetabular components were placed within the safe zone for inclination and anteversion. A meta-analysis including 7 clinical trials and 485 patients compared THA with and without and imageless navigation, where desired position of anteversion deviated on average less in navigated cases and the authors found no differences in mean cup inclination and anteversion [5].

Leg length equality may be well restored with CAS with decreased outliers regarding leg length discrepancies, but there is no current scientific evidence that CAS may be superior regarding this aspect. There is also currently no evidence for significantly higher or specific risks related to CAS; results from a retrospective, small cohort study showed no differences after 5–7 years post-op evaluation regarding clinical outcomes (HOOS, HHS, range of motion), bone mineral density, or polyethylene wear when comparing navigated and non-navigated THA [6]. Image-based CAS has also been shown to be a valuable alternative to conventional THA, with highly precise and favorable measurements of cup alignment, less placement outside the safe zone, less dislocations, and similar survival rates [7].

A potential disadvantage of imageless navigation is the reliance on consistently accurate registration of bony landmarks for evaluation of the anterior pelvic plane (APP). The individual variability of soft tissue thickness overlaying landmarks such as the bilateral ASIS and the symphysis pubis may be challenging and lead to registration errors affecting cup positioning. It has been questioned whether the APP derived from the position of aforementioned landmarks as an anatomical reference plane for navigation may actually be inferior (especially in cases with difficulty to access the bony landmarks due to surrounding soft tissue) to the alternative supine coronal plane, which some systems allow to assess and use as a functional reference plane.

10.4 Cost-Effectiveness of CAS

Despite numerous positive reports regarding the safety, accuracy, and clinical outcomes, most surgeons have not yet adopted the technology citing high cost, the learning curve, and increased operative time. However, the complexity of current systems has significantly decreased throughout the past decade, and it allows for easier integration into the operating room (OR) workflow. Overall, there is a significant initial setup cost associated with the integration of computer navigation in the OR, so it has been postulated that lower priced systems may be crucial to justify setup and use of the technology for many facilities having to balance cost and efficiency [8]. This initial setup cost may be well compensated by the longer term efficacy; overall, there may be a smaller number of required instrumentation trays [1], and implants, and a decrease of other indirect costs. Other major factors determining cost effectiveness may be the overall case volume (with decreased efficiency associated with lower number of surgeries), efforts to decrease revision rates in comparison to existing methods, and reducing costs of the technology itself, additional equipment, and disposables. The use of image-based navigation requires additional presurgery imaging, which further increases costs, and there has been some concern about infection due to pins placed percutaneously at the iliac crest, thus increasing risk for the patient. The latter has been identified and addressed by several navigation device manufacturers, as some devices either do not require the use of femoral trackers or use pinless technology where markers/trackers are attached to the limb surface without the need for incision or drilling. Alternatively, in certain systems, leg length may be acquired by positioning a probe on a distal femur landmark.

10.5 Some Current Navigation Systems

The imageless Intellijoint system (Intellijoint Surgical Inc., Waterloo, Canada) was developed to tackle current issues associated with conventional CAS, mainly the high per-patient costs, the increased surgical time, and the interruption of surgical workflow. This miniature tool acts as an intraoperative guidance tool that can provide information on cup position, leg length, offset, and hip center. The system is based on optical infrared technology described earlier and consists of a camera magnetically attached to a pelvic platform attached to the ipsilateral (contralateral in direct anterior approach arthroplasty) iliac crest with two screws, and a femoral disc tracking/registration point that is secured at the greater trochanter. The surgeon must also create an accurately reproducible tracking point at the distal femur, which can either be done via a small incision or some other surface marker that will not move.

This allows for a real-time evaluation of joint alignment and component positioning, and the magnetic array allows for easy adjustment of the camera-tracker setup, e.g., to attach the tracker to the bone impactor or a surgical probe. The native characteristics of the hip and femur are evaluated before dislocation; then during trial reduction, tracker measurements are conducted through the range of motion, and tracking then helps with selection of correct implant size and component placement (Fig. 10.1).

One major advantage of this system (apart from no requirements for additional imaging) is that the miniature-format system can be set up in the sterile field (with the camera sterilely draped and the monitor outside the sterile field) with no interruption of the surgical workflow. This also

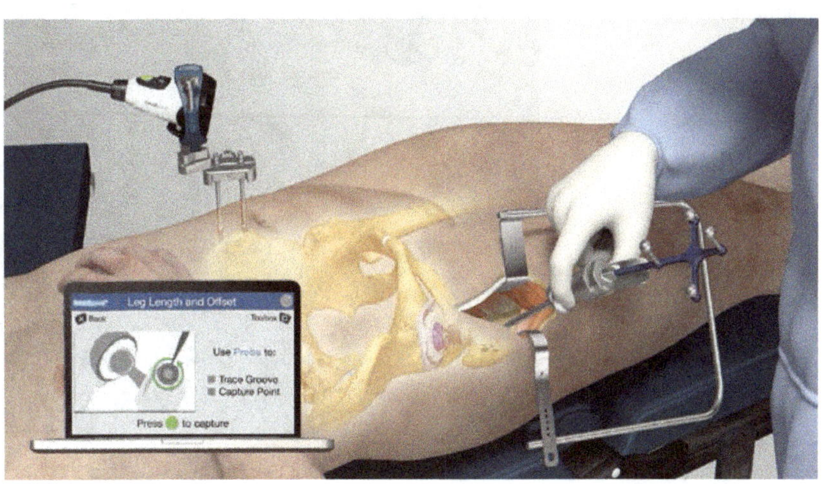

Fig. 10.1 Intraoperative monitoring of leg length and offset using the Intellijoint miniature navigation system. The digitizing probe is used to trace the groove of the disc attached to the femur to establish femoral position and orientation changes

minimizes any issues regarding visibility of the markers for the camera.

The imageless Brainlab Hip System (Brainlab, Munich, Germany) uses wireless technology and is a touchscreen-based planning and navigation module. A single camera unit (consisting of two cameras for 3D space) that is part of the navigation station outside the sterile field emits and detects infrared flashes. Just as with other similar systems, markers that are attached to reference arrays on patients' bony landmarks (and a pinless femur reference option), probes, and instrumentation reflect the infrared light back to the camera system where it is detected and processed by software to calculate the 3D positions of the different landmarks and instruments. Preoperatively, the operator measures ASIS distance and pelvic tilt. Then, after making the incision and preparing the bone, a landmark registering process follows, which provides the computer with reference landmarks in space relative to reference arrays and information about individual patient anatomy. Instrument adapters allow for the use of devices not provided by the manufacturer, but require additional calibration steps. Intraoperative planning can be conducted in regards to both cup and femoral component, and "leg situation analysis" allows for intraoperative evaluation of leg length and combined femoral and pelvic offset (Fig. 10.2). It also allows for intraoperative range of motion and, depending on approach, impingement analysis.

Stryker's OrthoMap imageless system (Stryker Corporation, Kalamazoo, MI, USA) allows for registration in both supine and lateral position for different approaches, intraoperative evaluation of leg offset, leg length, ROM, and joint stability, and enables the user to intraoperatively plan both the cup and stem. Users may utilize the Stryker instruments or compatible instruments from several other cup manufacturers. A single infrared light-emitting and detecting unit is used in combination with markers/tracker attached to the pelvis and the femur, whereas leg length assessments can also be done without the use of a femoral tracker by using skin marker digitization at the distal femur. Cup positioning is based on the anatomical definition of cup alignment and allows for the determination of inclination, anteversion, and hip center shift (translation of the cup relative to the hip center in 3D space). Stem alignment and position can be assessed (e.g., anteversion, leg length, and femoral offset).

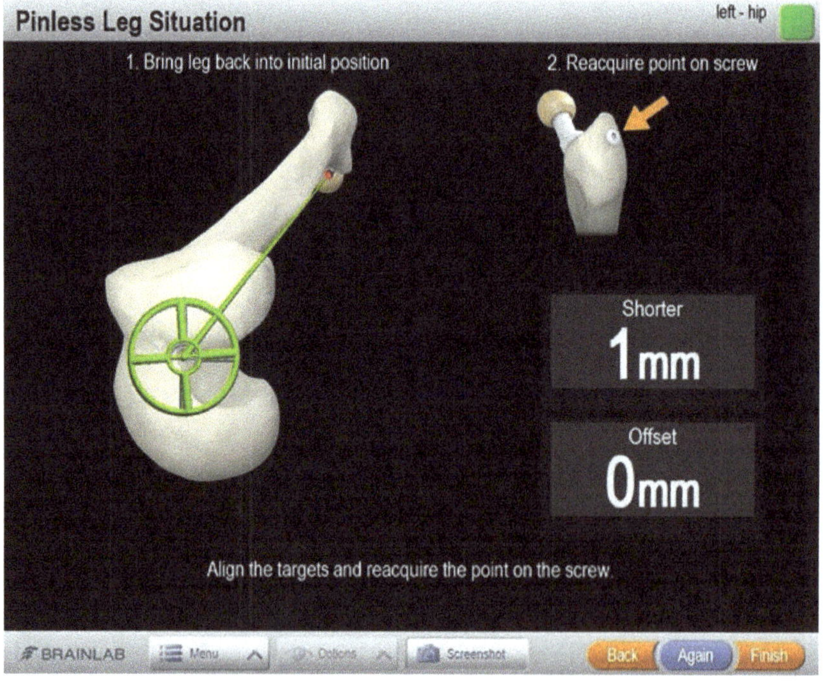

Fig. 10.2 The Brainlab system for THA uses a proximal femoral screw/tracker that can be reacquired throughout the procedure for assessment of the leg length and offset

10.6 Robotic Assistance

It has been proposed that every industry, including modern medicine and ultimately total joint arthroplasty, follows a similar set of steps of maturation with the final phases being automation and computer integration [9]. Hence, the development of robotic assistance for orthopedic surgery is not surprising. Robotic assistance in joint surgery has been around since the 1990s, with William Bargar and Howard Paul developing the technique in 1992 for hip arthroplasty. Robotic devices such as the pioneering ROBODOC (Curexo Technology, Fremont, CA and Think Surgical Inc., Fremont, CA) have the robot navigate based on mechanical, computer-assisted navigation, and meticulous preplanning/templating before surgery.

Surgical robots can be classified as active, semi-active, and passive systems. Passive systems assist in parts of the surgery, under complete guidance from the surgeon, e.g., keeping a guide in position while the surgeon performs the bone preparation. Semi-active systems require intervention from the surgeon in form of manipulation of the cutting tool, while the system provides the operator with either haptic, visual, and/or auditory feedback regarding predetermined (preplanned) spatial constraints associated with the cutting process (i.e., "active constraint"). The Mako system (Stryker Corporation, Kalamazoo, MI, USA) is an approved and well-known semi-active system providing haptic guidance throughout the cutting procedure. Active robots execute tasks such as cutting without dependence on guidance from the surgeon, and once initiated, conduct the bone preparation autonomously.

The first robot of this kind was the aforementioned ROBODOC built on the platform of a traditional computer-assisted manufacturing system [10]. Another system is the TSolution One (Think Surgical, Inc., Fremont, CA), which is built on the foundation of ROBODOC technology. The overall strongest argument for the use of robotic assistance is the improved accuracy of bone milling in combination with 3D planning of the surgery for optimal bone preparation and implant placement.

10.7 Benefits, Complications, and Specific Risks of Robotics

Most of the existing studies comparing robotic surgery and traditional THA include only small cohorts, allowing only for preliminary conclusions about efficacy and safety. However, a recent meta-analysis of 178 articles (eight studies included in quantitative synthesis) and including only studies from 2005 to 2017 provided more insight regarding this topic [11]. Their analysis of intraoperative complications (femoral fractures/cracks) and postoperative complications (infection, nerve palsy, deep vein thrombosis, and dislocation) showed a significantly higher intraoperative complication rate for manual THA and similar postoperative complication rates between manual and robotic-assisted THA. The total complication rates were significantly higher in manual THA, including in the three included randomized-controlled trials. There were no significant differences between the THA methods for several outcome measures (Japanese Orthopaedic Association Score, Harris Hip Score, Merle d'Aubigne Hip Score, Western Ontario and McMaster Universities Osteoarthritis Index). Radiographic data analyses showed no differences in leg length discrepancy, but a higher rate of optimal cup placement (within the safe zone) for robotic THA. This efficient and consistent placement within the margins of the safe zone is, in turn, associated with a decreased risk for dislocation, instability, and revisions. The authors found no significant differences regarding surgical time in the pooled analysis but an overall trend toward shorter surgery times for conventional THA. This factor may be related to each surgeon's individual experience and the learning curve, and more research is required to investigate how much surgeon experience can affect shortening of robotic surgery times. Blood loss was only evaluated in two studies, with one favoring robotic THA, and one finding no differences. Additionally, it has been suggested that there has been an increased number of litigations related to earlier robotic devices, potentially due to patients' perception that the use of robots indicates a lack of human oversight or decreased human control and involvement during the surgery [4].

Robots are designed to execute a plan, and a current obstacle or limitation is the inability of active robot systems to adjust this plan intraoperatively (intraoperative modifications are much less of an issue in semi-active robotic assistance THA), since there is a dynamic environment whose variables may change in an instant. For example, if there is an intraoperative finding that requires adjustments or if there is a fracture occurring, the surgeon has to stop the robot and manually finish bone cuts as there is no flexibility of the robotic technology at this present time in case of unforeseen events. This current problem of active robotics will most likely be solved in the future with progress in artificial intelligence and improved control software.

10.8 Cost-Effectiveness

A major issue regarding the current lack of cost efficiency is the high cost of purchasing the robotic system and its hardware and software components, and associated costs such as cost of disposables, training of staff, and maintaining the system, that is, (re-)calibrations, upgrades. Conventional THA has an advantage regarding intraoperative time as a major cost evaluation aspect, but with current developments in robotic technology, we can expect intraoperative time to further decrease, e.g., with development of simpler bone registration methods and improved OR workflow. Another very significant aspect are potential cost savings associated with robotic surgery related to the significant reduction of instruments needed and potential elimination of inventory in the field. To realize these cost savings, it will require a close collaboration between the individual stakeholders such as hospitals, OR facilities, device representatives, and physicians. Since there are still unanswered questions and a lack of long-term studies related to potential advantages/disadvantages of robotic THA, more research is needed to make valid statements about the overall cost-effectiveness. Ultimately, the market will decide whether the use of robotic technology is justified and the cost-effectiveness calculations will require constant updates and reevaluations, since the technology is still being further developed and refined.

10.9 Personalizing Hip Replacement and the Role of CAS and Robotics

The usefulness of Lewinnek's "safe zone" as a standard for cup orientation in THA has been questioned more and more in the past few years [12–14]. This is due to patients' individual muscular and bony anatomical differences that may affect lumbo-pelvic kinematics and spine–hip relationship throughout the range of motion. These individual differences have been proposed to be crucial for finding accurate cup positioning to ensure optimal postoperative function and prevention of dislocation, instability, and premature failure. The general "safe zone" does not account for such individual differences, but there are efforts to take these aspects into consideration for THA. One promising approach is a preoperative evaluation of the patients' joint kinematics and lumbo-pelvic interactions, as provided by Corin's Optimized Positioning System (OPS, Corin, Cirencester, UK). The system uses preoperative imaging to investigate the individual dynamics of the lumbo-pelvic complex (Fig. 10.3). The kinematic information is then used to create an operative plan including suggestions for optimal cup inclination and anteversion (Fig. 10.4). The software also provides a preview of the planned osteotomy and the cup placement (Fig. 10.5). Such individualized systems for THA are likely to be useful for improving postoperative outcomes, but a solid created plan is only as good as its execution in the OR. For this specific system, Corin provides personalized jigs that are used to perform the suggested osteotomy/bone preparation on the acetabular and femoral side.

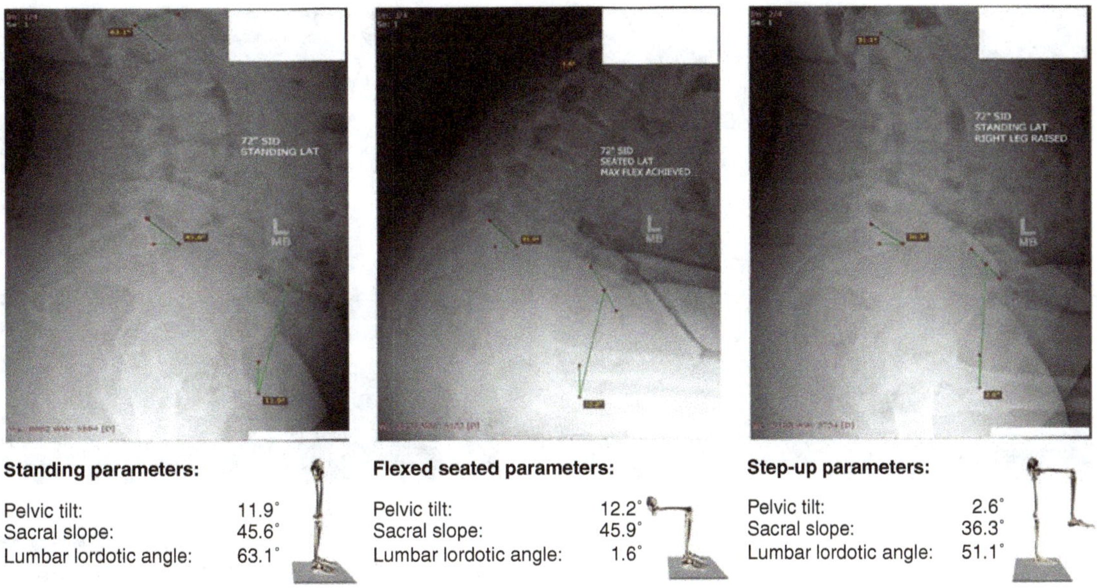

Fig. 10.3 Preoperative functional imaging for evaluation of individual kinematics and personalized cup orientation using the Optimized Positioning System (Corin OPS, Cirencester, UK)

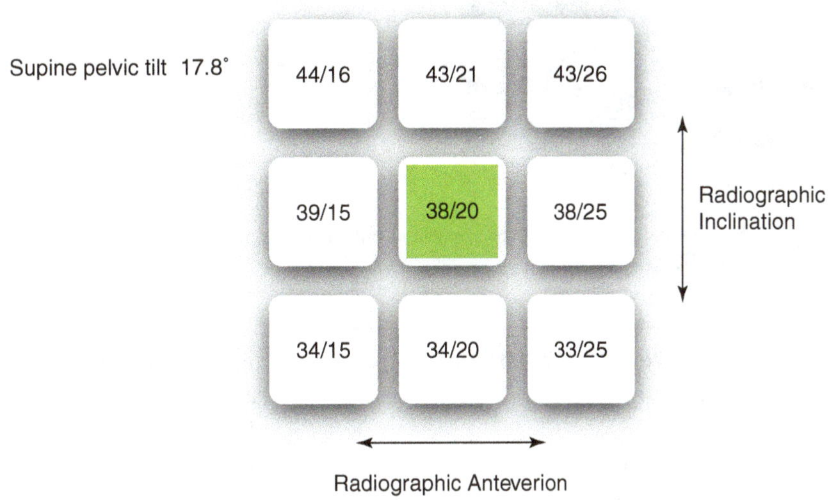

Fig. 10.4 Operative plan for individualized cup orientation based on preoperative functional evaluation. (Corin OPS, Corin, Cirencester, UK)

However, for high-precision intraoperative navigation, the system could be combined and integrated with CAS, i.e., with the use of the Intellijoint system. This would allow the surgeon to use both a personalized approach through thorough preoperative planning in combination with high precision and accuracy operative execution with the help of CAS.

The value of this combination of preoperative planning and CAS may be further enhanced by concurrent developments in robotic assistance technologies. Hence, the functional assessment of native joint anatomy and kinematics in combination with CAS and the precision of robotic assisted bone preparation could lead to a paradigm shift in regards to THA standard of care; the technological progress and fine-tuned combination of the described tools could lead to significant improvements of orthopedic care.

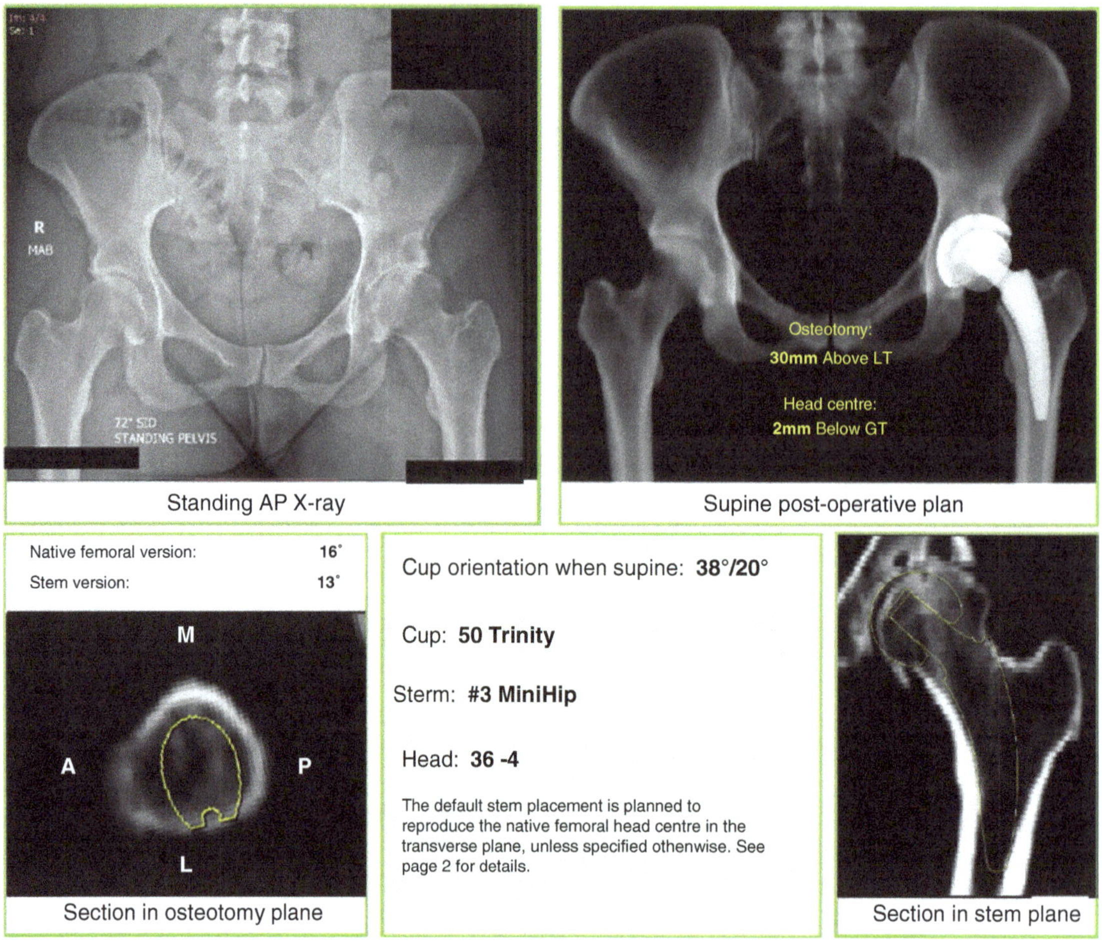

Fig. 10.5 Preview of planned osteotomy and cup placement with the Optimized Positioning System (OPS, Corin, Cirencester, UK)

10.10 Future of CAS and Robotic Surgery

"The only current limitation in the application and adoption of these technologies is the imagination and understanding of what can be accomplished in the future" [15]. Overall, the potential developments in CAS and robotic surgery could include improved preoperative and intraoperative planning and streamlined workflow, improved time efficiency, accuracy, and more flexibility. The aforementioned combination of preoperative functional hip analyses and operative plan execution may be beneficial to make THA more efficient and minimize the number of patients dissatisfied with their treatment. Navigated THA and robotic surgery have benefitted greatly from the technological advancements of the past two decades, specifically in the areas of computation, optical positioning/motion capturing, and industrial robotics. While it is difficult to predict the future, the past has indicated which path future innovations could take. On a sensor/imaging level, the use of ultrasound for defining a reference plane, or 3D laser scanning could become more important once the technologies are introduced in the workflow.

Whereas it is impressive how precisely robots perform their given tasks, future developments in artificial intelligence and sensor technology as part of the "Industry 4.0" phase may allow robots to be more efficient than they are currently; more advanced robots could be able to adjust to changing intraoperative variables and be able to perform modified bone cuts without requirements for intervention of the surgeon. Once robots will be able to distinguish between tissue types, they may assist both in soft tissue preparations and balancing and also be less likely to injure bone-surrounding ligaments, tendons, or blood vessels.

In their outlook regarding the future potential of robotic innovation, Jacofsky and Allen [9] suggest that a recreation of the former kinematics of the native joint with less emphasis on imaging will be a potential next step, and there are recently initiated efforts to develop highly sophisticated customized and personalized implants that potentially will not even be implantable without the use of robotic assistance.

Automation and robotics will not be excluded from future THA developments, and most likely play a larger role than today. "...one thing is clear: robotics appears to be here to stay" [9].

Case Report

This particular case was a 26-year-old Caucasian woman with a Crowe IV dysplastic hip and pseudo-acetabulum (Fig. 10.6), who reported having had symptoms since the age of 12 years. The patient had previously undergone Chiari pelvic osteotomy, femoral osteotomy, and femoral lengthening, which were unsuccessful in improving pain and function in the longer term.

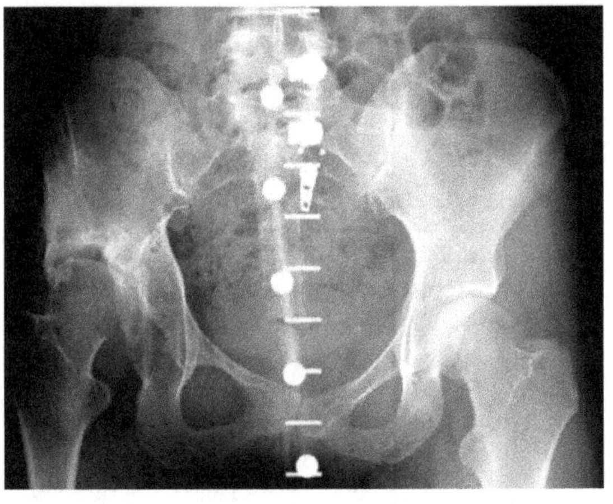

Fig. 10.6 Preoperative X-rays of 26-year-old patient with a Crowe IV dysplastic hip and pseudo-acetabulum

Considering the history of the patient in terms of disease progression, pseudo-acetabulum, deformities, and earlier treatments, preoperative planning would have been extremely difficult without CAS and robotic assistance. The semi-active robotic assistance also allowed for intraoperative plan modifications regarding cup placement to recreate the true acetabulum and femoral preparation to reproduce the proximal femur anatomy. We used the MAKOplasty Robotic Arm Interactive Orthopedic (RIO) robotic arm (MAKO Surgical Corp., Ft. Lauderdale, FL, USA) and surgery-planning software, which allowed us to preoperatively plan the placement of the acetabular shell into the severely dysplastic true acetabulum based on patient-specific anatomical characteristics (based on three-dimensional [3D] reconstructions of patient computed tomography [CT] scans, Fig. 10.7). Also, a small femoral tracker was placed on the proximal femur and a small electrocardiogram (ECG) lead was attached to the kneecap, so the system's digitizer could be used to register those points for intraoperative evaluation of leg length and combined offset. This provided the opportunity to make intraoperative modifications when necessary. The use of the robotic arm helped to optimize accuracy and to execute the surgery plan with high levels of precision.

A Trinity shell (Corin, Cirencester, UK) was fixated using two screws and a neck-preserving MiniHip (Corin, Cirencester, UK) femoral stem was used. The surgery led to the reconstruction of the true acetabulum, which was associated with a decrease in leg length discrepancy (Fig. 10.8). The use of a neck-preserving short-stem implant in combination with use of the MAKO system helped to recreate the proximal femur anatomy. The patient followed up over 18 months and reported no issues related to her hip in the postoperative phase.

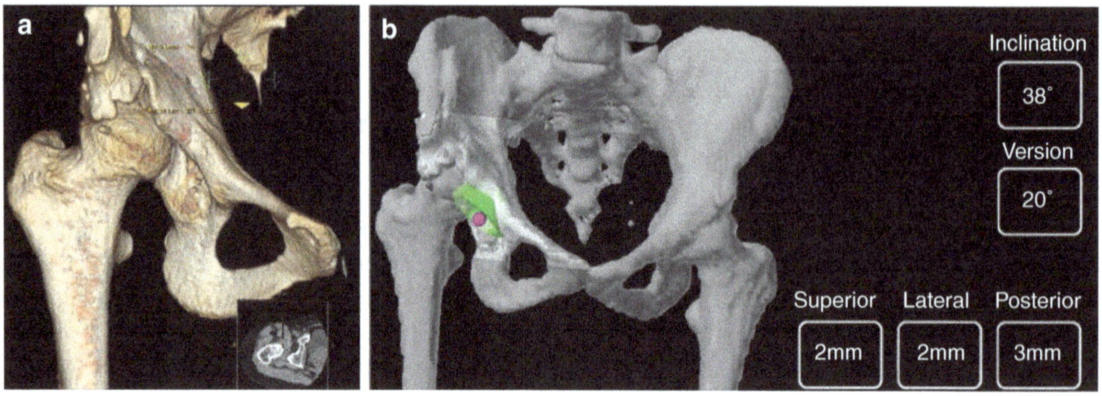

Fig. 10.7 (**a**) 3D model of the hip showing pseudo-acetabulum and (**b**) planned position of the shell in the dysplastic true acetabulum

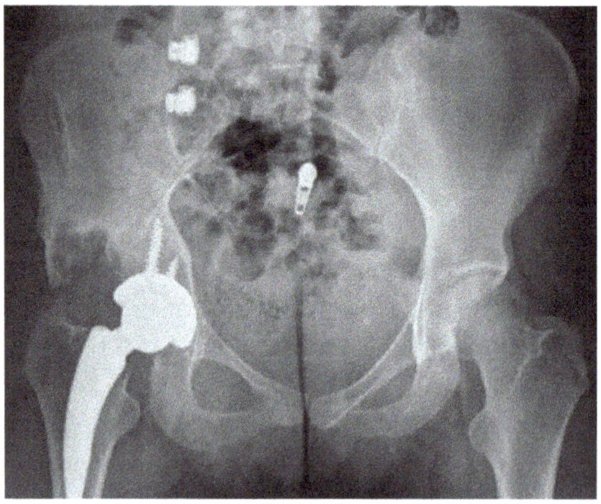

Fig. 10.8 Postoperative X-rays showing recreated true acetabulum and short-stem femoral implant

References

1. Deep K, Shankar S, Mahendra A. Computer assisted navigation in total knee and hip arthroplasty. Sicot J. 2017;3:50. http://www.sicot-j.org/10.1051/sicotj/2017034.
2. Steppacher SD, Kowal JH, Murphy SB. Improving cup positioning using a mechanical navigation instrument. Clin Orthop Relat Res. 2011;469(2):423–8.
3. Lewinnek GE, Lewis JL, Tarr R, Compere CL, Zimmerman JR. Dislocations after total hip-replacement arthroplasties. J Bone Joint Surg Am. 1978;60(2):217–20. http://www.ncbi.nlm.nih.gov/pubmed/641088.
4. Lang JE, Mannava S, Floyd AJ, Goddard MS, Smith BP, Mofidi A, et al. Robotic systems in orthopaedic surgery. J Bone Joint Surg Br. 2011;93(10):1296–9. http://www.ncbi.nlm.nih.gov/pubmed/21969424
5. Liu Z, Gao Y, Cai L. Imageless navigation versus traditional method in total hip arthroplasty: a meta-analysis. Int J Surg. 2015;21:122–7. https://doi.org/10.1016/j.ijsu.2015.07.707.
6. Keshmiri A, Schröter C, Weber M, Craiovan B, Grifka J, Renkawitz T. No difference in clinical outcome, bone density and polyethylene wear 5–7 years after standard navigated vs. conventional cementfree total hip arthroplasty. Arch Orthop Trauma Surg. 2015;135(5):723–30.
7. Waddell BS, Carroll K, Jerabek S. Technology in arthroplasty: are we improving value? Curr Rev Musculoskelet Med. 2017:378–87.
8. Inaba Y, Kobayashi N, Ike H, Kubota S, Saito T. The current status and future prospects of computer-assisted hip surgery. J Orthop Sci. 2016;21(2):107–15. https://doi.org/10.1016/j.jos.2015.10.023.
9. Jacofsky DJ, Allen M. Robotics in arthroplasty: a comprehensive review. J Arthroplasty. 2016;31: 2353–63.
10. Dungy DS, Netravali NA. Active robotics for Total hip arthroplasty. Am J Orthop. 2016;45(4):256–9.
11. Chen X, Xiong J, Wang P, Zhu S, Qi W, Peng H, et al. Robotic-assisted compared with conventional total hip arthroplasty: systematic review and meta-analysis. Postgrad Med J. 2018;2:335–41.
12. Abdel MP, von Roth P, Jennings MT, Hanssen AD, Pagnano MW. What safe zone? The vast majority of dislocated THAs are within the Lewinnek safe zone for acetabular component position. Clin Orthop Relat Res. 2016;474(2):386–91.
13. Tezuka T, Heckmann ND, Bodner RJ, Dorr LD. Functional safe zone is superior to the Lewinnek safe zone for total hip arthroplasty: why the Lewinnek safe zone is not always predictive of stability. J Arthroplast. 2018;34(1):3–8. https://doi.org/10.1016/j.arth.2018.10.034.
14. Reina N, Putman S, Desmarchelier R, Sari Ali E, Chiron P, Ollivier M, et al. Can a target zone safer than Lewinnek's safe zone be defined to prevent instability of total hip arthroplasties? Case-control study of 56 dislocated THA and 93 matched controls. Orthop Traumatol Surg Res. 2017;103(5):657–61.
15. DiGioia AM, Jaramaz B, Colgan BD. Computer assisted orthopaedic surgery. Image guided and robotic assistive technologies. Clin Orthop Relat Res. 1998;354:8–16.

Part IV

Total Hip Arthroplasty

11

Total Hip Replacement: Kinematic Alignment Technique

Charles Rivière, Ciara Harman, Oliver Boughton, and Justin Cobb

Key Points

- Kinematically aligning hip components consists of restoring the native hip anatomy, plus or minus adjusting cup orientation and design to account for an abnormal spine–hip relationship.
- By restoring close-to-physiological hip biomechanics and preventing poor dynamic component interaction, the KA technique may be advantageous by improving prosthetic function, patient satisfaction and reducing the risk of revision surgery.
- The individual spine–hip relationship, which is radio-clinically defined, is now becoming a new parameter to consider when planning a hip replacement.
- Defining the spine-hip relationship of each patient is more informative than just assessing their sagittal lumbo-pelvic kinematics, and is likely to result in more refined surgical planning.
- The kinematic implantation may be performed freehand, and therefore at low cost, by relying on intra-articular anatomical landmarks.

C. Rivière (✉)
The MSK Lab-Imperial College London, White City Campus, London, UK

South West London Elective Orthopaedic Centre, Epsom, UK

C. Harman
South West London Elective Orthopaedic Centre, Epsom, UK

O. Boughton · J. Cobb
The MSK Lab-Imperial College London, White City Campus, London, UK
e-mail: o.boughton@imperial.ac.uk; j.cobb@imperial.ac.uk

11.1 Introduction

11.1.1 The Concept

The concept was developed as a consequence of the increasing awareness that dynamic function is, in addition to improved arthroplasty materials and component positioning, a significant factor in total hip arthroplasty stability and lifespan [1–4].

The kinematic alignment (KA) technique for hip replacement consists of restoring the native hip anatomy, plus or minus adjusting the cup orientation and design to account for an abnormal spine–hip relationship (SHR) [1, 5, 6] (Fig. 11.1). In other words, it is a combination of both an anatomical hip reconstruction (proximal femur, acetabular anteversion and hip centre of rotation) and a kinematic cup alignment technique [7]. While the former enables a close-to-physiological peri-prosthetic soft tissue balance for optimum prosthetic function and patient satisfaction, the latter could reduce the risk of poor dynamic

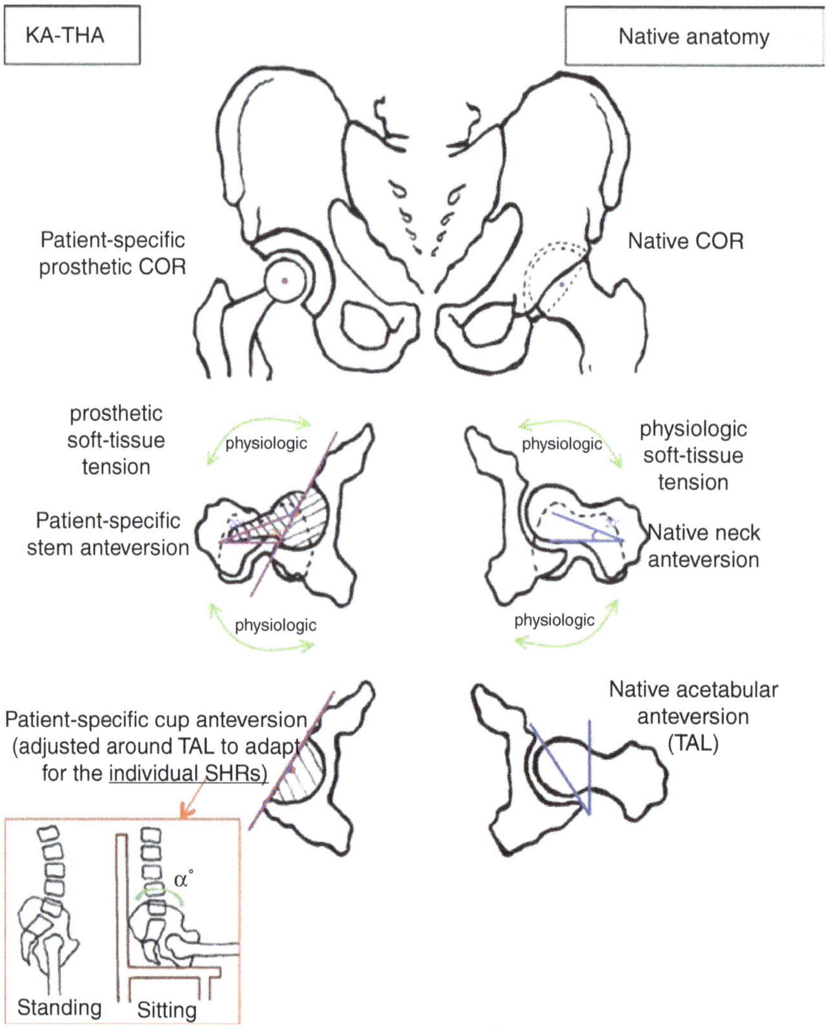

Fig. 11.1 Figure illustrating the restoration of the native anatomy (right) when kinematically aligning (KA) total hip components (left). *COR* centre of rotation, *TAL* transverse acetabular ligament, *SHR* spine–hip relationship

component interaction during activities of daily living (ADLs) for optimal implant lifespan. By generating a component interaction that is the best compromise between the standing and sitting positions, kinematically aligned hip components hopefully prevent the occurrence of an aberrant component interaction during ADLs, which may be clinically advantageous. This personalized technique applies to both stemmed (THR) and resurfacing (HR) implants, and is even more pertinent at a time when arthroplasty patients are becoming younger, with higher demands and expectations, in addition to a longer life expectancy [8].

The KA concept takes the individual SHR into consideration in order to determine a targeted adjustment of an anatomical cup positioning [6] (Fig. 11.2). The subsequent plan can be well executed without the need for costly technology. Several reported strategies exist for taking the individual lumbo-pelvic sagittal kinematics into consideration when implanting hip components [9, 10], however they differ slightly from the reported KA concept presented here [1, 5, 6]. With other strategies, following radiographic estimation of the individual lumbo-pelvic kinematics, a targeted cup orientation is defined and then executed with the use of intraoperative technological tools [9, 10]. The radio-clinical definition of the individual SHR provides information on the patient's lumbo-pelvic kinematics, the presence of a spine–hip and/or hip–spine syndrome [11], the spinal sagittal balance status and, lastly, the constitutional biomechanical spine

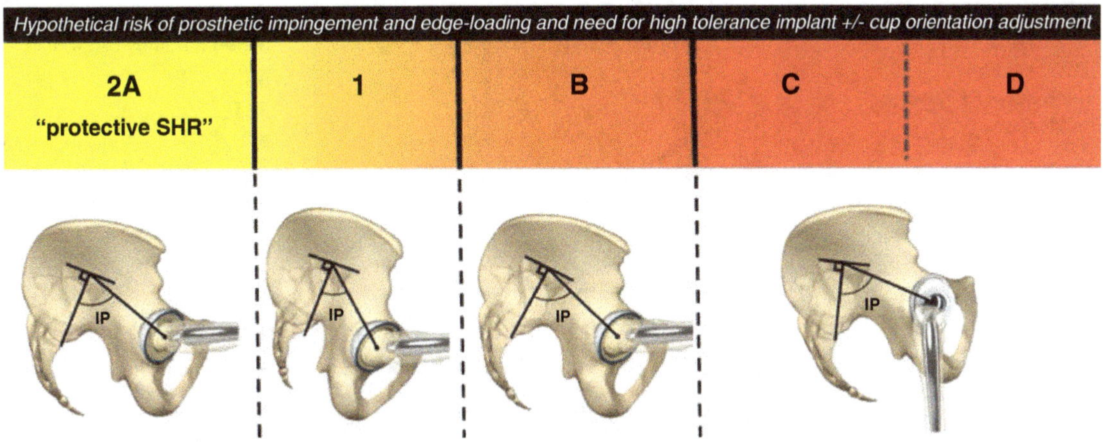

Fig. 11.2 Simplified Bordeaux classification of spine–hip relationship (SHR) with types 2A, 1, B, C and D. The risks of poor functional component interaction and the need for cup adjustment (design and orientation) are likely to increase from left (yellow colour) to right (red colour)

profile (this depends on the pelvic incidence value and whether the patient is a spine or hip user) [1]. Kinematically aligning hip components is therefore a sophisticated concept that leads to more refined THR planning.

11.1.2 The Rationale

Gold-standard techniques for implanting hip components have generated good long–term outcomes, but have failed to solve the common residual complications affecting modern prosthetic hip patients [8]. Those conventional techniques are designed to be biomechanically sound, do not aim to accurately reproduce the native hip anatomy [12], and traditionally involve either systematic [12] or combined component orientation [13] approaches. Despite successful reports, complications related to poor component interaction such as edge loading [14], articular impingement [15–17] and prosthetic instability [18] remain. Interestingly, the higher surgical precision achieved by means of technological assistance (computer navigation and robotics) has failed to significantly improve clinical outcomes of conventional THA [19]. Another interesting finding is the poor correlation observed between the static standing/supine radiographic cup orientation and the risk of conventional THA instability [20–22]. Those last observations challenge the accuracy of such conventional implantation philosophies.

Alternative anatomic alignment techniques for implanting hip prostheses have successfully been promoted over the past few decades, but they have also failed to lessen the burden of residual complications from which prosthetic hip patients suffer [23–25]. These techniques aim to restore the native hip anatomy (with the exception of the acetabular inclination), and are best characterised through the following examples: use of the transverse acetabular ligament (TAL) for aligning the cup [23], hip resurfacing [26] and neck-sparing total hip replacement (neck anchorage short femoral stem designs) [27]. The rationale for anatomical implantation lies in the following:

1. The limited ability to calculate an ideal cup orientation from preoperative images due to the multiple acetabular functional orientations and femoro-acetabular interplay combinations that individuals display during ADLs [28, 29].
2. Most hip pathologies causing degeneration (e.g. cam impingement, most pincer impingements, low-grade dysplasia, avascular necrosis, genetic, protrusio, all causes of hip arthritis, synovial diseases) are automatically corrected when modern high-tolerance (high

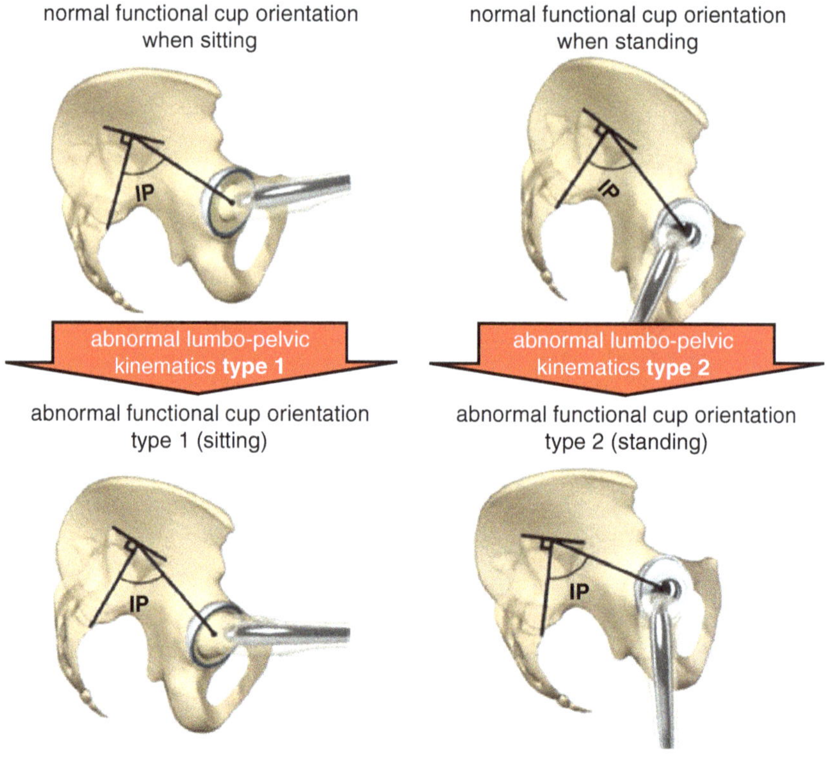

Fig. 11.3 Classification of abnormal lumbo-pelvic sagittal kinematics. *PI* Pelvic incidence

head-neck ratio) hip components are anatomically positioned.

3. The fact that restoring the native hip anatomy improves prosthetic hip function and patient satisfaction through the generation of a more physiological peri-prosthetic soft tissue balance and prosthetic hip kinematics [16, 30, 31].

Similar to conventional techniques, despite having been reported as safe and suitable for the majority of patients, several complications remain with anatomically implanted hip prostheses, primarily related to poor dynamic interaction of components [23, 27, 32]. Many of these may be explained by a lack of consideration for the functional aspect of the acetabular orientation, or in other words, through neglecting the individual lumbo-pelvic sagittal kinematics/SHR [32].

The presented kinematic alignment technique takes into consideration the functional acetabular orientation to allow more refined THA planning, and hopefully improved clinical outcomes of prosthetic hip patients [1, 5, 6]. Neglecting the sitting component interaction, along with the fact that many complications occur when sitting, probably partly explains the poor correlation observed between the static standing/supine radiographic cup orientation and the risk of conventional THA instability [20–22].

The classification of abnormal lumbo-pelvic kinematics (Fig. 11.3) and SHRs (Table 11.1) [1], along with methods for defining the individual SHR (Fig. 11.4) and for determining the amount of cup adjustment needed (design [1] and orientation [6]) (Table 11.2) has previously been published. There are primarily two abnormal lumbo-pelvic kinematics (Fig. 11.3), the first being related to individuals who sit without sufficiently retroverting their pelvis (type 1 abnormal lumbo-pelvic kinematics – SHR B), and the second is the result of an ageing process with a stiff degenerated spine, locking the pelvis in a chronic retroverted position when the patient stands (type 2 abnormal lumbo-pelvic kinematics – SHR C/D) [1]. Both abnormal lumbo-pelvic kinematics (type 1 [32, 33] and type 2 [34–37]) adversely affect prosthetic hip patient outcomes (spine–hip syndrome), as they alter the sitting (type 1) or standing (type 2) acetabular orientation

Table 11.1 Simplified Bordeaux classification of spine-hip relationship and their diagnostic criteria

	Simplified Bordeaux classification of SHR					
LPC	Flexible LPC	Stiff LPC				
SHR	A	1	B	C	D	Fused spine
Diagnosis	PI >30° No standing PI-LL mismatch > 10° delta SS from standing to sitting	PI <30°	No standing PI-LL mismatch < 10° delta SS from standing to sitting	Standing PI-LL mismatch Normal SVA	Standing PI-LL mismatch Abnormal SVA	Instrumented or biologically fused spine

SHR Spine–Hip Relationship, *LPC* Lumbo-Pelvic Complex, *PI* Pelvic Incidence, *LL* Lumbo-Lordosis, *SS* Sacral Slope, *SVA* Sagittal Vertical Axis distance

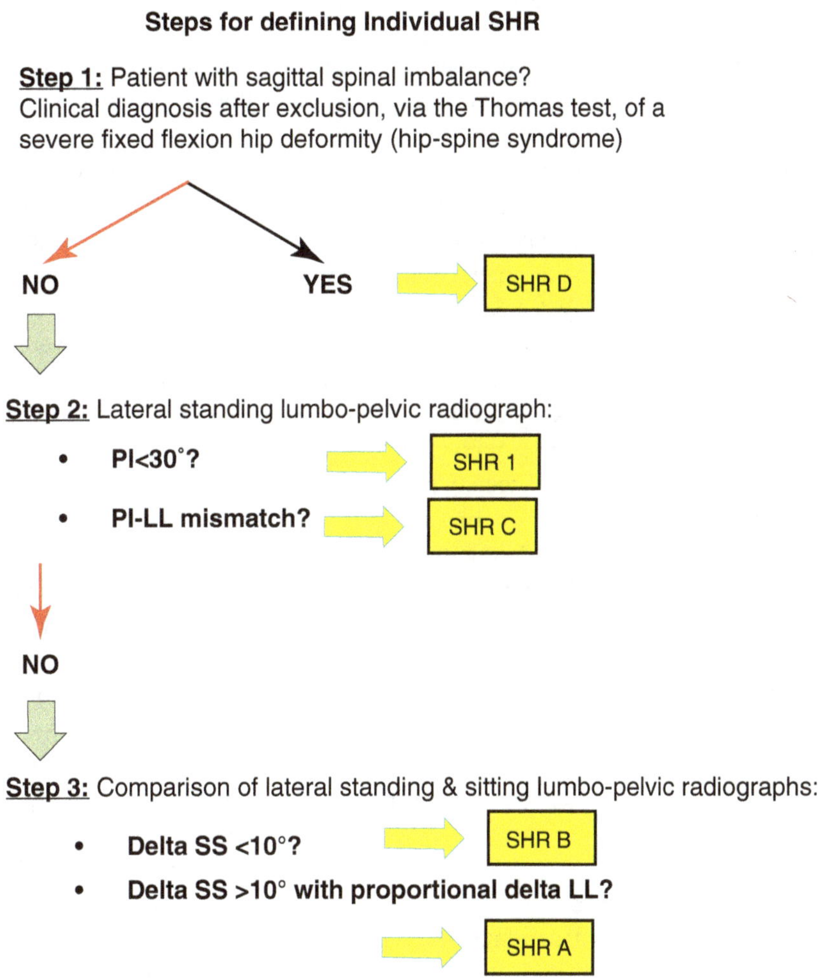

Fig. 11.4 Algorithm for defining the individual spine–hip relationship (SHR). *PI* pelvic incidence, *LL* lumbar lordosis, *SS* sacral slope

and component interaction. When implanting such patients, it is important to adjust the cup (orientation and design) in order to compensate for the abnormal functional acetabular orientation. The appreciation and understanding of the individual SHR is therefore critical for the next stage of improvements in hip arthroplasty.

11.1.3 Intended Benefits

Compared to conventional techniques for replacing a hip, kinematically aligned hip components may potentially *improve prosthetic hip function and lifespan* because of the potential for improved anatomical reconstruction and interaction of

Table 11.2 Algorithm for adjusting the cup orientation to account for the individual spine-hip relationship (SHR)

	Simplified Bordeaux classification of SHR					
SHR	A	1	B	C	D	Fused spine
Cup anteversion adjustment	None (cup parallel to TAL)	Increased cup anteversion by 3.5° (relative to TAL) for every 10° of lack of pelvic retroversion when sitting (normal pelvic retroversion when sitting = 20°)		Reduced cup anteversion by 3.5° (relative to TAL) for every 10° of excessive standing pelvic retroversion (normal standing SS = 75% of PI)		Idem B or C, depending on position of fusion and residual flexibility
Cup inclination adjustment	None (radiographic target: 40°)	Don't change your freehand technique for cup inclination as the additional cup anteversion will increase the radiographic cup inclination (radiographic target: 40° to 50°)				

TAL Transverse Acetabular Ligament, *APP* Anterior Pelvic Plane

components during ADLs, respectively. The anatomic reconstruction should generate a close-to-physiological peri-prosthetic soft-tissue balance and hip biomechanics, which may be clinically advantageous, and hopefully result in improved prosthetic hip function and patient satisfaction [16, 30, 31, 38]. The better interaction of components during ADLs may decrease the risk of complications related to articular impingement and edge loading (e.g. instability, liner breakage, accelerated wear, squeaking and cup loosening) in addition to reducing the risk of revision, thus benefiting both the patient and society [8]. The benefits are even more likely considering that kinematic implantation is reproducible due to the fact that articular anatomical landmarks (TAL, femoral length and offset measures) are used for setting the components' orientation [39]. The relevance of the KA technique is further accentuated by the fact that implanted patients are now becoming younger and therefore have higher demands and expectations, as well as a longer life expectancy.

11.1.4 Indications and Contraindications

The kinematic alignment technique for hip components is applicable to most patients, as anatomically reconstructed hips are known to be successful [23, 26], and the kinematic cup adjustment aims to compensate for clinically deleterious abnormal spine–hip relations (SHRs) [34, 35, 40]. A series of 41 unselected consecutive KA THA patients has shown acceptable radiographic supine cup orientation and excellent early-term clinical outcomes (no complications, high function and satisfaction) [6].

Determining which hip anatomical variants should not be reproduced, due to biomechanical inferiority, remains unclear. It seems unreasonable to restore hip pathoanatomies resulting from a post-traumatic malunion, a poorly performed acetabular or femoral osteotomy, a protrusio acetabulum or severe developmental hip disease (high-grade dysplasia or Legg–Calvé–Perthes), as those anatomies are not the result of the development of a harmonious interaction between the acetabulum and the proximal femur. Should we anatomically restore the fraction (≈15%) of osteoarthritic hip patients that have an atypical femoral neck and/or acetabular anatomical orientation [12, 41, 42]? The functionality of the acetabulum and femoral neck orientations [1, 12, 43], in addition to the complex femoro-acetabular interplay [44, 45], makes it difficult to predict which hip anatomies may or may not be suitable for anatomic implantation. The fact that good long-term clinical outcomes have been reported with anatomically reconstructed hip patients [23, 26], even in those with degeneration secondary to a low-grade dysplasia [46], indicates anatomical implantation is probably reliable in the vast majority of patients.

In patients with severely stiff, degenerated hip(s), accurate definition of the individual SHR may not be possible, thus compromising kinematic planning. In the former situation, a severely stiff hip is likely to dictate the spine motion (or lumbo-pelvic kinematics) required between standing and sitting positions, thus making post-implantation lumbo-pelvic kinematics difficult to predict [28, 47–49]. In the latter case, bilateral degenerated hips make it difficult to discriminate clinically between true (resulting from severe spine degeneration) and false (caused by bilateral fixed flexion deformity hip–spine syndrome) spinal sagittal imbalance [11]. In these clinical situations, the pre- and post-operative SHR may significantly differ as a result of the correction of the hip–spine syndrome. Given that the post-implantation SHR is difficult to predict, kinematically aligning hip components in these scenarios should be done with caution.

11.2 Planning a Kinematic Implantation

Radio-clinical definition of the individual SHR: A thorough *clinical examination* is the first step in defining the individual status for spinal sagittal balance and degenerated hip flexibility. As previously stated, patients with a severely stiff hip or bilateral degenerated hips may not be the best candidates for a kinematic implantation. The second step is *radiographic evaluation* based on the analysis of lateral lumbo-pelvic views in functional standing and sitting positions (Fig. 11.5). This enables the definition of the individual pelvic incidence (PI), the diagnosis of spine degeneration (standing PI–lumbar lordosis mismatch) and an estimation of the lumbo-pelvic kinematics (delta sacral slope and delta lumbar lordosis) (Fig. 11.5) [1]. Ideally, the imaging should be performed with EOS™ bi-dimensional images (Biospace, Paris, France), but, if not available, conventional radiographs are sufficient. The methods for defining the individual SHR and the subsequent cup adjustment (design and orientation) have previously

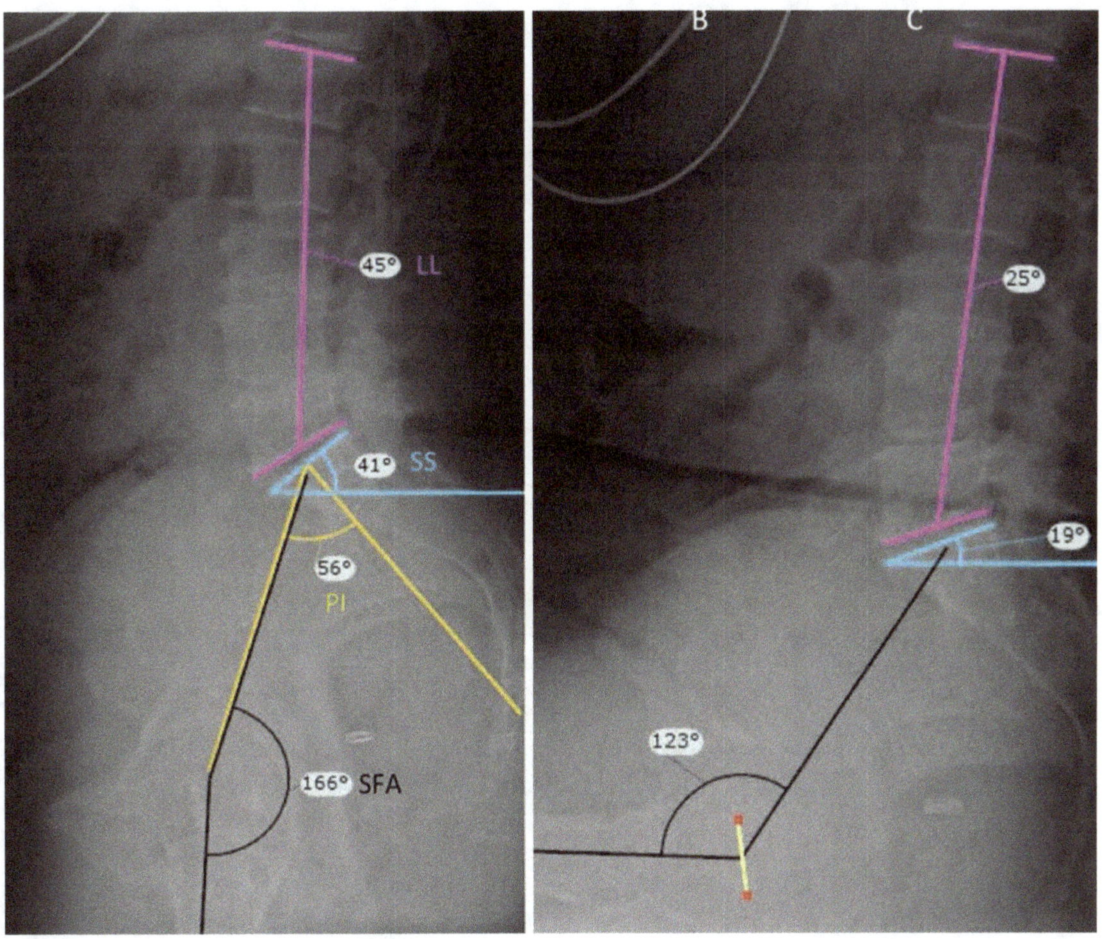

Fig. 11.5 Preoperative lateral lumbo-pelvic standing (left) and sitting (right) radiographs showing measurements of spino-pelvic parameters in both positions: *PI* pelvic incidence, *SS* sacral slope, *LL* L1–L5 lumbar lordosis and *SFA* – sacro-femoral angle

been published [1, 6] and are illustrated in Fig. 11.4 and Table 11.2, respectively.

Why take the individual pelvic incidence into consideration when planning a KA THA? The PI is an anatomical and biomechanical pelvic parameter that determines the sagittal spine morphology and kinematics (Fig. 11.6), in addition to the timing and severity of developing a spine–hip syndrome in the case of severe spine degeneration [1]. As a result, the PI has been shown to influence the functional acetabular orientation [42, 50] and the risk of prosthetic instability [34, 35]. There may be two explanations for this:

- Patients with an abnormally low PI (<30°) have a constitutionally low lumbar lordosis, and they are likely to primarily flex their hips (constitutional hip users – SHR type 1) when switching between standing and sitting positions (Fig. 11.6). This use of a large hip cone of mobility is likely to adversely affect prosthetic hip outcomes as a result of the increased

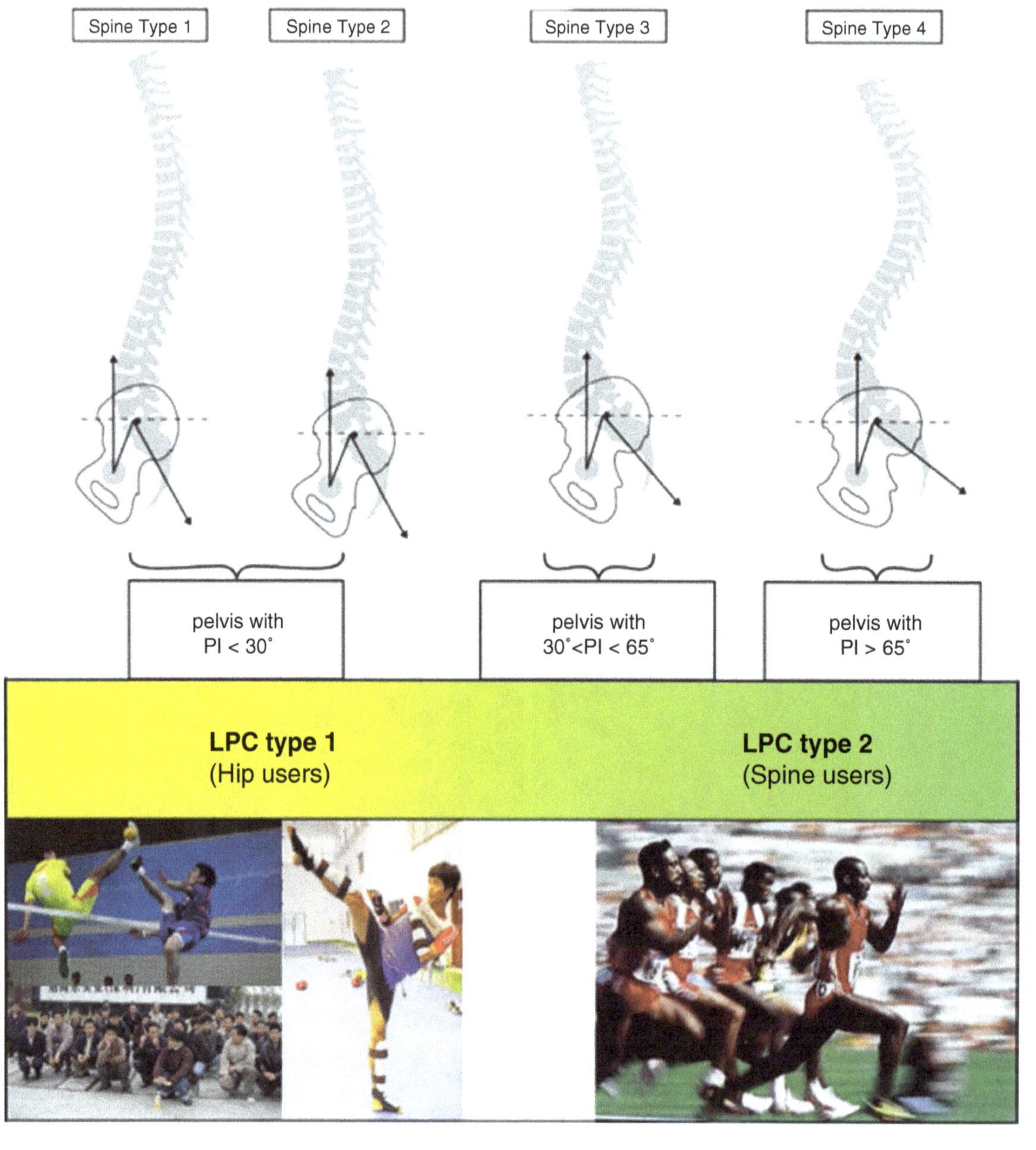

Fig. 11.6 Role of the pelvic incidence on the spine morphology and kinematics. *PI* pelvic incidence, *LPC* lumbopelvic complex

risks of articular impingement- and edge-loading–related complications. In the event of spine degeneration, these patients will rapidly decompensate their sagittal spinal imbalance but only moderately modify their hip biomechanics (slight deterioration of the standing acetabular orientation and standing femoro-acetabular interaction, plus slight increase of hip use, causing a moderate spine-hip syndrome). In the event of a hip replacement, such patients (SHR 1) may benefit from a high-tolerance cup design, plus or minus a slight adjustment of the cup orientation to compensate for the poor functional acetabular orientation resulting from the abnormal lumbo-pelvic kinematics (constitutionally stiff spine).

- Patients with a normal PI are likely to display more spine motion, and therefore less hip movement, when switching from a standing to sitting position (constitutional spine users). The use of a low hip range of motion for ADLs is likely to be protective with regard to the risks of prosthetic impingement, edge loading and instability [1]. However, in the situation of severe spine ageing, the loss of spine flexibility may have a severe clinical adverse impact as it significantly modifies the hip biomechanics: there is dramatic deterioration in the standing acetabular orientation and standing femoro-acetabular interaction, plus a significant increase in hip use, causing a severe spine-hip syndrome. This hypothesis may partly explain the higher PI [34, 35] and more severe spine degeneration (SHR types 2C and 2D) [35–37] that characterise unstable prosthetic hip patients. In the event of a hip replacement, such SHR 2D patients may benefit from a high-tolerance cup design in addition to a moderate cup orientation adjustment to compensate for their aberrant standing acetabular orientation.

Defining the cup adjustment (design and orientation) (Table 11.2): Planning a radiographic cup inclination below 50° is important to prevent poor standing and walking component interaction (superior edge loading). In contrast, the kinematic cup anteversion relative to the anterior pelvic plane cannot be planned as its value primarily depends on the TAL orientation, which cannot be estimated on simple preoperative radiographs. For this specific reason, the KA concept does not aim to plan cup orientation relative to the anterior pelvic plane, but rather the amount of cup orientation adjustment, relative to anatomical positioning (TAL), that is needed to compensate for an abnormal SHR [6]. The key points to understand the rationale supporting the adjustment are:

1. The adjustment should first target the cup orientation, as the restoration of the native proximal femur anatomy and hip centre of rotation is key to producing clinically advantageous, close-to-physiological prosthetic hip kinematics.
2. A cup orientation adjustment is made when, and in addition to, the use of a higher tolerance cup design (larger head [51, 52], dual mobility [53]) is likely to be insufficient in compensating for the poor functional acetabular orientation resulting from the abnormal lumbo-pelvic kinematics .
3. The cup orientation adjustment aims only to compensate for half of the functional acetabular orientation abnormality that results from the poor lumbo-pelvic kinematics (compromised orientation).
4. The algorithm for calculating the amount of cup adjustment needed (Table 11.2) was determined based on the following published observations: the average posterior pelvic tilt from standing to sitting for healthy patients is approximately 20° [54, 55], for every 10° of pelvic tilt there is a change of radiographic cup orientation by approximately 7° (anteversion) and 3° (inclination) [56], and the normal standing sacral slope angle approximates 75% of the PI angle [57].

11.3 Performing a Kinematic Implantation

Kinematically aligning hip components can be performed with or without technological assistance, the latter method having been shown to

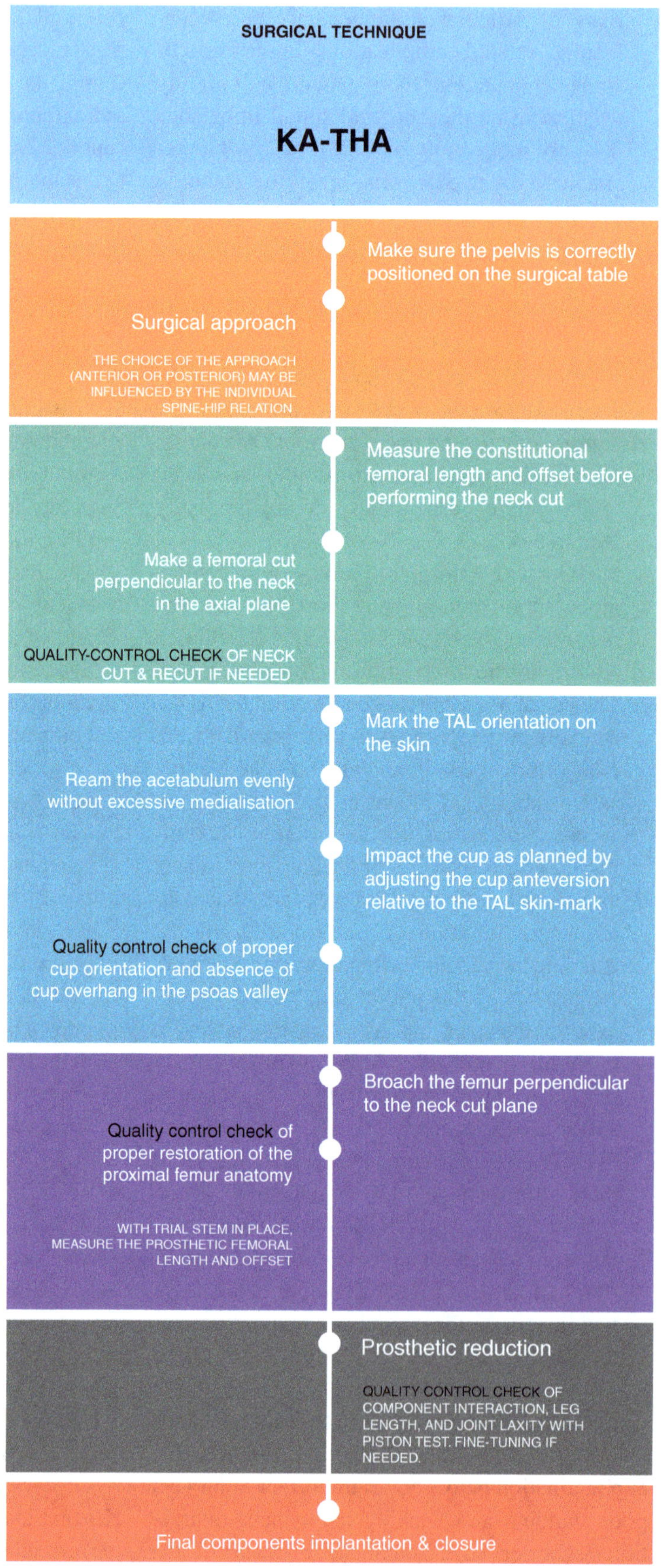

Fig. 11.7 Intraoperative steps for performing kinematic implantation of total hip components with manual instrumentation. *TAL* transverse acetabular ligament

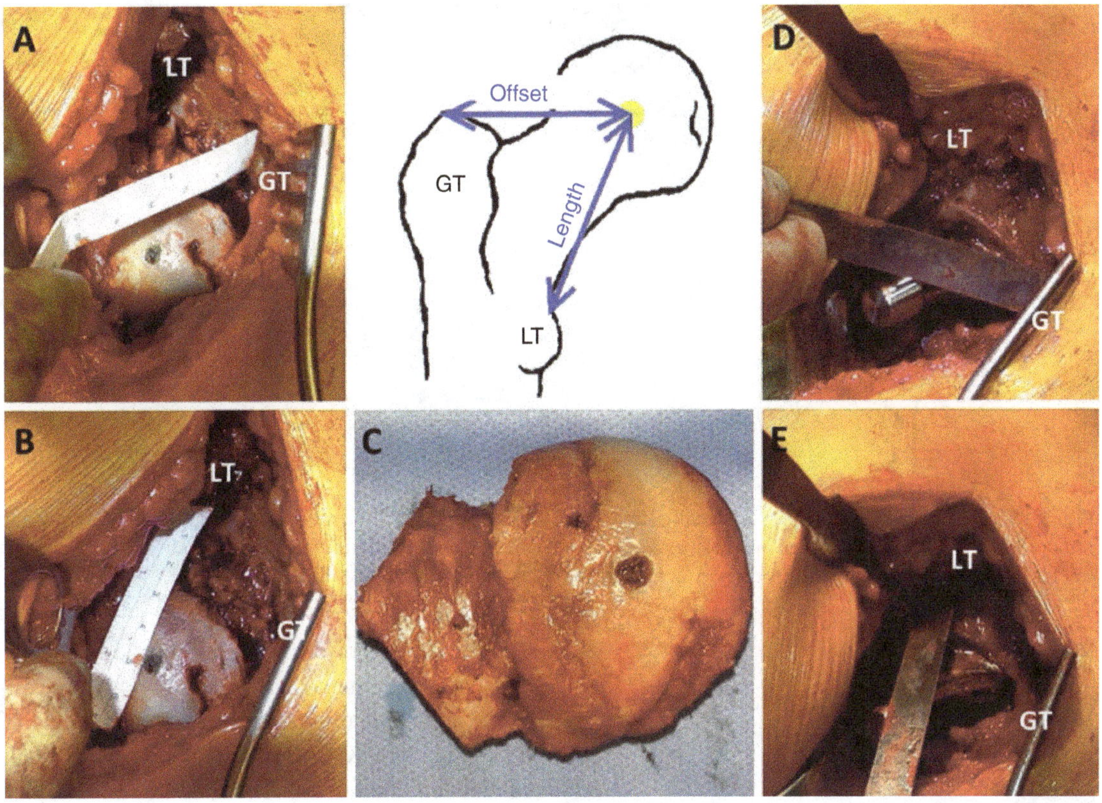

Fig. 11.8 Ruler technique for assisting restoration of femoral length and medial offset. The distances between the centre of the femoral head and the greater trochanter (GT– femoral neck offset – (**a**) and lesser trochanter (LT – femoral neck length – (**b**) are measured after dislocation, before the femoral neck cut. This serves to assess the quality of the femoral reconstruction with the trial stem in place (**d** and **e**). After the neck cut, ensure you accurately define the centre of the femoral head (**c**)

be reliable [6]. The freehand KA technique relies on intraoperative anatomical landmarks (e.g. TAL, femoral neck cut) and measurements (e.g. femoral offset and length), whilst following a precise stepwise execution as shown in Fig. 11.7. The *femoral reconstruction* aims to be anatomic, following a modified calliper technique as described by Hill et al. [58], which helps to restore the original femur length and medial offset (Fig. 11.8). Restoration of the constitutional femoral neck anteversion is done by ensuring a cut perpendicular to the neck (Fig. 11.9a, b) and broaching perpendicular to the neck cut (Fig. 11.9c). Regarding the *acetabular reconstruction*, the medio-lateral positioning (or depth) of the cup is adjusted by reaming the acetabulum not excessively medially, but rather sufficiently to restore the native hip centre of rotation as templated before the operation (Fig. 11.10). The cup inclination is adjusted with the use of the classic alignment rod, in addition to positioning the inferior and superior parts of the cup relative to the inner border of the TAL and the acetabular roof, respectively. The cup anteversion is set relative to the TAL orientation, which has been marked on the skin (Fig. 11.11), as previously described by Meftah et al. [59], and is impacted perpendicular to it (anatomic and kinematic cup positions are identical) unless slight adjustment is needed (anatomic and kinematic cup positions differ) (Fig. 11.11). Whilst freehand anatomic and kinematic implantations are unlikely to be technically demanding [39], it is probable that technology (3D planning, assistive devices for precise implantation and intraoperative quality control tools) would be of value in further improving its reliability.

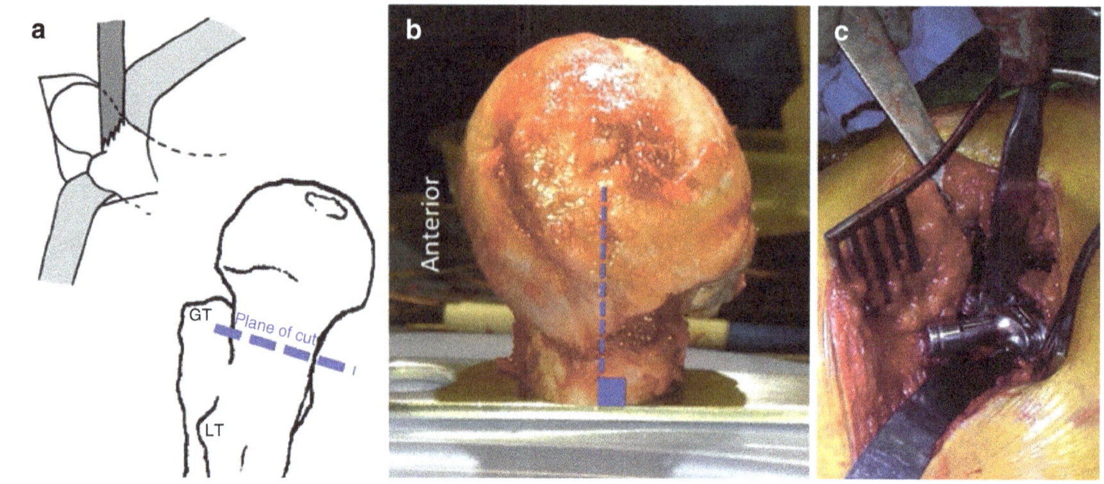

Fig. 11.9 The femoral cut is made perpendicular to the femoral neck in the frontal and axial planes (**a**). Following the neck cut, check the cut was properly executed in the axial plane (**b**). When broaching the femur and inserting the trial stem, ensure you are perpendicularly aligned to the femoral neck cut plane (**c**)

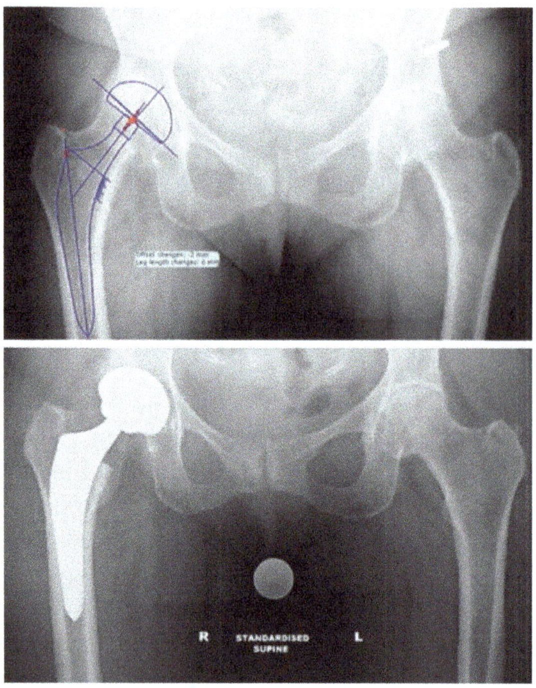

Fig. 11.10 Pelvic radiographs showing the planned (above) and performed (below) medio-lateral positioning of the cup

11.4 Clinical Evidence

A single clinical study [6], a matched case-control design on prospectively collected clinical data, concluded that KA-THAs were overall safe, efficacious and not inferior to the conventional THAs in the short term. The authors compared 41 consecutive freehand KA-THAs with 41 conventional mechanically aligned THAs with 1 year of follow-up. The KA patients had a more anatomical restoration and a higher supine radiographic cup anteversion, but with a similar proportion of cup orientations within the Lewinnek safe zone. Both techniques of alignment had similar excellent clinical outcomes with high function (mean Oxford Hip Score at 43), no instability or other aseptic complications and an average patient outcome satisfaction score of 95.4/100 and 89.5/100 for KA and MA patients, respectively.

11.5 Future Developments

The concept of kinematically aligning hip components is only at its early stage, with many refinements yet to be made. There are a few limitations which currently affect the quality of the kinematic planning, and thus need to be investigated through further research: firstly, the difficulty in accurately defining the preoperative individual SHR. This is due to the existence of various lumbo-pelvic kinematics in an individual between and within (intra-individual variability) multiple ADLs [29, 55, 60], and due to a frequent concomitance with a stiff osteoarthritic hip that may dictate some spine motion [11]. Secondly, it

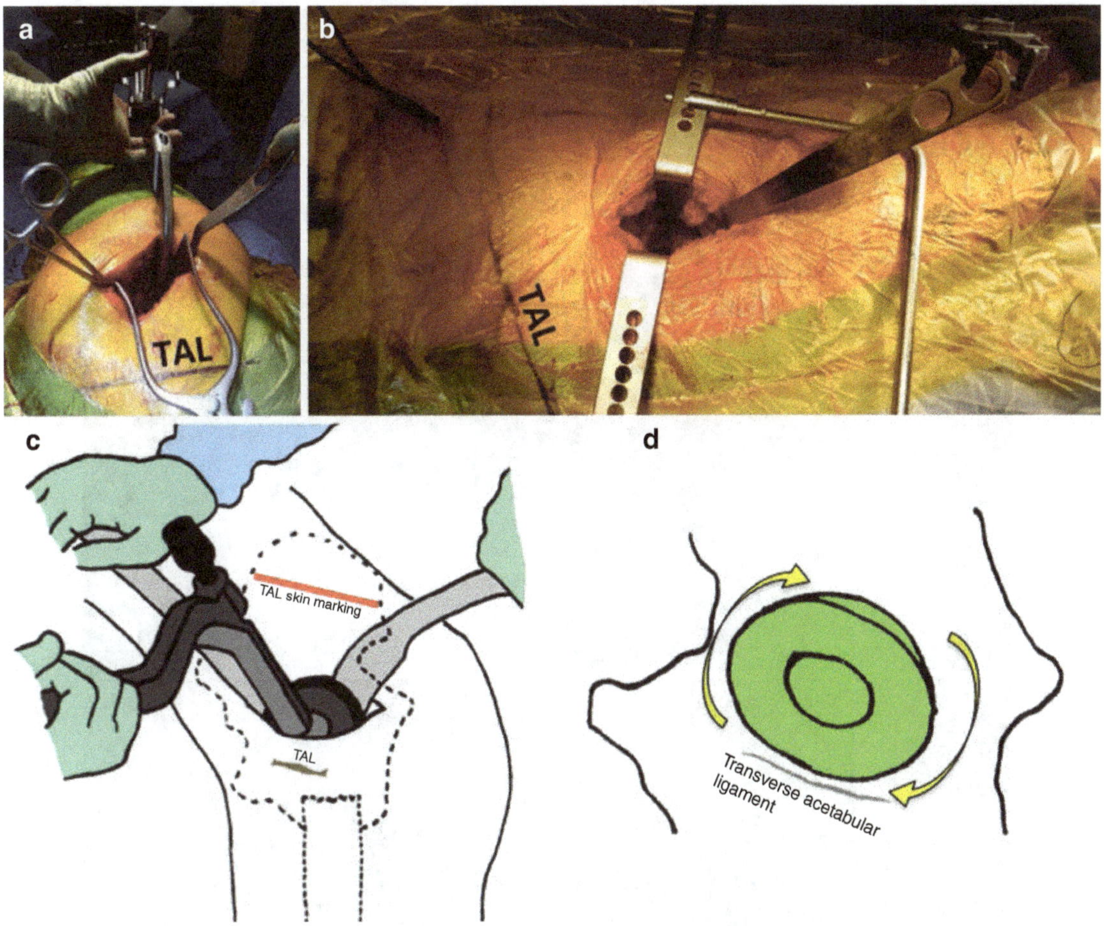

Fig. 11.11 Skin marking is made parallel to the transverse acetabular ligament (TAL) either through posterior (**a**) or direct anterior (**b**) approaches. The TAL skin mark serves to assist the kinematic cup implantation (**a** and **c**). Using the TAL skin mark, the surgeon can adjust the cup anteversion around the TAL orientation (**d**)

is difficult to anticipate the post-implantation individual SHR that will occur after correction of the hip soft tissue contracture [12, 28, 47, 49]. Lastly, it is the difficulty in anticipating the age-related SHR changes that will occur over years.

11.6 Conclusion

Kinematically aligning hip components involves restoring the native hip anatomy, plus or minus adjusting the cup (orientation and design) to account for an abnormal spine-hip relationship. By restoring close-to-physiological hip biomechanics and preventing poor dynamic component interaction, the KA technique may be advantageous by improving prosthetic function, patient satisfaction and reducing the risk of revision. The kinematic planning is based on the radio-clinically defined individual spine–hip relationship, and the implantation may be performed freehand by relying on intra-articular anatomical landmarks, incurring no additional technological costs. Further research is needed to refine the KA technique.

11.7 Case Illustration

Kinematic implantation on patients having SHR 2A, B and D are illustrated in Figs. 11.12, 11.13 and 11.14, respectively.

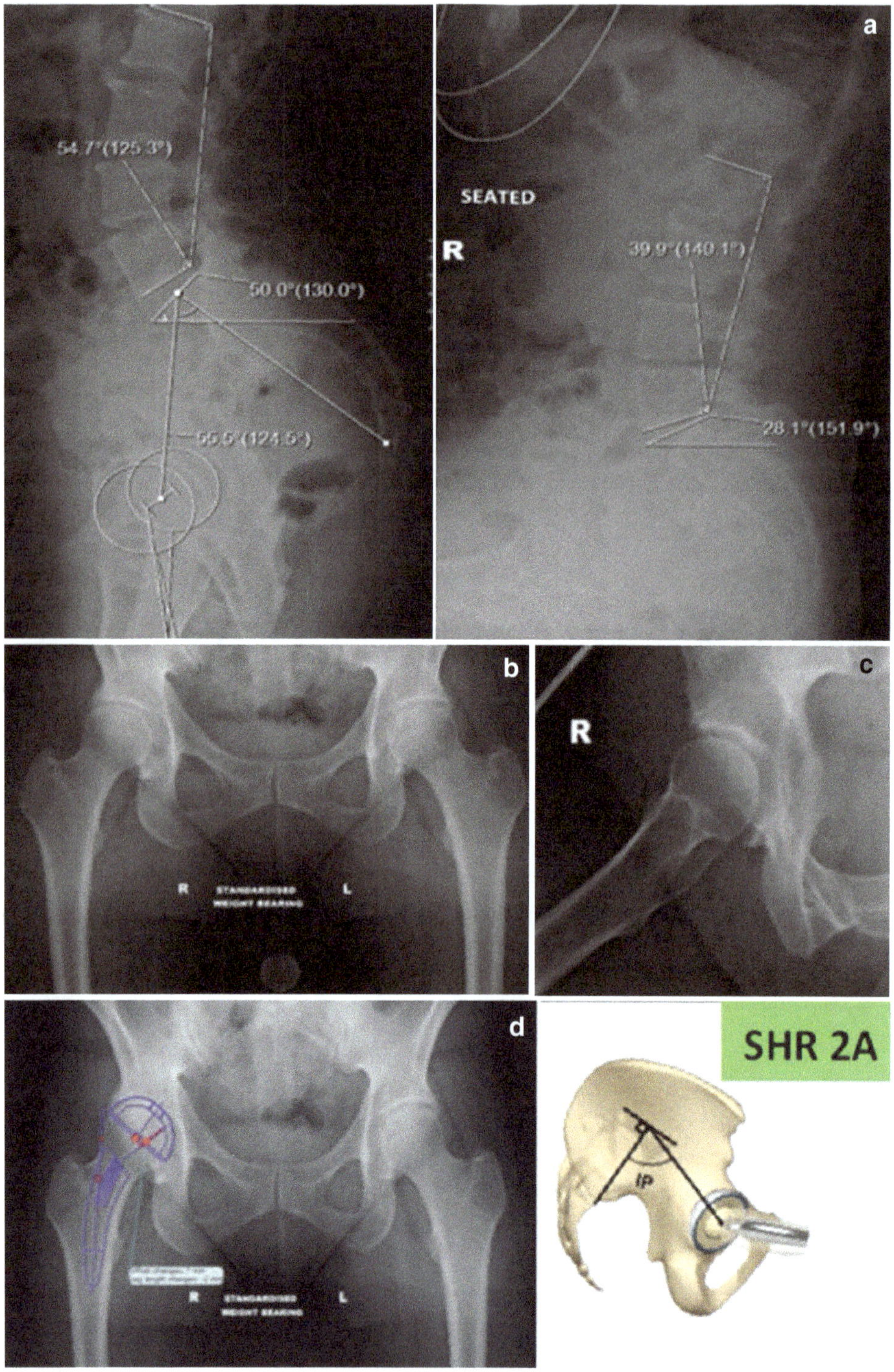

Fig. 11.12 A 58-year-old patient with a right osteoarthritic hip and a spine-hip relationship type 2A (normal pelvic incidence ≈ 56°, normal standing lumbar lordosis ≈ 55°, normal delta sacral slope ≈ 22°). The cup and stem (neck-sparing design for subsequent neck anchorage) were then kinematically implanted without the need for a cup orientation adjustment, and a 36 mm ceramic bearing was used. Pre-operative lateral lumbo-pelvic standing (left) and sitting (right) radiographs with spino-pelvic parameter measurements (**a**). Preoperative standing pelvic (**b**) and lateral cross-leg osteoarthritic hip views (**c**). Total hip replacement planning using Traumacad™ software (**d**). Post-operative supine pelvic (**e**) and lateral Dunn (**f**) radiographs with the kinematically implanted prosthetic hip

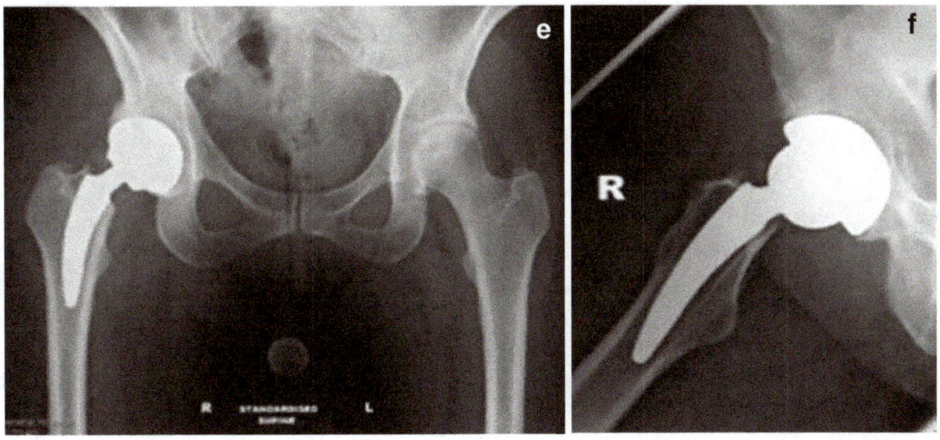

Fig. 11.12 (continued)

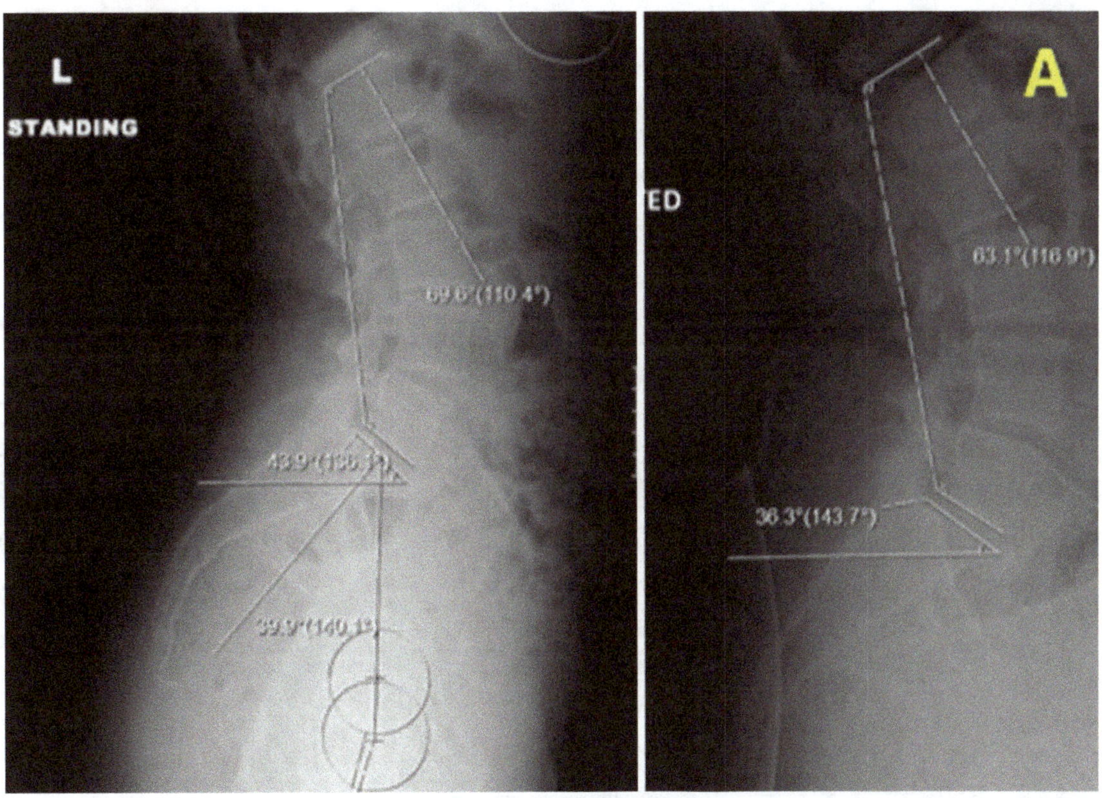

Fig. 11.13 A 62-year-old patient with bilateral osteoarthritic hips secondary to protrusio and a spine-hip relationship type B (normal pelvic incidence ≈ 44°, high standing lumbar lordosis ≈ 69°, low 8° delta sacral slope). In the event of a replacement, anatomically aligning components would have been suboptimal considering the risk of complications (posterior edge loading and posterior instability) related to poor interaction between components when sitting. In order to reduce those risks, the patient received a KA-THA performed through a direct anterior approach, preserving the integrity of posterior hip soft tissue. The stem was anatomically implanted; the cup orientation was slightly adjusted with an additional 4° of anteversion relative to the transverse acetabular ligament. On both hips, the centre of rotation was not lateralised and no medial acetabular bone grafting was performed; this is because the protrusion was slight and no significant bony overhang was observed at the periphery of the cups during trialing and after final implantation. Pre-operative lateral lumbo-pelvic radiographs (**a**) in standing (left) and sitting (right) positions. Pre-operative antero-posterior standing pelvic (**b**) and lateral left hip (**c**) radiographs. Digital KA-THA templating (**d**). Post-operative antero-posterior supine pelvic (**e**) and lateral hip (f) radiographs

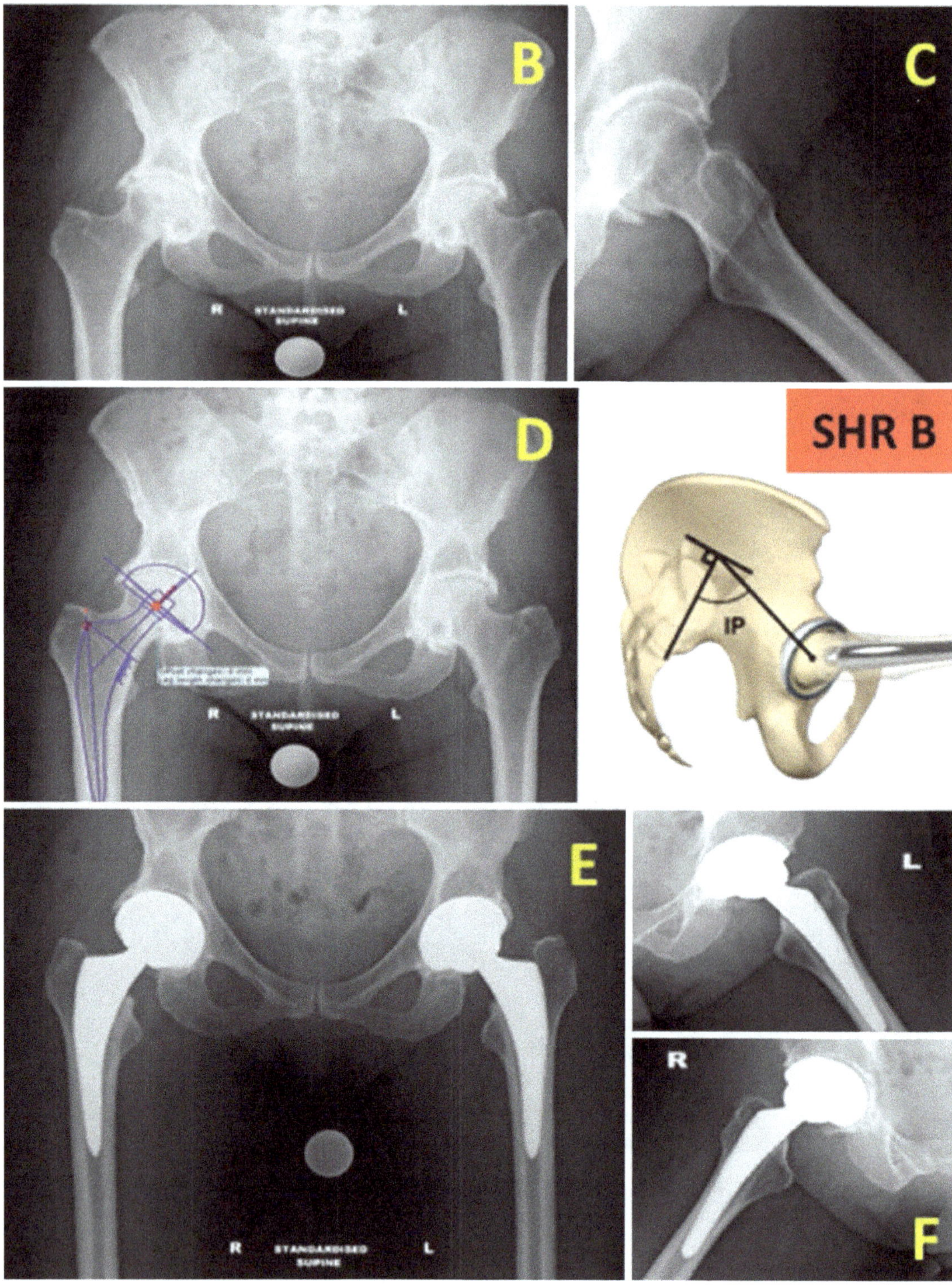

Fig. 11.13 (continued)

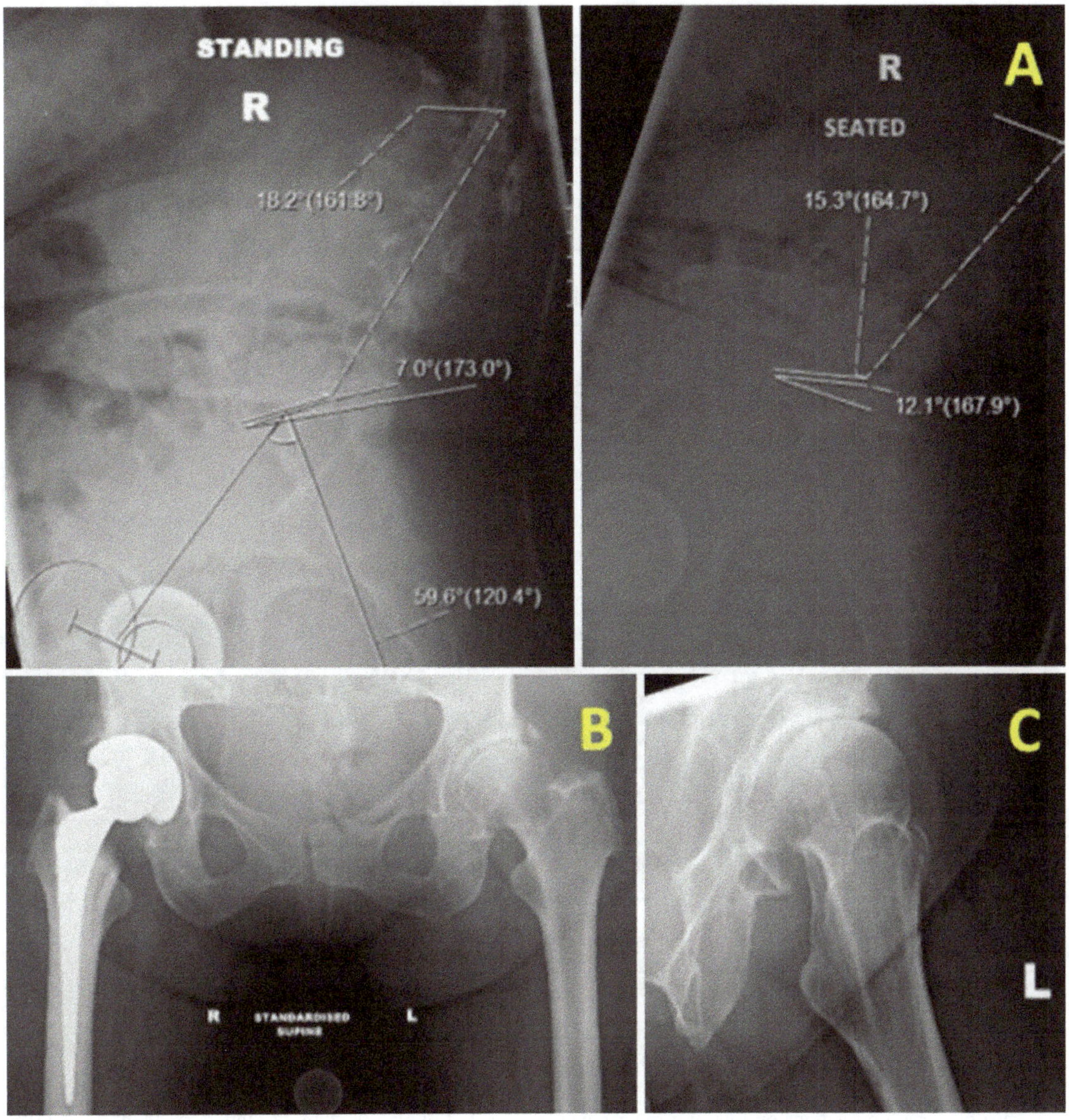

Fig. 11.14 A 79-year-old patient with severe spine degeneration and a spine-hip relationship type D (decompensated sagittal spinal imbalance). There is a normal pelvic incidence ≈ 60° and low standing lumbar lordosis ≈ 18° for 42° mismatch, 41° standing pelvic version (normally 20% of PI, which is approximately 12°) suggesting the patient has 29° excessive pelvic retroversion when standing. In the event of a replacement, anatomically aligning components would have been suboptimal considering the risks of poor standing component interaction (antero-superior edge loading and posterior prosthetic impingement) and anterior instability. In order to reduce those risks, the patient received a KA-THA performed through a mini-posterior approach, preserving the integrity of anterior hip soft tissue, and with an adjusted kinematically aligned dual mobility cup, 5° retroverted relative to the TAL. Pre-operative lateral lumbo-pelvic radiographs (**a**) in standing (left) and sitting (right) positions. Pre-operative antero-posterior standing pelvic (**b**) and lateral left hip (**c**) radiographs. Digital KA-THA templating (**d**). Post-operative antero-posterior supine pelvic (**e**) and lateral left hip (**f**) radiographs

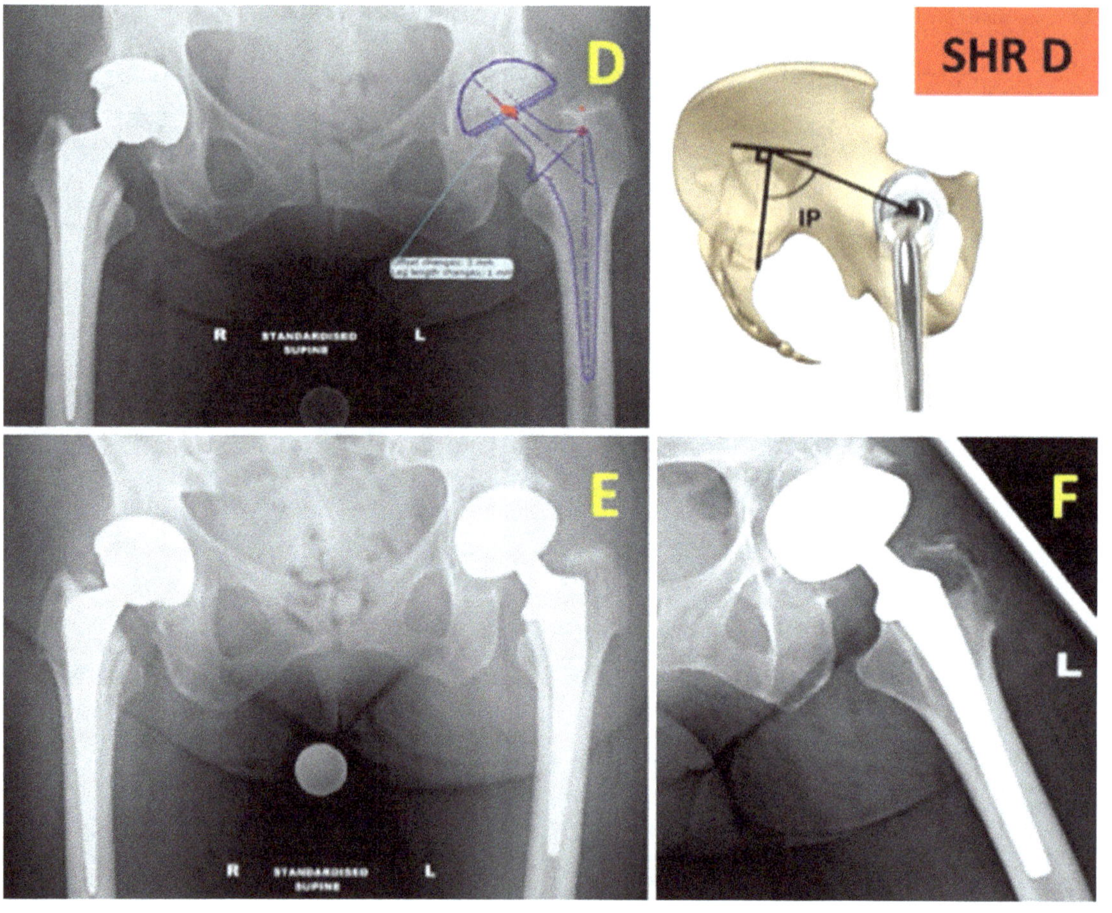

Fig. 11.14 (continued)

References

1. Rivière C, Lazennec J-Y, Van Der Straeten C, Auvinet E, Cobb J, Muirhead-Allwood S. The influence of spine-hip relations on total hip replacement: a systematic review. Orthop Traumatol Surg Res. 2017;103(4):559–68.
2. Sultan AA, Khlopas A, Piuzzi NS, Chughtai M, Sodhi N, Mont MA. The impact of spino-pelvic alignment on total hip arthroplasty outcomes: a critical analysis of current evidence. J Arthroplast. 2018;33(5):1606–16.
3. Phan D, Bederman SS, Schwarzkopf R. The influence of sagittal spinal deformity on anteversion of the acetabular component in total hip arthroplasty. Bone Jt J. 2015;97-B(8):1017–23.
4. Lum ZC, Coury JG, Cohen JL, Dorr LD. The current knowledge on Spinopelvic mobility. J Arthroplast. 2018;33(1):291–6.
5. Rivière C, Lazic S, Villet L, Wiart Y, Allwood SM, Cobb J. Kinematic alignment technique for total hip and knee arthroplasty: the personalized implant positioning surgery. EFORT Open Rev. 2018;3(3):98–105.
6. Riviere C. Kinematic versus conventional alignment techniques for total hip arthroplasty: a retrospective case control study. Orthop Traumatol Surg Res. 2019;105(5):895–905.
7. Maillot C, Harman C, Villet L, Cobb J, Rivière C. Modern cup alignment techniques in total hip arthroplasty: A systematic review. Orthop Traumatol Surg Res. 2019;105(5):907–13.
8. Bayliss LE, Culliford D, Monk AP, Glyn-Jones S, Prieto-Alhambra D, Judge A, et al. The effect of patient age at intervention on risk of implant revision after total replacement of the hip or knee: a population-based cohort study. Lancet. 2017;389(10077):1424–30.
9. Stefl M, Lundergan W, Heckmann N, McKnight B, Ike H, Murgai R, et al. Spinopelvic mobility and acetabular component position for total hip arthroplasty. Bone Joint J. 2017;99-B(1_Supple_A):37–45.
10. Spencer-Gardner L, Pierrepont J, Topham M, Baré J, McMahon S, Shimmin AJ. Patient-specific instrumentation improves the accuracy of acetabular component placement in total hip arthroplasty. Bone Joint J. 2016;98-B(10):1342–6.
11. Rivière C, Lazic S, Dagneaux L, Van Der Straeten C, Cobb J, Muirhead-Allwood S. Spine–hip relations in patients with hip osteoarthritis. EFORT Open Rev. 2018;3(2):39–44.
12. Lazennec JY, Thauront F, Robbins CB, Pour AE. Acetabular and femoral anteversions in standing position are outside the proposed safe zone after total hip arthroplasty. J Arthroplast. 2017;32(11):3550–6.

13. Dorr LD, Malik A, Dastane M, Wan Z. Combined anteversion technique for Total hip arthroplasty. Clin Orthop. 2009;467(1):119–27.
14. Hua X, Li J, Jin Z, Fisher J. The contact mechanics and occurrence of edge loading in modular metal-on-polyethylene total hip replacement during daily activities. Med Eng Phys. 2016;38(6):518–25.
15. Marchetti E, Krantz N, Berton C, Bocquet D, Fouilleron N, Migaud H, et al. Component impingement in total hip arthroplasty: frequency and risk factors. A continuous retrieval analysis series of 416 cup. Orthop Traumatol Surg Res. 2011;97(2):127–33.
16. Shoji T, Yamasaki T, Izumi S, Kenji M, Sawa M, Yasunaga Y, et al. The effect of cup medialization and lateralization on hip range of motion in total hip arthroplasty. Clin Biomech. 2018;57:121–8.
17. McCarthy TF, Alipit V, Nevelos J, Elmallah RK, Mont MA. Acetabular cup anteversion and inclination in hip range of motion to impingement. J Arthroplast. 2016;31(9):264–8.
18. Malkani AL, Ong KL, Lau E, Kurtz SM, Justice BJ, Manley MT. Early- and late-term dislocation risk after primary hip arthroplasty in the medicare population. J Arthroplast. 2010;25(6):21–5.
19. Parratte S, Ollivier M, Lunebourg A, Flecher X, Argenson JN. No benefit after THA performed with computer-assisted cup placement: 10-year results of a randomized controlled study. Clin Orthop. 2016; 474:2085–93.
20. Abdel MP, von Roth P, Jennings MT, Hanssen AD, Pagnano MW. What safe zone? The vast majority of dislocated THAs are within the Lewinnek safe zone for acetabular component position. Clin Orthop Relat Res. 2016;474(2):386–91.
21. Esposito CI, Gladnick BP, Lee Y, Lyman S, Wright TM, Mayman DJ, et al. Cup position alone does not predict risk of dislocation after hip arthroplasty. J Arthroplast. 2015;30(1):109–13.
22. Reina N, Putman S, Desmarchelier R, Sari Ali E, Chiron P, Ollivier M, et al. Can a target zone safer than Lewinnek's safe zone be defined to prevent instability of total hip arthroplasties? Case-control study of 56 dislocated THA and 93 matched controls. Orthop Traumatol Surg Res. 2017;103(5):657–61.
23. Archbold HAP, Mockford B, Molloy D, McConway J, Ogonda L, Beverland D. The transverse acetabular ligament: an aid to orientation of the acetabular component during primary total hip replacement. J Bone Joint Surg. 2006;88(7):4.
24. Girard J, Lons A, Ramdane N, Putman S. Hip resurfacing before 50 years of age: a prospective study of 979 hips with a mean follow-up of 5.1 years. Orthop Traumatol Surg Res. 2018;104(3):295–9.
25. Hill JC, Archbold HA, Diamond OJ, Orr JF, Jaramaz B, Beverland DE. Using a calliper to restore the centre of the femoral head during total hip replacement. The J Bone Joint Surg. 2012;94(11):1468–74.
26. Girard J, Lons A, Ramdane N, Putman S. Hip resurfacing before 50 years of age: a prospective study of 979 hips with a mean follow-up of 5.1 years. Orthop Traumatol Surg Res. 2018;104(3):295–9.
27. Shin Y-S, Suh D-H, Park J-H, Kim J-L, Han S-B. Comparison of specific femoral short stems and conventional-length stems in primary cementless total hip arthroplasty. Orthopedics. 2016;39(2):e311–7.
28. Nam D, Riegler V, Clohisy JC, Nunley RM, Barrack RL. The impact of total hip arthroplasty on pelvic motion and functional component position is highly variable. J Arthroplast. 2017;32(4):1200–5.
29. Mellon SJ, Grammatopoulos G, Andersen MS, Pandit HG, Gill HS, Murray DW. Optimal acetabular component orientation estimated using edge-loading and impingement risk in patients with metal-on-metal hip resurfacing arthroplasty. J Biomech. 2015;48(2):318–23.
30. Patel AB, Wagle RR, Usrey MM, Thompson MT, Incavo SJ, Noble PC. Guidelines for implant placement to minimize impingement during activities of daily living after total hip arthroplasty. J Arthroplast. 2010;25(8):1275–1281.e1.
31. Takao M, Nishii T, Sakai T, Sugano N. Postoperative limb-offset discrepancy notably affects soft-tissue tension in total hip arthroplasty. J Bone Joint Surg. 2016;98(18):1548–54.
32. Pierrepont JW, Feyen H, Miles BP, Young DA, Baré JV, Shimmin AJ. Functional orientation of the acetabular component in ceramic-on-ceramic total hip arthroplasty and its relevance to squeaking. Bone Jt J. 2016;98-B(7):910–6.
33. Bedard NA, Martin CT, Slaven SE, Pugely AJ, Mendoza-Lattes SA, Callaghan JJ. Abnormally high dislocation rates of total hip arthroplasty after spinal deformity surgery. J Arthroplast. 2016;31(12):2884–5.
34. DelSole EM, Vigdorchik JM, Schwarzkopf R, Errico TJ, Buckland AJ. Total hip arthroplasty in the spinal deformity population: does degree of sagittal deformity affect rates of safe zone placement, instability, or revision? J Arthroplast. 2017;32(6):1910–7.
35. Dagneaux L, Marouby S, Maillot C, Canovas F, Rivière C. Dual mobility device reduces the risk of prosthetic hip instability for patients with degenerated spine: A case-control study. Orthop Traumatol Surg Res. 2019;105(3):461–6.
36. Esposito CI, Carroll KM, Sculco PK, Padgett DE, Jerabek SA, Mayman DJ. Total hip arthroplasty patients with fixed spinopelvic alignment are at higher risk of hip dislocation. J Arthroplast. 2018;33(5):1449–54.
37. Fessy MH, Putman S, Viste A, Isida R, Ramdane N, Ferreira A, et al. What are the risk factors for dislocation in primary total hip arthroplasty? A multicenter case-control study of 128 unstable and 438 stable hips. Orthop Traumatol Surg Res. 2017;103(5):663–8.
38. Bonnin MP, Archbold PHA, Basiglini L, Fessy MH, Beverland DE. Do we medialise the hip Centre of rotation in total hip arthroplasty? Influence of acetabular offset and surgical technique. Hip Int. 2012;22(4):371–8.
39. Grammatopoulos G, Alvand A, Monk AP, Mellon S, Pandit H, Rees J, et al. Surgeons' accuracy in achieving their desired acetabular component orientation. J Bone Joint Surg. 2016;98(17):e72.

40. Pierrepont JW, Feyen H, Miles BP, Young DA, Baré JV, Shimmin AJ. Functional orientation of the acetabular component in ceramic-on-ceramic total hip arthroplasty and its relevance to squeaking. Bone Jt J. 2016;98(7):910–6.
41. Merle C, Grammatopoulos G, Waldstein W, Pegg E, Pandit H, Aldinger PR, et al. Comparison of native anatomy with recommended safe component orientation in total hip arthroplasty for primary osteoarthritis. J Bone Joint Surg. 2013;95(22):e172.
42. Thelen T, Thelen P, Demezon H, Aunoble S, Le Huec J-C. Normative 3D acetabular orientation measurements by the low-dose EOS imaging system in 102 asymptomatic subjects in standing position: analyses by side, gender, pelvic incidence and reproducibility. Orthop Traumatol Surg Res. 2017;103(2):209–15.
43. Uemura K, Takao M, Otake Y, Koyama K, Yokota F, Hamada H, et al. Can anatomic measurements of stem anteversion angle be considered as the functional anteversion angle? J Arthroplast. 2018;33(2):595–600.
44. Rivière C, Hardijzer A, Lazennec J-Y, Beaulé P, Muirhead-Allwood S, Cobb J. Spine-hip relations add understandings to the pathophysiology of femoroacetabular impingement: a systematic review. Orthop Traumatol Surg Res. 2017;103(4):549–57.
45. Mayeda BF, Haw JG, Battenberg AK, Schmalzried TP. Femoral-acetabular mating: the effect of femoral and combined anteversion on cross-linked polyethylene wear. J Arthroplast. 2018 [cited 2018 Sep 11]. https://linkinghub.elsevier.com/retrieve/pii/S0883540318305539.
46. Miyoshi H, Mikami H, Oba K, Amari R. Anteversion of the acetabular component aligned with the transverse acetabular ligament in total hip arthroplasty. J Arthroplast. 2012;27(6):916–22.
47. Piazzolla A, Solarino G, Bizzoca D, Montemurro V, Berjano P, Lamartina C, et al. Spinopelvic parameter changes and low back pain improvement due to femoral neck anteversion in patients with severe unilateral primary hip osteoarthritis undergoing total hip replacement. Eur Spine J. 2018;27(1):125–34.
48. Shah SM, Munir S, Walter WL. Changes in spinopelvic indices after hip arthroplasty and its influence on acetabular component orientation. J Orthop. 2017;14(4):434–7.
49. Berliner JL, Esposito CI, Miller TT, Padgett DE, Mayman DJ, Jerabek SA. What preoperative factors predict postoperative sitting pelvic position one year following total hip arthroplasty? Bone Joint J. 2018;100(10):8.
50. Zahn RK, Grotjohann S, Pumberger M, Ramm H, Zachow S, Putzier M, et al. Influence of pelvic tilt on functional acetabular orientation. Technol Health Care. 2017;25(3):557–65.
51. Ezquerra L, Quilez MP, Pérez MÁ, Albareda J, Seral B. Range of movement for impingement and dislocation avoidance in total hip replacement predicted by finite element model. J Med Biol Eng. 2017;37(1):26–34.
52. McCarthy TF, Nevelos J, Elmallah RK, Chughtai M, Khlopas A, Alipit V, et al. The effect of pelvic tilt and femoral head size on hip range-of-motion to impingement. J Arthroplast. 2017;32(11):3544–9.
53. Ohmori T, Kabata T, Maeda T, Kajino Y, Taga T, Hasegawa K, et al. Increase in safe zone area of the acetabular cup using dual mobility cups in THA. Hip Int. 2017;27(4):361–7.
54. Philippot R, Wegrzyn J, Farizon F. Pelvic balance in sagittal and Lewinnek reference planes in the standing, supine and sitting positions [Étude de l'équilibre sagittal pelvien et du plan de Lewinnek en orthostatisme, clinostatisme et position assise]. Orthop Traumatol Surg Res. 2009;95(1):70–6.
55. Ochi H, Homma Y, Baba T, Nojiri H, Matsumoto M, Kaneko K. Sagittal spinopelvic alignment predicts hip function after total hip arthroplasty. Gait Posture. 2017;52:293–300.
56. Maratt JD, Esposito CI, McLawhorn AS, Jerabek SA, Padgett DE, Mayman DJ. Pelvic tilt in patients undergoing total hip arthroplasty: when does it matter? J Arthroplast. 2015;30(3):387–91.
57. Le Huec JC, Hasegawa K. Normative values for the spine shape parameters using 3D standing analysis from a database of 268 asymptomatic Caucasian and Japanese subjects. Eur. Spine J. 2016;25(11):3630–7.
58. Hill JC, Archbold HAP, Diamond OJ, Orr JF, Jaramaz B, Beverland DE. Using a calliper to restore the Centre of the femoral head during total hip replacement. J Bone Joint Surg Br. 2012;94-B(11):1468–74.
59. Meftah M, Yadav A, Wong AC, Ranawat AS, Ranawat CS. A novel method for accurate and reproducible functional cup positioning in total hip arthroplasty. J Arthroplast. 2013;28(7):1200–5.
60. Ranawat CS, Ranawat AS, Lipman JD, White PB, Meftah M. Effect of spinal deformity on pelvic orientation from standing to sitting position. J Arthroplast. 2016;31(6):1222–7.

12

Spine–Pelvic–Hip mobility and its Effects on THA

Nathanael Heckmann, Nicholas A. Trasolini, Michael Stefl, and Lawrence Dorr

Key Points

- The Lewinnek safe zone has failed in its predictive limits of cup position for stability.
- The functional hip motion safe zone is measured by the combined sagittal index (CSI) and is the best measure of risk of impingement including dislocation.
- Excessive femoral motion measured by pelvic femoral angle (PFA) is the greatest reason for dislocation, not the acetabular position.
- Preoperative sagittal X-rays should be taken to determine if spinopelvic imbalance is present and if so the cup position is adapted to the imbalance. Postoperative sagittal X-rays will confirm the hip is safe from spinopelvic to hip impingement.
- Intraoperatively ideally the technique uses combined anteversion rather than just anteversion and targets the cup position with a smart tool for precision so the chance for the hip being in the functional safe zone is optimized.

N. Heckmann · N. A. Trasolini
Keck Medical Center of USC, Los Angeles, CA, USA
e-mail: Nicholas.Trasolini@med.usc.edu

M. Stefl
McFarland Clinic, Ames, IA, USA

L. Dorr (✉)
Pasadena, CA, USA

12.1 Introduction

Accurate and precise component positioning in total hip arthroplasty is a ubiquitous goal amongst hip surgeons and an important topic of research. Early studies defined a "safe zone" for placement of the acetabular cup, and divergence from the defined safe zone was shown to predispose patients to dislocation [1]. However, ideas regarding the position of the acetabular cup have continued to evolve beyond the initial description by Lewinnek in 1978 [1]. Murray et al. [2], in 1993, defined anatomic, operative, and radiographic parameters for inclination and anteversion. DiGioa et al. expanded upon this work by describing functional cup position, rather than just anatomical inclination and anteversion, as being the angles of the acetabulum that correlated to the axis of the body, using lateral radiographic measurements of the spine, pelvis, and hip [3]. This expanded definition was the first to consider spinal parameters as part of a functional spine–pelvis–hip relationship. Lazennec et al. [4], in France, used a new imaging modality (EOS, Biospace Med, Paris, France) to clearly demonstrate the interrelationship of spinal mobility to acetabular position during postural change of sitting to standing (Fig. 12.1). This research increased our understanding that spine–pelvis–hip motion is synchronized for the purpose of allowing the normal hip to move freely through its arc of motion without the greater trochanter

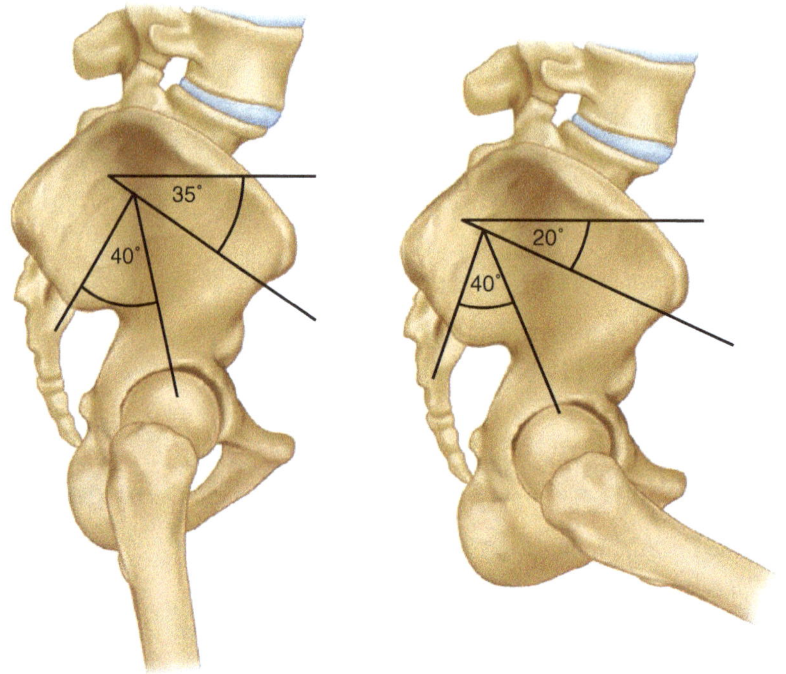

Fig. 12.1 Illustration of normal motion of spine–pelvis–hip during postural change from stand to sit. On left is standing and pelvis tilts anteriorly with sacral slope of 35°. The pelvic incidence is low at 40°. The femur is in extension, but pelvic femoral angle not measured here (see Fig. 12.2). On the right is sitting position with pelvis tilted posteriorly and sacral slope is 20°. PI is static and remains at 40°. The femur flexes but not to 90°. Normal sitting is a combination of posterior tilt of the pelvis and flexion of the femur of 55°–70°

impinging on the pelvis, or the lesser trochanter on the ischium. As hip surgeons learned more about the anatomy of this spine–pelvis–hip relationship, research shifted to studying the effect of this relationship on outcomes following total hip arthroplasty. The cumulative effect of that work has been to redefine the safe zone for acetabular component positioning (functional safe zone) and the influence of sagittal hip motion by taking into account spinopelvic motion. This chapter will focus on the evolving definition of an acetabular safe zone in the context of the spine–pelvis–hip construct, as well as how to personalize and optimize component positioning based on patient-specific spinopelvic parameters.

12.2 Normal Spine–Pelvis–Hip Motion

Understanding the relationship between spinopelvic motion and total hip arthroplasty requires a familiarity with normal pelvic movement in the sagittal plane. When one stands, the pelvis is tilted anteriorly and the lumbar spine assumes a normal lordotic curvature (Fig. 12.1). This positions the acetabulum over the femoral head, while the extended hip allows the spine to support the load of the anterior trunk mass over the pelvis [5]. The amount of anterior pelvic tilt and lumbar spinal lordosis is dependent on a measurement named pelvic incidence (PI) defined by Legaye [6]. High pelvic incidence means that the lordosis and sacral tilt are increased. With postural change, these patients have increased pelvic motion and less hip motion. Low pelvic incidence leads to decreased sacral tilt and a more kyphotic lumbar spine. This means the hip must flex more when a patient moves from a standing to seated position resulting in an increased risk of impingement [5]. It is unknown why people have more or less standing pelvic tilt, but it has been suggested that patients with low pelvic incidence are at greater risk of arthritis of the hip. They definitely have more hip flexion and higher risk of impingement.

With sitting, the pelvis tilts posteriorly as the lordosis of the lumbar spine straightens (Fig. 12.1). This change accommodates the necessary hip flexion and internal rotation of the femur by opening the acetabulum by increasing the functional anteversion of the cup [4, 7, 8]. The spinopelvic motion from standing to sitting is normally 20°, while the femur flexes only 55°–70° to accomplish sitting [4, 9]. To bend forward from the waist to pick up an object on the floor requires increased flexion of the hip to 85° combined with internal rotation of 12° [10]. The magnitude of spinopelvic mobility affects the amount of hip motion needed to perform these activities. With increased mobility of the pelvis, the hip does not need to flex as much to sit or extend as much to stand. To the contrary, when the spinopelvic construct is stiff, the hip must flex more to sit or bend and extend more to stand. Increased hip motion increases the risk for impingement (articular and extra-articular) [4, 11].

Measurements can be made to quantify the mobility of the spinopelvic construct and hip before and after THA (Table 12.1). The radiographic measurements derive from the lateral standing and sitting spinopelvic X-rays (Figs. 12.1 and 12.2). The spinal segments from

Table 12.1 Normal radiographic spinopelvic values

	Standing	Sitting	Δ
Pelvic incidence	53° ± 11°	53° ± 11°	–
Sacral tilt	40° ± 10°	20° ± 9°	11°–29°
Pelvic femoral angle	180° ± 15°	125° ± 12°	50°–75°
Anteinclination	35° ± 10°	52° ± 10°	–

Δ = difference between standing and sitting

Pelvic incidence is a static anatomic measurement and does change between standing and sitting. The other three measurements are dynamic positional parameters so they change between postural positions

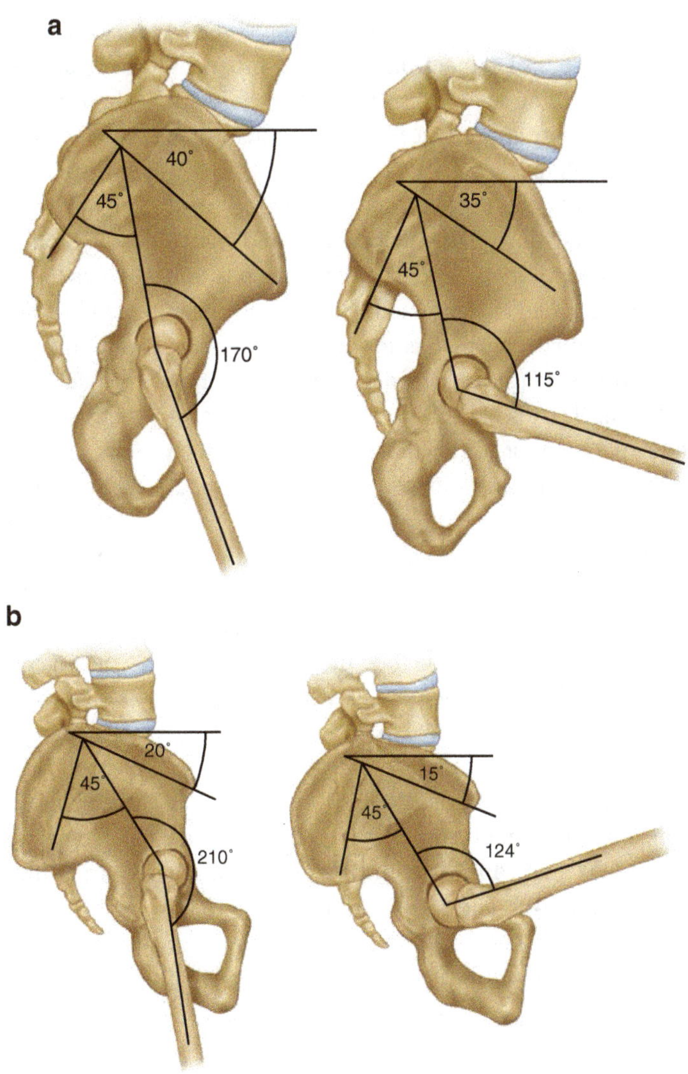

Fig. 12.2 (**a**) Illustration of a pelvis that is fixed in anterior tilt or "stuck standing." The lumbar spine is in lordosis. The pelvic incidence is 45° and the sacral slope is 40° standing and only 35° sitting which means it has only 5° of motion which means the spine is effectively fused. The pelvic femoral angle is 170° standing because of the anterior tilt, but with flexion goes to 115° which is excessive flexion and with the pelvis fixed with anterior tilt the acetabulum remains relatively closed so this flexion presents risk for anterior impingement and posterior dislocation. (**b**) Illustration of pelvis that is fixed in posterior tilt or "stuck sitting." The spine is straight standing and actually slightly kyphotic sitting. The pelvic incidence is 45° and fixed posterior tilt is more commonly associated with low pelvic incidence. The sacral slope goes from 20° standing (with normal motion, the standing sacral slope is above 30°); the sitting sacral slope is 15°, so again this is only 5° of motion which means the lower lumbar spine is effectively fused. With a stuck-sitting deformity, there is hyperextension of the femur and the PFA at standing is 210°. This creates risk of posterior impingement of the greater trochanter on the pelvis which presents some risk for anterior dislocation. With sitting there is normal flexion of the femur of 124°

L3 to S1 need to be visualized because this segment of the lumbar spine moves with the pelvis. The sacrum is fixed to the lower lumbar spine, so degenerative disease of this portion of the spine impacts the mobility of the pelvis (ΔSS), the mobility of the acetabulum (ΔAI), and the arc of motion of the hip (ΔPFA). The ratio of change between sacral slope and pelvic femoral angle is that 1° of SS is inversely correlated to 0.9° of PFA (i.e., for every 1° decrease in ΔSS, there is a 0.9° increase in PFA motion).

The sacral slope is the most accurate measurement of dynamic change [7, 11]. The change in sacral tilt (ΔSS) from standing to sitting (and vice versa) is normally 20° with a normal range of 11°–29° [11]. A measurement of <10° indicates stiffness; a fused construct has a ΔSS < 5°; and hypermobile spinopelvic construct has a ΔSS > 30° [11]. Pelvic femoral angle (PFA) is the measure of femoral motion, and the mean is 180° standing and 125° sitting. This femoral motion is more important for impingement than the acetabulum.

Ante-inclination is a sagittal measurement of the acetabulum that can be measured in the preoperative hip as well as the cup position following THA [7]. Ante-inclination is correlated to the coronal cup inclination and anteversion. The normal range for standing ante-inclination following THA is 42°–63°, which provides a sagittal safe zone for acetabular cup position which can be used to help estimate the risk of impingement [11].

Two other measurements are used. The first is the coronal combined anteversion of the stem and cup which is important because both sides of the joint must be included to fully understand hip impingement and stability [12]. The second measurement, Combined Sagittal Index, is a measure of the sagittal hip motion, and it predicts risk of and direction of dislocation. The combined sagittal index (CSI) is the sum of AI and PFA with outliers of standing values of ≥243° and sitting values of ≤151°. This measurement can be considered the functional hip motion safe zone because it is: CSI = AI+PFA.

12.3 Abnormal Spine–Hip–Pelvis Motion

Spinopelvic–hip imbalance is hypermobility or stiffness of the spinopelvic construct. When the pelvic motion during postural change is altered from normal, it impacts the sagittal acetabular angle (ante-inclination), and to compensate for abnormal pelvic motion, the femur as measured by the PFA must also change. Stiffness is almost always caused by degenerative disc disease or fusion surgery [11]. In a study of 160 patients, 30% of those below the age of 60 years had radiographic stiffness of the spine, while 55% of patients older than 60 were affected [11].

Stiffness of the spinopelvic construct means the sacral slope moves ≦10° with postural change between standing and sitting. But imbalance can also be categorized into patterns, and patterns help us understand how to compensate for spinopelvic abnormality when performing total hip replacement. Within a pattern, motion may or may not be stiff. Stefl et al. [11] define specific patterns of imbalance and the effect on acetabular position. Stefl's patterns are defined by the position in which the spinopelvic construct is fixed in both the standing and sitting postures. In the standing position, the pelvis is fixed in anterior tilt. Therefore, the subset of patients with posterior tilt <30° with sitting is classified as stuck-standing. With this pattern, the acetabulum does not completely open during sitting (and the less mobility of sacral slope between standing and sitting, the less it opens), so the hip has to flex more to allow sitting which increases the risk of anterior impingement of the greater trochanter on the pelvis [20, 22]. Conversely with stuck sitting, the pelvis is fixed in posterior tilt. In a subset of patients, it does not tilt anteriorly >30° with standing, and these patients are thus classified as stuck sitting [11]. Here, the femur must hyperextend (increased PFA) for the person to stand up straight, and the risk is posterior impingement of the greater trochanter on the pelvis, and lesser trochanter on the ischium.

There is a pattern of hypermobility (ΔST > 30°) that we consider a normal variant, and is found mostly in younger age and women patients. Hypermobility is considered to be imbalance when the increased mobility of the spine is a result of the spine tilting beyond flat with sitting. Kyphosis as a spinopelvic motion pattern occurs when hips are so stiff they do not bend enough to allow sitting so the pelvis must tilt excessively posteriorly. This is most common in patients with stiffening collagen vascular disease and in patients with a BMI over 40 because the trunk mass, with sitting, forces the balance center posteriorly.

Spinopelvic–hip imbalance occurs in 40% of patients who are undergoing primary THA [11]. The occurrence of each pattern of spinopelvic imbalance has been determined [11]. Stiffness alone (<10° ST mobility) without a pattern is 3%, and each of the stuck standing and stuck sitting patterns are 14%. Kyphotic deformity occurs in 11% of patients [11, 23, 24].

12.4 Clinical Significance of Spinopelvic–Hip Imbalance

The loss of the smooth transition of the spine–pelvis–hip movement can cause hip impingement, and with THA can affect the usual cup positions the surgeon selects. Patients presenting for primary THA with normal spine–pelvis–hip mobility are at low risk of prosthetic impingement with cups that are: in the Lewinnek safe zones [2], combined anteversion safe zone [12], and have restoration of the physiological biomechanical balance (center of rotation, hip length, and offset). In these patients, hip impingement is caused by component malposition (prosthetic impingement) or a short hip length and/or offset (extra-articular impingement) [13]. Sadhu et al., [14] recently confirmed that dislocations in primary THA occur more often in hips with cups outside the Lewinnek safe zones. However, correct coronal cup position does not always protect patients with sagittal hip motion outside the normal range. Our data shows 14% of hips having the cup aligned inside the Lewinnek zone are not in the normal sagittal hip motion zone. The primary predictive factor is increased hip motion, the second is a stiff Sacral Slope ($\Delta SS \leq 10°$) and the third is low pelvic incidence. We agree with the futility of the Lewinnek safe zone and have declared it as meaningless with the functional safe zone more predictable [23, 24]. Pathologic stiffness is the biggest threat for impingement because of increased hip flexion, and the classic example is patients with a surgical spinal fusion who are known to have increased risk of dislocation [15].

12.5 What Does Imbalance Mean for THA?

Surgeons are used to viewing the hip replacement on coronal radiographs, and the science of sagittal cup position during postural change is new. Its contribution to the understanding of impingement with THA, which is a silent source of failure, is also new [4, 7, 11]. Surgeons cannot easily diagnose impingement because it is a clinical diagnosis, and no imaging or computer technique is available to identify it. Dislocation is the most recognized consequence, and it occurs when the collision of impingement, either component or bony, is severe enough that the mechanical constraint of the combined anteversion of stem and cup, and the biological constraint of the capsule and muscle tension, cannot prevent escape at the egress site [16], but other complications occur because of impingement. Pain is a known consequence but difficult to classify; wear debris and fluid in the joint may or may not be symptomatic or destructive (pseudotumors can be destructive) [17]; loosening of components occurs because of constant collision of impingement [16].

To reduce the risk of impingement with spinal imbalance, the THA cup must be positioned to compensate for sagittal change of acetabular mobility and maintain the hip inside the functional safe zone. It is for this reason that the suggestion has been made that personalization of the cup position for each patient with spinopelvic–hip imbalance is preferable [8, 11, 18]. The cup positions that keep the sagittal motion of the cup in the ante-inclination safe zone for each pattern of imbalance have been defined by Stefl et al. [11].

Cup inclination and anteversion used for normal pelvic motion is satisfactory for hips that are stuck sitting or stuck standing if the ST motion within that pattern is >10°. The dangerous hips are those that are both fixed with anterior or posterior tilt and have a stiff ST. The functional hip safe zone cannot be duplicated with use of femoral head size, risk of wear with inclination >45°, or the anterior hip approach. This creates the conundrum that the anatomic acetabular position cannot be used for the THA cup in patients with severe spinopelvic imbalance. With spinopelvic stiffness, the coronal inclination and anteversion of the cup need to be higher to mechanically open the cup, and with hypermobility the position needs to be more closed, so that it does not open too much.

Patients who have revision THA or late dislocations are older than those with primary THA and have a greater prevalence of spinopelvic stiffness. Pathologic stiffness creates risk of dislocation for both primary and revision THA, but in a study of patients 10 years after THA there were 60% with spinopelvic stiffness compared to 20% in those undergoing primary THA [11, 19]. In primary THA, the hips with dangerous stiffness can be controlled with a mechanically opened cup because the capsule adds biological constraint. In older patients with revision THA and those with late dislocation, dangerous stiffness is related to dislocation in 70–90% of cases because the impingement risk is compounded by loss of capsular integrity and abductor muscle strength [20].

12.6 Technical Changes for Spinopelvic Imbalance

Preoperative planning for patients with spinopelvic imbalance requires obtaining lateral spinopelvic-hip X-rays (see Case Report). But how does the surgeon define those patients? The easiest way is to X-ray all patients which we do. If selection is preferred, we recommend patients over 65 years of age; those with prior spine surgery; those with symptoms of stenosis; and particularly those with increased PFA in either direction [11, 23, 24]. From these stand and sit sagittal X-rays, the cup position can be planned according to the combined mobility and position of the spinopelvic construct as summarized in the previous section. Specific numbers are published according to this combination of the spinopelvic construct. Our data shows 14% of hips have no safe zone (even if inside the Lewinnek zone) because they are not within the functional safe zone, which is defined by the sum of the cup ante-inclination (AI) + PFA, and this is named the Combined Sagittal Index (CSI) [20, 23]. And this percentage of functional outliers was in a group of patients where 92% of hips were in the Lewinnek zones because we used computer navigation. The number of outliers might be higher if the percentage inside the Lewinnek zones were only 50% [21]. They are identified best on sitting sagittal X-rays and have low PFA (increased femoral flexion) as the primary predictor for outlier of CSI but are even more at risk if there is a stiff sacral slope combined with increased hip motion. Low PI was the third most prevalent predictor, and cup position is not in the top three. But the cup counts because these hips need optimal coronal cup position to optimize AI (which is part of CSI equation). Hips with abnormal PFA, ΔSS < 10° and low PI have no functional safe zone so should have additional mechanical support of dual mobility articulation at surgery because biological balance cannot be obtained.

Intraoperatively, we prepare the femur first because combined anteversion is more important than anteversion itself. If femoral anteversion is less than 5° to retroverted, a decision to change the femur to a modular design or cement the femoral stem at 10° anteversion (any more anteversion results in intoeing for patients) must be made. The cup is targeted to be within the combined anteversion safe zone of 25°–45° with stiff spinopelvic hips having a higher cup anteversion and thus a higher combined anteversion. Retroverted hips are not able to be anteverted sufficiently, so a decision must be made if the articulation is stable or a dual mobility is needed. Retroverted hips can be diagnosed preoperatively by the X-ray signs of crossover or ischial spine sign. Intraoperatively, the noncemented stem anteversion in the femur is 5° or less (and if zero or less, it is best to cement the stem), and the cup is difficult to anteversion more than 10° without prominent metal above the posterior rim of the acetabulum. Patients with pincer impingement commonly have retroversion of the acetabulum. If noncemented implants are chosen, it is better to use dual mobility articulation to increase mechanical stability. We use computer navigation to be accurate in cup positioning, but if the surgeon decides not to use a smart tool then he/she must validate the precision of their manual technique. This can be done by measuring the postoperative sagittal X-ray to verify the hip is within the normal CSI and the femoral head is centralized in the cup on the sitting X-ray.

12.7 Summary

The literature on spine–pelvic–hip mobility and its effects on THA continue to grow. It is important for hip surgeons to begin considering the spinopelvic construct in preoperative planning, intraoperative technique, and postoperative risk stratification. Understanding the patterns of spine–pelvic–hip anatomy and mobility helps the hip surgeon to optimize and personalized cup position. The Lewinnek safe zone [2] has been used for decades, but it is well known that dislocations occur both inside and outside that safe zone [14]. Its importance has been as a guide to improve our precision of cup placement. Likewise, the use of spinopelvic imbalance will guide hip surgeons toward proper patient-specific component positioning by focusing on the functional hip motion safe zone. The authors recommend performing lateral spinopelvic X-rays on all preoperative THA patients because recent data shows 40% of primary patients have spinal imbalance. Lateral spinopelvic X-rays from L3 to S1 are sufficient, and full-length films like EOS are not necessary because it is the lower lumbar segment (L3–S1) that is connected to the hip.

Spinopelvic mobility affects the dynamic cup position and should be considered during positioning of the acetabular cup. Consideration of the specific spinopelvic motion patterns described in this chapter can minimize the risk of impingement. In patients with spinopelvic hypermobility, the coronal cup position must be more closed so that the acetabulum does not open excessively with sitting. Conversely, if there is stiffness, the cup should be opened to prevent impingement with sitting. In the positional patterns of stuck standing or sitting without mobility stiffness, inclination of 40° and anteversion of 20° will almost always keep the sagittal cup position in the AI safe zone if the pattern is not stiff too. In the patient undergoing primary THA with pathologic spinal imbalance (fused spine or kyphosis with fixed posterior pelvic tilt), surgeons should consider adding constraint to the THA with a dual mobility articulation. It is also important to remove any bony impingement of the greater and lesser trochanter in patients with stiff constructs because mechanical constraint alone does not always provide sufficient protection from dislocation. This is necessary when stuck standing or stuck sitting pattern with stiffness is present (see Case Report). There is sufficient bone both anteriorly and posteriorly on the greater trochanter to do this with a high-speed drill. If this treatment will injure the gluteus medius, then the trochanter should be transferred.

Case Report

An 80-year-old female presented to our clinic after having two anterior dislocations out of her right total hip arthroplasty. She underwent an uncomplicated right total hip arthroplasty approximately 19 years ago and a left total hip arthroplasty 4 years ago, both through a posterior approach. Her left total hip arthroplasty has been asymptomatic since the time of surgery. However, her right total hip arthroplasty has dislocated twice—the first dislocation occurred approximately 15 years after her index procedure and was treated successfully with a closed reduction and; the second dislocation occurred approximately 19 years after surgery, and she underwent a closed reduction at an outside hospital. Both occurred while walking without any precipitating traumatic events. The patient reported apprehension while walking and intense fear of repeat dislocation that hindered her from performing daily activities.

Standard anteroposterior pelvic radiographs revealed excessive polyethylene wear and a well-fixed cementless acetabular cup and femoral stem on the right side (Fig. 12.3). Standing and sitting lateral spine–pelvis–hip radiographs revealed stiff spinopelvic motion as indicated by a delta sacral slope of 10° (Fig. 12.4). Given these radiographic findings, as well as her two previous dislocations, we recommended revision surgery to restore stability. At the time of revision surgery, the patient was found to have wear debris in her capsule that was debrided. The cup was measured using computer navigation and found to have 55° of inclination and 14° of anteversion. Her stem and cup were found to be well fixed and left in place; she was revised with a constrained liner and had excellent stability throughout a functional arc of motion (Fig. 12.5). However, 6 weeks following her revision surgery, she dislocated anteriorly while walking.

The patient underwent a second revision surgery. At the time of surgery, the patient's constrained ring was found to be dissociated from her liner. The patient's acetabular cup was removed, and a new acetabular cup was placed with a new

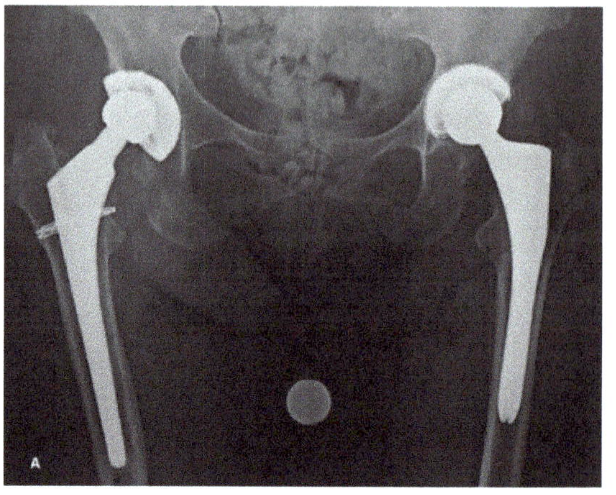

Fig. 12.3 Standard low AP pelvis of patient upon presentation. Note the excessive polyethylene wear and vertically oriented cup on the right side

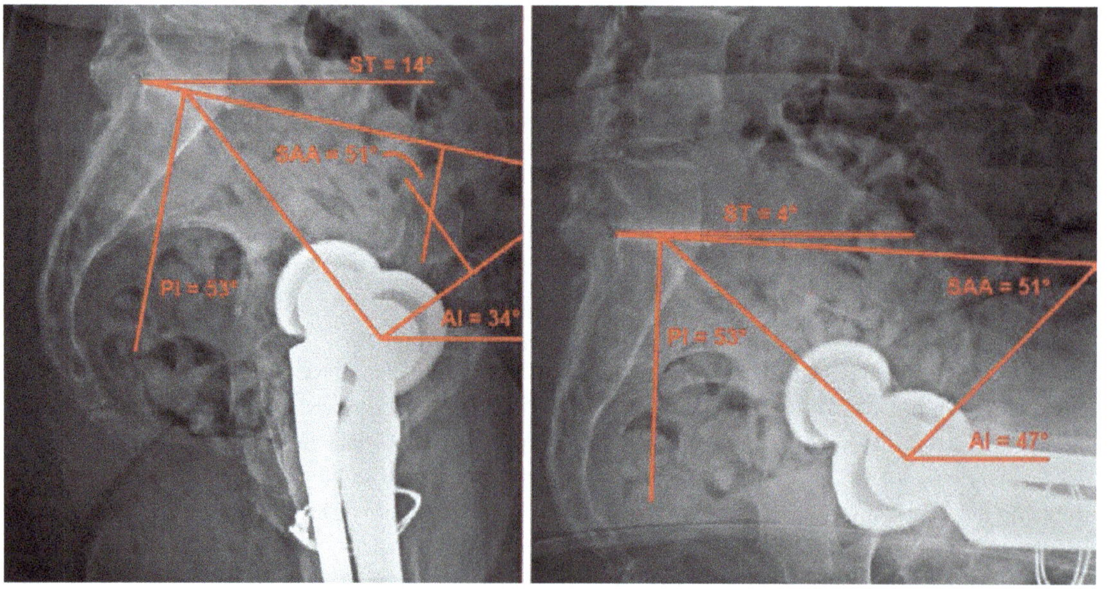

Fig. 12.4 Lateral standing and sitting spine–pelvis–hip radiographs, demonstrating a posteriorly tilted pelvis as indicated by a standing sacral tilt of 14°. Also, the change in sacral tilt (ΔST) is only 10°, indicating decreased spinopelvic motion

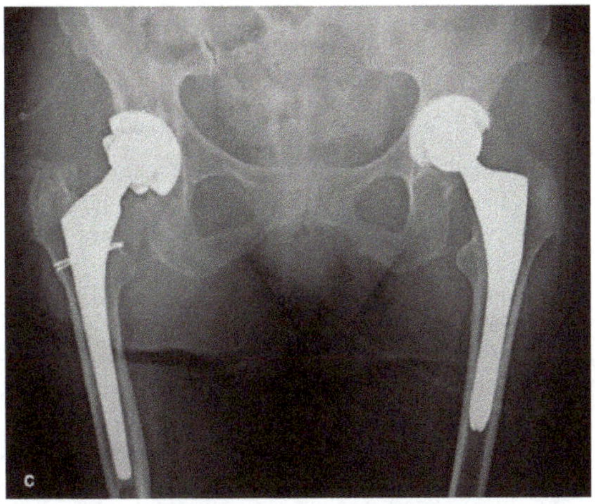

Fig. 12.5 Standard low AP pelvis, following first revision surgery to a constrained liner

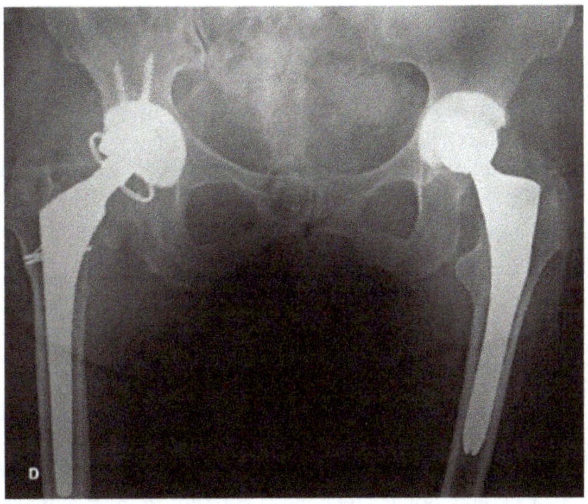

Fig. 12.6 Standard low AP pelvis, following second revision surgery with replacement of the acetabular cup and implantation of a new constrained liner

constrained liner and + 10-mm increased head length (Fig. 12.6). The patient's hip was stable throughout a functional arc of motion; however, with terminal extension and external rotation of her femur, her greater trochanter impinged on her ilium, and her lesser trochanter impinged on her ischium. To avoid future impingement, her lesser trochanter and the posterior portion of her greater trochanter were removed with care taken to not violate the gluteus medius tendon (Fig. 12.7). The patient had an uneventful recovery and had no further episodes of instability at her 2-year follow-up.

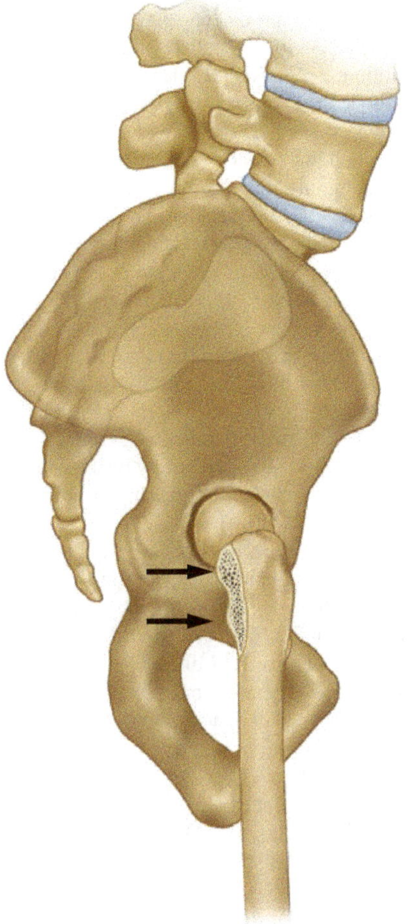

Fig. 12.7 An illustration depicting the portion of the greater trochanter, typically removed to avoid impingement. If the amount of bony excision required to avoid impingement is thought to disrupt the gluteus medius tendon, a trochanteric transfer can be performed

References

1. Lewinnek GE, Lewis JL, Tarr R, Compere CL, Zimmerman JR. Dislocations after total hip-replacement arthroplasties. J Bone Joint Surg Am. 1978;60(2):217–20.
2. Murray DW. The definition and measurement of acetabular orientation. J Bone Joint Surg Br. 1993;75:228–32.
3. DiGioia AM, Jaramaz B, Blackwell M, Simon DA, Morgan F, Moody JE, Nikou C, Colgan BD, Aston CA, Labarca RS, Kischell E, Kanade T. The Otto Aufranc Award. Image guided navigation system to measure intraoperatively acetabular implant alignment. Clin Orthop Relat Res. 1998;355:8–22.

4. Lazennec JY, Charlot N, Gorin M, Roger B, Arafati N, Bissery A, Saillant G. Hip-spine relationship: a radio-anatomical study for optimization in acetabular cup positioning. Surg Radiol Anat. 2004;26(2):136–44.
5. Philippot R, Wegrzyn J, Farizon F, Fessy MH. Pelvic balance in sagittal and Lewinnek reference planes in the standing, supine and sitting positions. Orthop Traumatol Surg Res. 2009;95(1):70–6.
6. Legaye J, Duval-Beaupère G, Hecquet J, Marty C. Pelvic incidence: a fundamental pelvic parameter for three-dimensional regulation of spinal sagittal curves. Eur Spine J. 1998;7(2):99–103.
7. Kanawade V, Dorr LD, Wan Z. Predictability of acetabular component angular change with postural shift from standing to sitting position. J Bone Joint Surg Am. 2014;6(12):978–86.
8. Phan D, Bederman SS, Schwarzkopf R. The influence of sagittal spinal deformity on anteversion of the acetabular component in total hip arthroplasty. Bone Joint J. 2015;97-B(8):1017–23.
9. Larkin B, van Holsbeeck M, Koueiter D, Zaltz I. What is the impingement-free range of motion of the asymptomatic hip in young adult males? Clin Orthop Relat Res. 2015;473(4):1284–8.
10. Sugano N, Tsuda K, Miki H, Tako M, Suzuki N, Nakamura N. Dynamic measurements of hip movement in deep bending activities after total hip arthroplasty using a 4-dimensional motion analysis system. J Arthrop. 2012;27:1562–8.
11. Stefl M, Lundergan W, Heckmann N, McKnight B, Ike H, Murgai R, Dorr LD. Spinopelvic mobility and acetabular component position for total hip arthroplasty. Bone Joint J. 2017;99-B(1 Supple A):37–45.
12. Dorr LD, Malik A, Dastane M, Wan Z. Combined anteversion technique for total hip arthroplasty. Clin Orthop Relat Res. 2009;467(1):119–27.
13. Dorr LD, Wan Z. Causes of and treatment protocol for instability of total hip replacement. Clin Orthop Relat Res. 1998;355:144–51.
14. Sadhu A, Nam D, Coobs B, Barrack TN, Nunley RM, Barrack RL. Acetabular component position and the risk of dislocation following primary and revision Total hip arthroplasty: a matched cohort analysis. J Arthroplast. 2017;32:987–91.
15. Buckland AJ, Hart RA, Mundis GM Jr, et al. Risk of total hip arthroplasty dislocation after adult spinal deformity correction. Spine J. 2016;16(10):S180. https://doi.org/10.1016/j.spinee.2016.07.086.
16. Brown TD, Elkins JM, Pedersen DR, Callaghan JJ. Impingement and dislocation in total hip arthroplasty: mechanisms and consequences. Iowa Orthop J. 2014;34:1–15.
17. Grammatopoulos G, Pandit H, Kwon YM, Gundle R, McLardy-Smith P, Beard DJ, Murray DW, Gill HS. Hip resurfacings revised for inflammatory pseudotumour have a poor outcome. J Bone Joint Surg Br. 2009;91(8):1019–24.
18. Pierrepont J, Hawdon G, Miles BP, Connor BO, Baré J, Walter LR, Marel E, Solomon M, McMahon S, Shimmin AJ. Variation in functional pelvic tilt in patients undergoing total hip arthroplasty. Bone Joint J. 2017;99-B(2):184–91.
19. Yukizawa Y, Dorr LD, Ward JA, Wan Z. Posterior mini-incision with primary total hip arthroplasty: a nine to ten year follow up study. J Arthroplast. 2016;31(1):168–7.
20. Heckmann N, Stefl M, Trasolini N, McKnight B, Ike H, Dorr LD. Late dislocation following total hip arthroplasty. JBJS. 2018;100:1845–53.
21. Callanan MC, Jarrett B, Bragdon CR, Zurakowski D, Rubash HE, Freiberg AA, Malchau H. The John Charnley Award: risk factors for cup malpositioning: quality improvement through a joint registry at a tertiary hospital. Clin Orthop Relat Res. 2011;469(2):319–29.
22. Ike H, Dorr LD, Trasolini N, Stefl M, McKnight B, Heckmann N. Spine-pelvis-hip relationship in THR functioning of a total hip replacement. J Bone Joint Surg Am. 2018;100:1606–15.
23. Tezuka T, Heckmann N, Bodner R, Dorr LD. Functional safe zone is superior to the Lewinnek safe zone for total hip arthroplasty: why the Lewinnek safe zone is not always predictive of stability. J Arthroplasty. 2019;34:3–8.
24. Dorr LD, Callaghan JJ. Death of the Lewinnek "safe zone". J Arthroplasty. 2019;34:1–2.

13

Total Hip Arthroplasty: Imaging and Radiographic Evaluation

Omar A. Behery, Lazaros Poultsides, and Jonathan M. Vigdorchik

Key Points

- Personalized component implantation in total hip arthroplasty aims to reproduce normal hip joint anatomy and improve functional outcomes and implant survivorship.
- Traditional radiographic evaluation for total hip arthroplasty consists of an anteroposterior view of the pelvis and a cross table lateral of the hip, and is useful to delineate anatomy and component sizing, but does not take into account the dynamic position of the hip joint in different postural positions.
- The conventional acetabular component "safe zone" does not account for the spino-pelvic relationship and the dynamic nature of acetabular component orientation, which impacts the function and stability of a total hip arthroplasty.
- Sitting and standing alignment radiographs have gained recent popularity and are important to routinely obtain and analyze to determine the best patient-specific component position, given the high concordance between hip and spine pathology.
- Three-dimensional cross-sectional imaging or 2-D/3-D reconstructions can also be useful to better delineate hip anatomy and template component size and position.
- Postoperatively CT imaging can be useful in assessing the accuracy and quality of personalized total hip component implantation.

13.1 Introduction

Successful total hip arthroplasty (THA) greatly depends on appropriate implant choice and accurate femoral and acetabular component positioning. Preoperative radiographic templating is crucial, and accurate intraoperative execution of the templated plan is important to maximize implant stability and bearing performance. Traditionally, plain radiographs have been used for preoperative planning, as well as postoperative follow-up and assessment of component position, with historically defined "safe zones"

O. A. Behery · L. Poultsides
NYU Langone Health, NYU Langone Orthopedic Hospital, New York, NY, USA
e-mail: Omar.Behery@nyulangone.org

J. M. Vigdorchik (✉)
Hospital for Special Surgery, New York, NY, USA
e-mail: VigdorchikJ@HSS.EDU

for component position. However, as our understanding of optimal implant positioning in the setting of spino-pelvic dynamics has expanded, more advanced methods of radiographic assessment of implant positioning have gained popularity. Given the variations in anatomy and functional kinematics of a patient's hip joint, the optimal THA component alignment and positioning may differ on a case by case basis, and therefore, advanced methods of assessing optimal patient-specific implant positioning are of prime importance.

13.2 Personalized Total Hip Arthroplasty

Personalized techniques for implanting hip components have been developed with the goal to solve residual complications that occur with conventionally implanted hip prostheses. One of the causes of failure in conventionally implanted hip prostheses is the suboptimal interaction between components (e.g., edge loading and prosthetic impingement). This is primarily related to the systematic and generalized approach for templating and implanting total hip components in the traditional technique (similar implants positioning for all patients), thereby disregarding the unique individual joint anatomy, biomechanics, and spino-pelvic dynamics. Personalized techniques for joint replacement have therefore been developed to address these issues and improve on the outcomes of THA. This represents a paradigm shift in the approach to THA.

Personalized techniques for THA aim to reproduce normal hip anatomy and biomechanics to generate a more physiological prosthetic hip to improve function, patient satisfaction, and implant survivorship. The growing knowledge surrounding the impact of spino-pelvic dynamics on the stability of a THA is an important discussion in the delivery of personalized total hip components. A more detailed description of the evolution of hip arthroplasty from traditional systematic to modern patient-specific kinematic techniques can be found in the Chap. 3 (hip replacement: development and future). This paradigm shift in the technique for implanting hip components from a traditional, systematic approach toward personalized component implantation necessitates developing reliable methods of postoperative radiographic evaluation and assessment of the accuracy and quality of personalized hip component implantation.

13.3 Traditional Radiographic Evaluation

Traditional radiographic evaluation consists of plain films. An array of different projections can be obtained to gain information regarding hip pathology, alignment, osseous anatomy and morphology, as well as bone quality. Following THA, plain films can demonstrate implant alignment, positioning, the presence of a periprosthetic fracture, as well as reactive bony changes such as osteolysis and stress shielding. Radiographs are typically easy to obtain, less expensive compared with advanced imaging, but may be somewhat limited in providing information on important anatomical relationships such as femoral neck anteversion and functional acetabular orientation.

13.3.1 Anteroposterior (AP) View of the Pelvis

This projection is obtained supine or weight bearing, with both legs internally rotated 15° to obtain a profile view of the femoral neck anatomy which is on average 15° anteverted. In order to properly assess implant positioning on an AP pelvis, it is important that the image is obtained with the proper technique and with a marker of a known size (typically 25 mm) present as close to the hip joint as possible for calibrating size and accurate magnification. The hip center of rotation is the center of the femoral head articulating within the acetabular cup. Leg lengths can be estimated by drawing a horizontal reference line connecting both teardrops (or ischial tuberosities) and comparing the perpendicular distance from that line to a similar reference point on the proximal femur, typically the lesser trochanter. On the acetabular side, the static supine or standing cup abduction angle can be measured by using the horizontal reference line connecting both tear drops and measuring the acute angle subtended by an intersecting line connecting the superior and inferior edges of the cup (Fig. 13.1a). The static supine or standing cup anteversion may also be measured on an AP pelvis using one of multiple methods such as the Lewinnek method which is based on a mathematical formula [1] (Fig. 13.1b) or using computer software based on the geometry of the ellipse created by the anterior and posterior lips of the cup. On the femoral side, stem size and fit can be evaluated based on knowledge of the implant and expected fixation pattern. The varus/valgus alignment of the stem can be assessed based on any deviation of the stem from the alignment of the femoral canal, and femoral offset can be measured from the center of rotation of the hip joint to a line traveling down the femoral canal. Furthermore, the static supine or standing femoral version can be estimated based on the AP pelvis radiograph as described by Weber et al. [2]. This technique relies on calculating the femoral version by rotation-based change in the measured neck—shaft angle of the stem, using the following formula: Stem version = arcos [tan (measured neck shaft angle)/tan (true implant neck shaft angle)]. An alternative technique of measuring femoral version has been described based on a specialized posteroanterior seated hip radiograph called a Budin view [3]. Computed tomography is the gold standard in measuring the anatomic femoral anteversion, which is made relative to the posterior condylar line of the knee.

13.3.2 Cross Table and Frog-Lateral Views

A cross table lateral is obtained in the supine position, with the leg internally rotated 15°, contralateral hip flexed, with the beam centered over the femoral head and aimed 45° in the coronal plane to avoid the contralateral hip. On this projection, the static supine acetabular anteversion can be measured by the angle created between a line over the face of the cup and a line that is perpendicular to the horizontal plane as described by Woo and Morrey. This measurement however is prone to inaccuracy as it can be affected by pelvic tilt, which changes as the contralateral hip is flexed. A more recent employment is the ischio-lateral method of estimating anteversion is based off of the longitudinal axis of the ischial tuberosity and can avoid this issue [4]. The femoral stem fit and anteroposterior angulation is also visualized on this view, but the proximal femur is better visualized on a frog-lateral radiograph, which is obtained by centering the beam

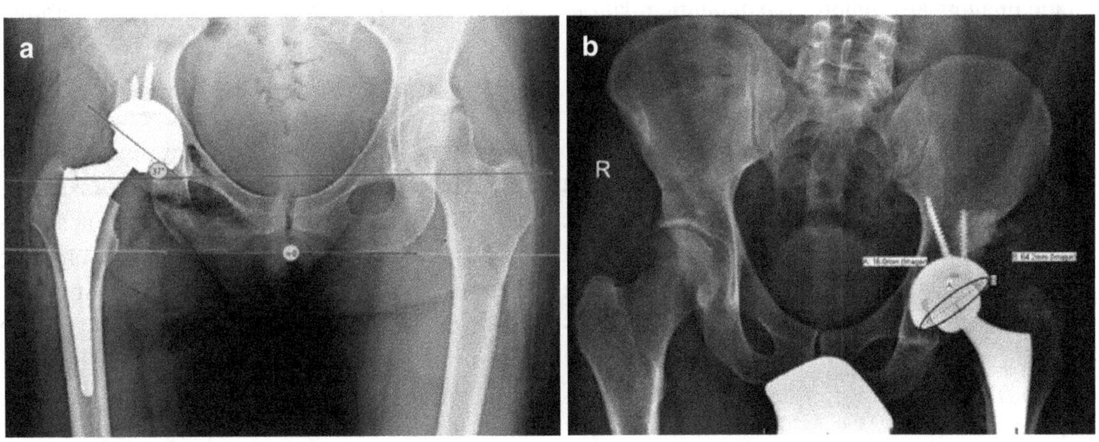

Fig. 13.1 (**a**) Acetabular component inclination may be estimated on this supine anteroposterior view of the pelvis based on a horizontal reference line connecting the tear drops. (**b**) Acetabular component anteversion calculated based on Lewinnek's method (Version = Arcsin (short axis/long axis)) to be approximately 25°

over the femoral head with the hip flexed and abducted 45°. Although this view is a lateral of the proximal femur, it is not a lateral view of the acetabular cup.

13.3.3 Shortcomings of Traditional Radiographic Assessment

There are some important considerations that are not completely evaluated using the traditional radiographic methods. For instance, plain films are two-dimensional, and an AP view of the pelvis only allows for coronal plane templating of the acetabular component. The thickness and width of the anterior and posterior walls are not visualized, and therefore unaccounted for when templating acetabular component size. Although knowing femoral head diameter may reproducibly allow deduction of a reliable cup size template, axial imaging may better visualize acetabular anterior and posterior wall bone stock and therefore more accurate component size templating.

Furthermore, plain radiographic assessment only provides static landmarks of acetabular inclination and anteversion, which assumes a constant position of the acetabulum. Changes in acetabular inclination and anteversion secondary to postural pelvic obliquity, tilt, or rotation in a weight bearing position may be completely missed on AP pelvis views (supine or standing). Static imaging also ignores the dynamic relationships between the acetabular position, the pelvis, and the spine, which change in different postural positions. Patients may have physiologically or pathologically different profiles of spino-pelvic mobility which can impact cup position and therefore their risks of instability, prosthetic impingement, and edge loading if these variables are ignored by using a universally defined "safe zone" target of cup position of 40 ± 10° of inclination and 15 ± 10° of anteversion as defined by Lewinnek [1]. In fact, in a large cohort of 9784 patients, 58% of THA dislocations occurred in patients with components placed in the classically defined "safe zone" [5].

Traditional plain radiography may be inadequate in judging the quality of personalized total hip component implantation. Postoperative radiographs have been shown to lack precision when assessing the quality of the restoration of the hip biomechanical parameters (femoral medial offset and femoral length) and cannot fully inform if the personalized implants have been positioned to reproduce the native hip anatomy and match the individual spino-pelvic dynamics. For instance, plain films do not inform the operator if the cup is oriented parallel to the native transverse acetabular ligament, nor if the adjustment of anteversion to accommodate a stiff lumbar spine has been precisely achieved, or whether the prosthetic neck anteversion has reproduced the native femoral anteversion. These limitations of static, 2-D plain radiographs in the postoperative evaluation of personalized component positioning compel the use of more advanced imaging techniques.

13.4 Modern Concepts and Radiographic Evaluation

The dynamic relationship between the pelvis and the lumbar spine affects acetabular cup position and can therefore profoundly impact the stability of THA. Hip pathology frequently coexists with lumbar spine pathology, and lumbar stiffness or fusion has been linked with increased instability following THA [6, 7]. This warrants thorough radiographic assessment and analysis of spino-pelvic parameters and determination of spino-pelvic motion when preoperatively planning the ideal acetabular implant and cup position, to estimate a "safe zone" that is specific to the patient evaluated. Traditionally, the transverse acetabular ligament has been used to guide patient-specific cup anteversion; however, given the dynamic nature of the hip joint, the functional anteversion of the acetabulum may differ based on pelvic tilt [8].

13.4.1 Sitting and Standing Alignment Radiographs

Although not routinely obtained, sitting and standing lateral full-length radiographs are often obtained to determine the changes in spino-pelvic parameters and become especially important to obtain in patients with lumbar spinal disease or fusion or to evaluate acetabular component position if presenting with recurrent total hip instability [9, 10]. It is known that patients with a stiff or fused spine, who experience prosthetic dislocation, have a tendency to demonstrate decreased spine flexion, smaller change in pelvic tilt, and increased hip flexion from standing to sitting position [11]. These sitting and standing films may be obtained on a 36-inch film cassette or if available, using EOS™ stereoradiographs (EOS™ Imaging, Paris, France) (Fig. 13.2a–d). More dynamic imaging including flexed-seated and single-leg step-up lateral images are gaining popularity as they may be better at assessing the functional position of the hip joint and spino-pelvic dynamics and have been used for an Optimized Positioning System™ used to preoperatively plan patient-specific target component position [12].

Several spino-pelvic parameters can be measured and analyzed on the lateral sitting and standing alignment films (Fig. 13.3):

(a) Pelvic tilt (PT) or pelvic version may be measured as the angle between the vertical axis and a line connecting the center of the S1 vertebral endplate and the center of the femoral head. Pelvic tilt increases as the pelvis retroverts when going from standing to a sitting position.
(b) Sacral slope (SS) can be measured as the angle between a horizontal reference line and a line parallel to the S1 endplate. This parameter decreases as the pelvis goes into retroversion.
(c) Pelvic incidence is the sum of SS and PT and can be measured as the angle between a line connecting the femoral head and the center of the S1 endplate and a line perpendicular to the S1 endplate. This parameter remains constant through pelvic motion; however, it can be used as a direct indicator of the ability to recruit pelvic tilt to compensate for spinal deformity.
(d) Lumbar lordosis (LL) is the Cobb angle between two lines parallel to the L1 and the S1 endplates. This value is typically within 10° of the PI in a normal lumbar spine.
(e) The anterior pelvic plane (APP) can be used to measure pelvic tilt as well. It is created by a line connecting both anterior superior iliac spines and the pubic symphysis, and the angle created between this plane and the vertical axis represents that anterior pelvic plane-pelvic tilt (APP-PT) angle.

In a normal and flexible lumbar spine, the pelvic tilt increases when going from standing to sitting, which increases acetabular anteversion and decreases the risk of impingement and posterior dislocation. Acetabular anteversion increases by 0.7° for each 1° increase in pelvic tilt [13]. However, in the case of a stiff or fused lumbar spine, the change in pelvic tilt markedly decreases from standing to sitting. This change is typically less than 20° [9], although it is not yet entirely clear what degree of angular difference in these parameters indicates a stiff spine. When the pelvic tilt does not adequately increase, there is consequently less acetabular anteversion when in a sitting position and, therefore, increased risk of impingement and posterior dislocation.

Patient-specific acetabular component position can be decided based on these standing/

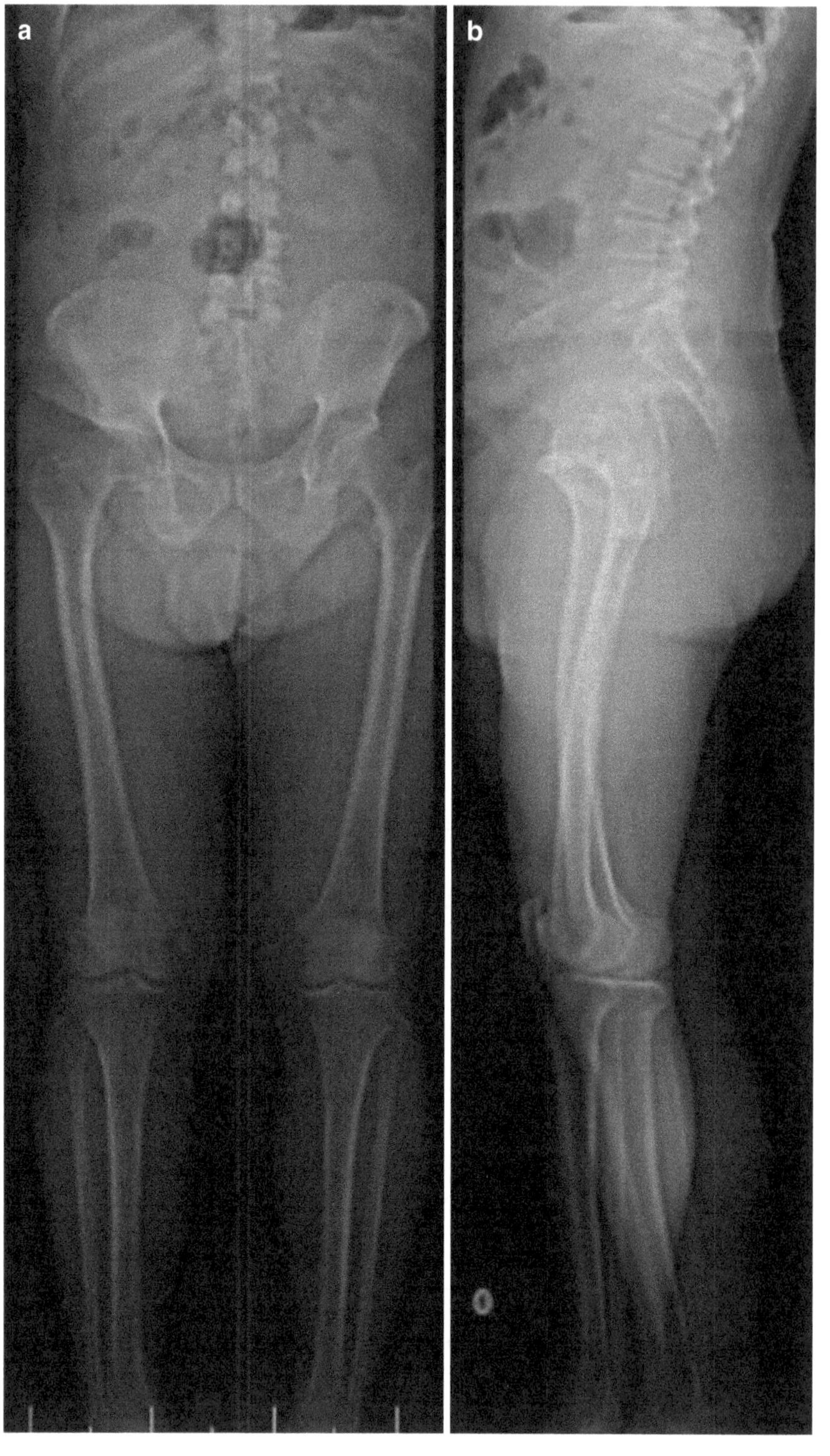

Fig. 13.2 Full leg-length standing anteroposterior (**a**) and lateral (**b**) and sitting anteroposterior (**c**) and lateral (**d**) films obtained on long cassette

Fig. 13.2 (continued)

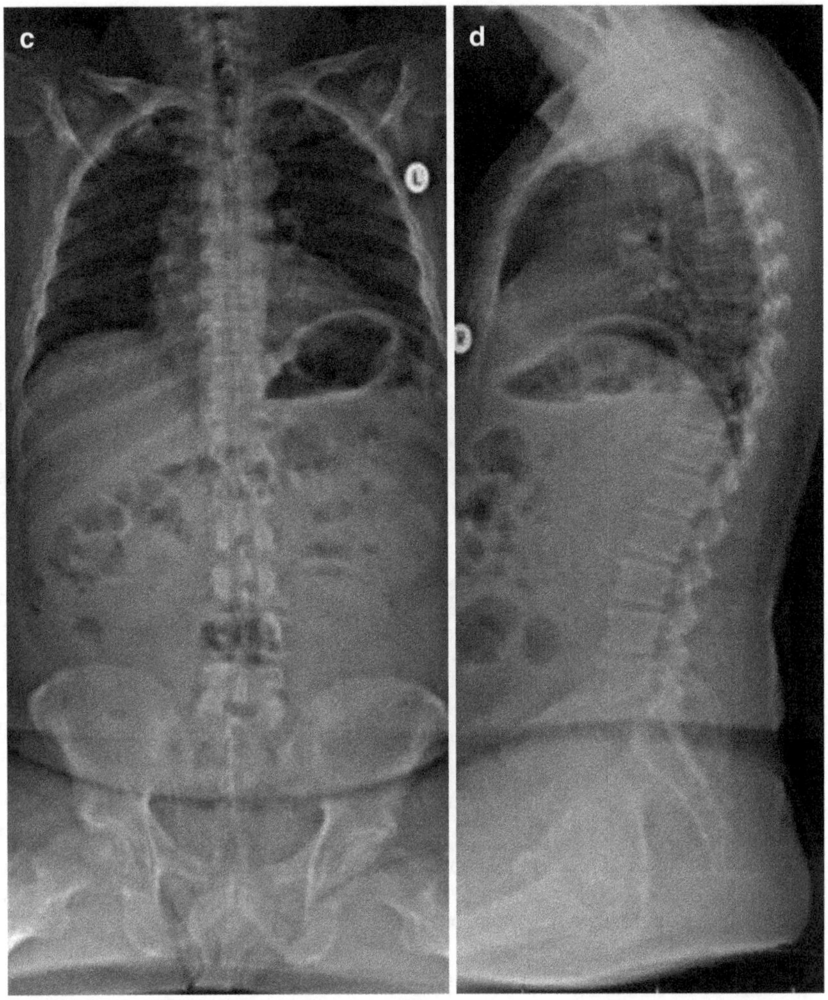

sitting alignment films and changes in spino-pelvic parameters. Increasing cup anteversion may be warranted in patients with a significantly stiff lumbar spine and very limited changes in pelvic tilt from standing to sitting. In higher-risk cases, dual mobility implants may be considered (Fig. 13.4). Without obtaining this radiographic assessment of the patient's spino-pelvic dynamics, it is difficult to identify who may be at a higher risk of dislocation, and choosing the same target cup position for all may lead to dislocation in those with stiff or fused lumbar spines.

13.4.2 Stepwise Evaluation of Acetabular Component Position in Total Hip Instability

When evaluating a patient with prosthetic hip instability for revision surgery or a patient at high-risk of dislocation following primary THA, it is critical to employ a stepwise radiographic assessment of component positioning to determine the optimal patient-specific functional implant position that minimizes the risk of instability.

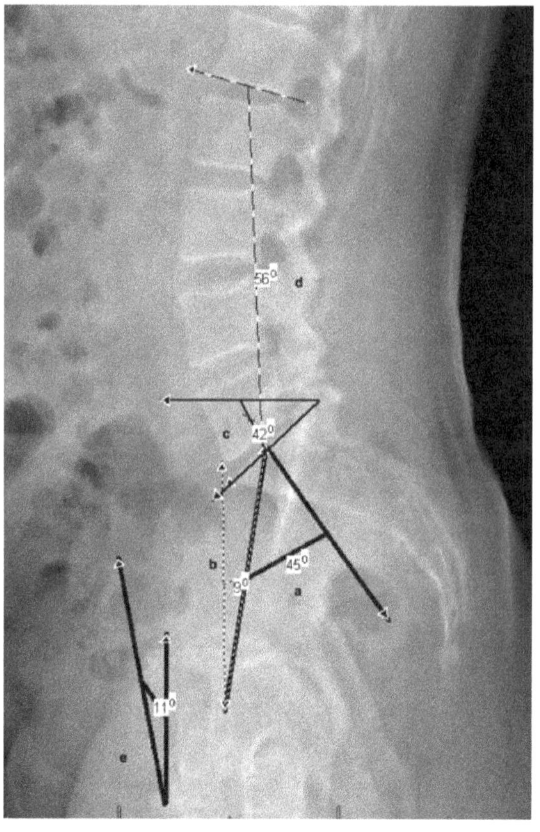

Fig. 13.3 Standing lateral radiograph demonstrating spino-pelvic parameter measurements. Pelvic incidence, a; pelvic tilt, b; sacral slope, c; lumbar lordosis, d; anterior pelvic plane, e

Initially a supine AP pelvis may be obtained, and the supine cup abduction and anteversion may be deduced as previously described. A standing or weight-bearing AP view of the pelvis can then be obtained for comparison with the supine view. This standing film offers an assessment of the cup abduction and anteversion in the patient's functional standing weight-bearing position. Pelvic obliquity, rotation, or tilt may affect the functional cup abduction or anteversion positions. For instance, patients with excessive anterior pelvic tilt will functionally have less cup anteversion in a standing position.

Subsequently, sitting and standing lateral full-length radiographs may then be obtained. Lumbar degenerative processes including spinal fusion, spondylosis, spondylolisthesis, or sagittal spinal imbalance or deformity can be assessed through these images. These lumbar pathologies significantly affect spino-pelvic motion and therefore have consequences that impact acetabular component position and therefore risks of instability, prosthetic impingement, and edge loading. The spino-pelvic parameters listed above can be assessed from these sitting to standing films, and based on changes in these parameters, the change in cup anteversion between these two functional

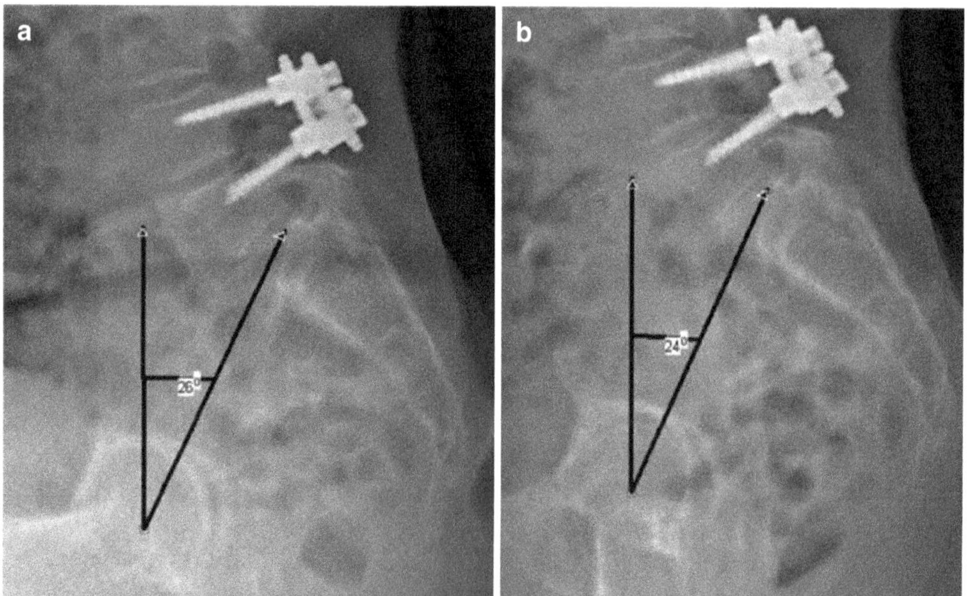

Fig. 13.4 Lateral sitting (**a**) and standing (**b**) plain films demonstrating minimal pelvic tilt change between the two functional positions in a patient with posterior L4-L5 spinal fusion for degenerative lumbar disease. The lack of pelvic tilt change limits cup anteversion in a sitting position, which increases the risk of dislocation

positions may be deduced as described by Lembeck [13]. In cases with limited changes in pelvic tilt, and therefore limited increase in cup anteversion when going from standing to sitting, it may be important to consider increasing the anteversion of the revision acetabular component to account for this limited pelvic mobility.

13.5 3-D Imaging to Assess Patient-Specific Component Position

13.5.1 Computed Tomography 3-D Imaging

Obtaining a CT scan prior to THA is not routine practice but is often done as part of the protocol of some robotic-assisted computer navigation tools. CT imaging can be used to template component positioning preoperatively and offers the advantage of axial imaging of the acetabular anteversion, anterior and posterior wall thickness, and a better delineation of the proximal femoral anatomy including femoral version. In complex cases of osteolysis and revision THA, CT imaging can better delineate bone loss and becomes even more important for preoperative planning and implant choice. However, CT imaging is still a static imaging modality that does not consider the dynamic changes in acetabular orientation between different functional positions. Furthermore, CT imaging may be used to determine femoral component version, which is useful when evaluating total hip instability.

13.5.2 Statistical Shape Modeling Method of Converting 2-D to 3-D Imaging

Although three-dimensional imaging is useful in preoperative planning and templating for patient-specific component positioning in THA, it is often derived from CT or MRI imaging which carry the inherent disadvantages of being expensive, time-consuming, and may expose the patient to significant ionizing radiation (CT).

A statistical shape model (SSM) reconstruction technique has been used to create a patient-specific 3-D surface model of the pelvis based on a single 2-D AP view of the pelvis [14]. This technique is predicated on landmark-based initialization and iterative matching of apparent image contours extracted from the 2-D radiograph to create a 3-D reconstruction. This method is a feasible technique to create patient-specific 3-D images, which may be used for preoperative planning without obtaining MRI or CT scan. This technique has also been successful in creating 3-D reconstructions of the lumbar vertebral anatomy [15].

13.5.3 The Use of CT Imaging in Assessment of Personalized Component Implantation

Precise assessment of conventionally implanted hip prostheses is possible with CT imaging by measuring component orientation relative to anatomical landmarks. For example, cup orientation and prosthetic neck anteversion are respectively measured relatively to the anterior pelvic plane and posterior condylar line. Similarly, CT imaging is useful in accurate assessment and quality control of personalized THA implantation, particularly if preoperative CT imaging is available for comparison (osteoarthritic vs. prosthetic anatomy). Comparisons of the pre- and postoperative imaging can indicate whether the native proximal femoral and acetabular orientations and the hip center of rotation have been appropriately reproduced and whether the components were implanted with accuracy compared to the preoperative template (Fig. 13.5). 3-D CT imaging of the native hip or the planned hip replacement and the executed THA can be overlaid to provide insight of the precision of the personalized implantation technique. If pre-operative 3-D imaging is unavailable, a direct comparison between the prosthetic and contralateral hip may be of utility. Nevertheless, this method is may be limited, as the symmetry index between the axial anatomical parameters (femoral neck and acetabular anteversion) of both hips in a given individual may be weaker than previously thought. Despite this utility in the postoperative evaluation of a personalized THA, CT imaging is a static modality, obtained in a supine position, and is best interpreted in conjunction with the previ-

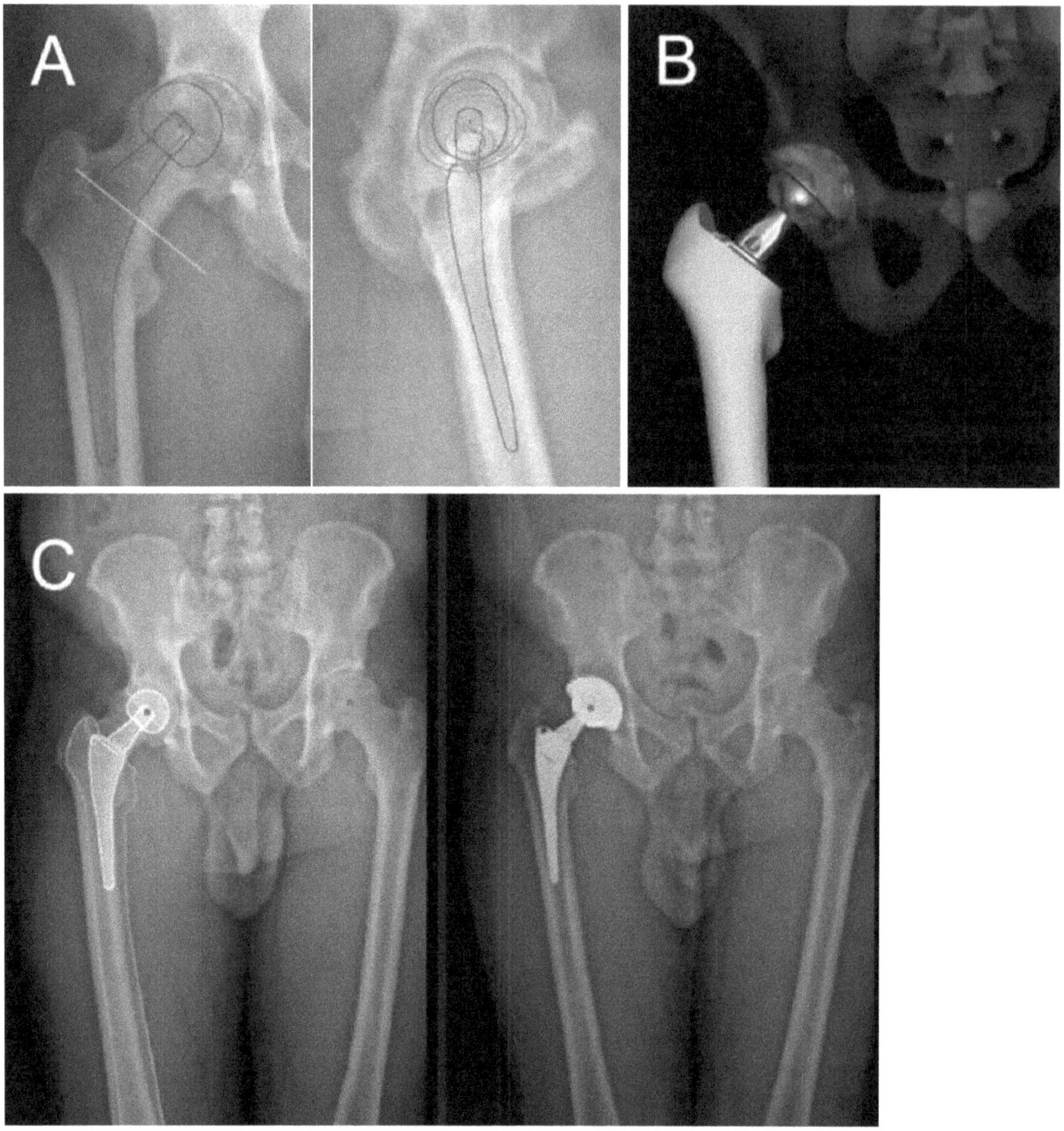

Fig. 13.5 This figure illustrates the planning of a total hip replacement on bi-dimensional EOS images (**a**), with tri-dimensional rendering (**b**) and relocation of postoperative pelvic radiograph (**c**) (With the courtesy and permission of E. Maury, MD, University Hospital of Montpellier, France)

ously mentioned dynamic radiographs assessing spino-pelvic dynamics for a given patient.

13.6 Conclusion

Traditional plain radiography in the form of an AP pelvis and frog or cross table lateral of the hip are useful but may not capture spino-pelvic dynamics, which are critical to stability of THA. Based on recent findings, the concept of a defined "safe zone" of component position has evolved to a more dynamic and functional definition. In order to determine this appropriate patient-specific "safe zone," modern imaging techniques such as sitting and standing alignment plain radiographs are necessary for improved understanding of spino-pelvic dynamics and more appropriate component positioning to minimize the risk of instability and maximize bearing performance in THA. Personalized total hip component implantation should aim to recreate normal hip joint anatomy, with a "safe zone" that matches an individual's spino-pelvic dynamics. Three-dimensional imaging systems can be useful in assessing the accuracy and quality of personalized hip implantation.

13.7 Case Presentation

A 75-year-old man with a history of lumbar radiculopathy initially underwent a primary right THA in 2014. He subsequently suffered two separate incidents of anterior right THA dislocation 4 years later, both in a position of hip extension. Preoperative evaluation of his total hip instability comprised of a supine AP pelvis, cross table lateral of the right hip, as well as sitting and standing AP and lateral alignment films (Fig. 13.6). Comparison of pelvic tilt from standing to sitting positions demonstrated limited change, signifying a stiff lumbar spine. Furthermore, in a standing position, the cup anteversion was found to be approximately 35°, while cup abduction was approximately 50° with respect to the coronal plane. Given this cup malposition, he was indicated for an acetabular component revision. Intraoperatively, stem version was found to be appropriate, and the stem was retained. However, the cup was revised to a dual mobility acetabular component, using computer navigation to place the new component in a position of less anteversion and inclination. Postoperatively, he recovered well, without further episodes of instability at 6 months of follow-up.

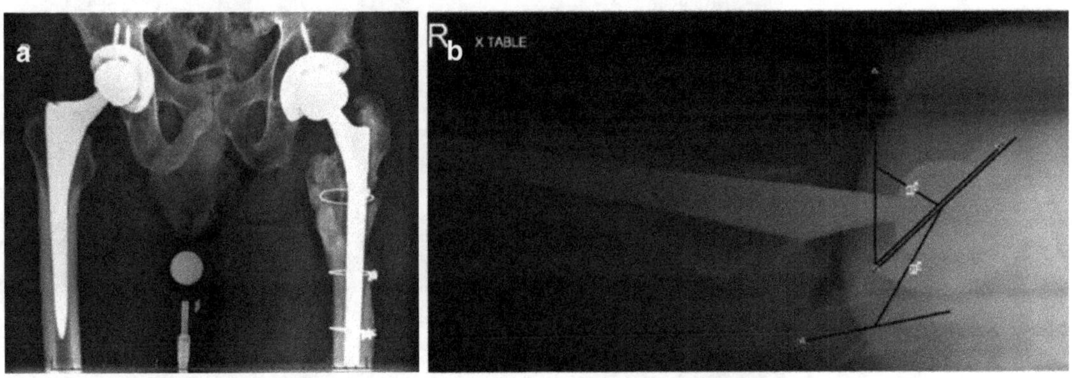

Fig. 13.6 Preoperative radiographic evaluation of a right total hip arthroplasty with anterior instability in the setting of degenerative lumbar stiffness. (**a**) Supine AP pelvis. (**b**) Supine cross table lateral view demonstrating the acetabular component anteversion measuring 48° using Woo and Morrey's method and 31° using the ischio-lateral method. This discrepancy can be attributed to this increased patient's tilt in a supine position. (**c**) AP and lateral sitting and standing alignment films were obtained. (**d**) Using software analysis (Intellijoint) of the sitting and standing alignment films, the anterior pelvic plane-pelvic tilt angle change from standing to sitting is noted to be limited, indicating stiffness in lumbar spino-pelvic mobility. Additionally, the acetabular component inclination and anteversion in the standing position were noted to be 51 and 35°, respectively

Fig. 13.6 (continued)

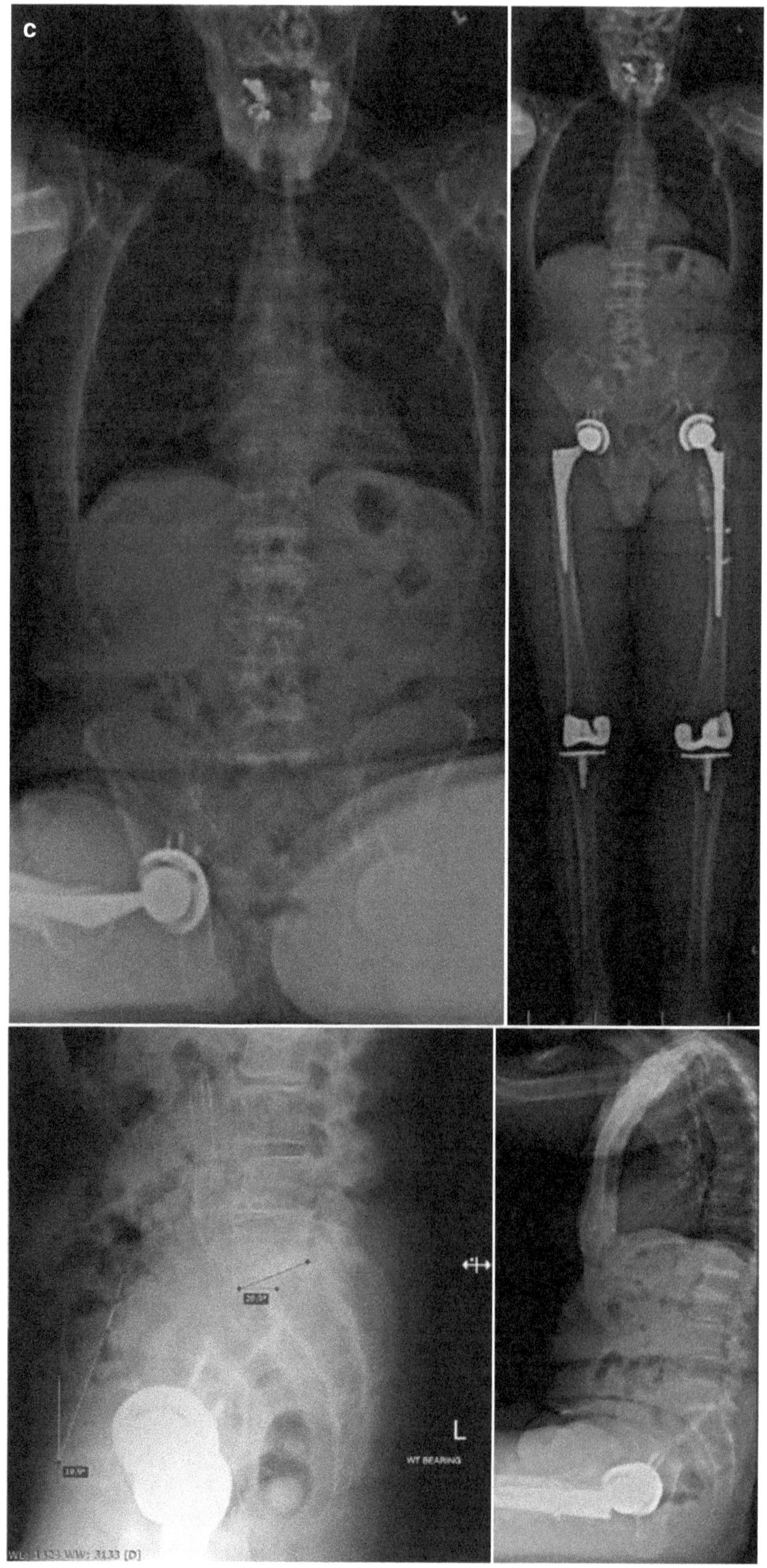

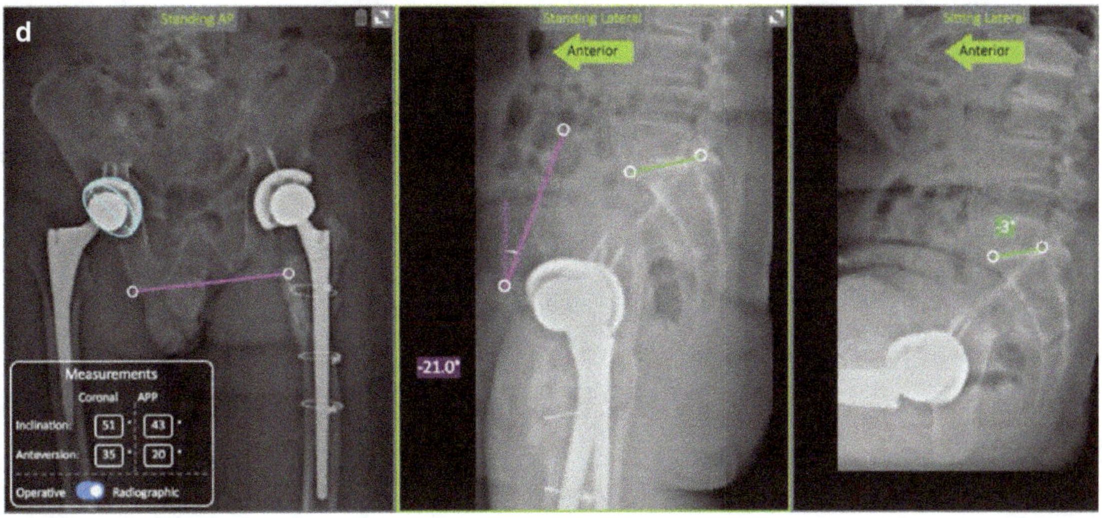

Fig. 13.6 (continued)

References

1. Lewinnek GE, Lewis JL, Tarr R, Compere CL, Zimmerman JR. Dislocations after total hip-replacement arthroplasties. J Bone Joint Surg Am. 1978;60(2):217.
2. Weber M, Lechler P, von Kunow F, Vollner F, Keshmiri A, Hapfelmeier A, Grifka J, Renkawitz T. The validity of a novel radiological method for measuring femoral stem version on anteroposterior radiographs of the hip after total hip arthroplasty. The Bone Joint J. 2015;97-B(3):306.
3. Woerner ML, Weber M, Craiovan BS, Springorum HR, Grifka J, Renkawitz TF. Radiographic assessment of femoral stem torsion in total hip arthroplasty-a comparison of a caput-collum-diaphyseal angle-based technique with the budin view. J Arthroplast. 2016;31(5):1117.
4. Pulos N, Tiberi Iii JV 3rd, Schmalzried TP. Measuring acetabular component position on lateral radiographs—ischio-lateral method. Bull NYU Hosp Jt Dis. 2011;69(Suppl 1):S84.
5. Abdel MP, von Roth P, Jennings MT, Hanssen AD, Pagnano MW. What safe zone? The vast majority of dislocated THAs are within the Lewinnek safe zone for acetabular component position. Clin Orthop Relat Res. 2016;474(2):386.
6. Buckland AJ, Puvanesarajah V, Vigdorchik J, Schwarzkopf R, Jain A, Klineberg EO, Hart RA, Callaghan JJ, Hassanzadeh H. Dislocation of a primary total hip arthroplasty is more common in patients with a lumbar spinal fusion. The Bone Joint J. 2017;99-B(5):585.
7. DelSole EM, Vigdorchik JM, Schwarzkopf R, Errico TJ, Buckland AJ. Total hip arthroplasty in the spinal deformity population: does degree of sagittal deformity affect rates of safe zone placement, instability, or revision? J Arthroplast. 2017;32(6):1910.
8. Fujita K, Kabata T, Maeda T, Kajino Y, Iwai S, Kuroda K, Hasegawa K, Tsuchiya H. The use of the transverse acetabular ligament in total hip replacement: an analysis of the orientation of the trial acetabular component using a navigation system. Bone Joint J. 2014;96-B(3):306.
9. Kanawade V, Dorr LD, Wan Z. Predictability of acetabular component angular change with postural shift from standing to sitting position. J Bone Joint Surg Am. 2014;96(12):978.
10. Stefl M, Lundergan W, Heckmann N, McKnight B, Ike H, Murgai R, Dorr LD. Spinopelvic mobility and acetabular component position for total hip arthroplasty. The Bone Joint J. 2017;99-B(1 Suppl A):37.
11. Esposito CI, Carroll KM, Sculco PK, Padgett DE, Jerabek SA, Mayman DJ. Total hip arthroplasty patients with fixed spinopelvic alignment are at higher risk of hip dislocation. J Arthroplast. 2018;33(5):1449.
12. Pierrepont JSC, Miles B, O'Connor P, Ellis A, Molnar R, Baré J, Solomon M, McMahon S, Shimmin A, Li Q, Walter L, Marel E. Patient-specific component alignment in total hip Arthroplasty. Reconstr Review. 2016;6(4):27.
13. Lembeck B, Mueller O, Reize P, Wuelker N. Pelvic tilt makes acetabular cup navigation inaccurate. Acta Orthop. 2005;76(4):517.
14. Zheng G. Statistical shape model-based reconstruction of a scaled, patient-specific surface model of the pelvis from a single standard AP X-ray radiograph. Med Phys. 2010;37(4):1424.
15. Zheng G, Nolte LP, Ferguson SJ. Scaled, patient-specific 3D vertebral model reconstruction based on 2-D lateral fluoroscopy. Int J Comput Assist Radiol Surg. 2011;6(3):351.

Part V

Patient Specific Knee Arthroplasty

14

Knee Arthroplasty: Anatomy and Biomechanics of the Knee

Vera Pinskerova and Pavel Vavrik

14.1 What Is the Normal Knee Biomechanics?

From the late 1960s to the early 1990s, when much of the original design work on knee replacement prostheses was carried out, the kinematics of the knee were universally understood to involve a rigid 4-bar link mechanism. It was understood that as the knee flexed, this mechanism caused both femoral condyles to roll back across the top of the tibia and then to roll forward with extension. Because this was thought to be a normal feature of knee flexion/extension, tibial components were made relatively unconstrained anteroposteriorly, thus permitting "roll back/forward." The concept of the 4-bar link mechanism originated with the work of Zuppinger [1]. The concept became part of received orthopedic knowledge, perhaps as a consequence of its appearance in a number of widely used textbooks.

In 1941 Brantigan and Voshell [2] reported that "the medial femoral condyle acts as the axis of rotation of the knee joint." They based this conclusion on their observation that the medial meniscus hardly moves anteroposteriorly in flexion, whereas the lateral meniscus moves backward. From the late 1990s onward, a number of investigators have used MRI and other techniques to demonstrate that Brantigan and Voshell were correct: the medial femoral condyle hardly moves anteroposteriorly between 0° and 120°, whereas the lateral femoral condyle moves about 20 mm anteroposteriorly over that arc. The arc from 120° to full flexion follows a different kinematic regime.

The shapes of the articulating surfaces: The sagittal and coronal shapes and modes of articulation observed using MRI have been confirmed by dissection and cryosection [3], by 3D digitization [4], and by CT [5]. The following description of the shape of the articulating bones is based on that work. The surface shapes in sagittal section are relevant to flexion/extension: when circular femoral surfaces contact the tibia, pure flexion may be thought to occur around their centers. *Medial femorotibial compartment:* The articular surface of the medial femoral condyle in sagittal section can be regarded as posteriorly circular (the flexion facet, FF, center: the FFC, see Fig. 14.1a) with an average radius of about 22 mm subtending an arc of 110°. The extreme posterior portion of the condyle (about 24° of arc) is of a smaller radius, but this portion contacts only the posterior horn (in extreme flexion), never the tibia itself, and is therefore not part of the direct tibiofemoral articulation (posterior horn facet, PHF). Anteriorly there is a second surface which may be approximated to a 50° arc of a second circle with a larger radius (32 mm), the extension facet (EF, center: the EFC). The

V. Pinskerova (✉) · P. Vavrik
1st Orthopaedic Clinic, 1st Faculty of Medicine, Charles University, Prague, Czech Republic
e-mail: vera.pinskerova@lf1.cuni.cz

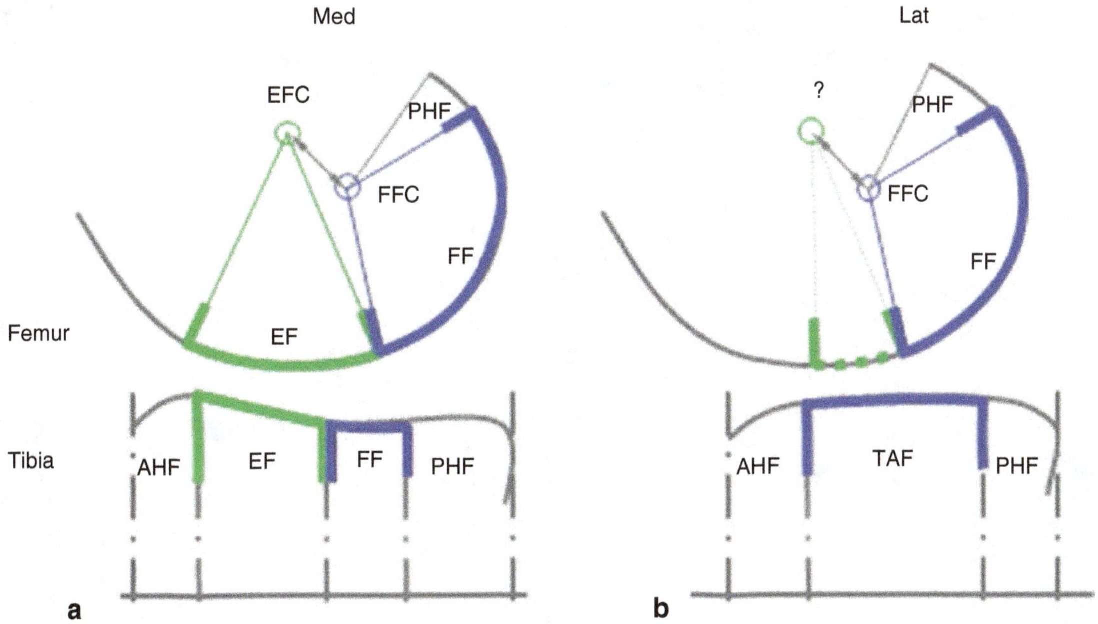

Fig. 14.1 Sagittal sections through the center of the medial (**a**) and lateral (**b**) compartments (see text)

medial tibial surface, if sectioned centrally, can be seen to be posteriorly flat and horizontal over approximately 25 mm (the flexion facet, FF). The posterior 15 mm of this surface always contacts the posterior horn of the meniscus (posterior horn facet, PHF). Anteriorly the surface slopes 11° upward and forward (the extension facet, EF) to contact the anterior circular surface of the femur in extension. *Lateral femorotibial compartment:* Laterally, the femur also has a posterior circular surface (FF, see Fig. 14.1b) subtending on average 114° with a radius of 21 mm. Anteriorly, the extension facet is much shorter compared to the medial condyle and therefore difficult to distinguish. The extreme posterior part of the femoral condyle (PHF) again contacts only the posterior horn of the meniscus, never the tibia. The extreme anterior end of the articular surface is relatively flat and contacts the anterior horn and the anterior extremity of the tibial articular surface in full extension (AHF). The central 24 mm of the lateral tibial surface is relatively flat (tibial articular facet, TAF). Anteriorly and posteriorly, the surface curves downward to receive the horns of the meniscus in extension and flexion (AHF, PHF), enhancing the impression of upward convexity, usually described as upwardly convex.

Collateral ligaments: Collaterals differ in the position of their attachment to the femur. The medial epicondyle with the medial collateral ligament (MCL) attachment coincides with the penetration point of the EFC. Medially, at first, contact occurs between the femoral and the tibial extension facets, the femur rotating on the tibia around the EFC axis and, therefore, around the MCL attachment (Fig. 14.2a). At about 30° flexion, contact "rocks" onto the flexion facets, and the femur then rotates around the FFC axis (Fig. 14.2b). From then on, the MCL attachment rotates upward and backward around the FFC. The lateral collateral ligament (LCL) is attached to the femur at the lateral epicondyle. This coincides with the center of the femoral flexion facet, i.e., the entry point of the transcondylar axis. At full extension, the LCL is tight. As the knee flexes, there is backward motion of the lateral femoral condyle. The LCL becomes more vertical with flexion up to about 90°, the ligament being visibly slack. With flexion to 120°, the femoral condyle "drops" as it rolls over the

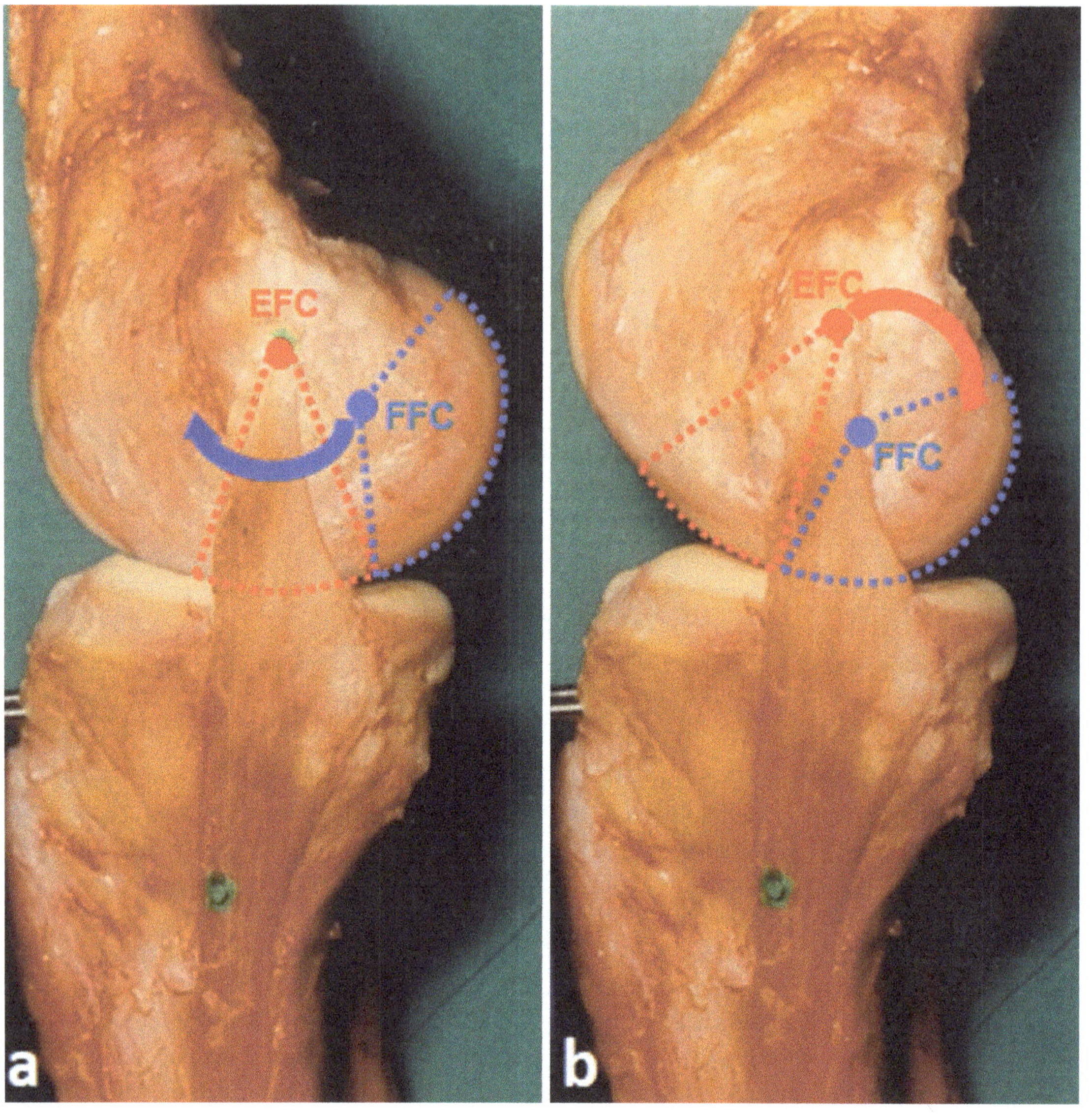

Fig. 14.2 Specimen viewed from the medial side in extension (**a**) and at 30° flexion (**b**), showing the position of the MCL femoral attachment (see text)

posterior round surface of the tibia, further relaxing the LCL. As a result, collaterals differ in that the MCL (at least its anterior superficial portion [6]) remains tight during flexion, whereas the LCL relaxes with flexion.

The relative movement of the condyles: The movement of the knee has been considered in this review in the context of the lower limb as a whole. Considered in isolation, descriptions of knee movement in terms of rotations, translations, and axes may be given either as the position of the contact areas or as the movement of the condyles. This section deals with the latter. The movement of the knee can be divided into three functional arcs: terminal extension [1], arc of active flexion [2], and arc of passive flexion [3].

Terminal extension: This begins at the subject's limit of passive extension. This varies from about 5° flexion to about 5° hyperextension. The arc has peculiarities: the contact surfaces differ from those in the arc of active flexion; there is thought to be a near-obligatory association between longitudinal rotation and flexion. There is always a tendency toward internal femoral rotation. MR images show that rotation, when it occurs, is due to continued forward movement of the lateral femoral condyle, while the medial femoral condyle does not move anteroposteriorly. To achieve full extension, the medial femoral condyle must "rock" up onto the upward-sloping tibial condyle (Fig. 14.3a); the lateral femoral condyle rolls forward onto the flat tibial surface (Fig. 14.3b). Finally, as terminal rotation ends with both condyles immobilized anteroposteriorly, it obviously helps to stabilize the knee.

Arc of active flexion: In the arc of active flexion, the medial femoral condyle can be viewed as a sphere which rotates to produce a variable combination of flexion, longitudinal rotation, and minimal varus (if lift off occurs laterally). It hardly translates and thus is analogous to a somewhat constrained ball-in-socket joint. The lateral condyle rolls but also "slides" anteroposteriorly. This permits longitudinal rotation around an axis passing through the center of the medial sphere (the FFC) and flexion around an axis penetrating the two FFCs (because the femoral surfaces are circular and remain in contact with the tibia). The medial femoral condyle translates no more than 7.1 mm anteroposteriorly, weight bearing and non-weight bearing [7]. The lateral femoral condyle also rotates around its FFC, but in contrast to the medial side, it tends to translate posteriorly about 15 mm by a mixture of rolling and sliding [7, 8]. As a consequence, between 10° and 120°, the femur tends to rotate externally (tibia internally) about 30° around a medial axis (Fig. 14.4). In the living weight-bearing knee during a squat, the general pattern of motion is again the same, although backward movement of the lateral femoral condyle may occur earlier [9]. At 90°, the tibia is free to rotate 20°–30° longitudinally without accompanying flexion.

Arc of passive flexion: This begins in a transition zone from 110° to 120° and continues to whatever may be the passive limit of the knee under study. The arc is entirely passive; the thigh muscles can flex the knee only to about 120° against gravity. In the range of flexion from 120° to 160°, the flexion

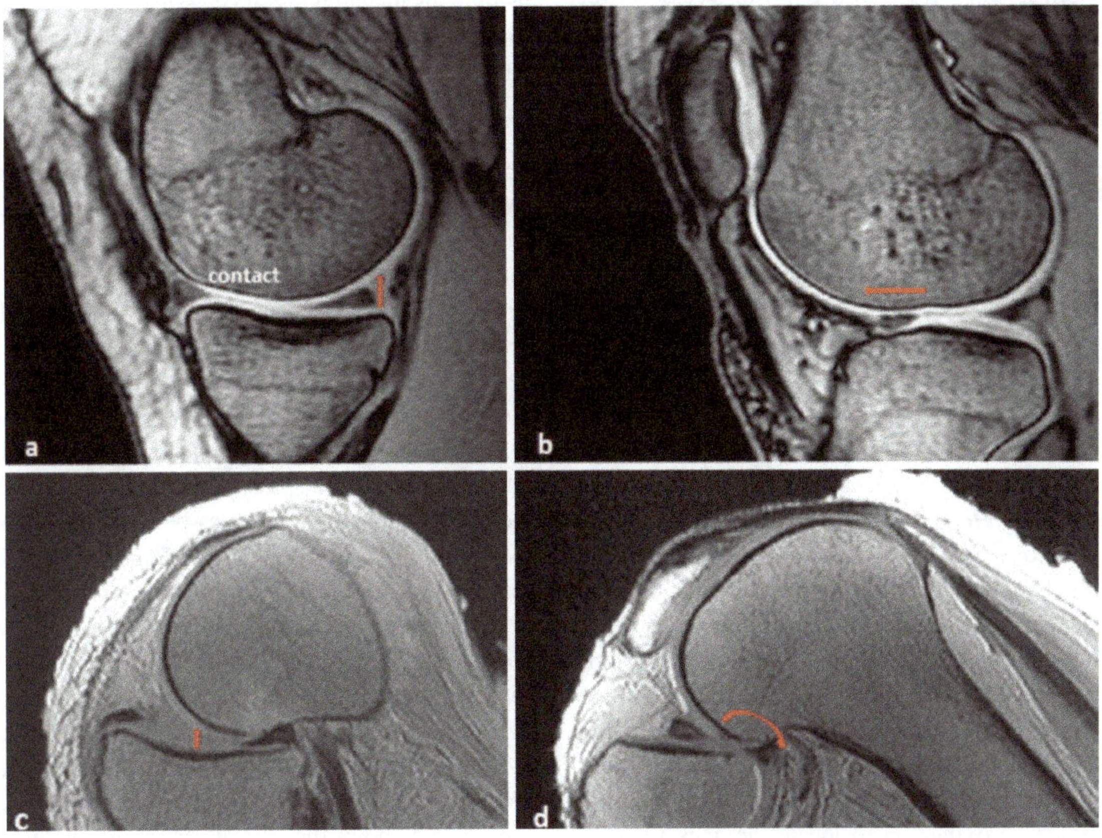

Fig. 14.3 Sagittal MRI through the medial (**a**) and the lateral compartments (**b**) in hyperextension (see text); sagittal MRI through the medial (**c**) and the lateral (**d**) compartments in 140° flexion (see text)

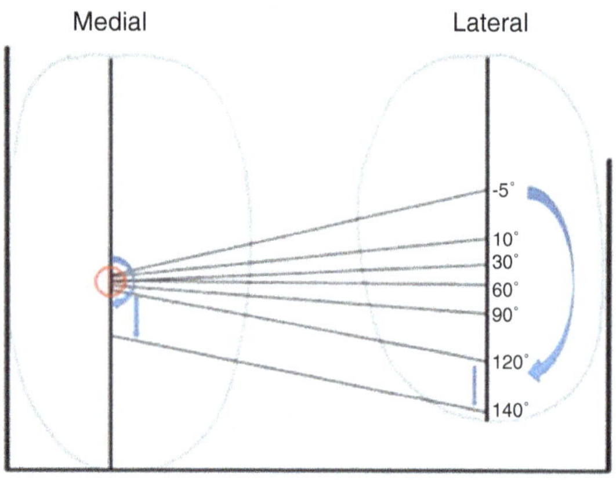

Fig. 14.4 Top of the tibia diagram showing the position of flexion axis from −5° to 140° flexion (see text)

facet center of the medial femoral condyle moves back about 5 mm and rises up on to the posterior horn of the medial meniscus. At 160°, the posterior horn is compressed in a synovial recess between the femoral cortex and the tibia (Fig. 14.3c). This limits flexion. The lateral femoral condyle also rolls back, with the posterior horn of the lateral meniscus moving with the condyle. Both move down over the curved posterior border of the tibia (Fig. 14.3d). Neither the events between 120° and 160° nor the anatomy at 160° could result from a continuation of the kinematics up to 120°. Therefore, hyperflexion is a separate arc of flexion. The anatomical and functional features of this arc suggest that it would be difficult to design an implant for total knee replacement that would enable physiological movement from 0° to 160° [10].

The Position of the Instant Axes from Full Extension to 160° Flexion: The femoral condyles are composed of two circular arcs (the EF and the FF), these arcs forming the articular surfaces. The instant axes of flexion pass through their centers (the EFC and the FFC). The anteroposterior orientation of the axes is measured as their vertical position relative to the posterior tibial cortex. *On the medial side*, from full extension to 120°, motion is 96% sliding which makes it a reasonable approximation to locate the axes vertically at the geometrical center of the contacting femoral facet (i.e., the EFC or the FFC). *Laterally*, from full extension to 120°, there is about 40% rolling, suggesting that the axis lies about halfway between the center and the contact point. Anteroposteriorly the penetration point of the axis will be vertically below the geometrical center, that is, on a line perpendicular to the tibial contact surface. In the arc of passive flexion (from 120° to 160°), as both femoral condyles roll back, the penetration points of the flexion axis appear to be at the posterior extremities of the medial and lateral femoral articular surfaces [10].

Longitudinal Rotation: Longitudinal rotation can be divided into that which accompanies flexion and that which occurs independently of flexion. We refer to rotation relative to the tibia of the femoral condyles, not to the flexion axes. The axis of longitudinal rotation is parallel to the long axis of the tibia. Zero might be defined as the rotational position of the femoral condyles at 0° flexion. Alternatively, zero might be defined as the rotational position of the femoral condyles relative to the frontal plane. From extension to 120° flexion, the medial femoral condyle does not move anteroposteriorly, while the lateral one moves posteriorly 18 mm. Figure 14.4 shows a diagram of tibial condyles with lines representing the connection of the medial and the lateral FFCs from −5° to 140° flexion. If the tibia is considered as fixed, the femur tends to rotate externally 20°. During the arc of the terminal extension, the femur rotates externally about 7°. There is thought to be a near-obligatory association between longitudinal rotation and flexion. In the arc of active flexion, the tibia (femur) is free to rotate 20–30° longitudinally without accompanying flexion. Thus the tibial IR which usually accompanies flexion is not obligatory. During the passive arc of flexion, as the medial femoral condyle moves back about 3 mm more than the lateral one, a little femoral internal rotation occurs from 120° to 160° of flexion [10].

Varus/Valgus Rotation: In full extension, both collateral ligaments are tight, and varus/valgus rotation is therefore hardly possible. *As the knee flexes*, the lateral collateral ligament becomes loose and enables not only longitudinal rotation around the medial axis but also varus rotation. Figure 14.5 shows the frontal section of the knee at 90° flexion with varus force applied to the tibia. The lateral joint space opens by a mean of 6.7°

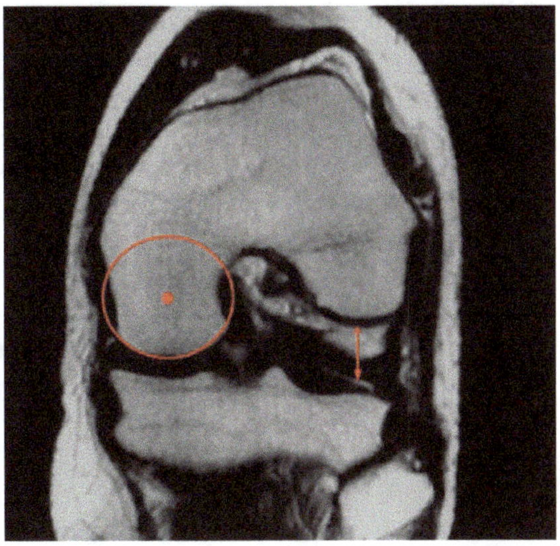

Fig. 14.5 Frontal MRI of a volunteer's knee at 90° flexion, with varus stress applied. For reasons explained in the text, the LCL is slack, and therefore the femur can be separated from the tibia laterally

(so-called lift off). The medial joint gap under valgus stress opens only by a mean of 2.1 mm [11]. There is therefore a clear asymmetry between the lateral and medial flexion gaps. This asymmetry can be explained both by the laxity of the LCL and by the shapes of the articulating bones. In the coronal plane, the posterior portion of the medial femoral condyle is also spherical; therefore, varus rotation occurs around the axis passing through the center of this sphere. *In full flexion*, valgus-varus movement was measured in volunteers whose knees were fully flexed and stressed manually into tibial valgus and varus [10]. No movement was detected on valgus stress, but the lateral compartment opened up to 10 mm under varus stress. These findings would be expected from the observed tensions in the collateral ligaments.

Finally, in the arc of active flexion, we can define three axes of motion (Fig. 14.6) which

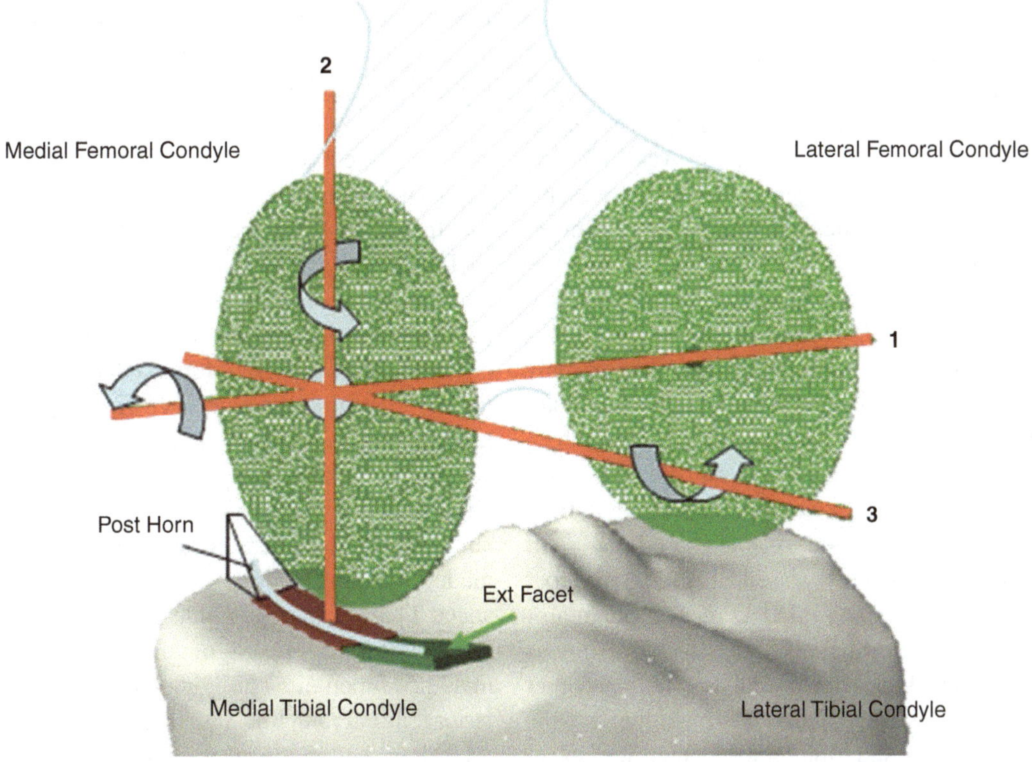

Fig. 14.6 Model of the knee showing the orientation of the three axes of motion in the active arc of flexion: 1, flexion axis; 2, longitudinal rotation axis; and 3, varus/valgus axis. They intersect roughly in the center of the posterior portion of the medial femoral condyle

are perpendicular to each other. They intersect around the center of the posterior portion of the medial femoral condyle (i.e., FFC).

14.2 How Inter-Individually Variable Is Knee Anatomy?

There is high individual variability in the tibiofemoral joint with respect to the anatomy, tissue properties, joint kinetics, and kinematics. It is influenced by both intra-articular and extra-articular parameters.

Increased attention has been paid to the shape, in particular, with respect to race and gender differences, of the distal femur. Data from the literature suggest that the female knee is narrower than the male knee, regardless of its size [12, 13]. It has been reported that standard TKA (total knee arthroplasty) used for a narrow female knee results in ML overhang of the femoral component [14]. Bellemans et al. [15] suggested that there are factors other than gender which also have an influence on the shape of the knee and that there is variability within each gender which could be explained by morphotypic variation. The morphotype characterization was based on the pelvis width/total leg length ratio. Patients with short and wide morphotype (endomorph) had, irrespective of gender, wider knees, whereas patients with long and narrow morphotype (ectomorph) had narrower knees. Morphotype significantly predicted the femoral aspect ratio but only weakly predicted the tibial aspect ratio. Lancaster and Nunley [16, 17] report a wide variation in the angle between extension and flexion facets of the medial tibial condyle (EFA) in normal knees that is unrelated to age. There is an association between an increased EFA (i.e., a steeper extension facet) and MRI evidence of anteromedial osteoarthritis. Although a causal link is not proven, Lancaster speculates that a steeper angle increases the duration of loading on the EF in stance and tibiofemoral interface shear. Eckhoff et al. [18] suggest there is a variation in the so-called "version" of the knee, defined as the static rotation of the tibia with respect to the femur in full knee extension. This angle, representing external rotation of the tibia relative to the femur, was increased significantly in patients with anterior knee pain. In conclusion, there is high individual variability in tibiofemoral joint conformity, and a wide range of TKA component sizes and shapes would be required to accurately replicate native joint conformity in most people.

14.3 When to Re-create and When Not to Recreate the Constitutional Knee Anatomy?

It follows that, firstly, when describing movement of the knee, care must be taken to define whether it is the contact points or the condyles that are under investigation since the two move differently and the movement of the bones cannot be deduced solely from the contact areas; secondly, that while it may be possible to design a total knee replacement implant which could replicate either the movement of the condyles or the contact areas, to replicate both, i.e., to produce normality, is probably impossible.

Key to a successful outcome of TKA is to achieve correct alignment, proper balance, and deformity correction.

Mechanical alignment in TKA introduced by Insall et al. [19] was used to achieve an even load distribution on the new joint line. However, part of the patients is still disappointed with the outcome. Bellemans [20] reports there is increasing evidence that for a number of patients, neutral alignment is not normal. For patients with so-called constitutional varus, restoring neutral alignment may not be the best option since it is abnormal to them. The development of a kinematic alignment aims to provide a properly balanced TKA during the whole arc of motion. The concept of kinematic alignment is to restore normal knee function by aligning the distal and posterior femoral joint line of the femoral component according the functional femoral transverse axes and joint line of the tibial component to those of the normal or pre arthritic condition.

This is possible in primary osteoarthritis without severe bone defects and ligament laxity.

Resurfacing the knee joint with kinematic alignment by preserving normal ligament laxities may be an attractive option in these cases.

However, certain circumstances such as post-traumatic arthritis or rheumatoid arthritis are often associated with severe deformities, significant bone defects, contractures, and instability. Such deformities are extremely difficult to balance with soft tissue release only and require additionally constrained prostheses even in primary TKA. To correct varus deformity, various techniques including step releases and multiple needle puncturing of the medial soft tissue structures during TKA are in common use. Correctly tensioned MCL represents the fundamental condition of restoring normal knee kinematics. Using anatomic designs after adequate medial release is therefore a method of choice because the primary stabilizer of the medial compartment is preserved.

Correction of fixed valgus deformity during TKA presents a challenging task. Multiple techniques to restore limb alignment and correct instability have been described, including various techniques of lateral soft tissue release, lateral femoral sliding, epicondylar osteotomy, reconstruction of the medial collateral ligament, and finally the use of a constrained condylar implant.

Little data exists to describe the kinematics of severe valgus knee. Baier [21] describes a paradoxical longitudinal rotation during flexion, suggesting that valgus knee rotates around the lateral axis. On the assumption that collateral ligaments behave conversely during flexion (i.e., MCL is loose and LCL remains tight), it would be extremely difficult, if not impossible, to restore natural knee kinematics using medially rotating knee designs. In such a situation, constrained condylar knee designs are the ultimate choice.

14.4 Can the Natural Knee Kinematics Be Reproduced in TKA?

Total knee arthroplasty has now been performed for more than five decades. The procedure has been successful in relieving patients', pain but both orthopedic surgeons and patients continue to seek a better functional outcome. However, a "forgotten" knee after TKA is unusual, whereas a "forgotten" hip after total hip replacement is commonplace.

It has been shown in multiple in vivo analyses that the kinematic patterns after mechanically aligned TKA differ considerably from those of the normal knee [22]. Pritchett [23] analyzed patients' preferences in mechanically aligned knee replacement. In a group of 688 of bilateral knee arthroplasty recipients (after excluding poor results), most of the patients thought one knee was worse than the other. They attributed this to the feeling of the inferior knee being less normal, weaker, on stairs, or less stable. It is interesting that the preferred knees all had a-p stable design: all of the patients preferred either the retention of both cruciates with the use of an ACL-PCL prosthesis or a substitution with medially pivoting designs.

Conventional designs of knee replacements, i.e., the posterior cruciate ligament (PCL) retaining and PCL substituting knees, failed to reproduce normal knee kinematics. Anterior cruciate ligament deficiency after TKA causes femoral forward motion during knee flexion, the so-called paradoxical motion. However, too much joint laxity is associated with persistent pain and poor long-term outcomes as a result of instability, causing premature polyethylene wear.

To improve anteroposterior stability, bicruciate-retaining total knee arthroplasty was introduced. However, it did not gain widespread popularity over recent decades because of unpredictable tensioning of the retained cruciate ligaments. Too high or low tension in the ACL can cause knee stiffness or instability after bicruciate-retaining TKA [24].

To reduce abnormal strains at the bone–implant interface during motion, mobile-bearing knee replacements based on a mobile polyethylene insert that articulates with a metallic femoral component and a metallic tibial tray were introduced.

However, relatively high rate of mechanical complications (including loosening of the femoral component, tibiofemoral dislocation in high flexion, and insert breakage) was described [25].

The stability and the kinematics of the knee depend on the musculature, the surrounding ligaments, the implants' orientation, and the geometry of the articular surfaces. Since the TKA procedure is nowadays performed on younger, more active patients, proper anteroposterior stability, and natural axial rotation patterns are essential for good patellar tracking and improved knee flexion.

TKA design should therefore provide anteroposterior stability and simultaneously allow longitudinal rotation, i.e., reproduce the pattern of movement of the natural knee. The concept, based on ball-in-socket geometry medially and with less constrained lateral surface, enables longitudinal rotation around the medial axis. This movement is possible because the LCL is loose in flexion. The combination of fully congruent medial compartment and flat lateral tibial surface, together with tight MCL and loose LCL, enables flexion accompanied with femoral external rotation around the stable medial condyle. The increased contact area reduces contact stresses and subsequent linear polyethylene wear.

Fully congruent medial designs reproduce neither the normal knee anatomy nor the motion toward full extension. Nevertheless, reproducing the anterior "rocking" of the medial femoral condyle onto the tibial extension facet toward full extension in TKA would increase the loading of the anterior lip of the tibial insert, causing excessive polyethylene wear. In deep flexion, the medially conforming articulation is beneficial in controlling the femoral AP position.

With the improvement of imaging and image processing technologies, the patient-specific cutting guides and patient-specific implants developed with the aim to create articular surfaces which closely mimic natural anatomy and kinematics of the knee.

In conclusion, providing stable and consistent knee kinematics in total knee replacement is an essential requirement of good long-term clinical results.

References

1. Zuppinger H. Die aktive flexion im unbelasteten Kniegelenk. Bergmann: Züricher Habil. Schr. Wiesbaden; 1904. p. 703–63.
2. Brantigan OC, Voshell AF. The mechanics of the ligaments and menisci of the knee joint. J Bone Joint Surg. 1941;23:44.
3. Iwaki H, Pinskerova V, Freeman MAR. Tibio-femoral movement 1: the shapes and relative movements of the femur and tibia in the unloaded cadaver knee. J Bone Joint Surg. 2000;82B(8):1189–95.
4. Martelli S, Pinskerova V. The shapes of the tibial femoral articular surfaces in relation to tibiofemoral movement. J Bone J Surg. 2002;84B:607–13.
5. McPherson A, Karrholm J, Pinskerova V, Sosna A, Martelli S. Imaging knee motion using MRI, RSA/CT and 3D digitization. J Biomech. 2005;38(2):263–8.
6. Gardiner JC, Weiss JA, Rosenberg TD. Strain in the human medial collateral ligament during valgus loading of the knee. Clin Orthop Rel Res. 2001;391:266–74.
7. Johal P, Williams A, Wragg P, Gedroyc W, Hunt M. Tibio-femoral movement in the living knee. An in-vivo study of weight bearing and non-weight bearing knee kinematics using 'interventional' MRI. J Biomech. 2005;38(2):269–76.
8. Kurosawa H, Walker PS, Abe S, Garg A, Hunter T. Geometry and motion of the knee for implant and orthotic design. J Biomech. 1985;18(7):487–99.
9. Hill PF, Vedi V, Iwaki H, Pinskerova V, Freeman MAR, Williams A. Tibio-femoral movement 2: the loaded and unloaded living knee studied by MRI. J Bone Joint Surg. 2000;82B(8):1196–8.
10. Pinskerova V, Samuelson KM, Stammers J, Maruthainar K, Sosna A, Freeman MAR. The knee in full flexion an anatomical study. J Bone Joint Surg. 2009;91B(6):830–4.
11. Tokuhara Y, Kadoya Y, Nakagawa S, Kobayashi A, Takaoka K. The flexion gap in normal knees: a MRI study. J Bone Joint Surg. 2004;86B:1133–6.
12. Dargel J, Joern WPM, Feiser J, Ivo R, Koebke J. Human knee joint anatomy revisited: morphometry in the light of sex-specific Total knee arthroplasty. J Arthroplast. 2011;26(3):346–53.
13. Guy SP, Farndon MA, Sidhom S, Al-Lami M, Bennett C, London NJ. Gender differences in distal femoral morphology and the role of gender specific implants in total knee replacement: a prospective clinical study. Knee. 2012;19(1):28–31.
14. Koninckx A, Deltour A, Thienpont E. Femoral sizing in total knee arthroplasty is rotation dependent. Knee Surg Sports Traumatol Arthrosc. 2014;22(12):2941–6.
15. Bellemans J, Carpentier K, Vandenneucker H, Vanlauwe J, Victor J. The John Insall Award. Both morphotype and gender influence the shape of the knee in patients undergoing TKA. Clin Orthop Relat Res. 2010;468:29–36.

16. Lancaster BJA, Cottam HL, Pinskerova V, Eldridge JDJ, Freeman MAR. Variation in the of the tibial plateau. A possible factor in the development of anteromedial osteoarthritis of the knee. J Bone Joint Surg. 2008;90B(3):330–3.
17. Nunley RM, Nam D, Johnson SR, Barnes CL. Extreme variability in posterior slope of the proximal tibia: measurements on 2395 CT scans of patients undergoing UKA. J Arthroplast. 2014;29:1677–80.
18. Eckhoff DG, Brown AW, Licoyne RF, Stamm ER. Knee version associated with anterior knee pain. Clin Orthop Relat Res. 1997;339:152–5.
19. Insall JN, Binazzi R, Soudry M, et al. Total knee arthroplasty. Clin Orthop Relat Res. 1985;192:13–2.
20. Bellemans J. Neutral mechanical alignment: a requirement for successful TKA: opposes. Orthopedics. 2011;34:e507–9.
21. Baier C, Benditz A, Koeck F, Keshmiri A, Grifka J, Maderbacher G. Different kinematics of knees with varus and valgus deformities. J Knee Surg. 2018;31(3):264–9.
22. Blakeney W, Clément J, Desmeules F, Hagemeister N, Rivière C, Vendittoli PA. Kinematic alignment in total knee arthroplasty better reproduces normal gait than mechanical alignment. Knee Surg Sports Traumatol Arthrosc. 2019;27(5):1410–7.
23. Pritchett JW. Patient preferences in knee prostheses. J Bone Joint Surg. 2004;86B(7):979–82.
24. Okada Y, Teramoto A, Takagi T, et al. ACL function in bicruciate-retaining total knee arthroplasty. J Bone Joint Surg Am. 2018;100:e114(1-7) d.
25. Chang CW, Lai KA, Yang CY, et al. Early mechanical complications of a multidirectional mobile-bearing total knee replacement. J Bone Joint Surg. 2011;93-B(4):479–83.

15

Total Knee Arthroplasty: Future Perspectives

William G. Blakeney and Pascal-André Vendittoli

Key Points

- After five decades of knee joint replacement development, we still do not reliably provide a forgotten knee joint to our patients.
- A better understanding of human anatomy will help to define the surgical goal during prosthetic implantation.
- Precise surgical tools like computer navigation, personalized instruments or robotics will be valuable to achieve each patient's individualised target.
- More anatomic surgical procedures and implants may better reproduce native joint kinematics.
- Improving perioperative care and reducing adverse events will remain major factors for success in knee joint replacement.
- The future of knee joint replacement relies on our capacity to restore patient-specific knee anatomy and function.

15.1 Introduction

Although total knee arthroplasty (TKA) is considered to be a cost-effective intervention, most patients do not experience natural joints, and it is reported that up to 20% of them are dissatisfied [1, 2]. A systematic review of gait analysis after TKA indicates that patients display significant kinematic differences from normal controls [3]. Due to the significant deficiencies in both our knowledge and technology in the past, we were far from replicating normal knee kinematics with TKA. These limitations in TKA function and patient satisfaction should stimulate us to restart the entire development process. Enhancements in our understanding of knee anatomy and biomechanics may suggest ways of improving TKA outcomes. Implant design needs to be advanced to reproduce the anatomy and kinematics of native knees. More precise surgical techniques with navigation, patient-matched instrumentation and robotics need to be further refined. The future of TKA is to produce more natural knee joints, with resultant improved patient satisfaction and ultimately a forgotten joint.

15.2 Historical Perspectives

The anatomy of the knee and its kinematics are complex and remain poorly understood. The normal anatomy varies widely, and pathological changes increase its variability further [4–6]. Instrument precision was poor, and implantation errors were frequent when TKA surgery was introduced in the 1970s [7]. The focus was therefore on implant survivorship rather than

W. G. Blakeney · P.-A. Vendittoli (✉)
Department of Surgery, Montreal University, CIUSSS-de-L'Est-de-L'Ile-de-Montréal, Hôpital Maisonneuve Rosemont, Montréal, QC, Canada

Department of Surgery, Albany Health Campus, Albany, WA, Australia reproducing normal knee anatomy and function. To simplify operations, surgeons selected neutral femoral and tibial cuts to create rectangular flexion and extension gaps and a neutral mechanical axis. Individual patient anatomy was not reproduced, with the focus on standardisation of the procedure. Bony anatomy modifications created by mechanical alignment are linked to mediolateral and flexion-extension joint gap imbalances [8]. Multiple soft tissue release techniques were developed to force the patient's soft tissues to adjust to the non-anatomical bone cuts.

There is a very large variation in the anatomy of the knee across individuals. The precise restoration of this anatomy during total knee arthroplasty (TKA) may improve knee stability, kinematics and clinical function. The future of TKA should therefore look to restore individual anatomy with a personalized joint replacement. Currently, there is a developing interest in new methods of alignment for TKA. In the future, this is likely to expand with a move away from traditional mechanical alignment to an individualised or kinematic alignment [9] (Fig. 15.1). In Chaps. 24, 25 and 26, a detailed description of these alignment philosophies are discussed. The authors feel a restricted kinematic alignment protocol offers the advantages of the restoration of the patient's constitutional limb anatomy but within a safe margin, which avoids reproducing the extreme pathologies that may result in early failure.

Conventional TKA instrumentation restricts the surgeon to standardised alignment, so new techniques and technologies are required to allow a patient-specific alignment.

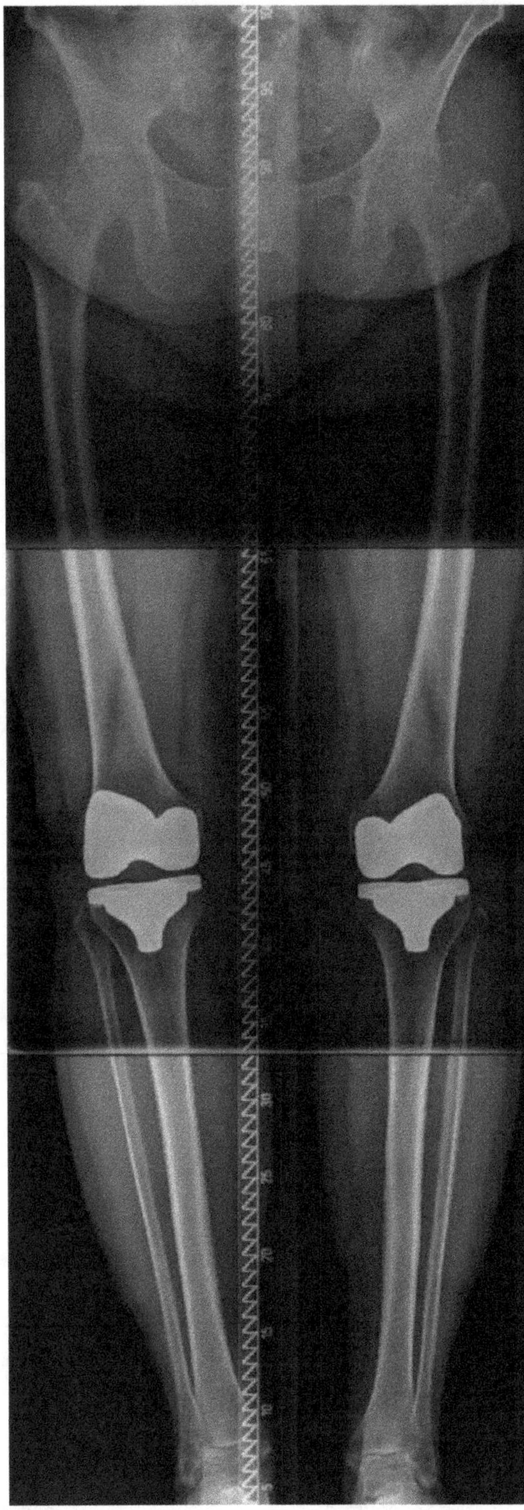

Fig. 15.1 Case example where the patient had the same TKA implant on both knees but the right knee implanted with MA and the left with KA. The patient achieved earlier ROM and higher clinical scores and preferred his left knee

15.3 Precision Technologies

Greater precision in surgery is now possible due to newer techniques using computer navigation, patient-specific instrumentation (PSI) and robotics. These technologies allow the surgeon to individualise the alignment of the knee replacement to replicate individual anatomy. Further study and refinement of these technologies will determine which will be the best to use going forward.

There is an abundance of evidence that computer navigation produces better precision than conventional instrumentation [10] but only limited evidence that this translates into better clinical outcomes [11]. The use of robotics in orthopaedic surgery is much more recent, so there is little evidence of efficacy in the literature at present. One benefit of PSI is standardisation of the procedure with all the planning done preoperatively, compared to computer navigation or robotic surgery where the planning is done at the time of surgery. This may lead to shorter operating times.

There is no doubt that greater accuracy in surgery is an important goal. Perhaps the reason why this greater accuracy has not always resulted in better clinical outcomes [12] is that we were aiming for the wrong target (Fig. 15.2). Accurately achieving a neutral HKA is of limited value if such implant orientation is not linked with improved patient satisfaction. With a new target in mind, being a personalized alignment goal for each patient, improved precision may reveal its value.

In a recent study, we compared the parameters of kinematics during gait of 36 TKA (single radius, CR) implanted using computer navigation with either kinematic alignment or mechanical alignment technique, with a group of 170 healthy controls [13]. Eighteen kinematically aligned TKAs were matched by gender and age to 18 mechanically aligned TKAs. Knee kinematics were assessed with the Knee KG™ (Emovi, Laval, Canada) frame and software (Fig. 15.3). The kinematic alignment group showed no significant knee kinematic differences compared to healthy knees in sagittal plane range of motion, maximum flexion, abduction-

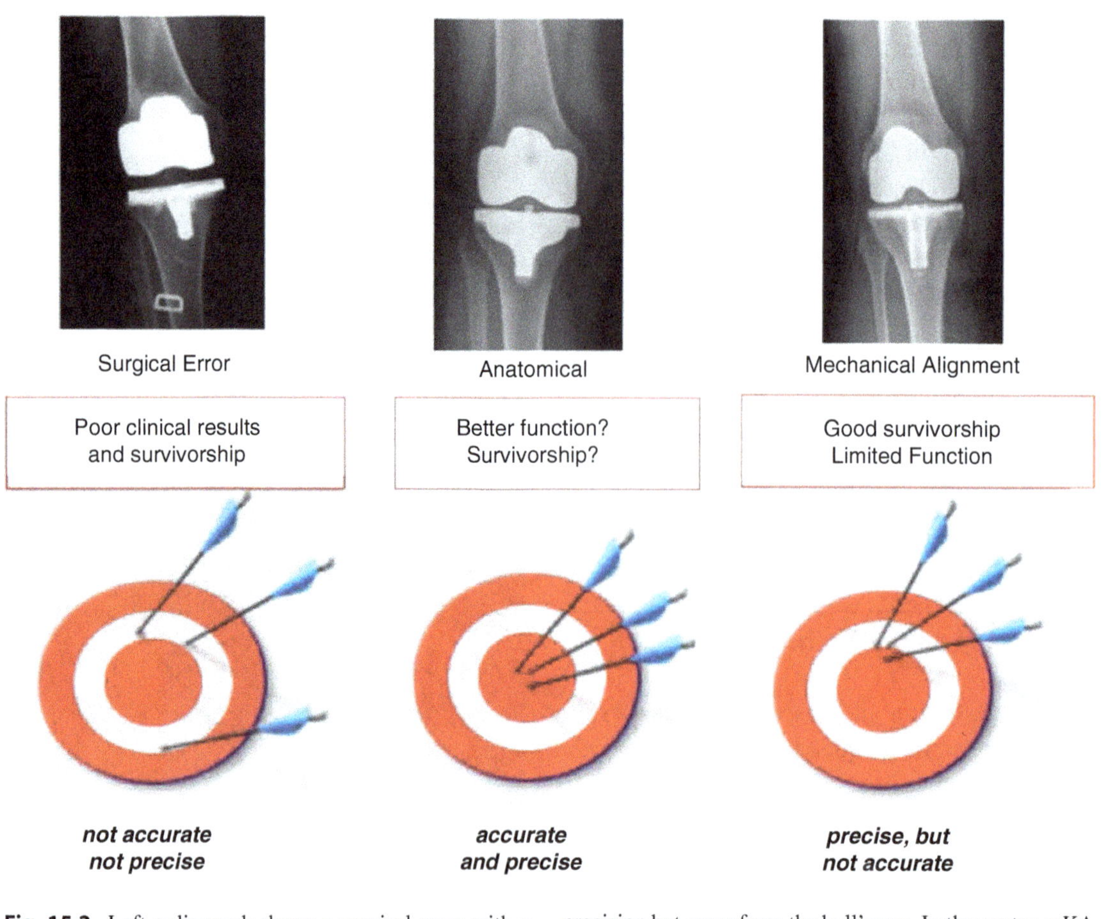

Fig. 15.2 Left radiograph shows a surgical error with a lack of precision on the target below. The right radiograph represents a well-performed MA TKA implanted with precision but away from the bull's eye. In the centre, a KA TKA precisely achieving the patient's anatomy restoration

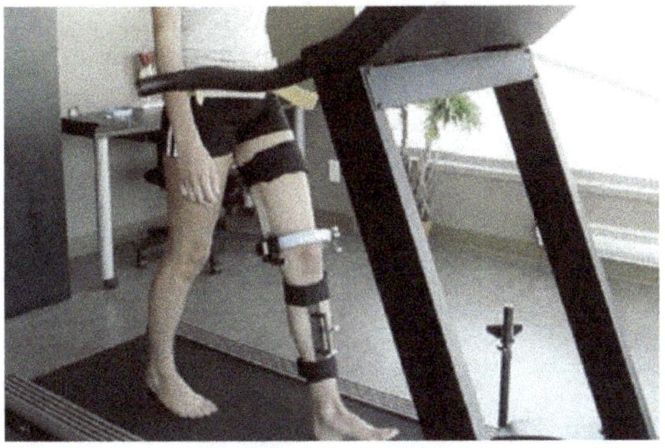

Fig. 15.3 Knee KG™ device on the left knee of a patient walking on a treadmill to assess knee kinematics

adduction curves or knee external tibial rotation. Conversely, the mechanical alignment group displayed several significant knee kinematic differences to the healthy group: less sagittal plane range of motion (49.1° vs. 54.0°, $p = 0.020$), decreased maximum flexion (52.3° vs. 57.5°, $p = 0.002$), increased adduction angle (2.0–7.5° vs. −2.8–3.0°, $p < 0.05$) and increased external tibial rotation (by a mean of 2.3 ± 0.7°, $p < 0.001$). The postoperative KOOS score was significantly higher in the kinematic alignment group compared to the mechanical alignment group (74.2 vs. 60.7, $p = 0.034$). Such results demonstrate that a better restoration of the individual's knee anatomy and ligament tension led to improved knee kinematics and clinical outcomes and greater patient satisfaction.

On the other hand, achieving a patient-specific implant implantation with a non-anatomic prosthesis design makes little sense either. The next logical step on this road forward would be to have a personalized implant to reproduce individual anatomy.

15.4 Customised Implants

Re-establishing the native knee anatomy and kinematics using custom implants has recently been developed as a novel technology in TKA. Matching the bony anatomy with the implant geometry should facilitate restoration of the native pre-arthritic limb alignment. Belzile et al. and Bonnin et al. in Chaps. 19 and 22 discuss the advantages of such patient-specific implants. These include an optimised implant fit to the native bone, avoiding prosthetic overhang or under-coverage. Improved ligament balancing may be achieved by avoiding resection laxity due to asymmetric bone cuts. Restoring the native radii of curvature of the knee may improve mid-flexion stability and kinematics. Restoring the native femoral rotation and a customised trochlea may lead to improved patellofemoral tracking.

The anatomy of the knee has been shown to vary by gender, ethnicity and body type [14, 15]. Furthermore, within these groups, there is substantial variation such that every individual has a unique anatomical geometry [16]. This would suggest that a customised implant would be advantageous to try to replicate this individual variation.

Although these customised implants are reproducing the bony anatomy and native knee alignment, they still resect the cruciate ligaments. Resecting the cruciate ligaments will affect the knee kinematics. Perhaps, the path to a more natural, forgotten joint should start with preservation of the cruciate ligaments.

Bi-cruciate-preserving TKA is not a new procedure, but as Pritchett et al. point out in Chap. 23, there are a number of new implant designs. There have been high failure rates of some historical designs of these knee replacements. This is in part because preservation of the cruciate ligaments is technically difficult. However, if done correctly, there is evidence of good long-term survivorship with excellent functional outcome.

Preservation of the cruciate ligaments mandates the correct tension of all of the knee's ligaments. There is more natural transmission of weight-bearing forces with more natural kinematics. Traditional CR design TKAs often exhibit paradoxical anterior slide and reverse rotation of the femoral component with increasing flexion [17, 18].

This consistent motion pattern is thought to be a result of the absence of the ACL, with the resultant inability to counterbalance the PCL properly and account for the changed geometry of the prosthesis [19].

Patient-specific/custom designs of bi-cruciate-preserving TKA that facilitate implantation and reduce the risks of specific complications such as fracture of the tibial eminence may be a possible solution to reproducing normal knee kinematics.

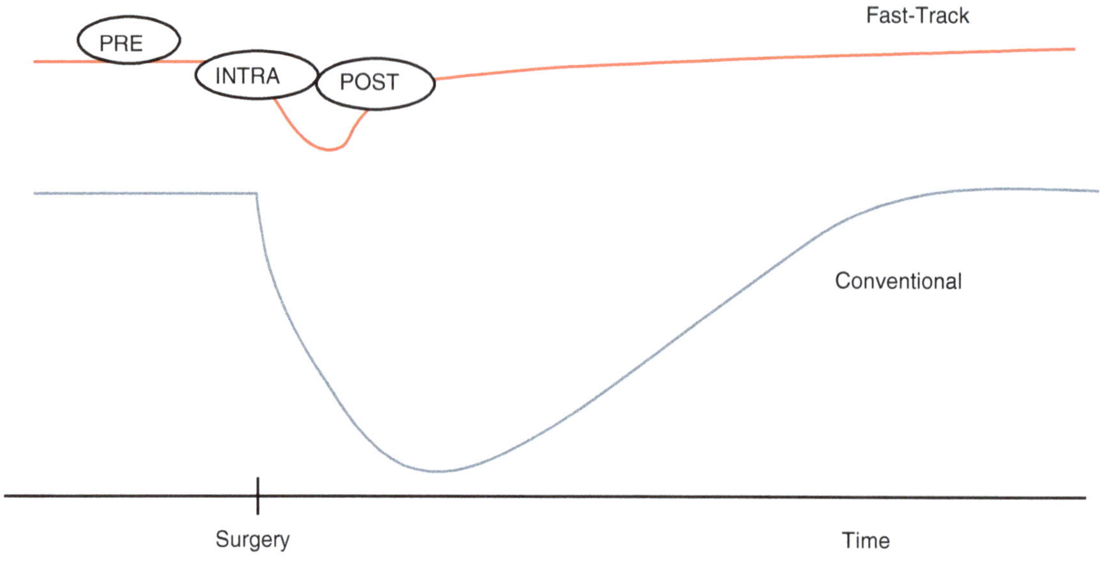

Fig. 15.4 An ERAS protocol aim at reducing the impact of surgery on patient's function. Patients will return to their preoperative status faster

15.5 Optimized Perioperative Care

Many of the advances in TKA surgery have been around the optimization of the perioperative care. This has seen a large reduction in the number of inpatient days following a joint replacement. The introduction of principles of enhanced recovery after surgery (ERAS) in TKA surgery has improved patient's well-being to a level allowing them to return home the same day (Fig. 15.4).

Implementation of an ERAS protocol in our facility had a dramatic impact on patient outcomes. We compared the complications rated according to the Clavien-Dindo scale, hospital LOS and costs of the episode of care between our first 120 ERAS short-stay THA or TKA and a matched historical control group of 150 THA or TKA [20]. ERAS cases had lower rate of Grade 1 and 2 complications compared with the standard group (mean 0.8 vs. 3.0, $p < 0.001$). No difference was found between the two groups for Grade 3, 4 or 5 complications. The mean hospital length of stay for the ERAS short-stay group decreased by 2.8 days for the THAs (0.1 vs. 2.9 days, $p < 0.001$) and 3.9 days for the TKAs (1.0 vs. 4.9 days, $p < 0.001$). The mean estimated direct healthcare costs reduction with the ERAS short-stay protocol was 1489 CND per THA and 4206 CND per TKA. Implementation of an ERAS short-stay protocol for patients undergoing THA or TKA at our institution resulted not only in reduced hospital length of stay but also in improved patient care and reduced direct healthcare costs.

A successful ERAS program requires multidisciplinary collaboration among anaesthesiologists, surgeons, physiotherapists, nurses and hospital administrators. The future of knee arthroplasty, is to improve perioperative care to obtain the ultimate goal of a "pain- and risk-free operation" [21].

15.6 Conclusion

It is an exciting time for surgeons to be performing knee replacements. The initial aim of TKA surgery in providing a reliable prosthesis with good survivorship has been met. The focus has therefore shifted to improving patient function, kinematics and satisfaction. New precision technologies, replication of native alignment and anatomy with preservation of soft tissues and ligaments are the areas of current and future developments in the field. The future of knee arthroplasty will rely on a personalized joint reconstruction. A patient-specific/custom prosthetic implanted with precision to match patient anatomy, coupled with a holistic perioperative care model will hopefully lead to the holy grail of joint replacement surgery: a forgotten or natural knee joint.

References

1. Collins M, Lavigne M, Girard J, Vendittoli PA. Joint perception after hip or knee replacement surgery. Orthop Traumatol Surg Res. 2012;98:275–80.
2. Bourne RB, Chesworth BM, Davis AM, Mahomed NN, Charron KDJ. Patient satisfaction after total knee arthroplasty: who is satisfied and who is not? Clin Orthop Relat Res. 2010;468:57–63.
3. McClelland JA, Webster KE, Feller JA. Gait analysis of patients following total knee replacement: a systematic review. Knee. 2007;14:253–63.
4. Bellemans J, Colyn W, Vandenneucker H, Victor J. The Chitranjan Ranawat award: is neutral mechanical alignment normal for all patients? The concept of constitutional varus. Clin Orthop Relat Res. 2012;470:45–53.
5. Almaawi AM, Hutt JRB, Masse V, Lavigne M, Vendittoli P-A. The impact of mechanical and restricted kinematic alignment on knee anatomy in total knee arthroplasty. J Arthroplast. 2017;32:2133–40.
6. Eckhoff DG, Bach JM, Spitzer VM, et al. Three-dimensional mechanics, kinematics, and morphology of the knee viewed in virtual reality. J Bone Joint Surg Am. 2005;87(Suppl 2):71–80.
7. Robinson RP. The early innovators of today's resurfacing condylar knees. J Arthroplast. 2005;20:2–26.
8. Blakeney W, Beaulieu Y, Puliero B, Kiss MO, Vendittoli PA. Bone resection for mechanically aligned total knee arthroplasty creates frequent gap modifications and imbalances. Knee Surg Sports Traumatol Arthrosc. 2019. https://doi.org/10.1007/s00167-019-05562-8.
9. Rivière C, Vigdorchik JM, Vendittoli PA. Mechanical alignment: The end of an era! Orthop Traumatol Surg Res. 2019;105(7):1223–6.
10. Hetaimish BM, Khan MM, Simunovic N, Al-Harbi HH, Bhandari M, Zalzal PK. Meta-analysis of navigation vs conventional total knee arthroplasty. J Arthroplast. 2012;27:1177–82.
11. de Steiger RN, Liu YL, Graves SE. Computer navigation for total knee arthroplasty reduces revision rate for patients less than sixty-five years of age. J Bone Joint Surg Am. 2015;97:635–42.
12. Abdel MP, Ollivier M, Parratte S, Trousdale RT, Berry DJ, Pagnano MW. Effect of postoperative mechanical axis alignment on survival and functional outcomes of modern total knee arthroplasties with cement: a concise follow-up at 20 years. J Bone Joint Surg Am. 2018;100:472–8.
13. Blakeney W, Clement J, Desmeules F, Hagemeister N, Riviere C, Vendittoli PA. Kinematic alignment in total knee arthroplasty better reproduces normal gait than mechanical alignment. Knee Surg Sports Traumatol Arthrosc. 2019;27(5):1410–7.
14. Leszko F, Hovinga KR, Lerner AL, Komistek RD, Mahfouz MR. In vivo normal knee kinematics: is ethnicity or gender an influencing factor? Clin Orthop Relat Res. 2011;469:95–106.
15. Bellemans J, Carpentier K, Vandenneucker H, Vanlauwe J, Victor J. The John Insall Award: both morphotype and gender influence the shape of the knee in patients undergoing TKA. Clin Orthop Relat Res. 2010;468:29–36.
16. van den Heever DJ, Scheffer C, Erasmus P, Dillon E. Classification of gender and race in the distal femur using self organising maps. Knee. 2012;19:488–92.
17. Yoshiya S, Matsui N, Komistek RD, Dennis DA, Mahfouz M, Kurosaka M. In vivo kinematic comparison of posterior cruciate-retaining and posterior stabilized total knee arthroplasties under passive and weight-bearing conditions. J Arthroplast. 2005;20:777–83.
18. Cates HE, Komistek RD, Mahfouz MR, Schmidt MA, Anderle M. In vivo comparison of knee kinematics for subjects having either a posterior stabilized or cruciate retaining high-flexion total knee arthroplasty. J Arthroplast. 2008;23:1057–67.
19. Zeller IM, Sharma A, Kurtz WB, Anderle MR, Komistek RD. Customized versus patient-sized cruciate-retaining total knee arthroplasty: an in vivo kinematics study using mobile fluoroscopy. J Arthroplast. 2017;32:1344–50.
20. Vendittoli PA, Pellei K, Desmeules F, Lavigne M, Massé V, Loubert C, Fortier L-P. Enhanced recovery short-stay hip and knee joint replacement program improves patients outcomes while reducing hospital costs. Orthop Traumatol Surg Res. 2019;105(7):1237–43.
21. Kehlet H. Enhanced recovery after surgery (ERAS): good for now, but what about the future? Can J Anaesth. 2015;62:99–104.

16

TKA: Kinematic Alignment Surgical Technique

Charles Rivière, Ciara Harman, Oliver Boughton, and Justin Cobb

Key Points

- Kinematic alignment (KA) is a relatively new surgical technique for implanting total knee components.
- The vast majority of patients are eligible for a kinematic implantation, and this may be achieved with most primary implant designs.
- Kinematically aligning the femoral component is relatively easy and straightforward; following this first step, the kinematic tibial implant positioning is made reproducible by a combination of measured resection and ligament referencing techniques. As the surgical technique is not demanding and complex cases are rare, the KA technique is overall reliable.
- KA implantation results in high prosthetic joint function, in a large range of preoperative deformity, and whether the postoperative alignment of the tibial component, knee and limb is in the varus and valgus outlier range of mechanical alignment criteria.
- Due to an improvement in knee biomechanics, it is expected that component lifespan will also be improved. A prospective study of 222 successive unselected KATKAs has reported excellent implant survival at 10-year follow-up. Nevertheless, long-term outcomes of KA patients still need to be defined.
- In the event of severe constitutional limb deformity, kinematic component positioning may be adjusted in order to reduce the limb deformity and hopefully improve prosthetic biomechanics. This defines the restricted kinematic alignment concept.
- Development of new implant designs adapted to KA implantation needs to be undertaken.

C. Rivière (✉)
South West London Elective Orthopaedic Centre, Epsom, UK

The MSK Lab-Imperial College London, White City Campus, London, UK

C. Harman
South West London Elective Orthopaedic Centre, Epsom, UK

O. Boughton · J. Cobb
The MSK Lab-Imperial College London, White City Campus, London, UK
e-mail: o.boughton@imperial.ac.uk; j.cobb@imperial.ac.uk

16.1 Introduction

16.1.1 What Is It? The Concept

The kinematic alignment technique (KA) for total knee arthroplasty (TKA) is a surgical technique recently developed that aims to anatomically position and kinematically align total knee components [1]. The kinematic implantation aims to resurface the knee joint by removing a cartilage and bone thickness equivalent to the implant thickness and where the knee implants are aligned on the knee kinematic axes that dictate motion of the patella and tibia around the distal femoral epiphysis [2–4]. Similar to unicompartmental knee replacement, kinematically aligning total knee components restores the constitutional knee joint line orientation and the physiological knee laxity without the need for soft-tissue release [5] (Fig. 16.1).

16.1.2 Why Has This New Surgical Technique Been Developed? The Rationale

The KA technique for TKA has been developed following the observations that mechanically aligned (MA) TKAs are affected by residual complications that have not been solved by technology, and the rationale for the MA technique is being challenged.

MA-TKAs are affected by residual complications that have not been solved by technology [6–10], thus suggesting intrinsic technical limitations. The proportion of residual knee symptoms (e.g. pain, instability, effusion) and patient dissatisfaction after MA-TKA has been reported to be as high as 50% and 20%, respectively [6–10]. Interestingly, neither the multiple modern TKA designs nor the many technological assistive devices (e.g. computer assistance, robotics, personalized instrumentation) have solved the issues [6–10]. The mechanical alignment technique is a technically challenging [11–13], systematic technique of implantation [5] that generates non-physiological prosthetic knee anatomy [5, 11, 14], balance [11, 15] and biomechanics [16–18]. Aiming at a similar component implantation alignment goal, it does not recreate the high variability in knee anatomy [14, 19] and laxity [20] between individuals. This may be responsible for

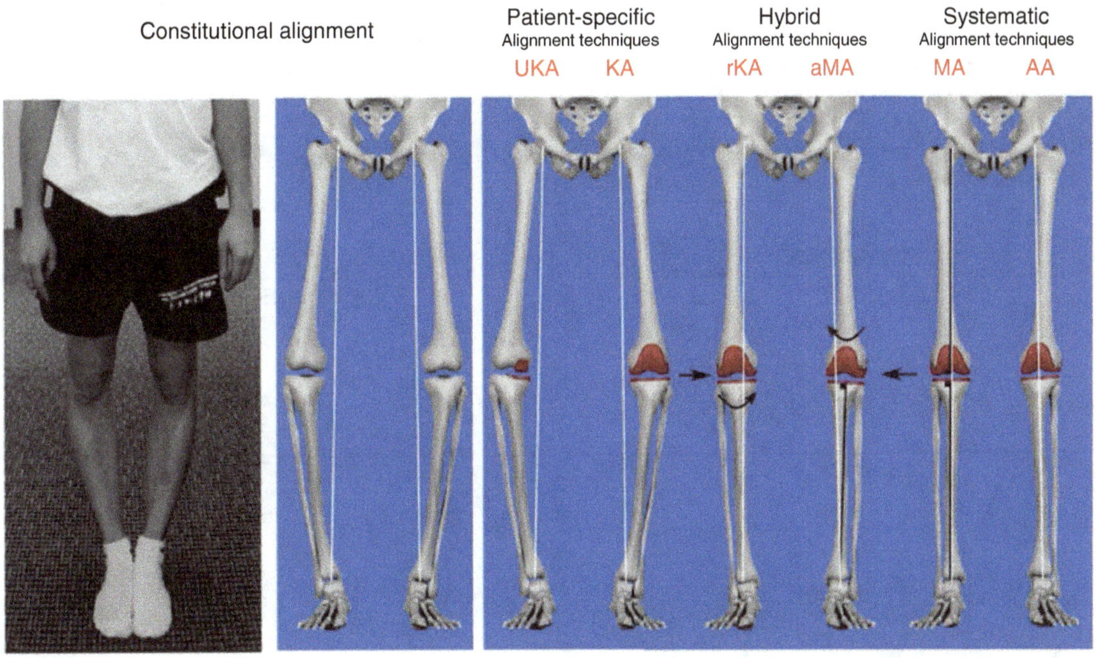

Fig. 16.1 The multiple philosophies for aligning knee components. Mechanical alignment (MA) and kinematic alignment (KA) are two different techniques for positioning knee components. MA and KA may have their component positioning adjusted in order to generate a more physiological (adjusted MA, aMA) or biomechanically sound (restricted KA, rKA) prosthetic knee. Only the unicompartmental knee replacement (UKA), KA and rKA are personalized techniques for implanting knee components

non-physiological knee ligament laxities and residual instability [10, 11, 15] and abnormal knee kinematics [13, 16, 17]. To illustrate these points, the MA technique was linked to:

1. Frequent prosthetic overstuffing of the distal lateral femoral condyle [11] which leads to abnormal stretching of the lateral retinaculum ligament during knee flexion.
2. Frequent, uncorrectable collateral ligament imbalance when performed with a measured resection technique (approximately 40% imbalance ≥2 mm) [11, 12] or gap-balancing (knee flexion gap tighter than physiological) [15] techniques.

The **rational of mechanically positioning knee implants is being challenged**:

- *The first pillar* of the MA technique is to align knee components systematically, perpendicular to femoral and tibial mechanical axes. In fact, a bulk of evidence now suggests that knee kinematics is dictated by three main axes (Fig. 16.2) [2], and the cylindrical (or trans-condylar) axis is the one upon which the tibia effectively rotates around the femur from 10° to 120° of knee flexion [4].
- *The second pillar* of the MA technique is the assumption that generating a neutrally aligned knee when standing creates a biomechanically friendly knee component environment that would persist even during gait. By reducing the prosthetic joint reaction force, this would optimise the lifespan of the components. In fact, many studies have now challenged this dogma, after having found that static standing limb alignment (hip knee ankle (HKA) angle) poorly predicts the risk of long-term MA-TKA failure [21, 22]. This may be due to the fact the HKA angle is a dynamic (or functional) value that changes when weight bearing [23] and walking [24] and that only partly predicts the knee adduction moment [24, 25] and the medial femoro-tibial joint reaction force [26].
- *The last pillar* of the MA technique is the assumption that generating rectangular and identical extension and flexion gaps would be clinically beneficial. However, some recent studies suggest that preserving the physiological ligament laxity difference between the medial and lateral compartments and between the flexion and extension spaces may in fact be clinically advantageous [27].

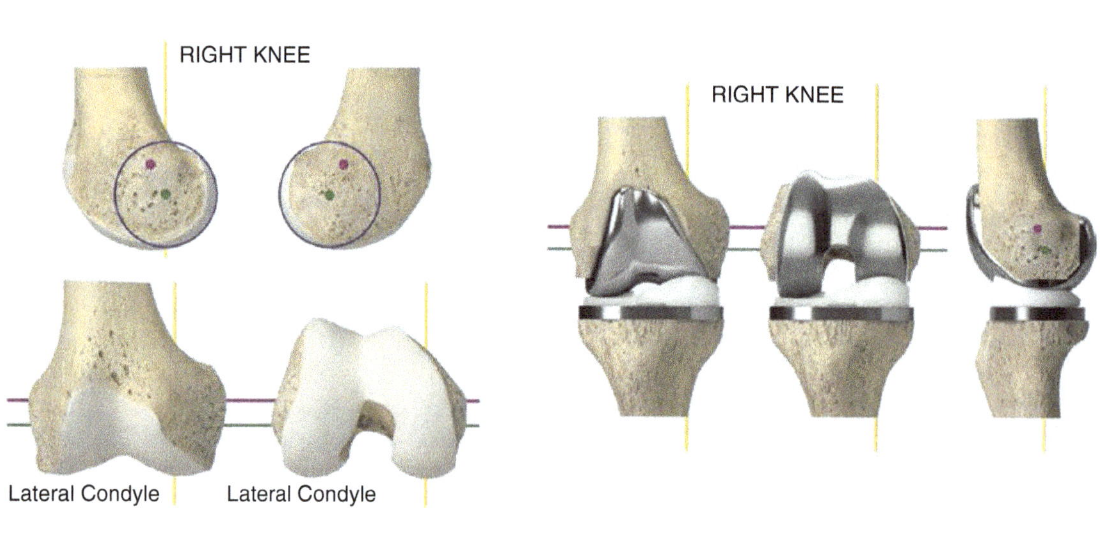

Fig. 16.2 Kinematically implanted knee components are aligned on the three main knee kinematics axes, which dictate physiological knee motion. This is achieved by anatomically positioning knee components or, in other words, by performing a true total knee resurfacing. Trans-condylar or cylindrical axis (green); patellar axis (purple); tibial longitudinal axis (yellow)

16.1.3 What Are the Intended Benefits?

By aiming for a more physiological and more reproducible implantation, the KA technique aims to improve prosthetic knee function, patient satisfaction and component lifespan, compared to conventional techniques for knee replacement. The anatomic knee reconstruction has been shown to be clinically beneficial [28] by means of the generation of a close to physiological peri-prosthetic soft-tissue tension [29, 30] and prosthetic knee biomechanics [31–34]. Interestingly, the kinetic aspect of a KA-TKA may also be advantageous (reduced prosthetic joint reaction force) compared to MA [31, 33, 34]. Those functional and biomechanical advantages with KA would hopefully contribute to counter the raising burden of revision in patients who are having joint replacement younger, with higher demands and expectations, and a longer life expectancy [7, 8].

16.2 Planning a Kinematic Implantation

16.2.1 Which Patient Can Be Kinematically Implanted?

Primary replacements requiring revision knee implants to treat a deficient knee soft-tissue envelope (e.g. MCL stretching and severe valgus knee) or severe bone loss are not eligible for KA. This is due to the design of revision implants, where the stem-implant angle dictates the implant orientation (often 6° for femur and 0° for tibia).

There is currently no evidence that osteoarthritic knees that require a primary replacement with sliding components lead to the preclusion of a surgeon using KA. Out of 219 consecutive unselected KA-TKAs prospectively followed for 10 years, prosthetic knees resulting in varus or valgus limb alignment (>3°) performed similarly as the ones neutrally aligned knees. Only three aseptic revisions (1.6%) were observed and were related to technical error in component positioning [35]. Similarly, the fact that only 13 cases of patella instability were reported out of 3212 consecutive KA-TKAs indicates that the vast majority of patella-femoral joints and axial femoro-tibial rotations may be safely reproduced when kinematically implanting total knee components [36].

Nevertheless, it is likely that certain types of constitutional anatomy may be biomechanically inferior and thus clinically detrimental if reproduced (osteoarthritic knee types 2, 3 and 5; Table 16.1).

- The safe range for frontal kinematically positioned total knee components is yet to be determined [5]. This explains why some authors use KA unless the patient is an outlier, with excessive deviation from the average constitutional knee anatomy [37, 38]. In this event, those authors would adjust the kinematic components positioning, by slightly deviating from the native anatomy, in order to fit an arbitrarily defined, range of component positioning and limb alignment [37, 38]. This defines the concept of restricted kinematic alignment, best illustrated by the Montreal protocol (see Chap. 17) [37, 38]. The outlier constitutional knee/limb anatomies must not be confused with extra-articular deformities resulting from trauma (e.g. femoral diaphysis malunion), which are not physiological. These more often need to be corrected with an additional osteotomy at the time of TKA (one stage) or before (two stages) the TKA.
- Similarly, the safe range for axially kinematically positioned total knee components is unknown [5]. Kinematically implanting patients having an antecedent of patella instability (osteoarthritic knee type 5; Table 16.1) may seem unreasonable as reproducing a poor anatomy (e.g. excessive Q angle or trochlea groove-tibial tuberosity distance) may lead to failure. As stated above, with solely 13 cases of patella instability out of 3212 consecutive unselected KA-TKAs [36], the vast majority of patella-femoral joint anatomies and axial femoro-tibial rotations may, apparently, be safely reproduced.

Table 16.1 Table illustrating different types of knee that make a kinematic implantation simple, complex or not indicated

	Simple KA-TKA	Complex KA-TKA				No KA-TKA
Knee type	1	2	3	4	5	6
Definition	None of the criteria defining the types 2, 3, 4, 5, 6	>5° constitutional varus	>5° constitutional valgus	Severe bone loss	Antecedent of patella instability	Deficient soft-tissue envelope
Surgical planning	KA	KA **or** 'KA + realignment osteotomy' **or** rKA		KA (unless revision implant needed)	KA ±MPFL reconstruction ±lateral retinaculum release and VMO plasty ±extensor mechanism realignment	**Constrained implants needed, KA technique not indicated**

Knee types 2, 3, 4 and 5 represent situations of complexity that are important to preoperatively recognise for refining the planning of the kinematic implantation

16.2.2 Which Implant Design May Be Kinematically Implanted?

It is likely that the majority of traditional primary implant designs (symmetrical sliding designs) available on the market such as medial pivot and cruciate(s) retaining or substituting designs may be suitable for a kinematic implantation. As kinematic prosthetic implantation aims to restore close to physiological knee kinematics, implant designs that promote unconstrained, physiological femoro-tibial kinematics and that preserve or replicate cruciate ligament(s) function are probably the most sensible for use. For this reason, kinematic implantations have traditionally been reported with fixed bearing cruciate-retaining implant designs [35–37, 39–42]. Nevertheless, successful kinematic implantation with mobile bearing postero-stabilised implant design has also been reported [43]. After having used cruciate-retaining and postero-stabilised designs, the author (CR) is now performing kinematic implantation with a medial pivot TKA component design [44]. By offering anteroposterior stability (substitution of both cruciate ligaments and medial meniscus) and medial implant congruency (ball in socket), medial pivot TKA design may be clinically advantageous by providing improved knee stability and reduced linear polyethylene wear. There is no study having compared the value of the multiple implant designs when kinematically positioned. Further research is therefore needed.

Asymmetric components with built-in joint line obliquity (e.g. Journey™, Genesis™—Smith & Nephew), because of asymmetry in the thicknesses of their medial and lateral compartments, are specifically designed for mechanical implantation (thus creating the effect of an anatomical alignment - see Fig. 16.1) and are inappropriate for kinematic alignment.

16.2.3 Which Instrumentation to use?

Conventional gap-balancing techniques, serving to define the femoral axial rotation, are inappropriate for KA. This is because a kinematic femoral component is always implanted parallel to the posterior condylar line (neutral rotation) in order to be adequately aligned with the cylindrical (trans-condylar) axis. This is easily achieved with a posterior referencing resection guide.

KA can be performed manually [45, 46] or with the use of assistive technology [35, 37, 39–41, 43]. Successful implantations have been reported using measured-resection manual instrumentation (Chap. 24) [45, 46], navigation systems (Chap. 26) [37, 43] and personalized cutting guide (Chap. 25) [35, 39–42]. A modified gap-balancing technique for performing the tibial cut is also being assessed [47].

Technological assistance (e.g. computer, robotics or PSI) is probably most of interest with the *restricted KA concept* [5, 37, 38, 48], by informing the surgeon about the patient's knee anatomy and the ability to precisely execute anatomy adjustment when needed. The restricted KA concept consists of restricting the use of the pure kinematic technique only for individual with HKA deviation above 3° and/or distal femoral/proximal tibia joint line obliquity higher than 5° (Montreal protocol, see Chap. 17) [38]. Outlier patients will have their component positioning adjusted by slightly deviating from their constitutional knee anatomy (adjusted kinematic implant orientation). When performing a pure kinematic implantation (no adjustment), it remains to be seen whether technological assistance is of any clinical advantage as the kinematic components positioned with manual instrumentation have been shown to be highly reliable in terms of reproducibility of implant positioning [46, 49, 50] and clinical outcomes [45, 46]. This is the result of using reliable intra-articular anatomical landmarks to set the level and orientation of the bone cuts, knowing the expected bone resection thicknesses, controlling their quality with a calliper (measured resection technique; Fig. 16.3) and by assessing the collateral ligaments tension with spacer block and/or trial implants (ligament referencing technique) and easily refining the cuts with specific user-friendly recut guides (Fig. 16.4, and see Chap. 24).

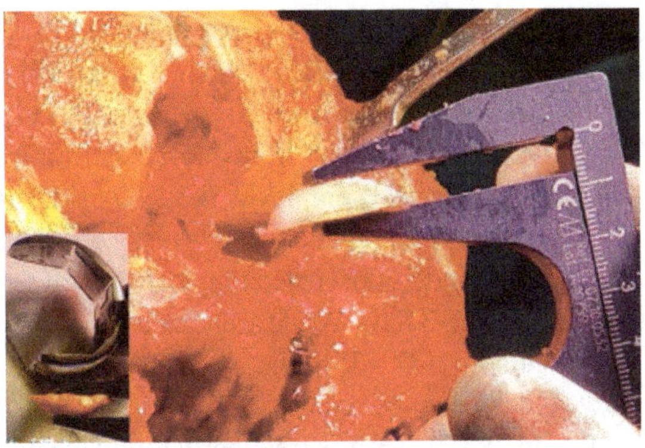

Fig. 16.3 The calliper is the key tool for successful KA implantation. Distal and posterior femoral cuts and the tibial cut must always be measured. The resection thicknesses should match those of the components, after compensating for cartilage and bone wear and the 1 mm kerf from the saw cut

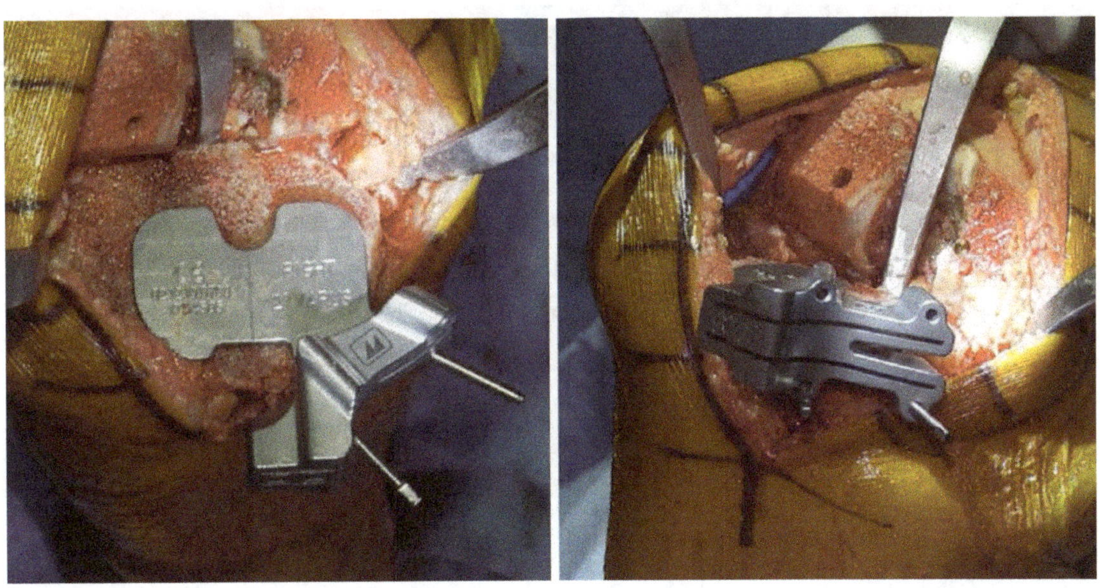

Fig. 16.4 Recently launched specific KA instrumentation™ (Medacta, Switzerland). It helps to compensate for cartilage loss on the femoral side as well as easing the refinement of the tibial cut through the various recut guides (additional tibia varus or valgus or slope). This figure illustrates the varus/valgus recut guide

16.2.4 Resurface the Patella or Not?

There is unfortunately no evidence to help with this choice. As MA and KA implantations significantly differ from each other, the evidence accumulated for the former technique can't be translated to the latter one.

MA frequently generates lateral femoral condyle prosthetic overstuffing that affects the patella balance (lateral retinaculum stretching) and biomechanics (lateral patella tilt/shift and increased lateral facet joint reaction force) when flexing the knee [11] and is sometimes responsible for MA-TKA failures [35, 36, 42]. In contrast, this significant alteration of the lateral femoral condyle anatomy does not occur when knee components are KA [11, 51, 52] and probably explains the more physiological patella biomechanics [33, 34] and the rare anterior knee pain [42, 53] and patella instability [35, 36] after KA-TKA. The improved patella environment after KA-TKA, relative to MA-TKA, may have a protective effect on it, whether it has been replaced or not. This would hopefully be clinically beneficial by reducing the risk of patella-femoral joint-related complications [35, 36, 42].

16.2.5 Recognising a Complex Case for KA Implantation

As KA and MA implantation significantly differ, both techniques are complex in different situations. A classification of the most frequent conditions that would make KA-TKA complex is illustrated in Table 16.1.

In contrast to MA, the frontal limb deformity is generally not a source of technical complexity with the KA technique [11, 12, 29, 30]. This is because the anatomical joint reconstruction given by KA reliably restores the physiological knee soft-tissue balance whatever the constitutional limb alignment of the patient [11, 12, 29, 30]. Therefore, constitutional frontal limb deformity does not add surgical complexity unless considered excessive and needing attenuation (restricted KA) or correction (additional osteotomy before or at the time of the KA-TKA). While arbitrarily defined by some authors [37, 38], the optimal deformity threshold is yet to be scientifically defined.

Complex KA-TKA is frequently found in situations of substantial articular surface bone loss. The assessment of the medial (valgus stress) and lateral (varus stress) femoro-tibial spaces before any cuts (Fig. 16.5) gives an idea of the

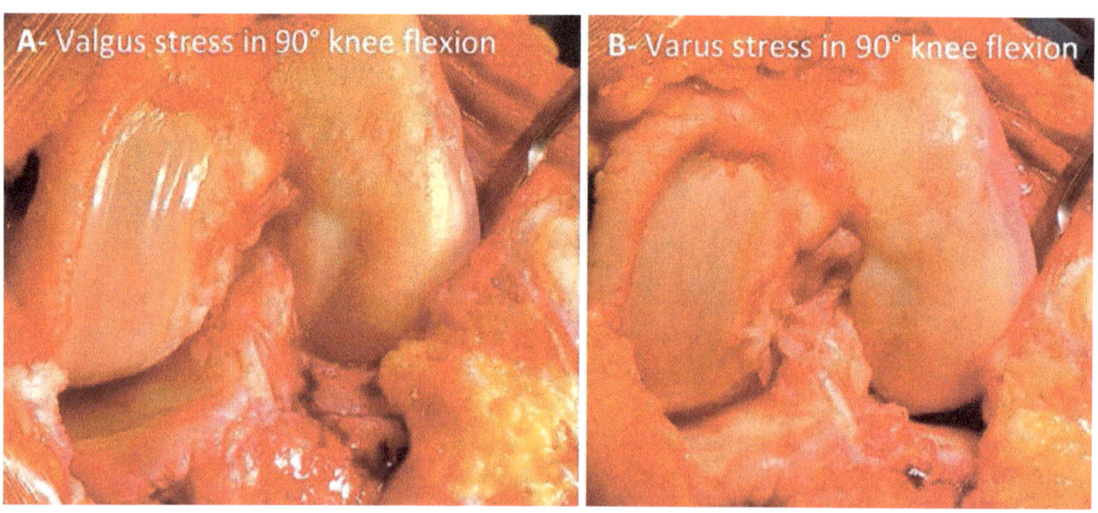

Fig. 16.5 Before performing any bone cuts, it is important to estimate the physiological knee laxity and amount of bone loss by doing varus (**b**, **d**) and valgus (**a**, **c**) stress tests in 90° (**a**, **b**) and 10° knee flexion and at full extension (**c**, **d**). In this case, there is a 3 mm to 4 mm physiological lateral laxity in flexion (**b**) but none at full extension (**d**) when doing a varus stress test. In contrast, there is excessive medial laxity when doing a valgus stress test, around 5 mm in flexion (**a**) and 10 mm in extension (**c**), which suggests significant medial compartment bone loss

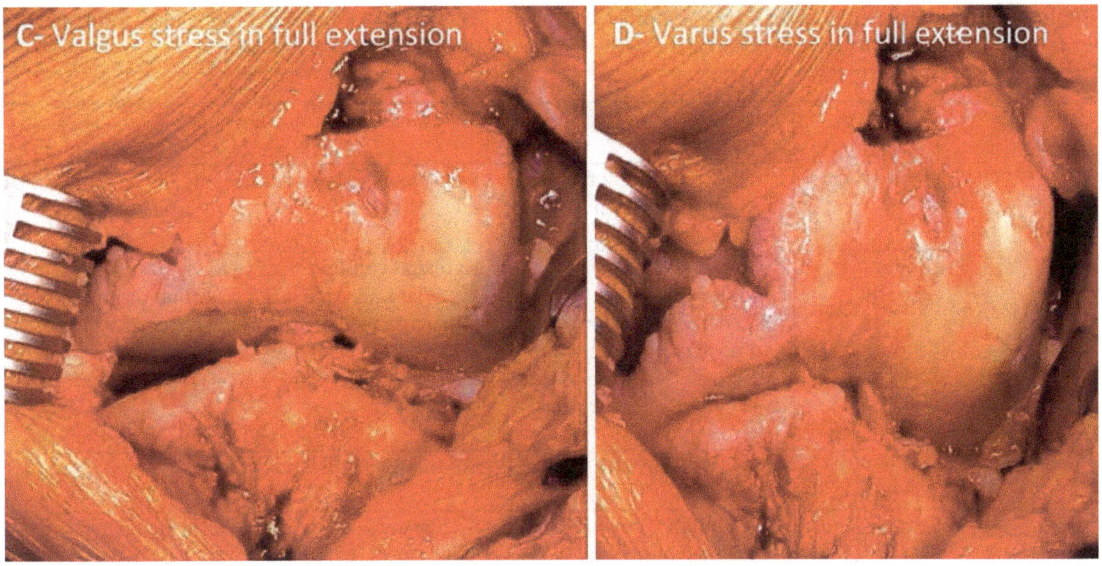

Fig. 16.5 (continued)

physiological femoro-tibial laxity and amount of bone loss and helps with planning the bone resection thickness. Then, by respecting the stepwise approach of a KA technique, with economic bone cuts followed by calliper-based quality control and potential recuts, KA in cases of substantial articular surface bone loss is usually relatively straightforward.

Patients with patella maltracking and/or a previous history of patella-femoral instability may need additional surgical correction (e.g. MPFL reconstruction, tibial tuberosity mobilisation) at the time of KA-TKA in order to optimise the patella tracking. Also, because the lateral retinaculum is often retracted in these cases, performing a lateral para-patellar arthrotomy, in addition to a plasty of the lateral retinaculum (Keblish style), may be advisable.

16.3 Key-Points for Performing a Kinematic Implantation

This section will only highlight key points of the KA technique. More details are provided in Chap. 24. The KA surgical technique significantly differs from the conventional MA technique. The only similarity between the techniques is in the execution and goal for sagittal femoral component positioning (Table 16.2) [5, 54]. The knee bony landmarks traditionally used for MA implantation are of little use when positioning implants using the KA technique [55, 56]. This is because the KA technique pays attention to intra-articular anatomical reference landmarks and strives to recreate the constitutional knee joint line orientation and knee laxity. In contrast, the MA technique focuses primarily of extra-articular long-bone mechanical axes and aims for mechanical component positioning [5, 54].

The KA technique follows a step-wise execution with the main steps being listed in Fig. 16.6. The KA implantation is traditionally a measured resection, femur first technique [45]. There are a few helpful tricks:

- First, *always estimate the individual physiological knee laxity and amount of bone loss* before performing any bone cuts, by varus/valgus stressing the knee throughout the knee range of motion (Fig. 16.5).
- Second, *always check the quality of the bone resection with a calliper* (Fig. 16.3). The expected thickness of the bone cut is easily

Table 16.2 Kinematic alignment (KA) and mechanical (MA) alignment are two different techniques for implanting knee components that only have in common the sagittal positioning of the femoral component

		KA technique	MA technique
Femoral component positioning	Flexion	Follows distal femoral bowing	Follows distal femoral bowing
	Varus-valgus	Parallel to the distal **femoral joint line** (considering articular surface wear)	Systematic and perpendicular to the femoral **mechanical axis**
	Rotation	Parallel to the **posterior condylar line** **Always measured resection and posterior referencing** techniques for a compromise done only on the trochlear offset	**External rotation** relative to the posterior condylar line. **Measured resection or gap-balancing** techniques. **Posterior or anterior referencing** techniques for a compromise done either on the flexion gap or on the trochlear offset, respectively
	Medio-lateral	Centred on the notch	**Slightly lateralised**
Tibial component positioning	Varus-valgus	Parallel to the proximal **tibial joint line** (considering the wear)	Systematic and perpendicular to the tibial **mechanical axis**
	Slope	Parallel to the **medial plateau slope**	**Systematic** and varies between 2° and 7° relative to the sagittal tibia mechanical axis
	Rotation	Parallel to **lateral plateau long-axis**	Towards the medial third of the **anterior tibial tuberosity**
Soft-tissue release	Femoro-tibial joint	**None**—close or physiological knee laxity automatically restored after bone cuts	**Frequent** for creating identical rectangular flexion and extension gaps
	Lateral retinaculum	**Rarely**—only in case of preoperative abnormal patella tracking with retracted lateral retinaculum ligament	**Often** performed to palliate the frequent prosthetic overstuffing of the lateral femoral condyle

calculated by deducting 1 mm from the implant thickness for the saw blade (kerf) thickness and by estimating the amount of articular surface wear. The cartilage thickness is frequently approximately 2 mm on the distal and posterior parts of the femoral condyles [57].

- Last, unless using technological assistance, *perform an economical tibial cut on the worn side* (Fig. 16.7) as the amount of bone loss is difficult to estimate precisely and it is easy to secondarily refine the tibia cut by using user-friendly KA-dedicated recut guides (Figs. 16.4 and 16.7).

If you face a femoro-tibial soft-tissue imbalance (tightness and/or excessive laxity) and the integrity of the knee soft-tissue envelope is still respected (no MCL or popliteal section), this is often because the tibial cut is improper. This is because performing a kinematic femoral component implantation is relatively straightforward and highly reproducible [49]. The solution is therefore to perform bone recuts by using specific recut guides that easily enable additional degrees of varus/valgus/slope to be made or an additional two millimetres of tibia to be cut. In summary, the kinematic tibial implant positioning is made reproducible by a combination of measured resection and ligament referencing techniques. The decision tree for solving imbalance while performing a kinematic implantation is illustrated in Fig. 16.8.

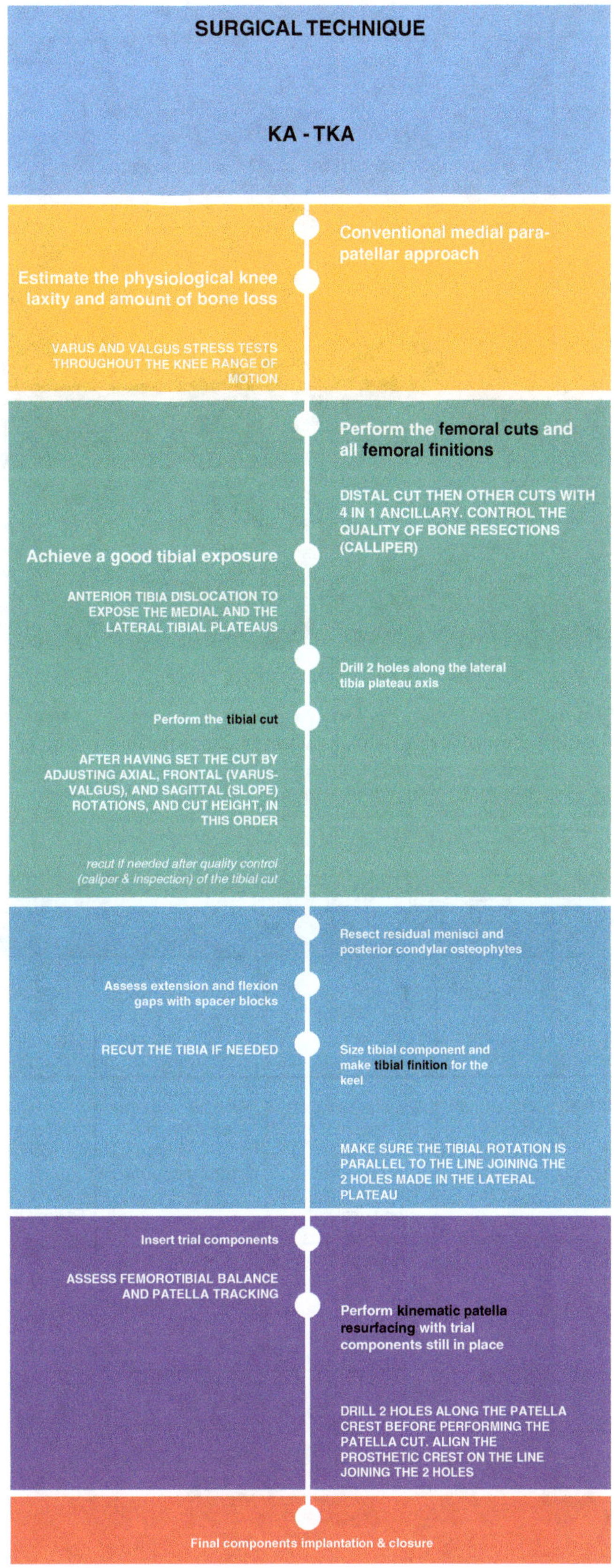

Fig. 16.6 The kinematic alignment technique for implanting total knee components follows a step-wise process that helps at making the implantation reliable

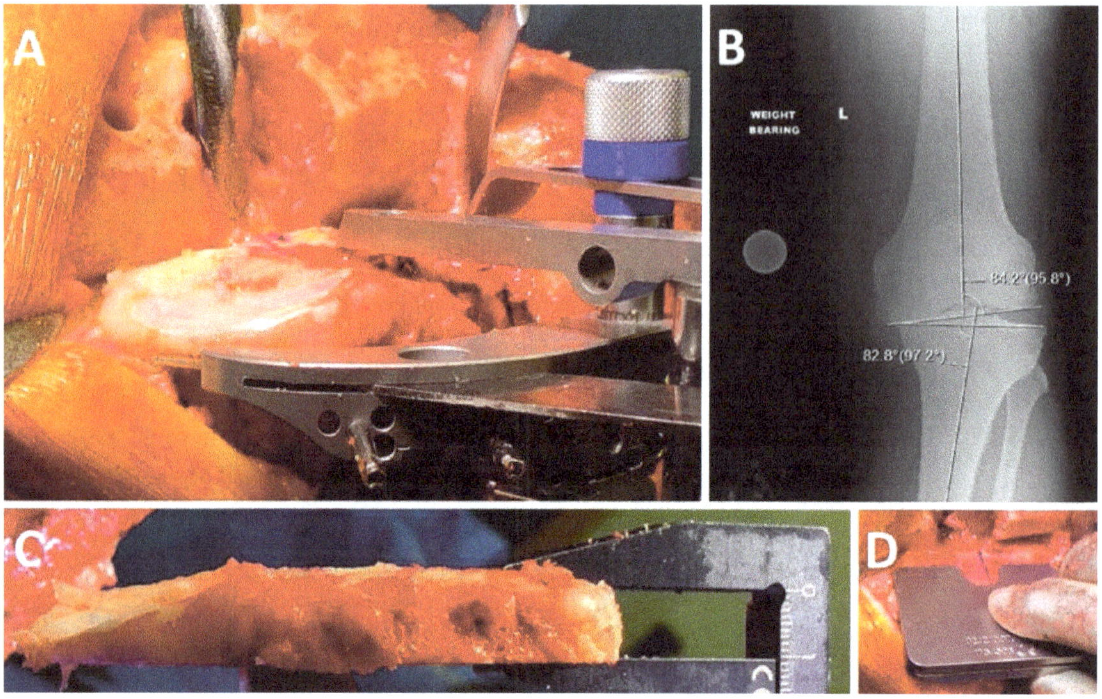

Fig. 16.7 Performing a conservative tibial bone resection on the worn medial side (**a**, **c**) is recommended as it is not easy to precisely estimate the amount of bone loss (**a**, **b**). If the knee feels tight when assessing the flexion and extension gaps (spacer block), refinement of the tibial cut will be easily executed with the use of specific recut guides (**d**)

DECISION-TREE FOR BALANCING A CALIPERED KINEMATICALLY ALIGNED MEDACTA **GMK SPHERE CS** TKA					
Tight in Flexion & Extension	Tight in Flexion Well-Balanced in Extension	Tight in Extension Well-Balanced in Flexion	Well-Balanced in Extension and Loose in Flexion	Tight Medial & Loose Lateral in Extension	Tight Lateral and Loose Medial in Extension
Recut tibia and remove 1-2 mm more bone.	Confirm complete resection of the PCL. Increase posterior slope until natural A-P offset is restored at 90° of flexion.	Remove posterior osteophytes. Strip posterior capsule. Insert trial components & gently manipulate knee into extension.	Add thicker insert and recheck knee extends fully. If still loose in flexion, then reduce slope or resect 1-2 mm bone from distal femur and add thicker **GMK Sphere CS** insert.	Remove medial osteophytes. Reassess. Recut tibia in 1-2° more varus. Insert 1 mm thicker insert.	Remove lateral osteophytes. Reassess. Recut tibia in 1-2° more valgus. Insert 1 mm thicker insert.

Fig. 16.8 Decision tree for balancing a kinematically aligned TKA

16.4 Current Evidence

The KA technique has been developed for trying to reduce the high proportions of dissatisfaction [6] and residual complications [7, 8, 10] that traditionally affect MA-TKA and are probably as a result of non-physiological (neglecting of unique individual knee anatomy and laxity) [5, 11, 14, 31, 33, 34] and unreliable (high rate of uncorrectable collateral ligament imbalance) [11, 12] implantation. Studies having assessed the value of KA-TKA have flourished over the last years, and the promises seem to have been met.

The KA technique generates high prosthetic knee function and a more natural feeling. Seven studies have compared KA and MA patients at short term (1–2 years), including five randomised controlled trials [39–42, 58] and two matched case-control study [32, 43]. All have reported better functional scores for KA patients, while this was statistically significant for only five studies [32, 41–43, 58]. In addition, a national multicentre survey in the USA found KA patients to be three times more likely to report their knee to feel "normal" [6]. Faster recovery for KA patients [40, 59], reduced risk of anterior knee pain [42, 53] and similar failure rates [39–43, 53, 58] were other interesting findings from those comparative studies. Three meta-analyses [28, 60, 61] concluded the superiority of the KA technique in terms of prosthetic function and recovery time, with a similar low failure rate. High functional scores have been shown to persist 10 years after implantation, with no difference between different groups of limb alignment (varus >3°, neutral, valgus >3°) [35]. The faster recovery of KA patients could be the consequence of a more physiological and soft-tissue-friendly prosthetic knee implantation. This superiority is even more emphasised when the excellent clinical outcomes for KA patients were achieved despite the use of recently recalled Otismed™ cutting guides [39–42, 53] and by surgeons likely in their learning curve for the KA technique. In contrast, MA implantations, which were often found to be inferior to KA implantation, were performed by surgeons familiar with the technique and sometimes using navigation assistance [39, 43, 58].

With short-term data, KA prostheses rarely failed. The early complication rates (initial 1–2 years after implantation) were reported to be similar between KA and MA patients [39–43, 53, 58]. The 10-year aseptic revision rate has been reported at 1.6% with 1 tibial component loosening and 2 patella recurrent instabilities out of 219 consecutive unselected KA-TKAs [35]. There were no differences between varus, neutral and valgus groups of limb alignment [35]. Also, only 13 cases of patella instability were reported out of 3212 consecutive kinematically implanted prosthetic knee patients during a 9-year period [36]. KA implantation, therefore, results in high implant survival at 10 years regardless of the level of preoperative deformity and whether the postoperative alignment of the tibial component, knee and limb are varus and valgus outlier ranges according to MA criteria.

The KA technique is reliable as it accurately kinematically positions the knee components [46, 49, 50]. Studies have demonstrated that KA components with manual instrumentation is highly reproducible for both femoral [46, 49] and tibial [46, 50] components. Also, the KA technique has been shown to properly restore physiological knee laxity [29, 30].

The KA technique is more physiological as it is generating close to native biomechanics. Many studies have shown that the femoro-tibial [31, 32, 62] and patellofemoral [33, 34] KA prosthetic kinematics and kinetics (or biomechanics) more closely resemble those of the native knee, when compared to mechanically aligned TKA. Interestingly, it seems that kinematic implantation may also be kinetically more advantageous than mechanical implantation by better aligning the knee joint line parallel to the ground in situations of weight bearing [48, 63], leading to reduced deleterious shear stress on the bearing surfaces and component fixation interface. KA alignment also reduces the joint reaction forces at the lateral patella-femoral facet [33, 34] and through the medial femoro-tibial compartment [31]. The improved patellofemoral kinetics [33, 34] may be explained by the prosthetic trochlea anatomy in the kinematically positioned femoral component being closer to the native trochlea groove alignment [52, 64]. The improved tibio-femoral kinetics [31] may be explained by the more physiological gait pattern after KA implantation that results in a lower knee adduction lever arm and, subsequently, a reduced knee adduction moment, despite the fact that lower limbs were slightly more varus [31]. This is not surprising when one realises that the frontal limb alignment (HKA angle) is a dynamic value [23, 24] that has been shown to poorly predict the knee adduction moment [24, 25] and the medial femoro-tibial joint reaction force [26]. The likely biomechanical advantage conferred to KA prosthesis may explain the very low rate of component failure that has been observed after KA [35].

16.5 Specific Component Designs for Kinematic Implantation?

Kinematically positioning contemporary knee components enables the restoration of the femoro-tibial joint line 3D orientation [46, 49], but it fails to accurately reproduce the individual trochlea anatomy [51, 52, 64]. This poor trochlea reconstruction is related to the fact that kinematic positioning of monoblock femoral components focuses on the reconstruction of the femoro-tibial joint line, with no possibility to fine-tune the prosthetic groove orientation. While this poor prosthetic trochlea anatomical reconstruction has not been responsible for catastrophic failure [5, 35, 36], it may nonetheless hinder optimal clinical outcomes of KA prosthetic knee. Some trochlea anatomy variations may therefore benefit from a more personalized reconstruction.

The native trochlea anatomy has been shown to be highly variable between people [3, 52] and poorly predicted by the frontal limb/knee anatomical parameters [65]. Therefore, potential solutions to a more personalized trochlea reconstruction are threefold:

1. New modular femoral component designs offer the possibility to intraoperatively fine-tune the groove orientation/radius and trochlea stuffing (Fig. 16.9).

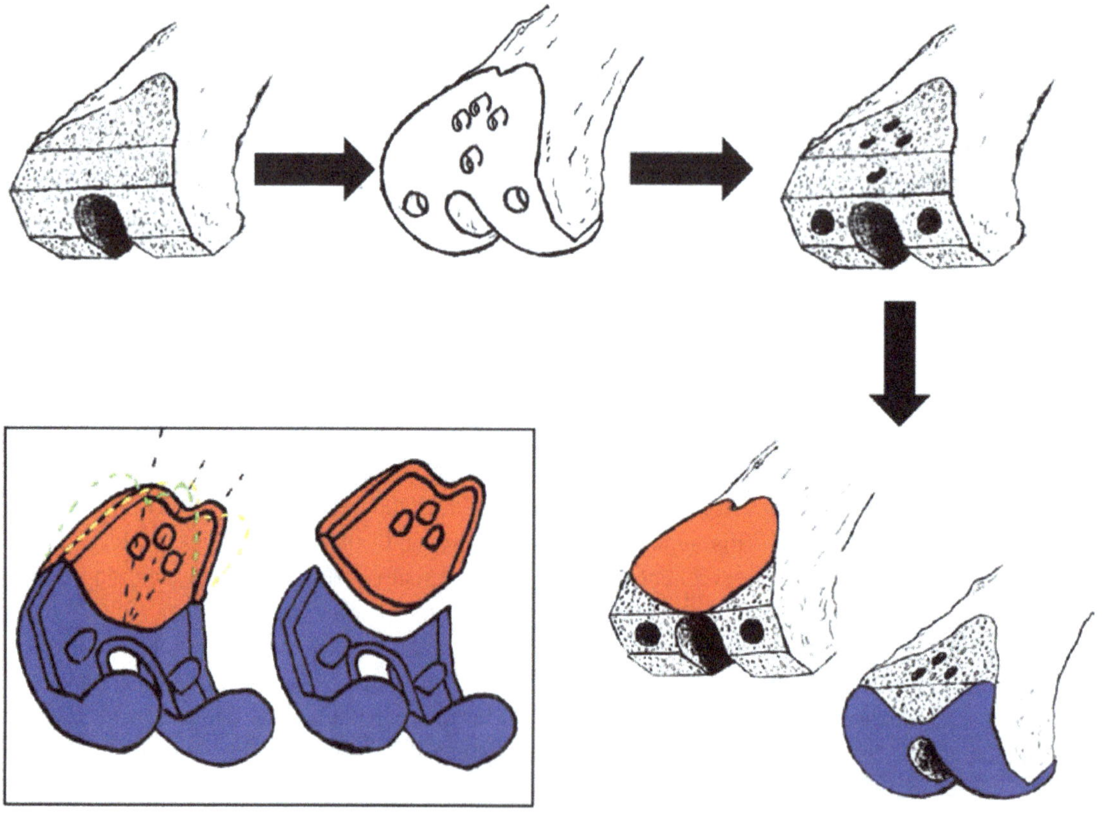

Fig. 16.9 A modular total femoral component may be one solution for restoring the individual femoro-tibial and patellofemoral joints anatomy and hopefully make clinical outcomes of KA patients even better. The surgeon would be offered the intraoperative ability to fine-tune the trochlea reconstruction (stuffing and groove orientation) and/or patella tracking by selecting through a wide range of modular trochlea designs that differ by their stuffing and groove orientation

2. Already existing custom femoral component (Origin™—Symbios, Yverdon-les-Bains, Switzerland—Fig. 16.10, Chap. 22).
3. New monoblock femoral component designs displaying various trochlea anatomies. The cost-effectiveness of the last two options may be questioned considering the current economic trend.

16.6 Conclusion

KA-TKA is a surgical technique that may help better reproduce physiological knee function without the need for soft-tissue release. The vast majority of osteoarthritic patients are eligible for a KA-TKA. Because the surgical technique is not demanding and complex cases are rare,

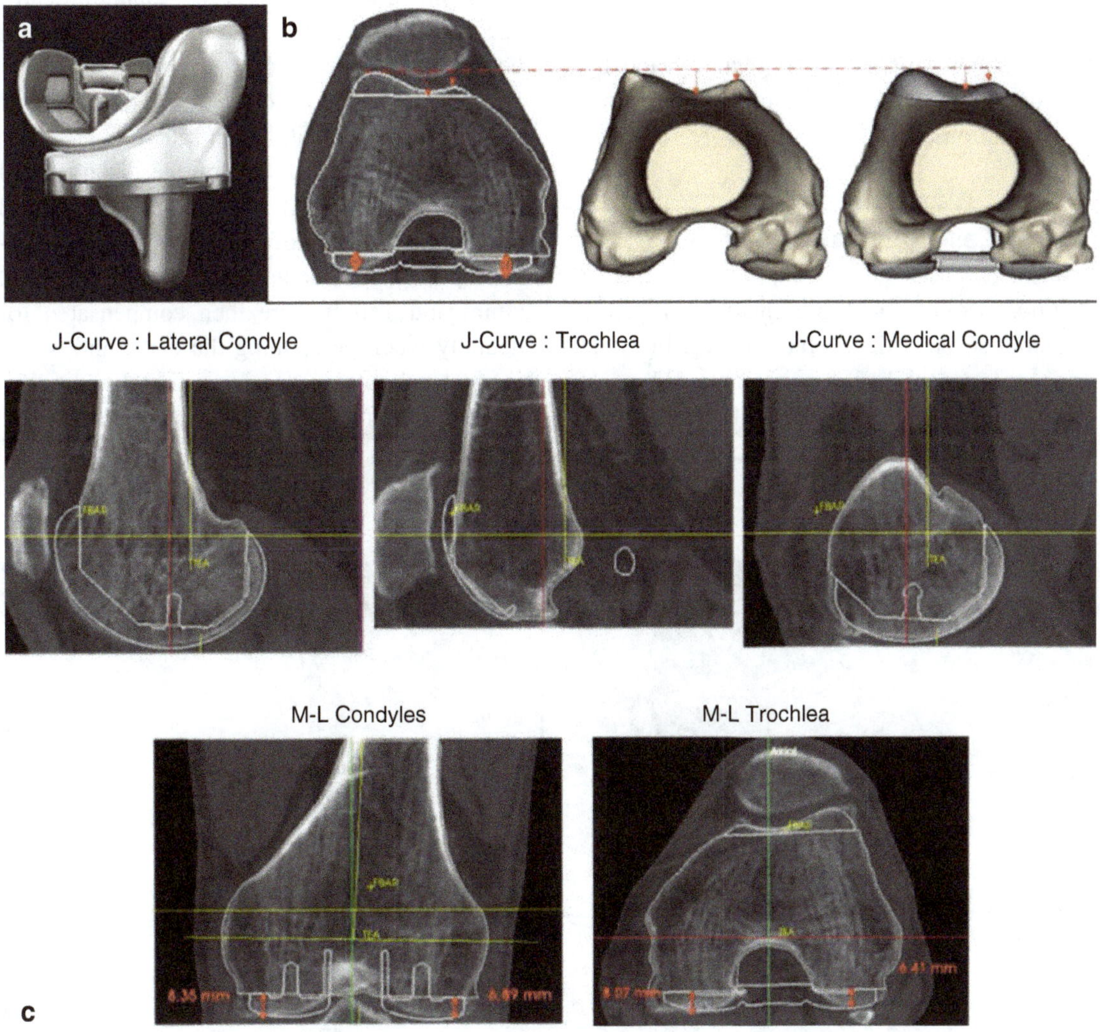

Fig. 16.10 The custom Origin™ total femoral component (Symbios, Yverdon-les-Bains, Switzerland) may be one solution for restoring the individual femoro-tibial and patellofemoral joints anatomy and hopefully make clinical outcomes of KA patients even better. The Origin™ (**a**) enables restoration of the individual trochlea (**b**) and femoro-tibial (**c**) anatomy

KA is reliable for most patients. KA implantation results in favourable implant survival and function at 10 years in a wide range of preoperative anatomies. Because the whole knee biomechanic environment is improved, it is hoped that component lifespan will also be improved. In the event of severe constitutional limb deformity, the kinematic component positioning may need to be adjusted in order to better suit the actual prosthetic fixation and bearing limitations; this defines the restricted KA concept. Long-term outcomes of KA patients still need to be defined. New TKA component designs that better match patients' knee anatomy and help replicate native knee kinematics may need consideration.

16.7 Case Illustration

A 66-year-old patient presented with painful, bilateral, severely degenerated knees. In the left knee, the patient had a correctable 10° to 15° varus deformity and a varus trust when walking. The knee range of motion was normal.

On plain radiographs (Fig. 16.11), there was bilateral, medial femoro-tibial bone-on-bone osteoarthritis. The left knee had a severe varus deformity with frontal femoro-tibial subluxation and some medial bone loss making the kinematic implantation slightly more complex than usual (knee type 5—Table 16.1).

Before performing any bone cuts on the left knee, the medial and lateral femoro-tibial laxities were assessed (Fig. 16.5), and an abnormal severe medial laxity was observed in full extension (Fig. 16.5b).

As shown in Fig. 16.12, the remaining cartilage thicknesses were assessed with a scalpel on the distal (Fig. 16.12a, b) and posterior (Fig. 16.12c, d) parts of each femoral condyle and on the lateral tibial plateau (Fig. 16.12e). There was no cartilage left on the distal medial condyle (Fig. 16.12a) and medial plateau and approximately 1 mm of cartilage loss on the posterior part of the medial condyle (Fig. 16.12c). 2 mm and 1 mm were then compensated for medially when performing the distal and posterior femoral cuts, respectively. Distal and posterior cuts were measured with a calliper and were within 0.5 mm of the plan.

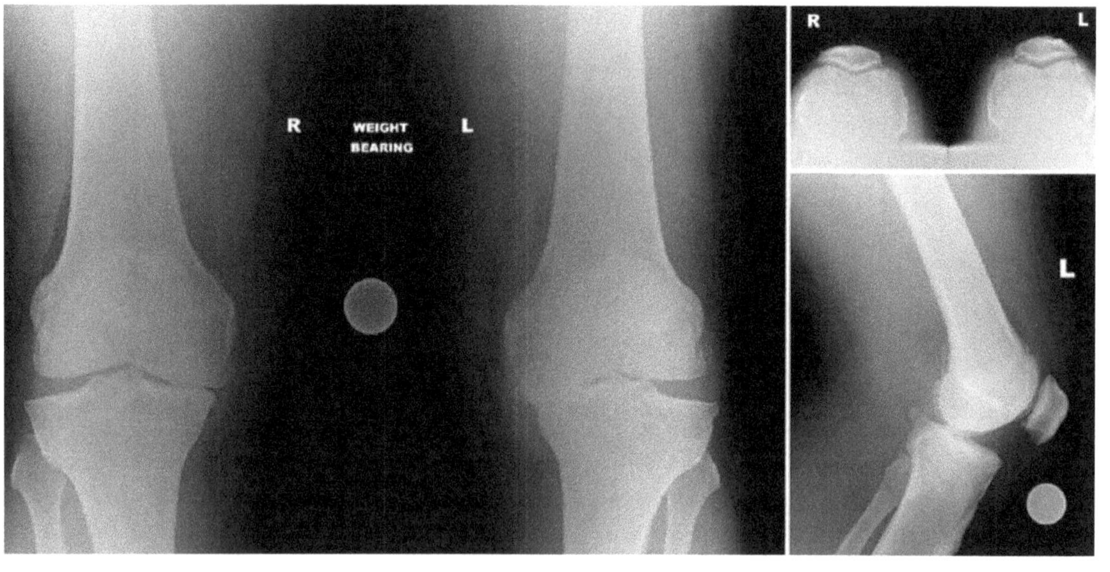

Fig. 16.11 Pre-operative knee radiographs

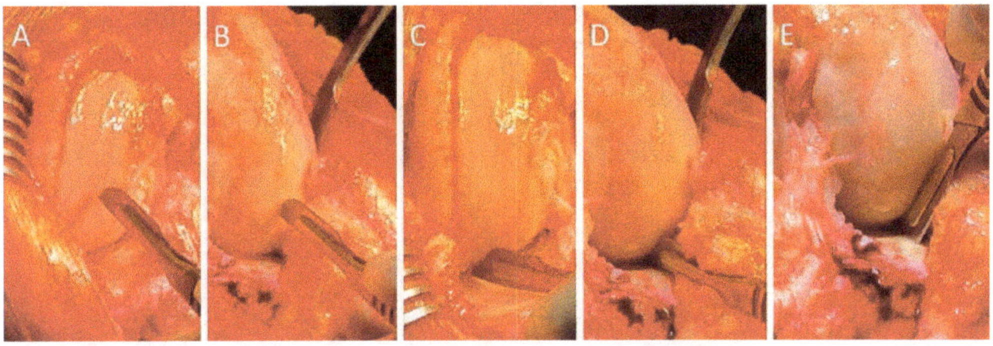

Fig. 16.12 Intra-operative estimation of cartilage thickness on the distal (**a**) and posterior (**c**) parts of the medial femoral condyle, the distal (**b**) and posterior (**d**) parts of the lateral femoral condyle, and the lateral tibia plateau (**e**)

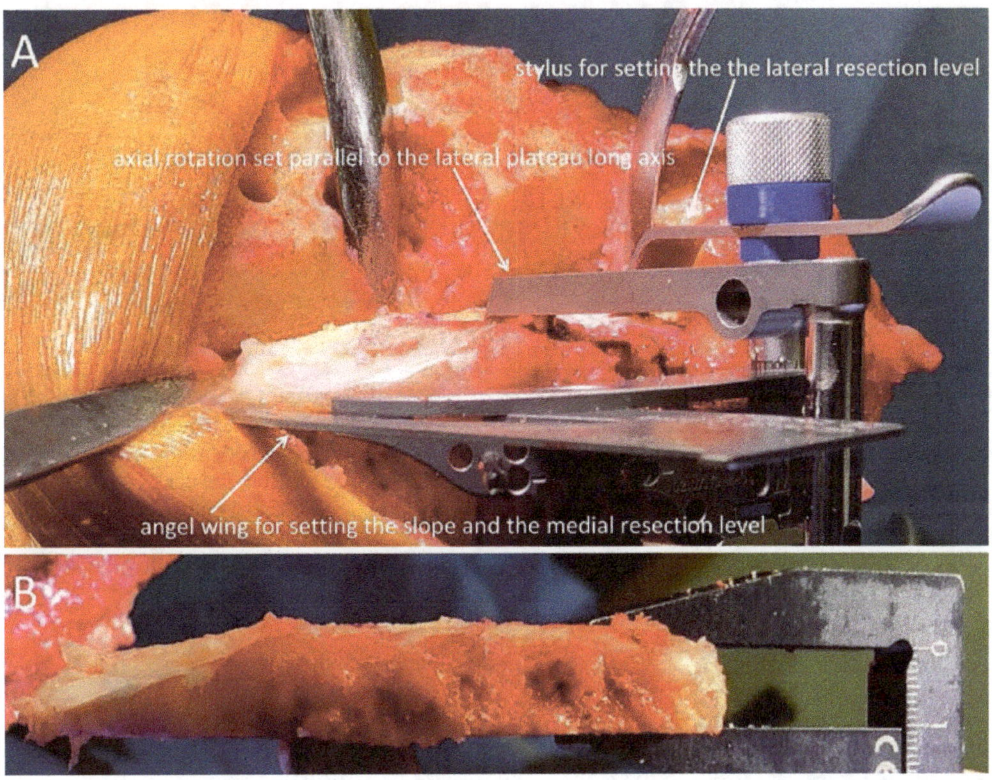
A
stylus for setting the the lateral resection level
axial rotation set parallel to the lateral plateau long axis
angel wing for setting the slope and the medial resection level
B

Fig. 16.13 Intra-operative photos illustrating the instrumentation setting to perform a kinematic tibial cut (**a**) and the quality assessment of the tibial cut with use of a caliper (**b**)

The extra-medullary alignment guide was used to stabilise the tibial cutting guide (Fig. 16.13a) while setting its orientation with the use of an angel wing and stylus. The tibial cut was done economically medially as the exact amount of medial plateau bone loss was unknown. The tibial cut was measured, revealing 10 mm was cut laterally and 3 mm medially (Fig. 16.13b).

The flexion and extension gaps were assessed with the use of spacer block (Fig. 16.14). The 90° flexion gap was found tighter, notably medially (Fig. 16.14a), than the gap at 10° of knee flexion (Fig. 16.14c). A recut of the tibia for an additional 2° of slope was performed.

After cementation of the final components (Fig. 16.15), patella tracking was judged

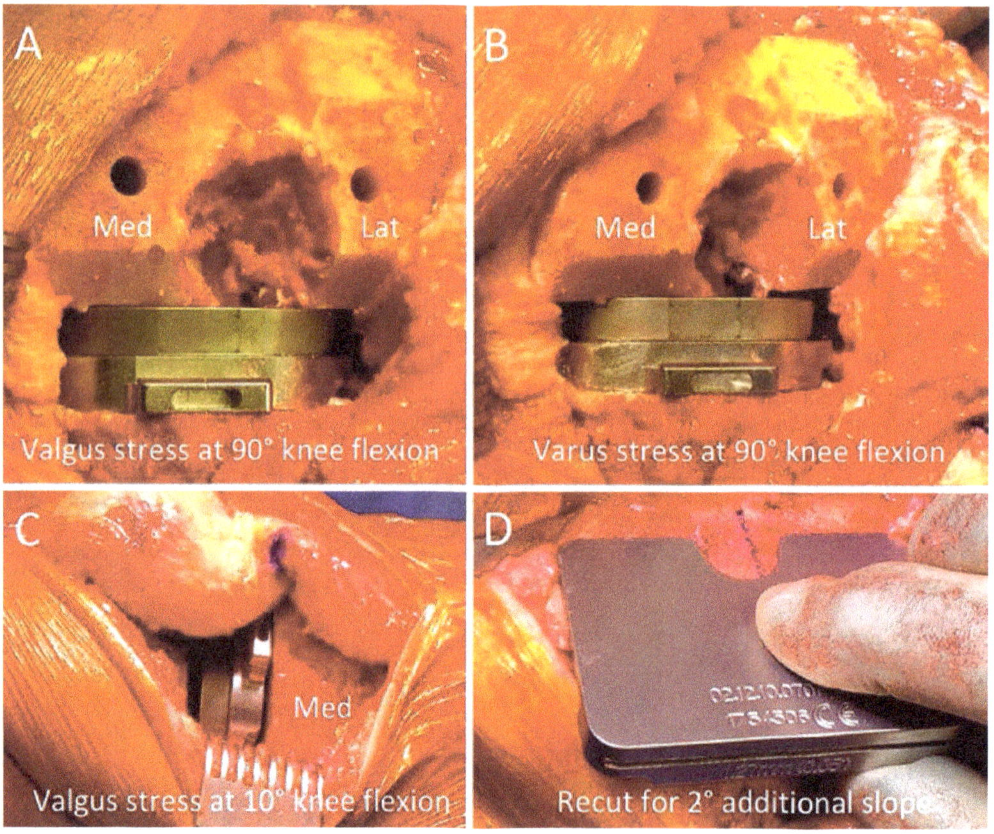

Fig. 16.14 Intra-operative photos illustrating the assessment of the residual femoro-tibial laxity with use of spacer block: medial (**a**) and lateral (**b**) knee compartment laxity in 90 degrees flexion, medial knee compartment laxity in 10 degrees flexion (**c**). As the adequacy of the femoral kinematic cuts was easily confirmed by quality check (calliper) and the femoro-tibial flexion gap was found excessively tight both medially and laterally, it was decided to recut the tibia inorder to slightly increase the slope (**d**)

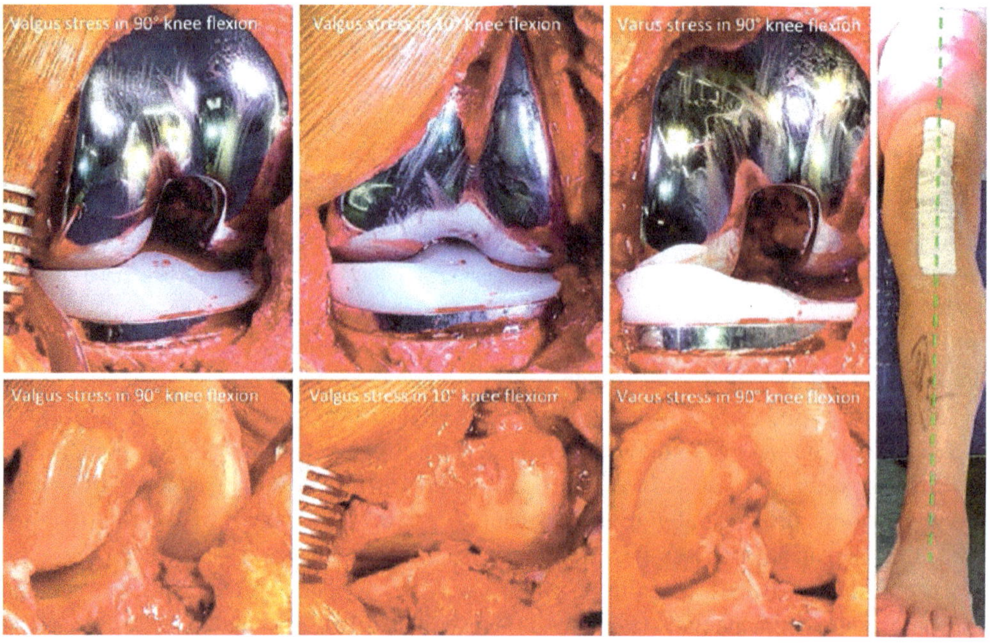

Fig. 16.15 Intra- and post-operative photos illustrating the pre- and post-implantation femoro-tibial laxities and the prosthetic lower limb alignment, respectively

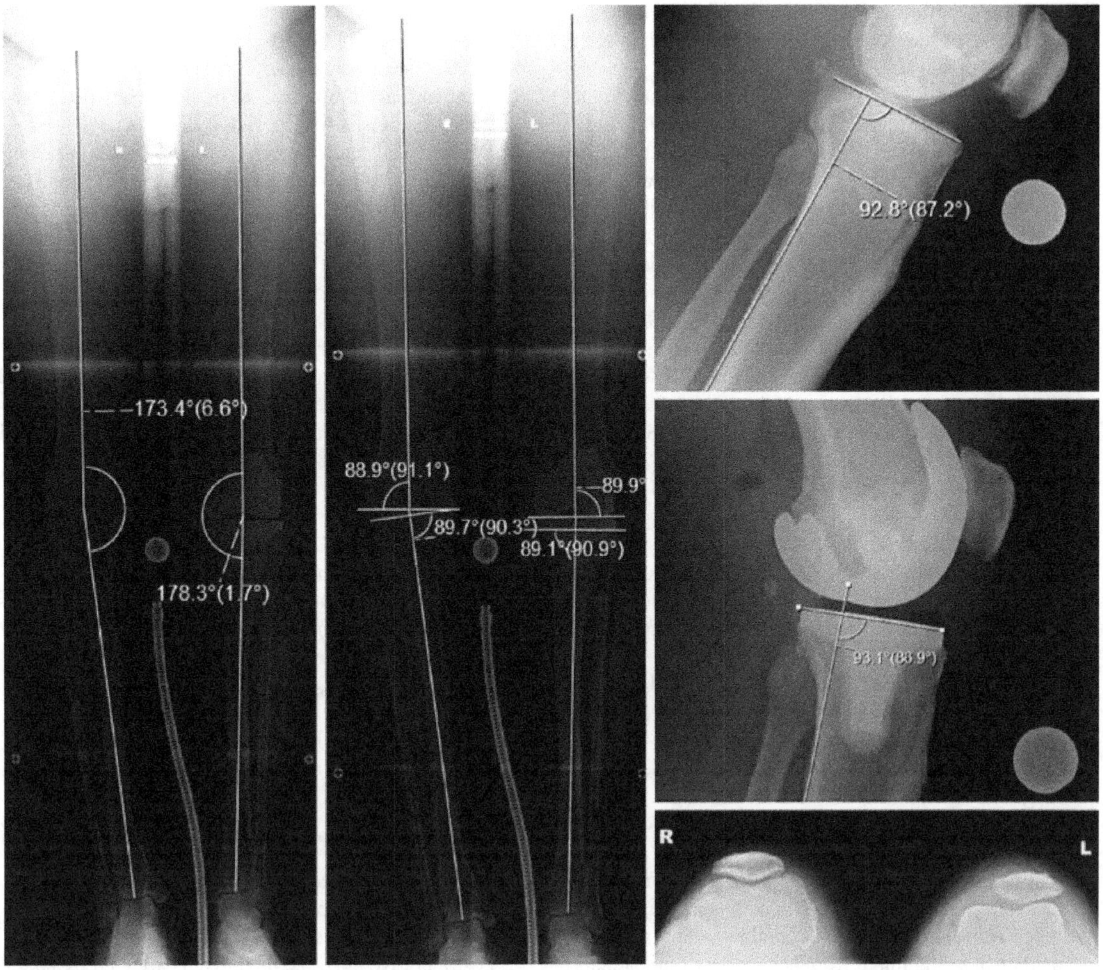

Fig. 16.16 Limb and knee radiographs. Post-operative long-leg radiographs with measurment of limb alignment (left long-leg radiograph) and components alignment relative to the femoral and tibial mechanical axis (right long-leg radiograph) suggesting adequat restoration of the constitutional frontal limb and knee alignment. Pre- and post-operative lateral knee radiographs confirming the adequat restoration of the individual tibia slope. Post-operative skyline view showing slight lateral patella shift at early knee flexion

excellent with no tilt or shift, full knee range of motion was restored, the limb looked neutrally aligned, and assessment of knee laxities showed a constant 2 mm medial and 4 mm lateral laxity throughout the all range of motion. There was no mid-flexion excessive laxity, and no residual laxity was present in full extension. The prosthetic and preoperative knee laxities were close (Fig. 16.15).

On postoperative radiographs (Fig. 16.16), the limb frontal alignment was 178°, and the distal femoral and proximal tibial articular surfaces orientations were restored within 1° from native orientations. On the skyline view, there was a slight lateral shift of the unresurfaced patella.

At 6 months follow-up, the patient was pain-free with an Oxford Knee Score at 42 and a satisfaction at 95/100.

References

1. Howell SM, Hull ML. Kinematically aligned TKA with MRI-based cutting guides. In: Thienpont E, editor. Improving accuracy in knee arthroplasty. New Delhi: Jaypee Brothers Medical Publishers (P) Ltd; 2012. p. 207–32.
2. Eckhoff DG. Three-dimensional mechanics, kinematics, and morphology of the knee viewed in virtual reality. J Bone Jt Surg Am. 2005;87(suppl_2):71.

3. Iranpour F, Merican AM, Dandachli W, et al. The geometry of the trochlear groove. Clin Orthop Relat Res. 2010;468(3):782–8.
4. Yin L, Chen K, Guo L, et al. Identifying the functional flexion-extension axis of the knee: an in-vivo kinematics study. PLoS One. 2015;10(6):e0128877.
5. Rivière C, Iranpour F, Auvinet E, et al. Alignment options for total knee arthroplasty: a systematic review. Orthop Traumatol Surg Res. 2017;103(7):1047–56.
6. Nam D, Nunley RM, Barrack RL. Patient dissatisfaction following total knee replacement: a growing concern? Bone Jt J. 2014;96-B(11_Supple_A):96–100.
7. Meehan JP, Danielsen B, Kim SH, et al. Younger age is associated with a higher risk of early periprosthetic joint infection and aseptic mechanical failure after total knee arthroplasty. J Bone Jt Surg Am. 2014;96(7):529–35.
8. Price AJ, Alvand A, Troelsen A, Katz JN, Hooper G, Gray A, et al. Knee replacement. Lancet. 2018;392(10158):1672–82.
9. Le DH, Goodman SB, Maloney WJ, Huddleston JI. Current modes of failure in TKA: infection, instability, and stiffness predominate. Clin Orthop Relat Res. 2014;472(7):2197–200.
10. Song SJ, Detch RC, Maloney WJ, Goodman SB, Huddleston JI. Causes of instability after total knee arthroplasty. J Arthroplast. 2014;29(2):360–4.
11. Rivière C, Iranpour F, Auvinet E, et al. Mechanical alignment technique for TKA: are there intrinsic technical limitations? Orthop Traumatol Surg Res. 2017;103(7):1057–67.
12. Gu Y, Roth JD, Howell SM, Hull ML. How frequently do four methods for mechanically aligning a total knee arthroplasty cause collateral ligament imbalance and change alignment from normal in white patients? J Bone Jt Surg Am. 2014;96(12):e101–19.
13. Barrack RL, Schrader T, Bertot AJ, et al. Component rotation and anterior knee pain after total knee arthroplasty. Clin Orthop. 2001;392:46–55.
14. Bellemans J, Colyn W, Vandenneucker H, et al. The Chitranjan Ranawat Award: is neutral mechanical alignment normal for all patients?: The concept of constitutional varus. Clin Orthop Relat Res. 2012;470(1):45–53.
15. Roth JD, Howell SM, Hull ML. Native knee laxities at 0°, 45°, and 90° of flexion and their relationship to the goal of the gap-balancing alignment method of total knee arthroplasty. J Bone Jt Surg Am. 2015;97(20):1678–84.
16. Stoddard JE, Deehan DJ, Bull AMJ, et al. No difference in patellar tracking between symmetrical and asymmetrical femoral component designs in TKA. Knee Surg Sports Traumatol Arthrosc. 2014;22(3):534–42.
17. McClelland JA, Webster KE, Feller JA, et al. Knee kinematics during walking at different speeds in people who have undergone total knee replacement. Knee. 2011;18(3):151–5.
18. Fitzpatrick CK, Rullkoetter PJ. Influence of patellofemoral articular geometry and material on mechanics of the unresurfaced patella. J Biomech. 2012;45(11):1909–15.
19. Eckhoff DG, Jacofsky DJ, Springer BD, et al. Bilateral symmetrical comparison of femoral and tibial anatomic features. J Arthroplast. 2016;31(5):1083–90.
20. Deep K. Collateral ligament laxity in knees: what is normal? Clin Orthop Relat Res. 2014;472(11):3426–31.
21. Bonner TJ, Eardley WGP, Patterson P, et al. The effect of post-operative mechanical axis alignment on the survival of primary total knee replacements after a follow-up of 15 years. J Bone Joint Surg Br. 2011;93-B(9):1217–22.
22. Abdel MP, Ollivier M, Parratte S, et al. Effect of postoperative mechanical axis alignment on survival and functional outcomes of modern total knee arthroplasties with cement: a concise follow-up at 20 years. J Bone Jt Surg. 2018;100(6):472–8.
23. Deep K, Eachempati KK, Apsingi S. The dynamic nature of alignment and variations in normal knees. Bone Jt J. 2015;97-B(4):498–502.
24. Rivière C, Ollivier M, Girerd D, et al. Does standing limb alignment after total knee arthroplasty predict dynamic alignment and knee loading during gait? Knee. 2017;24(3):627–33.
25. Nagura T, Niki Y, Harato K, et al. Analysis of the factors that correlate with increased knee adduction moment during gait in the early postoperative period following total knee arthroplasty. Knee. 2017;24(2):250–7.
26. Kutzner I, Trepczynski A, Heller MO, et al. Knee adduction moment and medial contact force—facts about their correlation during gait. PLoS One. 2013;8(12):e81036.
27. Nakano N, Matsumoto T, Muratsu H, et al. Postoperative knee flexion angle is affected by lateral laxity in cruciate-retaining total knee arthroplasty. J Arthroplast. 2016;31(2):401–5.
28. Takahashi T, Ansari J, Pandit H. Kinematically aligned total knee arthroplasty or mechanically aligned total knee arthroplasty. J Knee Surg. 2018;31(10):999–1006.
29. Shelton T, Howell S, Hull M. A total knee arthroplasty is stiffer when the intraoperative tibial force is greater than the native knee. J Knee Surg. 2019;32:1008–14.
30. Shelton TJ, Nedopil AJ, Howell SM, Hull ML. Do varus or valgus outliers have higher forces in the medial or lateral compartments than those which are in-range after a kinematically aligned total knee arthroplasty?: limb and joint line alignment after kinematically aligned total knee arthroplasty. Bone Jt J. 2017;99-B(10):1319–28.
31. Niki Y, Nagura T, Nagai K, et al. Kinematically aligned total knee arthroplasty reduces knee adduction moment more than mechanically aligned total knee arthroplasty. Knee Surg Sports Traumatol Arthrosc. 2018;26(6):1629–35.
32. Blakeney W, Clément J, Desmeules F, et al. Kinematic alignment in total knee arthroplasty better reproduces normal gait than mechanical alignment. In: Knee Surg Sports Traumatol Arthrosc, vol. 27; 2019. p. 1410–7.

33. Keshmiri A, Maderbacher G, Baier C, et al. Kinematic alignment in total knee arthroplasty leads to a better restoration of patellar kinematics compared to mechanic alignment. In: Knee Surg Sports Traumatol Arthrosc, vol. 27; 2019. p. 1529–34.
34. Koh IJ, Park IJ, Lin CC, et al. Kinematically aligned total knee arthroplasty reproduces native patellofemoral biomechanics during deep knee flexion. In: Knee Surg Sports Traumatol Arthrosc, vol. 27; 2019. p. 1520–8.
35. Howell SM, Shelton TJ, Hull ML. Implant survival and function ten years after kinematically aligned total knee arthroplasty. J Arthroplast. 2018;33:3678–84.
36. Nedopil AJ, Howell SM, Hull ML. What clinical characteristics and radiographic parameters are associated with patellofemoral instability after kinematically aligned total knee arthroplasty? Int Orthop. 2017;41(2):283–91.
37. Hutt JRB, LeBlanc M-A, Massé V, et al. Kinematic TKA using navigation: surgical technique and initial results. Orthop Traumatol Surg Res. 2016;102(1):99–104.
38. Almaawi AM, Hutt JRB, Masse V, et al. The impact of mechanical and restricted kinematic alignment on knee anatomy in total knee arthroplasty. J Arthroplast. 2017;32(7):2133–40.
39. Young SW, Walker ML, Bayan A, et al. The Chitranjan S. Ranawat Award: no difference in 2-year functional outcomes using kinematic versus mechanical alignment in TKA: a randomized controlled clinical trial. Clin Orthop Relat Res. 2017;475(1):9–20.
40. Waterson HB, Clement ND, Eyres KS, et al. The early outcome of kinematic *versus* mechanical alignment in total knee arthroplasty: a prospective randomised control trial. Bone Jt J. 2016;98-B(10):1360–8.
41. Calliess T, Bauer K, Stukenborg-Colsman C, et al. PSI kinematic versus non-PSI mechanical alignment in total knee arthroplasty: a prospective, randomized study. Knee Surg Sports Traumatol Arthrosc. 2017;25(6):1743–8.
42. Dossett HG, Estrada NA, Swartz GJ, et al. A randomised controlled trial of kinematically and mechanically aligned total knee replacements: Two-year clinical results. Bone Jt J. 2014;96-B(7):907–13.
43. Niki Y, Kobayashi S, Nagura T, et al. Joint line modification in kinematically aligned total knee arthroplasty improves functional activity but not patient satisfaction. J Arthroplast. 2018;33(7):2125–30.
44. Fitch DA, Sedacki K, Yang Y. Mid- to long-term outcomes of a medial-pivot system for primary total knee replacement: a systematic review and meta-analysis. Bone Jt Res. 2014;3(10):297–304.
45. Howell SM, Papadopoulos S, Kuznik KT, et al. Accurate alignment and high function after kinematically aligned TKA performed with generic instruments. Knee Surg Sports Traumatol Arthrosc. 2013;21(10):2271–80.
46. Nedopil AJ, Singh AK, Howell SM, et al. Does calipered kinematically aligned TKA restore native left to right symmetry of the lower limb and improve function? J Arthroplast. 2018;33(2):398–406.
47. Calliess T, Karkosh R, Windhagen H, et al. Concept of a femur-first-extension-gap-balancer for optimized manual kinematic alignment in total knee arthroplasty. Poster ESSKA Academy 2018.
48. Hutt J, Massé V, Lavigne M, et al. Functional joint line obliquity after kinematic total knee arthroplasty. Int Orthop. 2016;40(1):29–34.
49. Rivière C, Iranpour F, Harris S, et al. The kinematic alignment technique for TKA reliably aligns the femoral component with the cylindrical axis. Orthop Traumatol Surg Res. 2017;103(7):1069–73.
50. Nedopil AJ, Howell SM, Rudert M, et al. How frequent is rotational mismatch within 0°±10° in kinematically aligned total knee arthroplasty? Orthopedics. 2013;36(12):e1515–20.
51. Rivière C, Dhaif F, Shah H, et al. Kinematic alignment of current TKA implants does not restore the native trochlear anatomy. Orthop Traumatol Surg Res. 2018;104(7):983–95.
52. Rivière C, Iranpour F, Harris S, et al. Differences in trochlear parameters between native and prosthetic kinematically or mechanically aligned knees. Orthop Traumatol Surg Res. 2018;104(2):165–70.
53. Dossett HG, Swartz GJ, Estrada NA, et al. Kinematically versus mechanically aligned total knee arthroplasty. Orthopedics. 2012;35:e160–9.
54. Rivière C, Lazic S, Villet L, et al. Kinematic alignment technique for total hip and knee arthroplasty: the personalized implant positioning surgery. EFORT Open Rev. 2018;3(3):98–105.
55. Ng CK, Chen JY, Yeh JZY, et al. Distal femoral rotation correlates with proximal tibial joint line obliquity: a consideration for kinematic total knee arthroplasty. J Arthroplast. 2018;33(6):1936–44.
56. Brar AS, Howell SM, Hull ML. What are the bias, imprecision, and limits of agreement for finding the flexion–extension plane of the knee with five tibial reference lines? Knee. 2016;23(3):406–11.
57. Nam D, Lin KM, Howell SM, et al. Femoral bone and cartilage wear is predictable at 0° and 90° in the osteoarthritic knee treated with total knee arthroplasty. Knee Surg Sports Traumatol Arthrosc. 2014;22(12):2975–81.
58. Matsumoto T, Takayama K, Ishida K, et al. Radiological and clinical comparison of kinematically *versus* mechanically aligned total knee arthroplasty. Bone Jt J. 2017;99-B(5):640–6.
59. Dossett HG, et al. Kinematically versus mechanically aligned total knee arthroplasty. Orthopedics. 2012;35(2):e160–9.
60. Woon JTK, Zeng ISL, Calliess T, et al. Outcome of kinematic alignment using patient-specific instrumentation versus mechanical alignment in

TKA: a meta-analysis and subgroup analysis of randomised trials. Arch Orthop Trauma Surg. 2018;138(9):1293–303.
61. Courtney PM, Lee G-C. Early outcomes of kinematic alignment in primary total knee arthroplasty: a meta-analysis of the literature. J Arthroplast. 2017;32(6):2028–2032.e1.
62. McNair PJ, Boocock MG, Dominick ND, et al. A comparison of walking gait following mechanical and kinematic alignment in total knee joint replacement. J Arthroplast. 2018;33(2):560–4.
63. Ji H-M, Han J, Jin DS, Seo H, Won Y-Y. Kinematically aligned TKA can align knee joint line to horizontal. Knee Surg Sports Traumatol Arthrosc. 2016;24(8):2436–41.
64. Lozano R, Campanelli V, Howell S, Hull M. Kinematic alignment more closely restores the groove location and the sulcus angle of the native trochlea than mechanical alignment: implications for prosthetic design. Knee Surg Sports Traumatol Arthrosc. 2019;27:1504–13.
65. Maillot C, Riviere C, Ciara H. Poor relationship between frontal tibiofemoral and trochlear anatomic parameters: implications for designing new knee implants for kinematic alignment. Knee. 2019;26:106–14.

17

A Comprehensive Study of Restricted Kinematic Alignment

William G. Blakeney and Pascal-André Vendittoli

Key Points

- The normal knee anatomy varies widely, and the more extreme ones may be inherently biomechanically inferior which may have deleterious effects on the TKA biomechanics and wear patterns.
- The restricted kinematic alignment protocol (rKA) has been developed as an alternative solution to the "true" KA technique in situations of patients with atypical knee anatomy.
- The rKA protocol limits the femoral and tibial prosthesis coronal alignment to within ±5° of neutral, with the overall combined lower limb coronal orientation within ±3° of neutral.
- 50% of patients fit within the rKA safe range allowing a pure KA technique. Minimal corrections are needed for one third, and more important anatomy changes are needed for the rest (1/6).
- rKA protocol offers a satisfactory compromise, avoiding the important anatomy modifications and ligamentous releases required with MA but preventing the extremes of implant positioning that true KA technique may produce.

W. G. Blakeney
Department of Surgery, CIUSSS-de-L'Est-de-L'Ile-de-Montréal, Hôpital Maisonneuve Rosemont, Montréal, QC, Canada

Albany Health Campus, Albany, WA, Australia

P.-A. Vendittoli (✉)
Department of Surgery, CIUSSS-de-L'Est-de-L'Ile-de-Montréal, Hôpital Maisonneuve Rosemont, Montréal, QC, Canada

Department of Surgery, Université de Montréal, Montréal, QC, Canada

17.1 Mechanical Alignment: The End of an Era

Most patients following conventional total knee arthroplasty (TKA) do not experience a natural joint [1]. One fifth of patients are dissatisfied [2], over half may have residual symptoms [3], and up to a quarter would, in retrospect, not undergo the same surgery again [4]. Gait analysis studies have demonstrated that patients following TKA walked with less total range of knee motion and significant kinematic discrepancies [5].

When TKA was first introduced, instrument precision was poor, and implantation errors were frequent. There were many pitfalls to overcome; hence the focus was on implant survivorship, rather than reproducing normal knee function [6]. To achieve this, surgeons introduced the mechanical alignment (MA) technique. By selecting a neutral femoral and tibial cut with femoral rotation adapted and ligamentous releases to create equal femoral and extension gaps, a simpler method for alignment was created. This "one size fits all" approach, whilst reproducible, does not respect the wide range of normal anatomy of the knee [7]. Although the mean hip-knee-ankle angle (HKA) of patients scheduled for TKA is near neutral, a study of 4884 patients found only 0.1% of patients had both medial proximal tibial angle (MPTA) and lateral distal femoral angle (LDFA) at neutral, which is what MA aims to generate. Furthermore, a study on 1000 knee CT scans found that a systematic use of MA for TKA leads to many cases with gap asymmetries [8, 9]. Mediolateral imbalances >3 mm were created in 25% of varus and 54% of valgus knees. Using the trans-epicondylar axis for femoral rotation, only 49% of varus and 18% of valgus knees had <3 mm of imbalance in both mediolateral and flexion-extension gaps. Some imbalances may not be correctable surgically and may explain residual TKA instability and poor results.

With a better understanding of normal knee joint anatomy and function, kinematic alignment (KA) technique has been introduced to improve clinical results following TKA. The KA technique for TKA aims to restore the pre-arthritic patient's constitutional lower limb alignment and joint surface orientations. It is a joint resurfacing procedure with only exceptional soft tissue release [10, 11]. We believe it is the end of the MA Era [12].

17.2 Are All Anatomies Physiologic?

The normal knee anatomy varies widely, and pathological changes increase its variability further [7, 13, 14]. In 4884 knees scheduled for TKA, HKA was >3° in 40%, >5° in 19%, and >10° in 3% of them [7]. The MPTA range was from 20.5° varus to 20.5° valgus, with a mean of 2.9° varus. The LDFA range was from 11° varus to 15.5° valgus with a mean of 2.7° valgus. The wide ranges demonstrate the huge variability in patient's anatomy (Fig. 17.1).

The more extreme anatomies may be inherently biomechanically inferior and may have been altered by factors that might predispose to degenerative disease such as trauma, tumours, childhood deformity, or previous surgery (Fig. 17.2). A strong argument for the existence of patho-anatomies is the unilateral occurrence in some patients. We believe that surgeons should not blindly reproduce the same anatomy in these outlier patients as it may have deleterious effects on the TKA biomechanics and wear patterns. On the other hand, creating a neutral mechanical axis in these patients would be a significant anatomic modification and likely cause adjustments in soft tissue balance, differences in joint line orientation, variation of the femoral flexion axis, and alteration of knee kinematics.

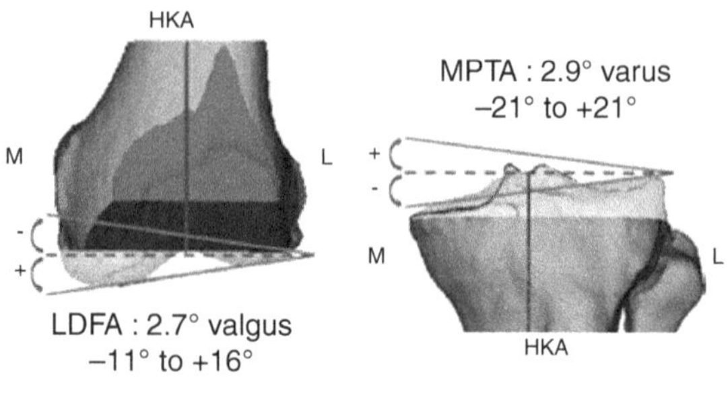

Fig. 17.1 Anatomic modification linked to mechanical alignment technique on the distal femur and proximal tibia

A computer simulation study looking at the effects of MA or KA in TKA on a single knee model found that KA TKA produced near-normal knee kinematics (with greater femoral rollback and more external rotation of the femoral component) [15]. However, there were also increased contact stresses, raising concerns about long-term outcomes. A retrieval study of 178 MA TKA revisions found that knees with greater varus alignment had increased total damage on the retrieved polyethylene inserts [16]. They also found that these MA TKAs tended to drift back towards the preoperative varus deformity before revision surgery, away from a neutral mechanical alignment. Other clinical [17] and simulator [18, 19] studies have similarly found an association between polyethylene wear and varus alignment. Greater tibial varus has also demonstrated a weak correlation ($r^2 = 0.45$) with tibial baseplate migration at 10-year follow-up, in an RSA study [20]. Interestingly, overall limb alignment, from an HKA of 1.3° valgus to over 10° varus, did not affect baseplate migration. There was

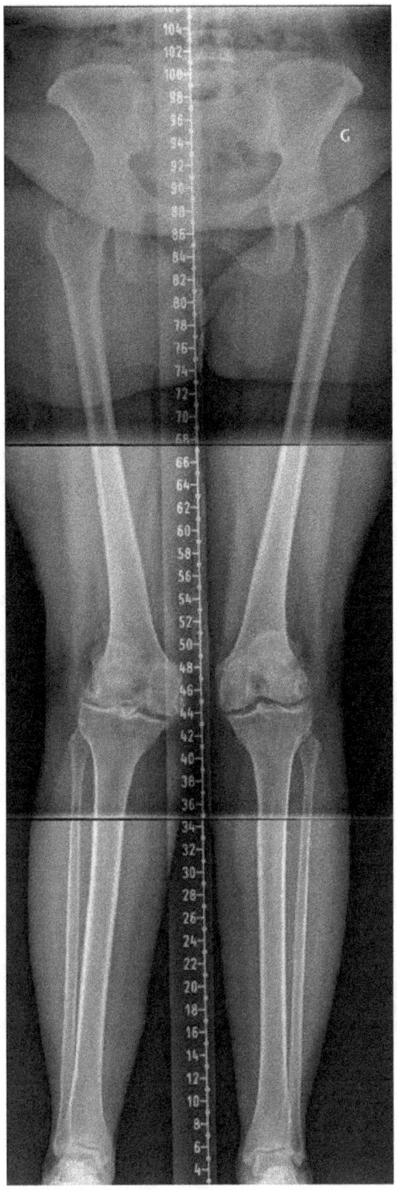

Fig. 17.2 Lower limb full-length radiographs show bilateral valgus lower limbs with severe right knee OA with LDFA of 11° and MPTA of 6°. Reproducing her right lower limb alignment with systematic KA would leave her lower limb HKA in 5° of valgus. We consider her right lower limb anatomy to be pathologic. One argument in favour of this assumption is the difference between the two lower limbs, with the left side being less extreme. Applying our protocol, we would reduce the LDFA to 5° valgus and the MPTA to 2° varus, resulting in a combined HKA of 3° valgus

no difference between those within ±3° of neutral and those >3°. These studies would suggest that systematically reproducing patients' pathoanatomy might not be suitable for implant survivorship using current TKA materials and fixation methods.

17.3 Restricted Kinematic Alignment Protocol (rKA)

The restricted kinematic alignment protocol (rKA) has been developed as an alternative solution to the "true" KA technique [11] in situations of patients with atypical knee anatomy. The concept of rKA is to reproduce the patient's constitutional knee anatomy within a safe range, avoiding the extreme pathological anatomies that have been demonstrated to exist [7]. The rKA protocol limits the femoral and tibial prosthesis coronal alignment to within ±5° of neutral, with the overall combined lower limb coronal orientation within ±3° of neutral (e.g. placing a femur in 4° of valgus with a tibia in 5° of varus would result in an overall combined coronal orientation of 1° varus). To resurface the posterior condyles, a posterior referencing guide is set to neutral rotation, thus resecting only the implant thickness of the posterior condyles and matching each patient's native femoral orientation. Tibial baseplate rotation is set relative to the trial femoral component with the knee in extension.

The surgeon aims to reproduce the patient's normal anatomy as in the KA technique. This can be achieved using measured resection techniques with a calliper, intraoperative computer navigation or preoperative planning with patient-specific instrumentation. Resections are only modified from the patient's anatomy if the measured angles fall outside the predefined safe range. A study assessed the preoperative CT scans of 4884 knees undergoing TKA surgery to analyse the effect of the rKA technique [7]. This demonstrated that 51% of patients fell within the safe range allowing a pure KA technique. Allowing for minimal corrections (mean of 0.5° for the tibia and 0.3° for the femur), this was increased to 83% of all patients.

The protocol for performing these minimal corrections is as follows (Fig. 17.3). First, the surgeon

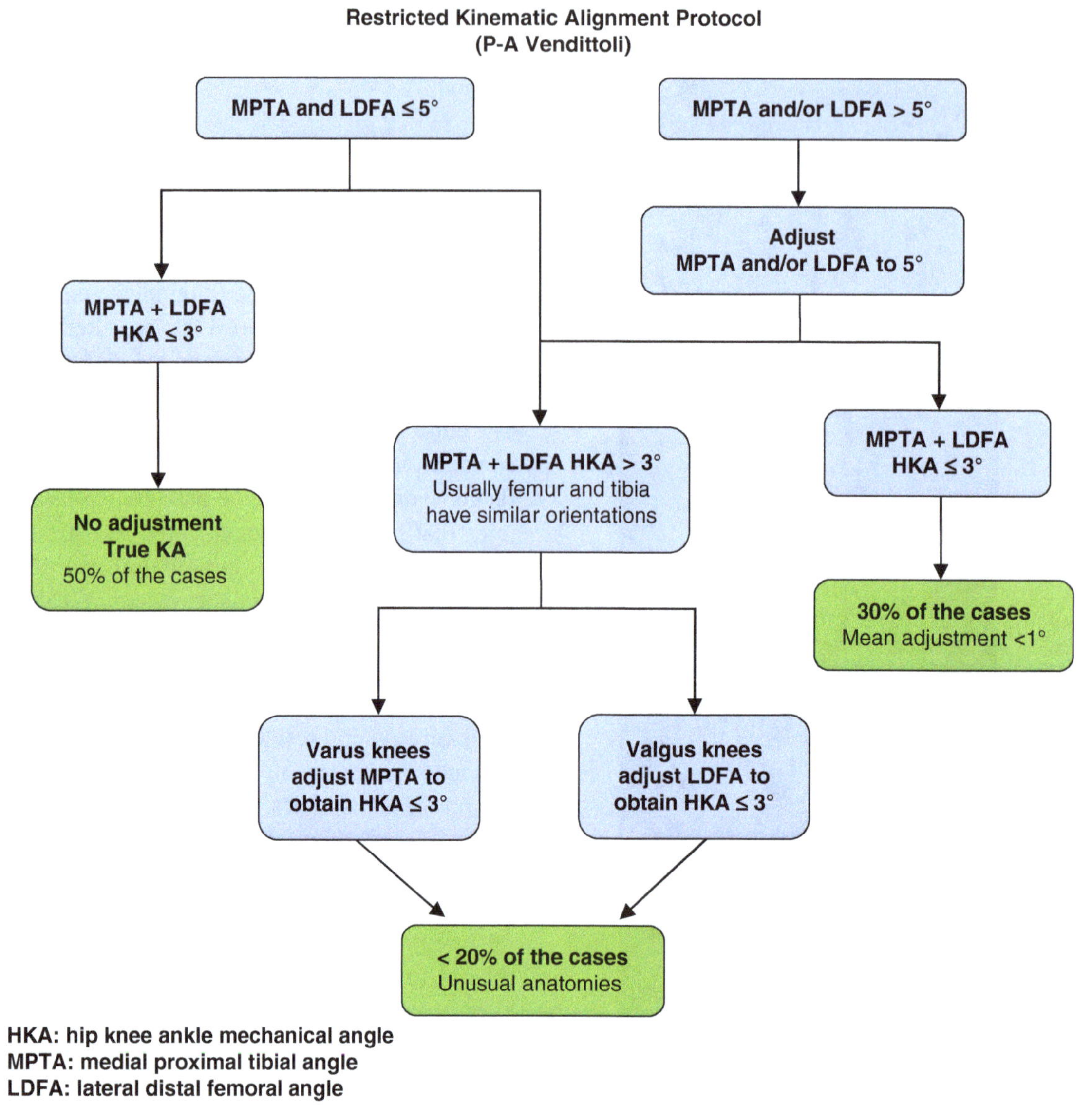

Fig. 17.3 rKA decision-making flow diagram

corrects the tibial and/or femoral bone cuts to fall within the 5° limit. This will then correct the overall HKA to within ±3° of neutral in a significant proportion (51%). In 8% of the cases, the patient maintained an HKA of >3° of varus (e.g. femur 1° valgus and tibia 5° varus = HKA 4° varus). In these cases, the tibial varus was further reduced until the HKA was 3° varus. In 7% of cases, the patient maintained an HKA of >3° of valgus (e.g. femur 5° valgus and tibia 1° varus = HKA 4° valgus). In these cases, the tibial varus was increased until the HKA was 3° valgus. When anatomic correction is needed, we prefer to modify the tibia to preserve as much as possible the femoral anatomy and its flexion axis. Ligamentous releases are usually not needed in cases with anatomic modifications of <3°. In larger corrections, minimal releases can be added (usually, to a much lesser degree compared to MA).

In our simulation study [7], 17% of knees had unusual anatomy, with both the femur and tibia articular orientations being in varus or valgus. As both bones contribute the same direction to the overall HKA deviation, the surgeon needs to decide which bone to correct to fall into the safe range. As stated earlier, we believe that the femoral flexion axis plays the more significant role in knee kinematics, our practice is to preserve femoral anatomy as closely as possible and perform greater modifications on the tibial side. For example, in a valgus knee with a femur in 9° valgus and a tibia with 1° valgus (overall HKA of 10° valgus), the femoral cut is modified to our maximum of 5° valgus and the tibial cut corrected to 2° varus, giving an overall HKA of 3° valgus. Similarly, in a severe varus knee with 2° varus femur and 6° varus tibia (overall HKA of 8° varus), the femoral orientation is maintained (2° varus), and the tibial varus is reduced to 1°, giving an overall HKA of 3° varus. One must consider that most of these cases have associated extra-articular deformities explaining these extremes HKAs. The severe valgus often has a tibia valga deformity in the diaphysis, and the severe varus may have a femoral bowing contributing to the lower limb alignment [21]. In these cases, resurfacing the knee joint (KA) will favour ligament laxities preservation but will not address the lower limb deviation linked to the extra-articular deformity. On the other hand, performing the rKA protocol will correct the extra-articular deformity with intra-articular cuts and may require ligament release/adjustment to avoid secondary instability.

The rKA protocol brings back the extreme anatomies towards acceptable values, modifying their deformities to allow an implant orientation compatible with current materials and fixation methods. On the other hand, simulating an MA technique in this same cohort of patients, significantly larger corrections were necessary [7]. The mean MPTA correction was 3.3° for MA versus 0.5° for rKA ($p < 0.001$). Similarly, the mean LDFA correction was 3.2° for MA versus 0.3° for rKA ($p < 0.001$). This highlights that across a large population, performing MA requires significant changes to normal anatomy. These greater anatomic modifications then necessitate larger soft tissue releases to balance the knee, which may have detrimental effects on normal biomechanics.

17.4 rKA Clinical Results

A clinical series of the first 100 patients operated on using the rKA protocol demonstrated satisfactory functional outcomes at early follow-up (mean 2.4 years, range 1–3.7). Only 5% of the knees required minor ligamentous release. A study of gait analysis comparing patients operated on with rKA compared to MA technique demonstrated that the rKA patients had knee kinematics that were significantly closer to healthy controls than MA patients [22]. The MA group displayed several significant knee kinematic differences to the healthy group: less sagittal plane range of motion (49° vs. 54°, $p = 0.020$), decreased maximum flexion (52° vs. 58°, $p = 0.002$), and increased adduction angle (2.0–7.5° vs. −2.8–3.0°, $p < 0.05$). These kinematic differences translated in significantly higher postoperative KOOS score in the KA group compared to the MA group (74 vs. 61, $p = 0.034$).

In a study of 1000 preoperative CT scans of patients undergoing TKA, bone cuts, we compared the mediolateral and flexion-extension gap asymmetry between measured resection MA and rKA protocol bone cut simulations. Two MA techniques were simulated for rotation: using the surgical transepicondyar axis (TEA) and 3° to the posterior condyles (PC). Extension space mediolateral (ML) imbalances (>2 mm) occurred in 33% of TKA with MA technique versus 8% of the knees with rKA; imbalances (>4 mm) were present in up to 11% of MA knees versus 1% rKA ($p < 0.001$). Using the MA technique, for the flexion space, higher ML imbalance rates were created by the TEA technique ($p < 0.001$). rKA again performed better than both MA techniques using TEA or 3° PC techniques ($p < 0.001$). Using MA with TEA or PC, there were only 49% and 63% of the knees respectively with < 3 mm of imbalance throughout the extension and flexion spaces and medial and lateral compartments versus 92% using rKA ($p < 0.001$). Other studies have similarly reported that the MA technique frequently results in significant anatomical modifications with a wide range of complex collateral ligament imbalances, which are not correctable by collateral ligament release [7, 23].

17.5 rKA Versus True KA: A Compromise?

Many surgeons worry about leaving too much varus or valgus with the KA technique. Howell et al. [24] observed 97.5% implant survivorship in a cohort of 208 KA TKAs at 6-year follow-up, with no increased failure in those with greater varus. In another study, radiostereometric analysis of TKAs randomised to MA or KA did not discern significant differences in implant migration between groups [25]. There are no long-term follow-up studies on KA TKAs, whereas MA TKAs have a long history of good survivorship [26–28]. Achieving a mechanical axis within 3° of neutral has been associated with better functional outcomes than malaligned TKAs in some studies [29–31]. Other studies have demonstrated increased aseptic loosening and rates of failure with malaligned components [32–34]. In contrast, more recent studies have failed to demonstrate greater survivorship or functional outcomes in well-aligned prostheses (within ±3° of neutral) compared to malaligned TKAs [35–38]. The results of these studies should be generalised to KA with caution. It must be understood that accurate KA, aiming for an HKA other than neutral, is very different from a malaligned TKA when aiming for neutral. There are no doubt other factors than coronal prosthesis alignment that affect how the knee will be loaded dynamically. Studies, both in asymptomatic patients [39] and in kinematic TKA patients [40], have demonstrated that despite a range in alignment, the joint line remains parallel to the ground when standing. The resultant functional joint line orientation may well be favourable for the overall load profile of the prosthetic joint.

In the absence of further evidence from long-term studies of KA TKAs, however, some authors have cautioned against widespread adoption of KA technique [41]. We believe the rKA protocol offers a satisfactory compromise, allowing recreation of normal patient anatomy for the majority of cases, avoiding the excessive corrections and ligamentous releases required with MA, but preventing the extremes of implant positioning that an unrestricted KA technique may produce.

17.6 Case Example

17.6.1 Case Example 1

A 65-year-old male, with severe varus right knee OA. Preoperative long leg radiographs (see Fig. 17.4) demonstrate right femoral varus (LDFA of 93°) with a valgus tibia (MPTA of 88°). The patient elected to undergo right TKA using our rKA protocol. In this case, as is the case with ~50% of cases, no modifications were required from his preoperative constitutional alignment allowing a pure KA approach. Although his resultant HKA is near neutral (1° varus), his joint surface orientations were maintained. With MA technique, both the femoral and tibial anatomies would have been significantly modified to neutral. This joint line orientation and flexion axis changes would affect knee kinematics. It is interesting to note that in such a case, using intramedullary rod alignment for the tibia would lead to an important error in valgus.

17.6.2 Case Example 2

An active 58-year-old female, with painful right knee OA and previous left knee MA TKA. Preoperative planning long radiographs demonstrate right femoral valgus (LDFA of 83°) with a neutral tibia (MPTA of 90°) (see Fig. 17.5). The patient elected to undergo right TKA using our rKA protocol. In this case, to stay within our rKA safe range, we increased her LDFA to 85° (reducing valgus from 7° to 5°) and reduced her MPTA to 88° (from neutral to 2° varus). Resultant HKA was valgus 3°. With such corrections, we tried to minimise femoral axis and femoral anatomy modifications. No ligament release was needed. The patient underwent an uneventful postoperative recovery. At 4 months post-surgery, she feels she has a right forgotten knee without restrictions. On the left MA TKA, even with a LDFA and MPTA at 90°, the resulting HKA is 3° varus. The patient prefers her right TKA.

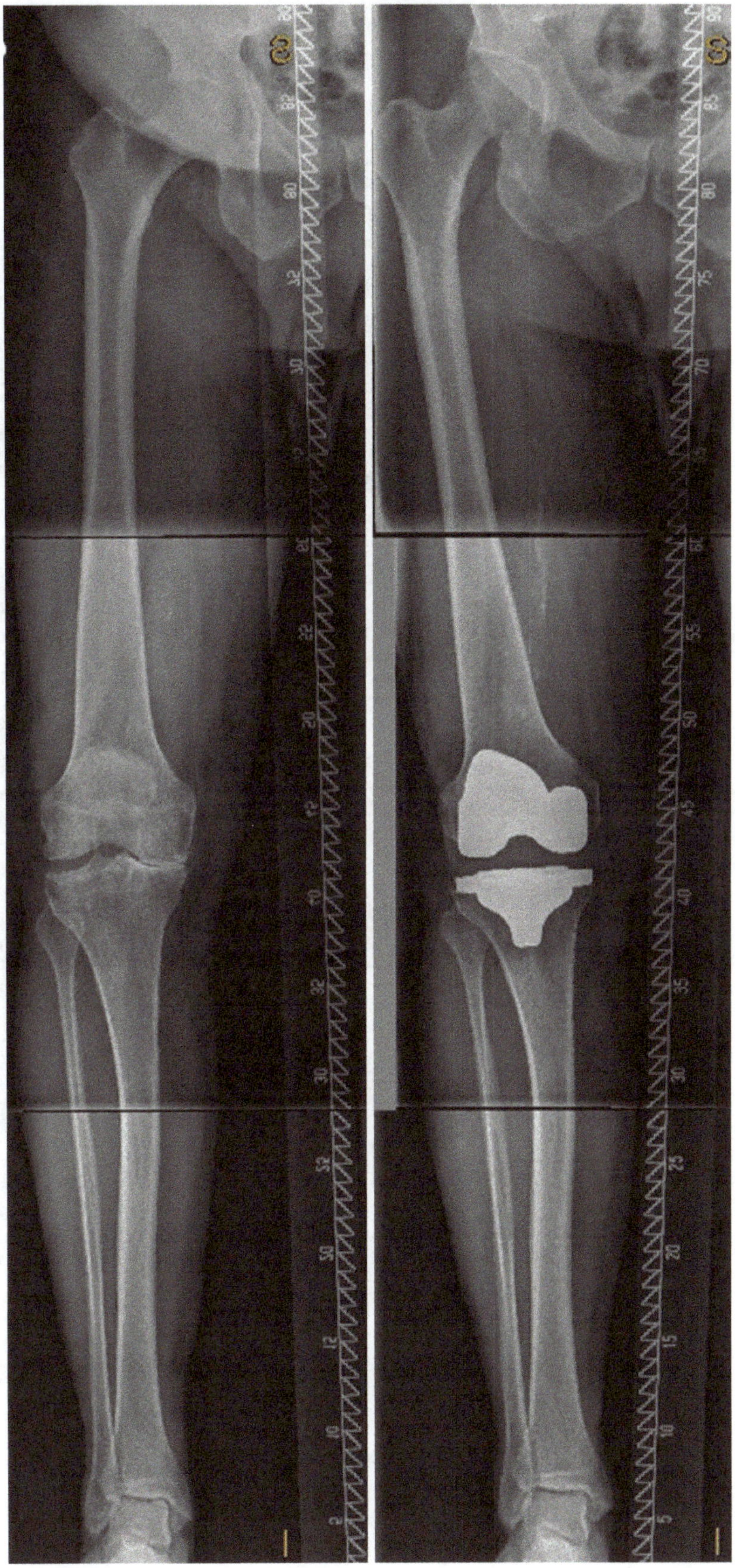

Fig. 17.4 Standing long radiographs of case example 1

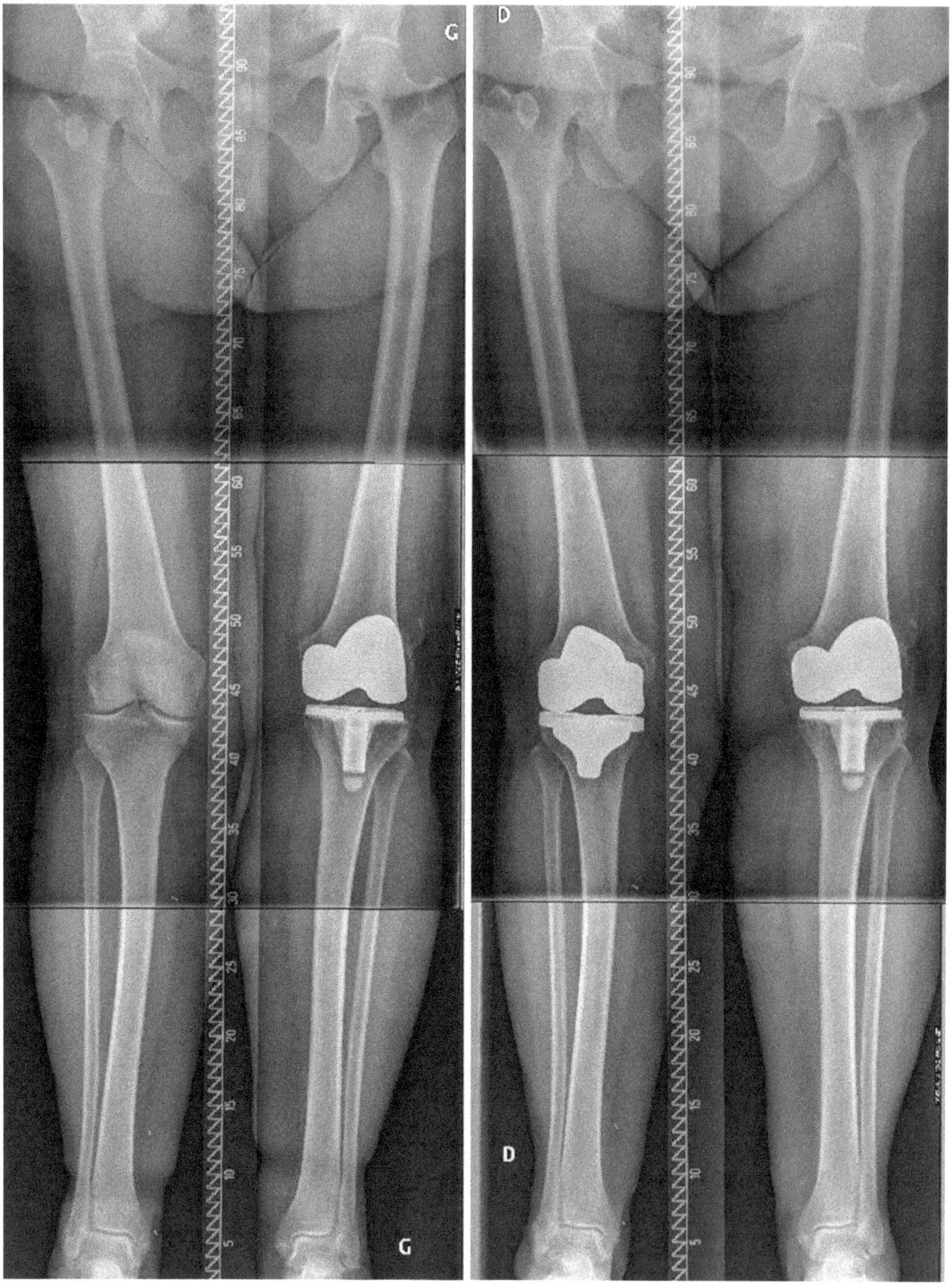

Fig. 17.5 Standing long radiographs of case example number 2

References

1. Collins M, Lavigne M, Girard J, Vendittoli PA. Joint perception after hip or knee replacement surgery. Orthop Traumatol Surg Res. 2012;98:275–80.
2. Bourne RB, Chesworth BM, Davis AM, Mahomed NN, Charron KDJ. Patient satisfaction after total knee arthroplasty: who is satisfied and who is not? Clin Orthop Relat Res. 2010;468:57–63.
3. Nam D, Nunley RM, Barrack RL. Patient dissatisfaction following total knee replacement: a growing concern? Bone Joint J. 2014;96-B:96–100.
4. Lingard EA, Sledge CB, Learmonth ID, Kinemax Outcomes G. Patient expectations regarding total knee arthroplasty: differences among the United States, United Kingdom, and Australia. J Bone Joint Surg Am. 2006;88:1201–7.
5. McClelland JA, Webster KE, Feller JA. Gait analysis of patients following total knee replacement: a systematic review. Knee. 2007;14:253–63.
6. Vendittoli PA, Blakeney W. Redefining knee replacement. Orthop Traumatol Surg Res. 2017;103:977–9.
7. Almaawi AM, Hutt JRB, Masse V, Lavigne M, Vendittoli P-A. The impact of mechanical and restricted kinematic alignment on knee anatomy in total knee arthroplasty. J Arthroplast. 2017;32:2133–40.
8. Blakeney W, Beaulieu Y, Puliero B, Kiss MO, Vendittoli PA. Bone resection for mechanically aligned total knee arthroplasty creates frequent gap modifications and imbalances. Knee Surg Sports Traumatol Arthrosc. 2019. https://doi.org/10.1007/s00167-019-05562-8.
9. Blakeney W, Beaulieu Y, Kiss MO, Rivière C, Vendittoli PA. Less gap imbalance with restricted kinematic alignment than with mechanically aligned total knee arthroplasty: simulations on 3-D bone models created from CT-scans. Acta Orthop. 2019;90(6):602–9.
10. Howell SM, Howell SJ, Hull ML. Assessment of the radii of the medial and lateral femoral condyles in varus and valgus knees with osteoarthritis. J Bone Joint Surg Am. 2010;92:98–104.
11. Hutt JRB, LeBlanc MA, Massé V, Lavigne M, Vendittoli PA. Kinematic TKA using navigation: surgical technique and initial results. Orthop Traumatol Surg Res. 2016;102:99–104.
12. Rivière C, Vigdorchik JM, Vendittoli PA. Mechanical alignment: The end of an era! Orthop Traumatol Surg Res. 2019;105(7):1223–6. https://doi.org/10.1016/j.otsr.2019.07.005.
13. Bellemans J, Colyn W, Vandenneucker H, Victor J. The Chitranjan Ranawat award: is neutral mechanical alignment normal for all patients? The concept of constitutional varus. Clin Orthop Relat Res. 2012;470:45–53.
14. Eckhoff DG, Bach JM, Spitzer VM, et al. Three-dimensional mechanics, kinematics, and morphology of the knee viewed in virtual reality. J Bone Joint Surg Am. 2005;87(Suppl 2):71–80.
15. Ishikawa M, Kuriyama S, Ito H, Furu M, Nakamura S, Matsuda S. Kinematic alignment produces near-normal knee motion but increases contact stress after total knee arthroplasty: a case study on a single implant design. Knee. 2015;22:206–12.
16. Li Z, Esposito CI, Koch CN, Lee YY, Padgett DE, Wright TM. Polyethylene damage increases with varus implant alignment in posterior-stabilized and constrained condylar knee arthroplasty. Clin Orthop Relat Res. 2017;475:2981–91.
17. Srivastava A, Lee GY, Steklov N, Colwell CW Jr, Ezzet KA, D'Lima DD. Effect of tibial component varus on wear in total knee arthroplasty. Knee. 2012;19:560–3.
18. Werner FW, Ayers DC, Maletsky LP, Rullkoetter PJ. The effect of valgus/varus malalignment on load distribution in total knee replacements. J Biomech. 2005;38:349–55.
19. D'Lima DD, Hermida JC, Chen PC, Colwell CW. Polyethylene wear and variations in knee kinematics. Clin Orthop Relat Res. 2001;392:124–30.
20. Teeter MG, Naudie DD, McCalden RW, et al. Varus tibial alignment is associated with greater tibial baseplate migration at 10 years following total knee arthroplasty. Knee Surg Sports Traumatol Arthrosc. 2018;26:1610–7.
21. Alghamdi A, Rahme M, Lavigne M, Masse V, Vendittoli PA. Tibia valga morphology in osteoarthritic knees: importance of preoperative full limb radiographs in total knee arthroplasty. J Arthroplast. 2014;29:1671–6.
22. Blakeney W, Clément J, Desmeules F, Hagemeister N, Rivière C, Vendittoli PA. Kinematic alignment in total knee arthroplasty better reproduces normal gait than mechanical alignment. Knee Surg Sports Traumatol Arthrosc. 2019;27(5):1410–7. https://doi.org/10.1007/s00167-018-5174-1.
23. Gu Y, Roth JD, Howell SM, Hull ML. How frequently do four methods for mechanically aligning a total knee arthroplasty cause collateral ligament imbalance and change alignment from normal in white patients? AAOS exhibit selection. J Bone Joint Surg Am. 2014;96:e101.
24. Howell SM, Papadopoulos S, Kuznik K, Ghaly LR, Hull ML. Does varus alignment adversely affect implant survival and function six years after kinematically aligned total knee arthroplasty? Int Orthop. 2015;39:2117–24.
25. Laende E, Richardson G, Biddulph M, Dunbar M. Implant fixation and gait analysis at one year following total knee arthroplasty with patient specific cutting blocks versus computer navigation. Bone Jt J. 2016;98-B:136.
26. Font-Rodriguez DE, Scuderi GR, Insall JN. Survivorship of cemented total knee arthroplasty. Clin Orthop Relat Res. 1997;345:79–86.
27. Gill GS, Joshi AB, Mills DM. Total condylar knee arthroplasty. 16- to 21-year results. Clin Orthop Relat Res. 1999;367:210–5.

28. Rodricks DJ, Patil S, Pulido P, Colwell CW. Press-fit condylar design total knee arthroplasty. Fourteen to seventeen-year follow-up. J Bone Joint Surg Am. 2007;89:89–95.
29. Choong PF, Dowsey MM, Stoney JD. Does accurate anatomical alignment result in better function and quality of life? Comparing conventional and computer-assisted total knee arthroplasty. J Arthroplast. 2009;24:560–9.
30. Blakeney WG, Khan RJK, Palmer JL. Functional outcomes following total knee arthroplasty: a randomised trial comparing computer-assisted surgery with conventional techniques. Knee. 2014;21:364–8.
31. Longstaff LM, Sloan K, Stamp N, Scaddan M, Beaver R. Good alignment after total knee arthroplasty leads to faster rehabilitation and better function. J Arthroplast. 2009;24:570–8.
32. Berend ME, Ritter MA, Meding JB, et al. Tibial component failure mechanisms in total knee arthroplasty. Clin Orthop Relat Res. 2004;428:26–34.
33. Fang DM, Ritter MA, Davis KE. Coronal alignment in total knee arthroplasty: just how important is it? J Arthroplasty. 2009;24:39–43.
34. Jeffery RS, Morris RW, Denham RA. Coronal alignment after total knee replacement. J Bone Joint Surg Br. 1991;73:709–14.
35. Abdel MP, Ollivier M, Parratte S, Trousdale RT, Berry DJ, Pagnano MW. Effect of postoperative mechanical axis alignment on survival and functional outcomes of modern total knee arthroplasties with cement: a concise follow-up at 20 years. J Bone Joint Surg Am. 2018;100:472–8.
36. Parratte S, Pagnano MW, Trousdale RT, Berry DJ. Effect of postoperative mechanical axis alignment on the fifteen-year survival of modern, cemented total knee replacements. J Bone Joint Surg Am. 2010;92:2143–9.
37. Morgan SS, Bonshahi A, Pradhan N, Gregory A, Gambhir A, Porter ML. The influence of postoperative coronal alignment on revision surgery in total knee arthroplasty. Int Orthop. 2008;32:639–42.
38. Bonner TJ, Eardley WGP, Patterson P, Gregg PJ. The effect of post-operative mechanical axis alignment on the survival of primary total knee replacements after a follow-up of 15 years. J Bone Joint Surg Br. 2011;93:1217–22.
39. Victor JM, Bassens D, Bellemans J, Gursu S, Dhollander AA, Verdonk PC. Constitutional varus does not affect joint line orientation in the coronal plane. Clin Orthop Relat Res. 2014;472:98–104.
40. Hutt J, Massé V, Lavigne M, Vendittoli P-A. Functional joint line obliquity after kinematic total knee arthroplasty. Int Orthop. 2016;40:29–34.
41. Abdel MP, Oussedik S, Parratte S, Lustig S, Haddad FS. Coronal alignment in total knee replacement: historical review, contemporary analysis, and future direction. Bone Jt J. 2014;96-B:857–62.

18

Diverse Facets of UKA

Justin Cobb and Charles Rivière

We aim to restore the kinematics of the knee in unicompartmental arthroplasty as it was being used by that individual before the arthrosis developed. The knee is used in compression when standing and squatting and in swing phase, where a competent anterior and posterior cruciate ligament complex allows efficient and congruent flexion after toe off, followed by extension leading to heel strike. This combination of ligament tension and joint congruence is the key to a natural and efficient gait at varying speeds and gradients. Following UKA, which restores both stability and congruence, this state can be approached, but it is very hard to achieve following TKA which inevitably involves ACL sacrifice [1].

However, human gait is not a single phenomenon—the varus knee is part of a human whose whole body movement differs substantially from a human with a valgus knee. Typically, the medial compartment of a varus knee can be considered fairly monodimensionally, in a horizontal coronal axis, while the lateral compartment of a valgus knee needs to rotate around both a coronal and a longitudinal axis. So any partial knee replacement must respect the way in which the knee was used and indeed wore out, correcting slightly, but importantly not trying to 'restore' a mechanical alignment that was never there.

18.1 Indications for Medial UKA (MUKA)

Pain is the dominant indication for MUKA, felt medially or anteromedially. Overloading the medial compartment results in arthrosis in the varus knee, causing painful overload of the bone surfaces. Pain may also be felt laterally, from soft-tissue tension. The pattern of pain is typical of arthrosis—start up pain, stiffness, swelling and loss of function.

The examination findings are also typical, with bone on bone articulation medially or anteromedially. Very strong data exists for the use of MUKA in this condition. Earlier intervention, performing a UKA after meniscal failure but before the onset of established arthrosis is more controversial, with poorer outcomes. The subchondral sclerosis that accompanies established arthrosis is a good substrate

J. Cobb (✉)
The MSk Lab, Imperial College London, London, UK
e-mail: j.cobb@imperial.ac.uk

C. Rivière
The MSk Lab, Imperial College London, London, UK

South West London Elective Orthopaedic Centre, Epsom, UK

for osseomechanical integration of the tibial component. In earlier interventions, before this reactive bone formation is established, there is a higher risk of tibial component loosening or migration. Importantly, there is a stable lateral meniscus. This can be demonstrated, by feeling for any meniscal extrusion on valgus stressing. A stable cruciate complex or central pivot must also be demonstrated using anteroposterior stressing with any varus deformity corrected into neutral.

Medial patella-femoral joint pain can be safely ignored, in a varus knee, as it is relieved by the correction of varus with MUKA [2]. Gross arthrosis of the patella-femoral joint should be addressed separately [3].

Indications for Lateral UKA (LUKA)
Pain is the dominant indication for LUKA, but the lateral compartment is loaded less than the medial compartment in extension, so pain is often less of a feature, with loss of function, and difficulty on stairs being a dominant feature. The pain is felt usually laterally, but often there is tension pain medially. Lateral arthrosis can be felt in the hip area, quite commonly reported either around the greater trochanter or buttock. This completely resolves following LUKA, but of course hip arthrosis can be felt in the knee, so the hip should be X-rayed as well as examined in these circumstances.

The examination findings include a knee that becomes progressively valgus on flexion and easily corrects towards neutral. On stressing the knee in varus, the medial meniscus should not extrude, and the cruciate complex should be stable to anteroposterior stressing. Once again, the patella-femoral joint can be ignored if the symptoms and signs are minor and laterally based [4].

18.2 Threshold for UKA vs. Osteotomy

Most surgeons would hesitate to proceed to knee arthroplasty in patients who want to run. In those who have bone on bone articulation on either the standing AP or Rosenberg views, in my hands the function of a UKA is more reliable than an HTO, which is borne out by one randomised trial [5] and clinical experience [6].

Threshold for UKA vs. Bi-UKA vs. TKA
In active people, who have medial arthrosis but also have an extruding lateral meniscus, a MUKA alone may not be sufficient. Knees like this may progress on the lateral side especially in the obese and in those who are not obviously varus. Currently a TKA is one option, while the more conservative option of a bi-UKA should be considered if the ACL/PCL complex is intact [7]. This bi-UKA is worth discussing in two groups, the young and active, who are likely to break up a TKA; the old and frail patient is another group for whom a bi-UKA may be attractive, as it is a very small operation, much less likely to result in systemic upset.

Device Choice: Mobile or Fixed
UKA is demonstrated to work very well indeed with either mobile [8] or fixed [9] bearings. Medium-term studies do not show major differences, so the choice will be more related to the surgeon and the patient in their regulatory environment. In my personal practice, I advise mobile bearings for those who are likely to wear out a fixed bearing, on both sides.

Fixation Method
Fixation using cement in partial knee replacement has good long-term outcomes in the fixed bearing devices. Cementless fixation is now well established in the mobile bearing implants [10]. In my personal experience, cementless mobile bearing devices have a very low rate of loosening, so they have significant attraction. The only issue in this regard is that of early periprosthetic fracture.

Anterior Cruciate Deficiency
In older or lower demand patients who have no symptoms of instability, a UKA can also be used in the absence of an ACL [11]. Typically in older patients, stiffness is common, while instability is an unusual symptom. So as long as the knee is

left in varus, the lateral compartment is unlikely to deteriorate, and the lack of ACL is seldom a problem.

18.3 Surgical Planning

Prior to surgery, the very minimum planning needed is an appreciation of the size of device required, confirming that neither the tibial plateau nor femoral condyle is too small or too big for the available device's range. From plain radiographs, the standing AP, schuss and lateral view will help in appreciating the amount of tibia vara and intra-articular bone loss. The amount of varus needed on the tibial cut can be envisaged and the depth of bone to be resected, to ensure the minimum thickness of bearing can be accommodated, while at the same time ensuring that the prosthesis is sited on the hardest subchondral bone possible.

Posterior slope of the tibial component and flexion of the femoral component can also be planned from the lateral plain radiographs to a significant extent. For smaller people from the subcontinent, in particular, a higher posterior slope is common and worth preserving to ensure even soft tissue tension. An absent or injured ACL may be better managed by reducing the posterior slope—some anterior tibial translation on the lateral view may confirm the clinical impression.

The last element of surgical planning is device specific. Depending on the design characteristics of the interface, varus slope of the tibial component must be matched with coronal plane and axial plane rotation of the femoral component. A spherical femoral component, on a wholly congruent meniscal bearing, will not need any adjustment from neutral, while a cam-type femoral component may need to be rotated in the coronal plane by a few degrees to ensure linear rather than point contact.

All these elements can be better addressed using 3D planning based upon either MRI or CT. The attraction of what appears to be an increase in complexity is that it allows almost all variables to be documented preoperatively, reducing the intraoperative procedure to a checklist, confirming the preoperative measurements. The best example of this is the tibial 'biscuit' which can be 3D printed and sterilised. The exact shape and size of the bone resection can then be compared with the plan, confirming that the resection is adequate in all dimensions.

18.4 Component Alignment

Kinematic alignment (KA) is a personalized technique for implanting knee components. The principles are to anatomically position (true resurfacing) and kinematically align (on the cylindrical femoral axis) the components, in order to restore the native articular surface level and orientation and improve prosthetic interaction (or biomechanics).

Interestingly, the Philippe Cartier's principles for implanting UKA components were consistent with those promoted by the KA technique but differently formulated (Fig. 18.1). In contrast, the mechanical alignment technique aims to systematically orientate the knee components (standardised implantation), relative to the long bone (femur and tibia) mechanical axes, thus neglecting individual medial knee compartment anatomy but thought to be beneficial for reliable implantation. The non-anatomic mobile bearing UKA Oxford® components have historically been recommended to be mechanically implanted while still reproducing the constitutional limb alignment (or hip-knee-ankle angle). The Oxford® femoral component is therefore oriented in the coronal plane parallel to the femoral mechanical axis; the tibial component is frontally positioned perpendicular to the tibia mechanical axis and with a 7° posterior slope. Personalizing the Oxford® components' orientation by performing kinematic alignment would reproduce the medial knee compartment anatomy and potentially be clinically advantageous by preserving tibia bone stock and by optimising the interactions between bone and prosthesis (more physiological loading of the supportive bone) and between bearing surfaces. It is therefore the authors' preference to perform kinematic implantation of UKA, regardless of whether the bearing is fixed or mobile (Fig. 18.2).

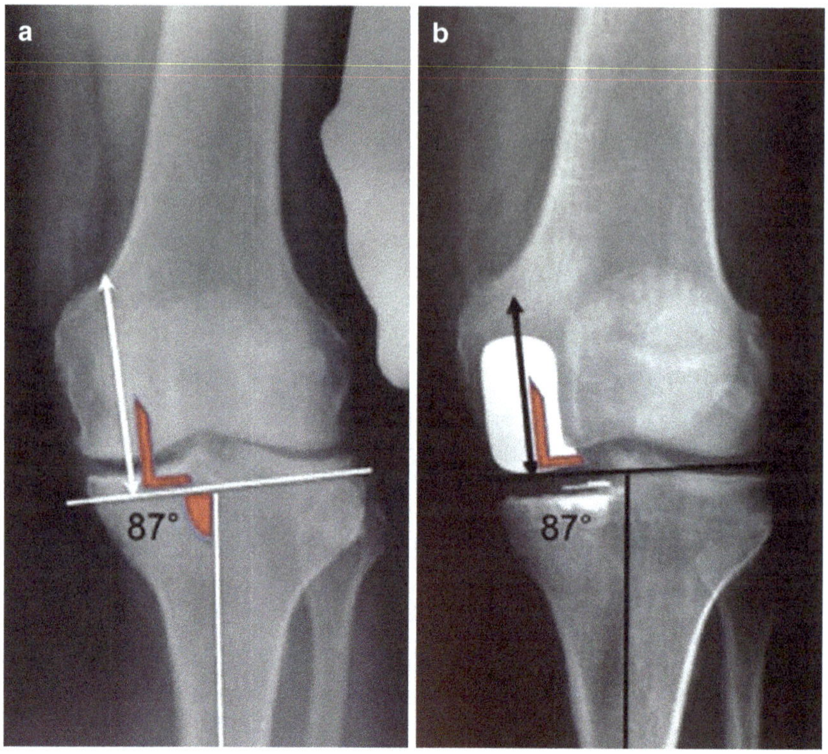

Fig. 18.1 Anteroposterior radiographs of a left knee before (**a**) and after (**b**) kinematic implantation of a fixed bearing medial UKA. The component alignment aims to reproduce the native orientation of articular surfaces (Image courtesy of Deschamps et al. [15])

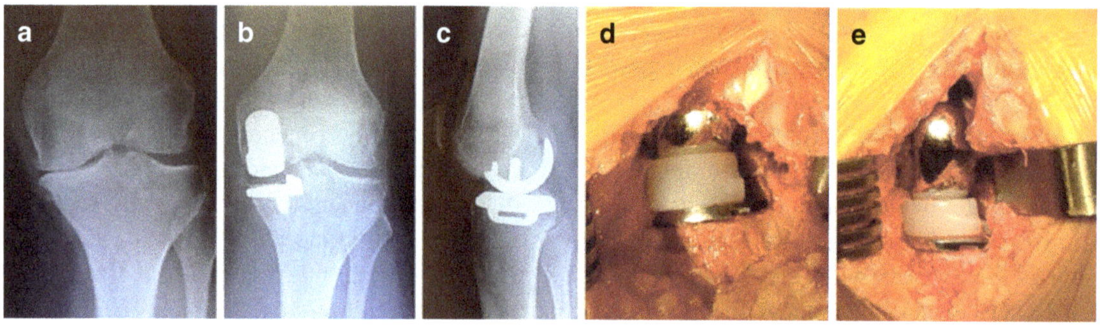

Fig. 18.2 Preoperative (**a**) and postoperative frontal (**b**) and lateral (**c**) radiographic views of a left knee implanted with a kinematically aligned mobile bearing Oxford® medial UKA. Intraoperative photos illustrating a good interaction between components in extension (**d**) and in flexion (**e**)

18.5 Technical Considerations

The patient can be set up in either the supine 'TKA' position or the 'dangle'. Both work well. The main reason for supine surgery is to allow conversion to TKA or if the addition of patella-femoral arthroplasty has been planned. The use of a tourniquet is not compulsory and is not needed if cementless fixation is planned but may help if cement is needed. Because the procedure should not last long, a tourniquet has few complications.

18.6 Medial

Following exposure and thorough clearance of osteophytes in the notch, the knee should extend well. Full flexion may not be possible until posterior osteophytes are removed, but flexion to 110° should now be easy, with gentle flexion beyond gravity alone. With the knee in 30° of flexion and with retractors in situ, there is no tension in the soft tissues, and the surgeon can confirm the amount of material lost to arthrosis. This will confirm the amount of bone that still needs to be resected, to ensure that only the minimum of bone is removed, and the orientation of the bone cut needed to reproduce the 'Cartier angle'.

Each degree of freedom should be addressed serially.

1. The tibia varus angle: this will have been chosen preoperatively but checked visually. Angle of 3° to 5° for the varus knee and of 1° to 3° for the valgus knee are approximately the respective populations mean values. A neutral or valgus metaphyseal angle is rare, and with UKA, it may increase the risk of tibial subsidence, by cutting into bone in the middle of the tibia that is markedly less stiff than the rest of the bone interface.
2. The posterior slope: this is device and patient specific. The surgeon's aim is to restore the joint line unless the slope is being reduced to compensate for some cruciate insufficiency.
3. Axial rotation: a precise definition of the front of the knee is hard. The flexion axis of the knee is fairly reliable and should be used for the first cut (sagittal cut).
4. Depth of resection: this should be minimal, based upon the amount of bone damage and the device minimum thickness.
5. Medial translation: the sagittal cut should be far up the tibial spine. This may not be possible without some osteophyte trimming of the condyle and retraction of both fat pad and patella. Some extension of the knee may help at this stage.

The tibial bony 'biscuit' is removed and then checked for depth and shape. Based upon its shape, adjustment may be needed. Commonly, the axial rotation may be adjusted, and a more lateral sagittal cut may be performed. The posterior slope should be noted.

The femur is then addressed with the tibial trial prosthesis in place. The knee will by now have a free range of motion between full extension and 100° of flexion. This is needed for femoral preparation. The femoral jigs are placed upon the knee, to ensure that adequate bone is removed in flexion. In medial arthrosis, the flexion gap is always preserved, so it is used as a datum point for ensuring that the flexion axis is restored without tension.

The alignment of the flexion gap is chosen based upon the preoperative analysis and plan including the device choice. Slight coronal plane rotation of the cutting block may be needed, if a fixed bearing device is used, to ensure that the bearing surface is congruent with the tibia. The extension gap is then assessed and compared with the expected gap on the plan. In medial arthrosis, it is always greater than the flexion gap, owing to material loss, while following surgery, the opposite will be the case: the flexion gap will be 1 mm greater than the extension gap, as it is in nature. Once again, subtle rotation and translation of the cutting block may be needed if a fixed bearing device is used, while for a mobile bearing, a neutral alignment is sufficient.

Two common errors occur with femoral block positioning: positioning the femoral block too medially if pushed outwards by a large patella in a large man and failing to flex the knee sufficiently when cutting the flexion gap. Too medial positioning of the femoral component may cause soft tissue impingement, while if the flexion gap is cut at less than 95°, the balance between the flexion and extension gaps will become problematic.

Fine-tuning of the balance between flexion and extension gaps can be achieved in several ways. Ideally, in full extension, the entire knee is snug, with just a single millimetre of play both in varus and valgus. By rocking the knee into valgus and varus, some laxity is felt, even in full extension. It is usually less than 1 mm. When balancing a medial uni, the medial compartment should feel snug in full extension. Checks should be made for any bony impingement in the notch—osteophytes on both tibial and femoral side may cause a block to full pain-free extension. In flexion, there should be no block to further flexion caused by the height of the tibial component. Preoperative analysis and planning will have revealed the presence of posterior osteophytes which may also need to be removed from the femoral condyle to enable full, impingement-free flexion.

18.7 Lateral

The surgical approach to the lateral compartment is broadly similar to the medial but differs in a few important ways.

After exposure and removal of meniscus anteriorly, a thorough osteophytectomy is performed, ensuring that the notch is clear and that any patella and trochlea osteophytes are also removed, so that full extension and flexion are possible.

The knee is then flexed and placed in 'figure-of-4' position. The tibial surface can be seen well in this position, and the tibial cutting block can then be attached. As with the medial side, tibial resection needs to be sufficient to restore the joint line with the minimal thickness of tibial component, to ensure that the strongest subchondral bone is preserved. The bone cut is made at the right orientation for the individual patient, usually in 1° or 2° of varus (mean tibial metaphyseal angle for valgus knees). The tibial 'biscuit' is then removed and inspected. On the lateral side, the common error is to leave the sagittal cut too lateral, pushed that way by the patella tendon and fat pad. By leaving the knee in figure of 4, and extending the knee to 45°, the tension is taken off the extensor mechanism, allowing the surgeon to sublux the patella medially and gain sagittal access.

When undertaking lateral UKA, the wear scar is greatest in the flexion facet, while the distal extension facet may still have full-thickness cartilage, so care must be taken to reduce the extension height sufficiently to ensure full extension without any medial tension. When the knee is rocked into varus in flexion, there should be at least 2 mm more gap than in extension, but in addition, at least 1 mm of opening should be possible in full extension, with no conflict between the edges of the components either in deep flexion or extension. With some ranges of devices, a long-standing valgus knee maybe wider than the range, so the sagittal cut may be more lateral, enabling the tibial component to be placed under the femur.

18.8 Postoperative Care and Outcome Measures

Following conservative arthroplasty of any sort, the postoperative course is not magical: the bone of the tibia, in particular, has to heal, and by leaving the varus knee in slight varus, the load across this interface can be critical. So weight bearing should be gradual and limited by pain. Because the cruciates are intact, joint kinematics are preserved, so the risk of requiring a manipulation under anaesthetic for inadequate range of motion is very small indeed, and no pressure is needed to encourage early range of motion. Physiotherapists will naturally encourage faster rehabilitation, but this is not advisable. The use of a walking aid for the first 3–4 weeks is mandatory.

Metrics of outcome for UKA are quite different from TKA. We recommend two different types of metric: one personal and one physical. The personal metric should revolve around one or two activities that the patient enjoys or used to enjoy. Use these as determinants of outcome. The web-based tool, www.jointpro.co.uk, is a simple way for a surgeon and patient to communicate how well those desired outcomes have been met or exceeded.

The physical dimension can be recorded using a variety of tools. Several pieces of software available for use on smart phones allow monitoring of the time taken for a known circuit, together with top speed, average speed, etc. Alternatively, a treadmill can be used, and measurements of top walking speed, cadence and stride length can be recorded as a measure of progress. Finally, the width of gait, and its consistency, is a sensitive measure, showing the extent to which a patient has returned towards normal. A healthy adult with normal strength and balance has quite a narrow gait, with little variation between steps. With increasing infirmity, the width of the gait increases as does the variability between steps. Preservation of the native joint line and cruciate ligaments enables the patient to retain these normal gait characteristics. This is hard following total joint replacement. These variables are more difficult to record without specialist equipment.

All these physical variables continue to improve postoperatively for at least 12 months, although more than 85% is achieved within 6 months.

18.9 Complications and Their Management

A well-performed, kinematically aligned UKA will seldom fail, but the 'reoperation rate' may well be higher than following total joint replacement for two reasons. First, because the knee feels normal, people do more and so are more prone to further mechanical events, so the lateral meniscus may fail 1 day if someone goes back to the tennis court or the gym. Secondly, it is easy to perform further surgery on a knee with a UKA, so small adjustments are possible. We also now know that they are successful at restoring function, often without the need for a total knee replacement. The last 100 s operations by my group included several causes of second surgery.

18.9.1 Bearing Wear or Fracture

Should a bearing wear out after more than a decade of high performance life, then this should be considered a success—the patient has clearly been having a great time! In this circumstance, a simple bearing change is all that is needed to restore function, and in all probability, there will be no need for a second bearing change as the patient will be that much older.

18.9.2 Bearing Dislocation

This is usually the consequence of excessive laxity or technical error. In either event, correct the error and consider revising the tibial component to a fixed bearing. The procedure is easy, and the cost in functional terms and durability is small, while second dislocations are hard to cope with psychologically.

18.9.3 Progressive Wear on the Contralateral Side

Should this occur within the first 2 years, it suggests that an error in decision-making was made preoperatively, in the diagnosis, or an error was made intraoperatively, by overstuffing the affected compartment. In either event, there are two options to discuss with the patient: immediate exchange to a total knee replacement or the addition of a second UKA. This latter intervention is a much smaller insult and should be considered in the same way as one would address a primary UKA. Most importantly, are the patella-femoral joint and the central pivot healthy? For both the young, and the old and frail, a second UKA is worth considering carefully, once again being sure to leave sufficient laxity in full extension to avoid ACL strain.

18.9.4 Infection

Deep infection is very rare indeed, presumably because the procedure does not involve extensive dissection and there is a correspondingly smaller surface area available for biofilm to develop. Aggressive early open lavage and exchange of plastic components are recommended. Should this fail, then a single stage or a two stages conversion to a primary TKA have good rationales, with the use of a home-made cement uni making life quite manageable with walking aids during the interim for the two stages.

18.9.5 Tibial Periprosthetic Fracture

This is more common if a patient has been on bisphosphonates and using cementless tibial components. Risks can be minimised by ensuring that the tibial resection is appropriately varus and that only minimal thickness of tibia is resected. If pain increases during the postoperative period, early repeat X-ray and CT if in any doubt will confirm the diagnosis. A crack, if detected early, can be treated with two screws and no plate at all. If there has been subsidence, then a buttress plate may be needed. If bone grafting and a plate fail, then consider using a custom condylar replacement. This will allow you to preserve the cruciates and the rest of the knee.

18.9.6 Conversion to TKA

When the rest of the joint has clearly failed, my preference is to use the same arthrotomy for the TKA. I personally use kinematic alignment for the TKA, as it was proven helpful in minimising the need for augments and stems and improved patients clinical scores [12]. The procedure is not difficult, and only two technical tips need to be considered:

Kinematic tibial resection: appropriate varus angle can be measured on pre-UKA radiographs if available or on the opposite knee. Then remove the tibial component with great care, and perform an initial cut removing the implant thickness from the intact side. It may then be necessary to recut, taking 2 mm more, if no bone was removed from the medial side.

Kinematic femoral resection: by maintaining the joint line obliquity of the tibia, femoral alignment will follow kinematic guidelines. Most TKA devices will require further bone resection than the bone implant interface of a UKA, so simply apply the cutting blocks on the knee before taking the femoral component off, and complete as much of the procedure as possible before removing the device very slowly and cautiously.

18.9.7 Why Not Go Straight for Kinematically Aligned TKA?

While TKA is safe and effective, in older people, UKA has the great advantage of safety: the risk of major complications such as infection or a stroke is halved by undergoing the much smaller intervention of UKA [13]. In younger patients, for whom higher-level function matters a great deal, UKA enables more normal gait at higher speeds and on different gradients, restoring function to a higher level than is possible using TKA [14].

Case Study

Mrs. GS presented as a 53-year-old woman, 30 years after ACL reconstruction following a skiing accident. Successive surgeons had suggested TKA, which she refused completely. GS has been very active in adulthood but now completely unable to play tennis or ski.

On examination, there was a significant varus thrust on weight bearing. The gross varus corrected substantially, with a firm medial end point. With gentle valgus pressure, there was no significant AP laxity.

Radiographs confirmed Ahlback grade V arthrosis, with substantial bone loss medially, extensive osteophytes, and a normal-looking lateral compartment (Fig. 18.3).

Preoperative planning confirmed the sizes and positions of the devices and showed the large and posterior wear scar on the tibia. The excessive tibial joint line varus of 11° was planned to be reduced to 5° (Fig. 18.4).

Intraoperatively, there was still some graft present. After correcting the varus, the knee was quite stable, as predicted preoperatively.

At 2 years post-op, function has improved steadily over a 2-year period, with excellent range of motion and return to skiing and tennis (Fig. 18.5). On examination at 1 year post-op, the knee is stable, with a leg that is still 1° or 2° varus. Post-op X-rays show a varus joint line, with good correction of the deformity, and a congruent lateral compartment (Fig. 18.6).

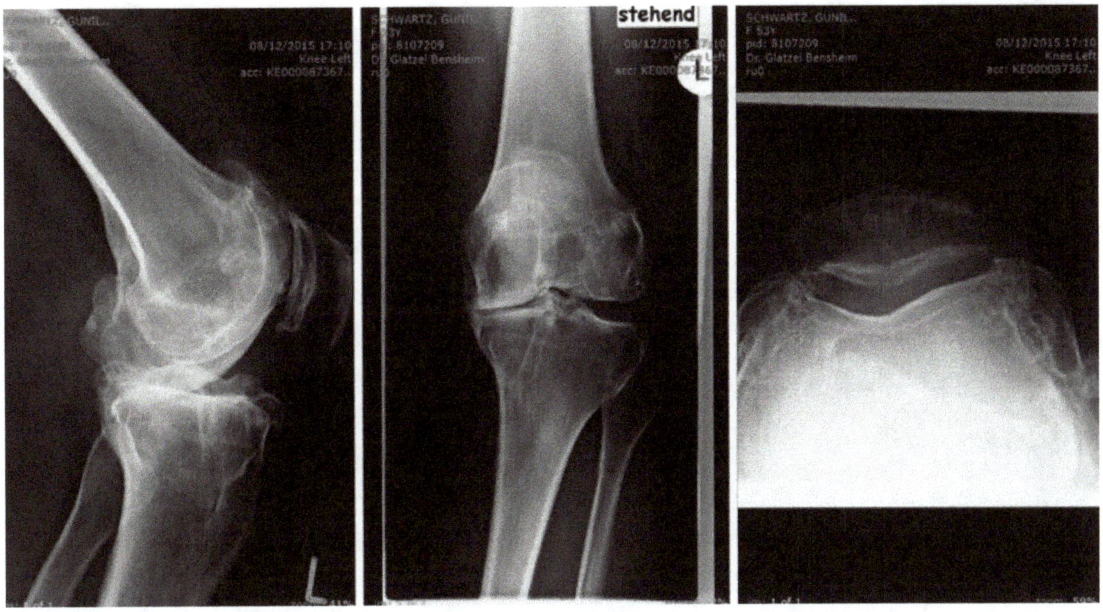

Fig. 18.3 Preoperative radiographs of a varus knee in a fit 53-year-old, 30 years post-ACL reconstruction. There is significant bone loss medially, while the lateral joint line is no longer congruent. There is extensive osteophytosis and some anterior translation of the tibia

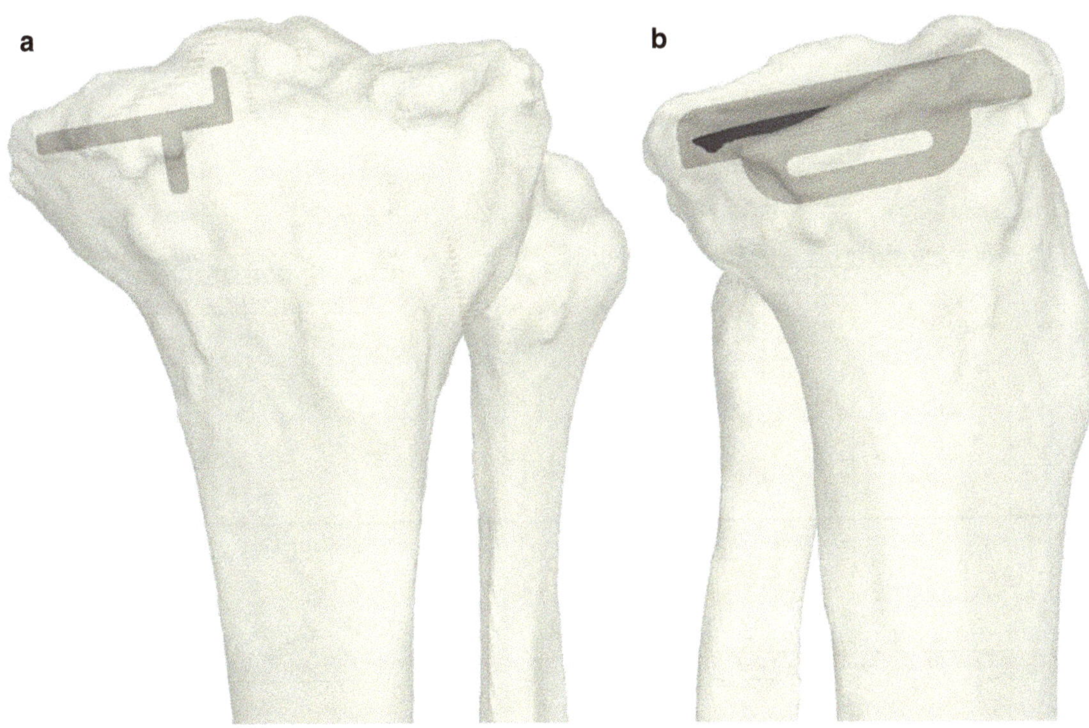

Fig. 18.4 Preoperative plans showing the size and position of the devices chosen. The tibia component was planned with (**a**) 5° of medial slope and (**b**) 8° of posterior slope. The femoral component was planned with (**c**) neutral frontal positioning and (**d**) 7° of flexion

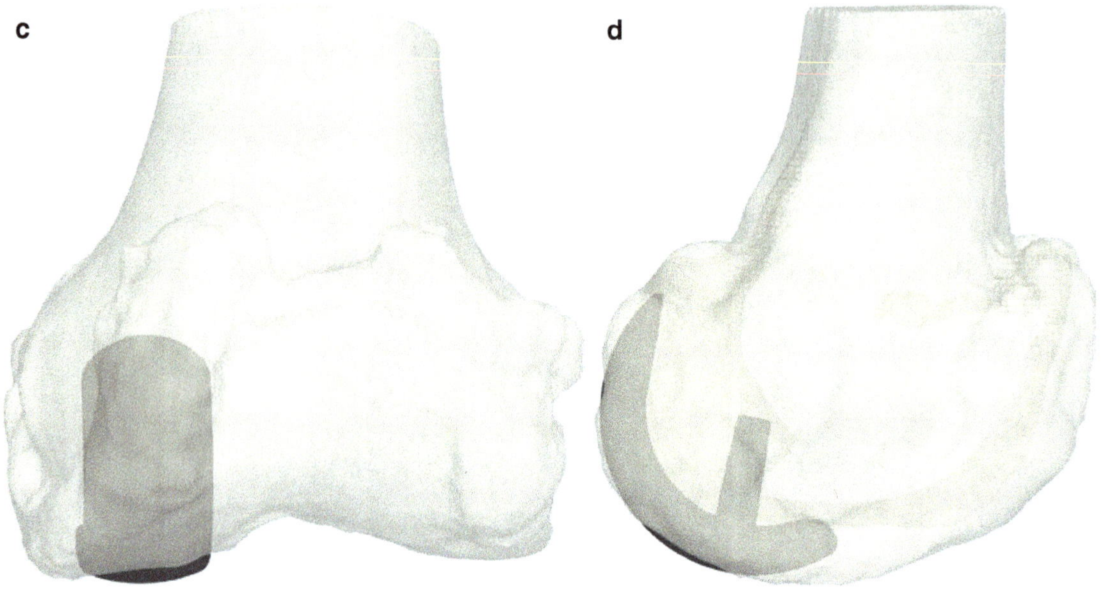

Fig. 18.4 (continued)

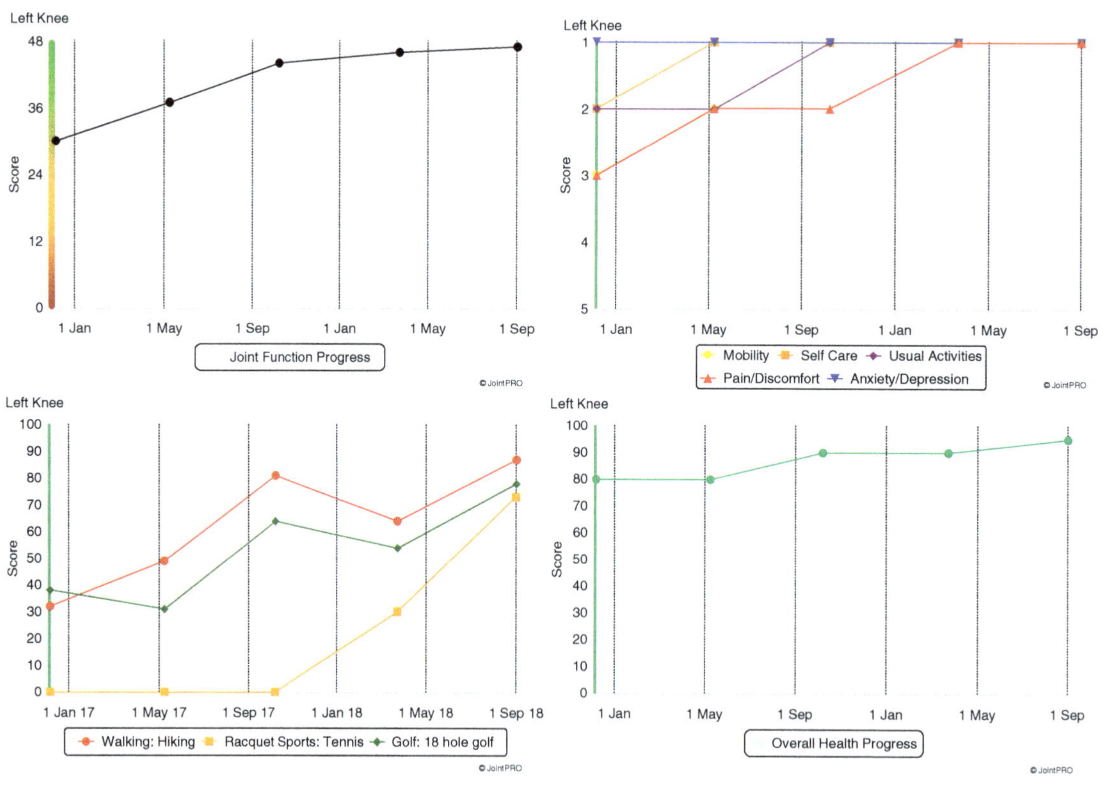

Fig. 18.5 Patient-reported outcome scores from pre-op to 20 months post-op, showing the ceiling effect of the Oxford Knee Score and EQ. 5D, while the functional scores continue to improve beyond 1 year

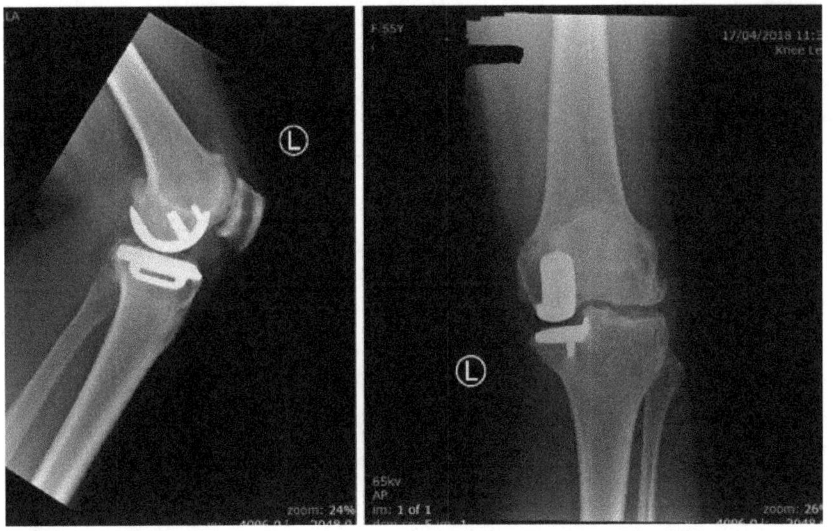

Fig. 18.6 Radiographs 1-year post-op showing that the knee is better aligned, with persisting varus limb alignment, and the planned joint line obliquity of 5°

References

1. Wiik AV, Manning V, Strachan RK, Amis AA, Cobb JP. Unicompartmental knee arthroplasty enables near normal gait at higher speeds, unlike total knee arthroplasty. J Arthroplasty. 2013;28(9 Suppl):176–8.
2. Beard DJ, Pandit H, Gill HS, Hollinghurst D, Dodd CA, Murray DW. The influence of the presence and severity of pre-existing patellofemoral degenerative changes on the outcome of the Oxford medial unicompartmental knee replacement. J Bone Joint Surg Br. 2007;89(12):1597–601.
3. Confalonieri N, Manzotti A, Montironi F, Pullen C. Tissue sparing surgery in knee reconstruction: unicompartmental (UKA), patellofemoral (PFA), UKA + PFA, bi-unicompartmental (bi-UKA) arthroplasties. J Orthop Traumatol. 2008;9(3):171–7.
4. Newman SDS, Altuntas A, Alsop H, Cobb JP. Up to 10 year follow-up of the Oxford domed lateral partial knee replacement from an independent centre. Knee. 2017;24(6):1414–21.
5. Stukenborg-Colsman C, Wirth CJ, Lazovic D, Wefer A. High tibial osteotomy versus unicompartmental joint replacement in unicompartmental knee joint osteoarthritis: 7–10-year follow-up prospective randomised study. Knee. 2001;8(3):187–94.
6. Krych AJ, Reardon P, Sousa P, Pareek A, Stuart M, Pagnano M. Unicompartmental knee arthroplasty provides higher activity and durability than valgus-producing proximal tibial osteotomy at 5 to 7 years. J Bone Joint Surg Am. 2017;99(2):113–22.
7. Confalonieri N, Manzotti A, Cerveri P, De Momi E. Bi-unicompartmental versus total knee arthroplasty: a matched paired study with early clinical results. Arch Orthop Trauma Surg. 2009;129(9):1157–63.
8. Price AJ, Waite JC, Svard U. Long-term clinical results of the medial Oxford unicompartmental knee arthroplasty. Clin Orthop Relat Res. 2005;(435):171–80.
9. Steele RG, Hutabarat S, Evans RL, Ackroyd CE, Newman JH. Survivorship of the St Georg Sled medial unicompartmental knee replacement beyond ten years. J Bone Joint Surg Br. 2006;88(9):1164–8.
10. Liddle AD, Pandit H, O'Brien S, Doran E, Penny ID, Hooper GJ, et al. Cementless fixation in Oxford unicompartmental knee replacement: a multicentre study of 1000 knees. Bone Jt J. 2013;95-B(2):181–7.
11. Boissonneault A, Pandit H, Pegg E, Jenkins C, Gill HS, Dodd CA, et al. No difference in survivorship after unicompartmental knee arthroplasty with or without an intact anterior cruciate ligament. Knee Surg Sports Traumatol Arthrosc. 2013;21(11):2480–6.
12. Toliopoulos P, LeBlanc MA, Hutt J, Lavigne M, Desmeules F, Vendittoli PA. Anatomic versus mechanically aligned total knee arthroplasty for unicompartmental knee arthroplasty revision. Open Orthop J. 2016;10:357–63.
13. Liddle AD, Judge A, Pandit H, Murray DW. Adverse outcomes after total and unicompartmental knee replacement in 101,330 matched patients: a study of data from the National Joint Registry for England and Wales. Lancet. 2014;384(9952):1437–45.
14. Wiik AV, Aqil A, Tankard S, Amis AA, Cobb JP. Downhill walking gait pattern discriminates between types of knee arthroplasty: improved physiological knee functionality in UKA versus TKA. Knee Surg Sports Traumatol Arthrosc. 2015;23(6):1748–55.
15. Deschamps G, Chol C. Fixed-bearing unicompartmental knee arthroplasty. Patient's selection and operative technique. Orthop Traumatol Surg Res. 2011;97:648–61.

Part VI

Utilization of Specific Implants for Personalized Knee Replacement

19

Custom Design UKA

Etienne L. Belzile, Michèle Angers, and Martin Bédard

Key Points

- Modern medicine now involves decreasing cost of surgical intervention while improving patient function and outcome.
- Renewed focus in kinematic alignment of the knee brought back the concept of minimizing biomechanical modifications during knee arthroplasty.
- A custom design UKA shows promising strategies exploiting knowledge from past designs and positioning its expected development in line with existing variability in functional knee phenotypes.

19.1 Introduction

Customization of a unicompartmental knee arthroplasty (UKA) implant is a new surgical philosophy aiming at reproducing the patient's anatomy and joint morphology while minimizing modifications in the biomechanics of the knee joint during reconstruction. Combining the advantages of single-use patient-specific instrumentation and custom implants led to the development of a unique UKA implant system. Custom UKA would offer clinician the opportunity to accurately restore each patient's femoral and tibial morphology while providing additive material to compensate for cartilage loss. Using this particular technique, better restoration of the natural knee kinematic is achieved through personalization of the implants.

Current modern off-the-shelf (OTS) UKA systems propose a joint mechanics based on standardized femoral and tibial morphologies of various sizes extracted from image banks obtained from cohort of normal knees. Most UKA designs have idealized or simplified knee joint biomechanics for the medial compartment. The surgical technique dictates to properly position that implant for optimal function on the medial or lateral compartment. Early results have shown 85% to 98% revision-free joint survival at 10 years [1–4]. Systematic reviews failed to show dominance of one design over another and rather promote equivalent clinical function and risk of revision surgery [5, 6]. Modern reports of fixed bearing devices account for similar implant survival rates [7, 8].

Despite attempts at summarizing femoral condyle morphology into a simple geometrical shape, one has to recognize that the medial and lateral condyles have different morphologies in terms of radius of curvature, j-curve definition and condyle width [9–11]. These differences may not be fully accommodated for by existing OTS implants [12]. The inventory requirements necessary to

E. L. Belzile (✉) · M. Angers · M. Bédard
Department of Surgery, Division of Orthopaedic Surgery, CHU de Québec-Université Laval, Quebec City, QC, Canada
e-mail: etienne.belzile@chudequebec.ca; michele.angers.1@ulaval.ca

cover all possible morphology or variability would be tremendous and therefore impossible to obtain. Instead, minor differences in femoral or tibial morphologies are averaged or ignored by the implant designers. In an era of increasing precision, patient-specific implants have shown statistically superior bone coverage [12]. Using statistical shape models, an estimate of what represents healthy distal femur has been recently conducted [13]. Patient-specific UKA have also been developed [14] and put to clinical use [15].

Why should we be looking for solutions? The most common reasons for failure of UKA today beside infections are polyethylene wear [6, 16], osteoarthritis progression and aseptic loosening [17, 18]. Malposition of implants has been identified as the most important cause leading to aseptic loosening in 559 UKAs with a survival of 83.7 ± 3.5% at 10 years in a multicentric retrospective study [19]. They concluded that a joint space height >2 mm, tibial component obliquity >3°, a tibial slope value >5° or a change in slope >2° and >6° divergence between the tibial and femoral components decreased significantly the prosthesis survival rate.

19.2 What Is the Rational for Custom UKA?

Most patients with medial knee osteoarthritis have a physiological varus aligned morphology before developing further degenerative changes. Thus, it is probably unnecessary to modify this alignment to neutral postoperatively. The custom design aims at 2° to 3° of hip-knee-ankle angle after implantation for a medial UKA [20–22].

The custom design software ensures proper preoperative planning of implant position which has been shown to be capital to optimize femoral to tibial contact stress area [23]. One may have the advantage, during preoperative planning, to measure and adjust such contact stress area. Furthermore, the height of the prosthetic joint space can also be built in the design of the components. This latter option allows implants to be seated *at or less than* 1 mm below the lateral compartment cartilage height [11] and avoids differences greater than 2 mm which have been shown to be detrimental to implant survival [19]. The surgeon should aim to use a 7 mm or 8 mm tibial polyethylene insert upon final implant cementation [16]. Using personalized cutting blocks, bone cut height can be accurately predicted and performed according to the optimal preoperative planning.

19.3 Which Problems Does It Solve?

Two problems are addressed by the custom UKA implant strategy. First, the exact reproduction of the patient's femoral condyle curvature and morphology combined with the natural patient's tibial slope should replicate native ligamentous tension throughout the full range of motion. Indeed, accurate ligamentous laxities across the full knee range of motion remains a challenge for the surgeon. A personalized knee implant design may offer a complete strategy to reach complete stress-free ligamentous range of motion across all variability in knee anatomy [24].

Secondly, precision in bone preparation is capital in order to position the implants according to the planned and measured location. Complications in implant positioning should be avoidable by improved instrumentation and surgical guidance. Obtaining proper implant positioning along with native morphological articular reconstruction will most likely lead to decreased premature implant loosening [14] and enhance gait pattern normalization [25].

19.4 For Who (Best Indications)?

Any patients presenting with unicompartmental knee pathology with intact cruciate and collateral ligaments would be ideal candidate to undergo custom UKA. Classic indications for OTS UKA have been well established [26], and custom UKA does not differ from these guidelines. Proper patient selection remains the best predictor of success for this type of surgery. Of mention, important osteonecrosis jeopardizing implant fixation, local malignancy, active infection, inflammatory arthritis, limited preoperative ROM, deformities greater than 10°, and more than 5 mm of unipolar bone defect would represent contraindications to this particular procedure.

19.5 What Is the Process?

After the traditional clinical encounter with a patient's history and complete physical exam, weight-bearing long-leg anteroposterior (AP) radiographs are obtained to evaluate the extent of the joint space narrowing and the femoro-tibial mechanical alignment. Once the patient is confirmed as a good candidate for a custom UKA, additional AP valgus stress views of the knee in extension are obtained [27]. This manoeuvre provides information on the unaffected compartment [28] and ensures relative quantification of the affected joint space gap when the collateral ligament is under full tension.

The patient is then required to undergo CT or MRI imaging of the affected knee. Images are converted to 3D volumes, and customization of the implant is prepared based on proprietary guidelines. Patient-specific instrumentation in the form of 3D-printed cutting guides for both the femur and tibia are then produced for every case. The femoral and tibial implants are manufactured according to the preoperative plan established by the surgeon in combination with a technician and an engineer. The treating physician has to accept the final preoperative planning before the custom cutting guides and implants can be manufactured. Polyethylene liners are produced in different thicknesses within a range of 5–9 mm. All components and cutting guides are made available between 2 and 6 weeks following the patient imagery and implant prescription.

19.6 Clinical Evidence Supporting This Concept?

The current literature regarding personalized UKA components is relatively scarce since this concept is emerging. Multiple studies are available on OTS UKA and show excellent 10- to 15-year survivorship [7, 8, 29]. Gait analysis following OTS UKA has shown a closer-to-normal gait restoration with UKA when compared to total knee arthroplasty (TKA) [30]. Unfortunately, OTS UKA do not necessarily restore normal gait patterns [25]. Customized 3D-printed UKA implants restore the normal knee anatomy and theoretically could restore normal gait patterns since physiological ligamentous tension should be obtained throughout the range of motion.

Researchers have worked with patient-specific instrumentation (PSI) for UKA implantation and have found 3.3% tibial fractures with 16.4% sagittal plane outliers [31]. While some authors propose no benefits [32, 33], others have demonstrated marked improvements with PSI [34]. Specifically relating to the BUKS™ (Bodycad, QC, Canada) custom UKA design, early reports are promising [35]. Since most of the technical errors in surgery are surgeon related [36], and surgical experience is capital in UKA surgical technique [37, 38], PSI may represent as an important tool for the inexperienced surgeon [39, 40].

19.7 What Is Its Cost-Effectiveness?

There are no published studies on custom UKA and no cost-effectiveness studies of PSI for UKA.

19.8 Clinical Case Presentation

A 56-year-old man presents with left knee pain and limping at activity. The patient evolved well after undergoing sessions of physical therapy and the use of some oral NSAIDs. He later developed progressive pain after prolonged walking and long days standing still. The patient is comfortable in the sitting position but reports having sharp pains in transitioning from the sitting to a standing position.

On physical exam, the patient displays a left-sided prolonged weight-bearing limp without a varus thrust. Clinically measured leg length is equal. Lower leg muscle strength is within

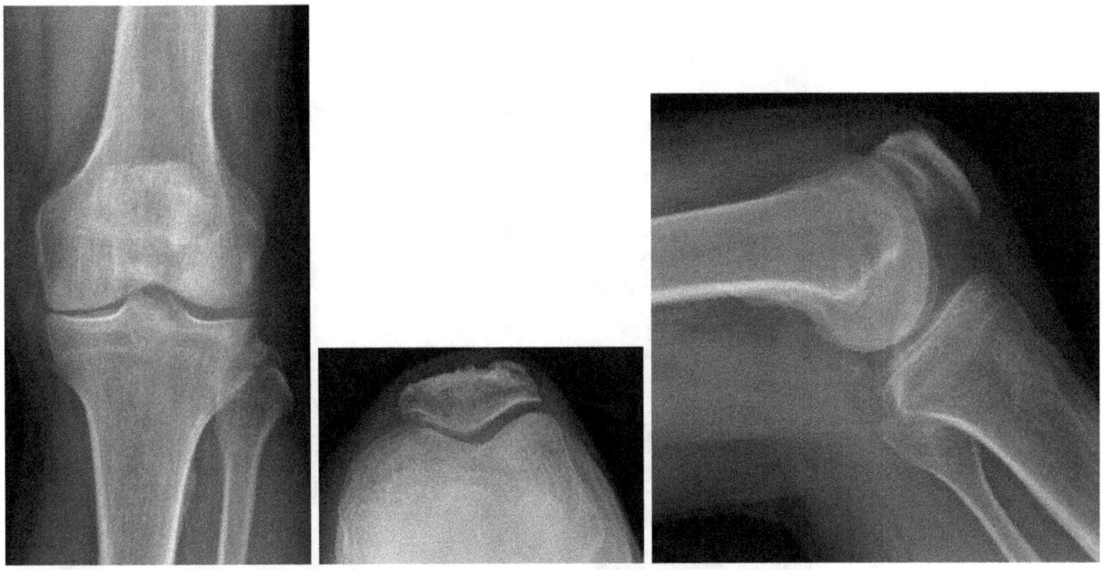

Fig. 19.1 Radiographic imaging confirms a joint space narrowing as shown medially

normal. Range of motion of the left hip shows pain-free and supple full range of motion. The left knee displays flexion from 5° to 110°. A valgus stress view at 0° of flexion demonstrated a 5 mm medial gap opening. All other ligamentous tests are within normal limits with a firm end feel.

19.9 Preoperative Radiographs

Radiographic imaging (Fig. 19.1) confirms a joint space narrowing as shown medially. Full-length films and stress view in valgus complete preoperative planning (Fig. 19.2).

19.10 Surgical Details

Similar to conventional UKA, a standard 8–12 cm skin incision is performed along the medial border of the patellar tendon (Fig. 19.3a). A quadriceps-sparing minimally invasive medial parapatellar arthrotomy is favoured in order to obtain adequate exposure to the medial compartment of the knee (Fig. 19.3b). Although the decision to perform a minimally invasive incision to limit soft-tissue trauma is the surgeon's own prerogative, this procedure can easily be performed using both the standard and minimally invasive approach.

The surgical technique first requires the subperiosteal exposure of the antero-medial proximal aspect of the tibial to allow adequate sitting of the patient-specific 3D-printed nylon cutting guides. Failure to obtain perfect sitting of the cutting block will result in malpositioning of the device and therefore produce inadequate and/or misaligned bone resection. The surgeon should not hesitate to obtain better exposure through a longer skin incision if perfect placement of the cutting block cannot be confirmed using the standard approach. The cutting block position should be assessed using the dentist hook to ensure that the periphery of the guide perfectly sits on the bone and that no voids are palpated. Once adequate positioning is confirmed, the cutting block can be secured to bone using two or three small 3.5 mm cortical screws (Fig. 19.3c).

Tibial bone resection can then be safely performed using a drill and making sure to drill every hole provided in the cutting guide (Fig. 19.3d) To enhance stability of the cutting block, a first drill bit can remain through the first drill hole, and the remaining holes can be drilled using a second drill bit. After drilling every holes, the cutting block can be fragmented using a cutter (Fig. 19.3e), and the remaining axial and sagittal

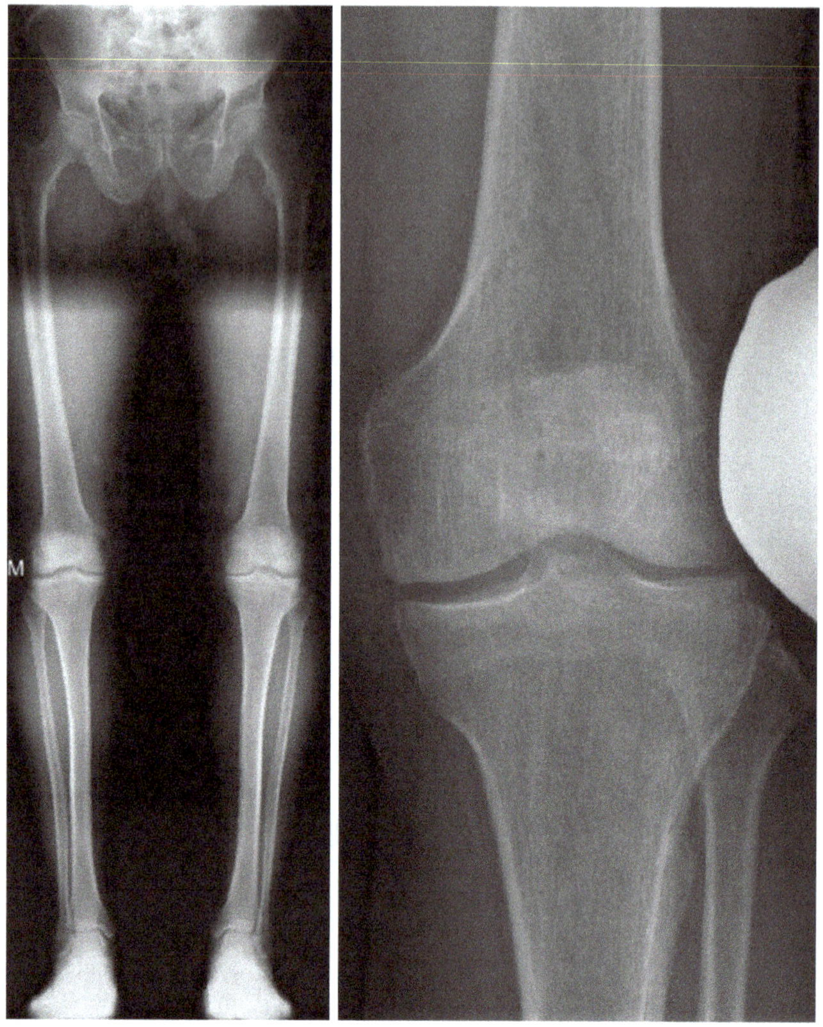

Fig. 19.2 Full-length films and stress view in valgus complete preoperative planning

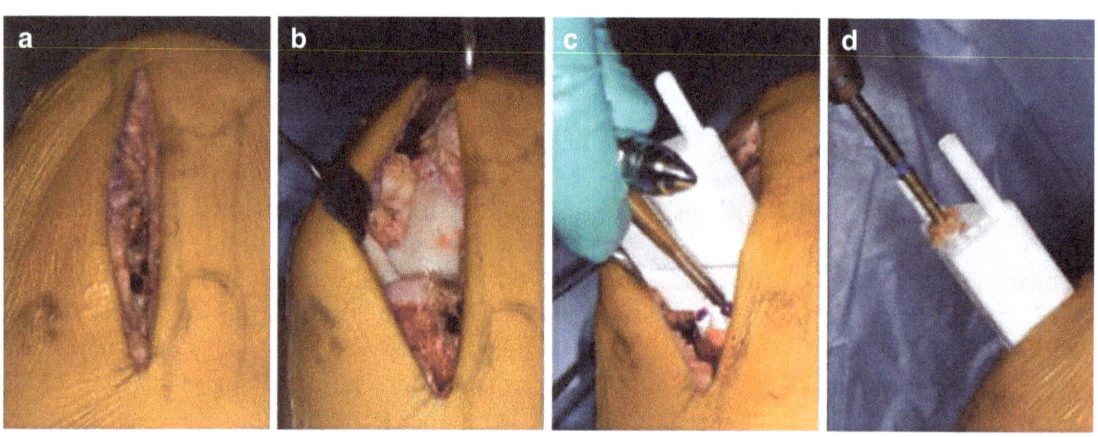

Fig. 19.3 Tibial bone resection starts with a medial incision on the left knee (**a**), medial arthrotomy (**b**), then the tibial cutting guide is stabilized with screws (**c**), bone is drilled (**d**), cutting guide is dismantled (**e**), a vertical pass is performed with a graduated osteotome (**f**), a horizontal pass with the osteotome, (**g**) and the cutting guide is removed (**h**)

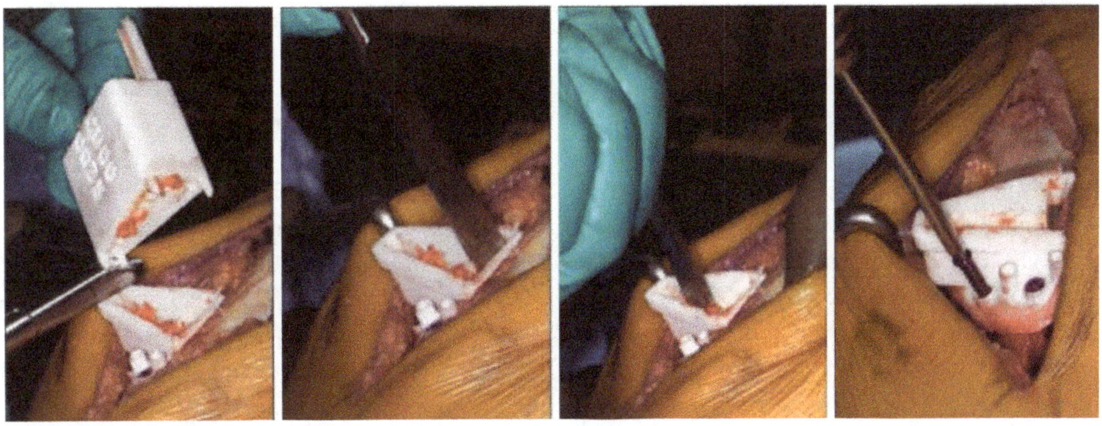

Fig. 19.3 (continued)

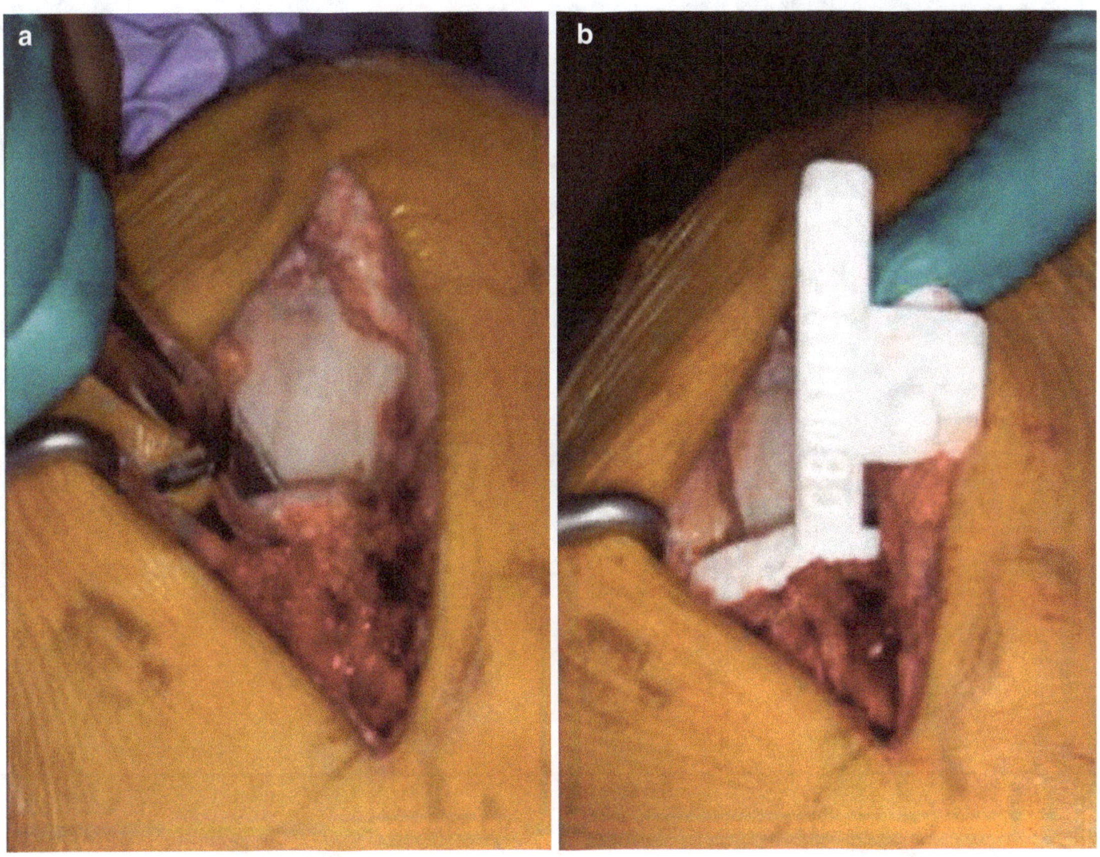

Fig. 19.4 The tibial bone is removed, (**a**) and a validator is used to verify resection (**b**)

tibial bone cuts can be completed using a graduated straight osteotome (Fig. 19.3f, g) The tibial cutting block is discarded after removing the screws (Fig. 19.3h).

The resected tibial bone is then removed using a grasping instrument (Fig. 19.4a). A tibial bone cut validator, provided for each case, is then placed on the proximal tibia in order to ensure that the amount of resected tibial bone matches the preoperative planned resection (Fig. 19.4b). The handle of the tibial validator also features an alignment hole allowing the surgeon to use a standard drop rod to validate tibial bone cut alignment if desired.

As for the femoral preparation, a custom femoral cutting block is required but should sit directly on hard sclerotic bone of the condyle. Therefore, a bone curette is used to scrape off any remaining cartilage left on the medial femoral condyle. Proper positioning of the femoral cutting block should also be assessed using a dentist hook, making sure once again that the periphery of the cutting block sits perfectly on the bone and that no voids are left underneath the cutting block.

The femoral cutting block is then secured to bone using 3.5 mm cortical screws (Fig. 19.5a). Sequential drilling (Fig. 19.5b), fragmentation of the cutting block (Fig. 19.5c), and osteotome passes (Fig. 19.5d) can be performed similarly to the tibial bone resection. After removal of the femoral cutting block, a nylon femoral component trial along with the tibial bone resection validator is inserted, and the femoral side is fixed with

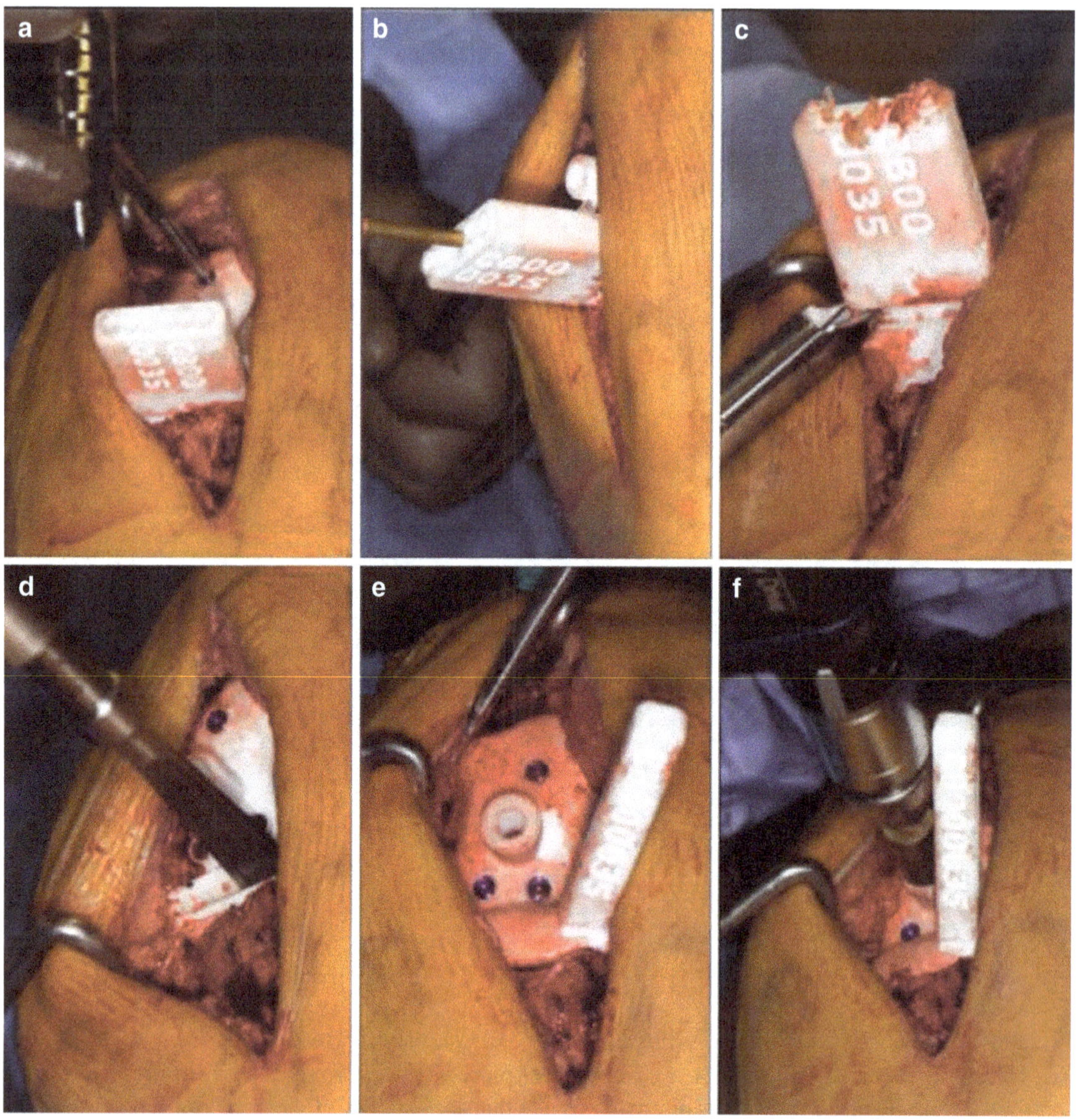

Fig. 19.5 Femoral bone resection starts by stabilizing the femoral cutting guide with screws (**a**) on exposed subchondral bone, bone is drilled (**b**), cutting guide is dismantled (**c**), passes are performed with a graduated osteotome (**d**), and the central peg hole is drilled (**e**, **f**) as the tibial bone resection validator is left in situ

screws. This allows for validation of the femoral component position before reaming of the peg hole using the provided femoral reamer through the base of the femoral trial (Fig. 19.5e, f).

After completing the bone resections, the surgeon should be able to proceed with trialing using the 3D-printed nylon components (Fig. 19.6a). At this stage, the proper polyethylene thickness should be assessed making sure ligamentous stability is perfectly achieved throughout the full range of motion. It is always preferable to leave a physiologic 2 mm medial compartment laxity to avoid overtensioning of the medial compartment and potentially inducing a mechanically valgus-aligned medial arthroplasty.

After completing trials and cleaning of bony surfaces, cementation and impaction of the final tibial implant are performed in a routine fashion. Excess cement is removed, and a 3.5 mm cortical bone screw is inserted in order to help in proper component positioning. The final femoral component is then cemented and impacted. Once again, one 4.0 mm cortical bone screw helps enhancing the final position of the femoral implant. Polyethylene thickness trialing can be repeated (Fig. 19.6b).

The final polyethylene is then inserted (Fig. 19.6c) and locked into the tibial baseplate using the provided locking pin (Fig. 19.6d). When cement has fully hardened, complete physical examination of the knee should be done to confirm full range of motion, ligamentous stability, proper patellar tracking, and the absence of soft-tissue impingement. Finally, the arthrotomy is closed using 1-0 absorbable sutures. Subcutaneous tissue is closed in a subcuticular fashion using 2-0 sutures. A sterile dressing is applied. Patient underwent an uneventful postoperative recovery (Fig. 19.7).

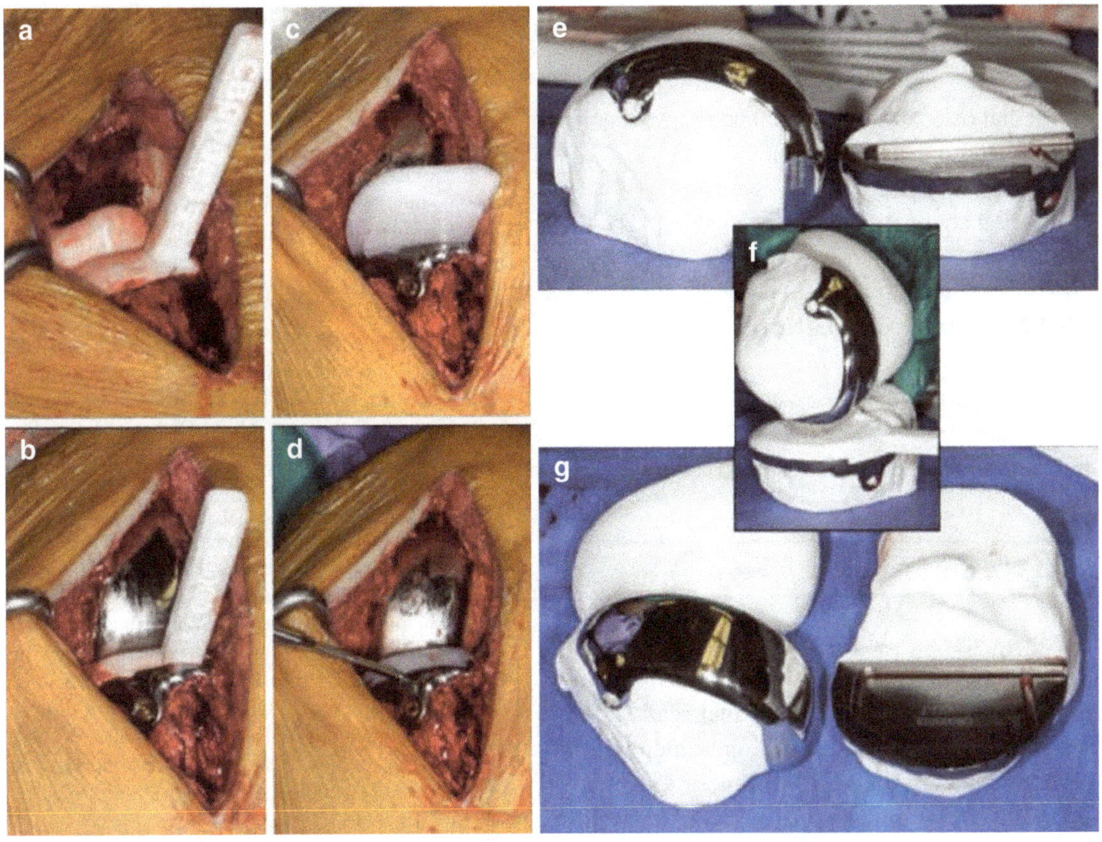

Fig. 19.6 Before the final implantation, 3D-printed nylon trial components are used for trialing (**a**), once implants are cemented, different thicknesses of polyethylene liners are trialed for proper ligament tensioning (**b**), and final liner is inserted and locked in place (**c**, **d**). Full-size 3D models are provided with the custom implants to allow for studying the implant position, size, and fit (**e**–**g**)

19.11 Follow-up Radiographs

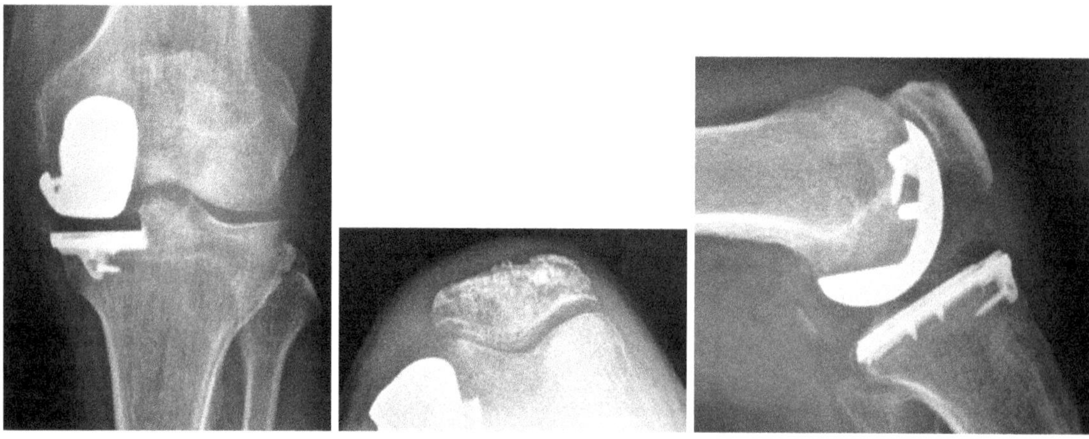

Fig. 19.7 Six months postoperative radiographs

19.12 Indications and Contraindications

19.12.1 Indications

- Medial osteoarthritis of the knee
- <15° coronal malalignment
- Efficient anterior cruciate ligament
- Flexion contracture <15° (debatable [41])

19.12.2 Contraindications

- Tricompartmental knee osteoarthritis
- Unstable knee
- Femoral condyle osteonecrosis

19.13 Conclusion

The next decade of knee implant designs will develop with amazing new technologies including navigation, robotics, and virtual reality. The innovating custom design UKA presented in this chapter shows promising strategies, exploiting knowledge from past designs and positioning its expected development in line with existing variability in functional knee phenotypes. Further adjustment in UKA custom designs may have to be aligned with clinical trial findings and implant biomechanical tests. The clinician has to remain vigilant about new technologies but critic in its introduction and initial use.

References

1. Murray DW, Goodfellow JW, O'Connor JJ. The Oxford medial unicompartmental arthroplasty: a ten-year survival study. J Bone Jt Surg. 1998;80-B(6):983–9.
2. Capra SW, Fehring TK. Unicondylar arthroplasty. A survivorship analysis. J Arthroplasty. 1992;7(3):247–51.
3. Berger RA, Nedeff DD, Barden RM, Sheinkop MM, Jacobs JJ, Rosenberg AG, et al. Unicompartmental knee arthroplasty. Clinical experience at 6- to 10-year followup. Clin Orthop Relat Res. 1999;(367):50–60.
4. Scott RD, Cobb AG, McQueary FG, Thornhill TS. Unicompartmental knee arthroplasty. Eight- to 12-year follow-up evaluation with survivorship analysis. Clin Orthop Relat Res. 1991;(271):96–100.
5. Peersman G, Stuyts B, Vandenlangenbergh T, Cartier P, Fennema P. Fixed- versus mobile-bearing UKA: a systematic review and meta-analysis. Knee Surg Sports Traumatol Arthrosc. 2015;23(11):3296–305.
6. Ko Y-B, Gujarathi MR, Oh K-J. Outcome of unicompartmental knee arthroplasty: a systematic review of comparative studies between fixed and mobile bearings focusing on complications. Knee Surg Relat Res. 2015;27(3):141–8.
7. Panni AS, Vasso M, Cerciello S, Felici A. Unicompartmental knee replacement provides early clinical and functional improvement stabilizing over time. Knee Surg Sports Traumatol Arthrosc. 2012;20(3):579–85.

8. Foran JRH, Brown NM, Valle Della CJ, Berger RA, Galante JO. Long-term survivorship and failure modes of unicompartmental knee arthroplasty. Clin Orthop Relat Res. 2013;471(1):102–8.
9. Nuño N, Ahmed AM. Sagittal profile of the femoral condyles and its application to femorotibial contact analysis. J Biomech Eng. 2001;123(1):18–26.
10. Zoghi M, Hefzy MS, Fu KC, Jackson WT. A three-dimensional morphometrical study of the distal human femur. Proc Inst Mech Eng H. 1992;206(3):147–57.
11. Du PZ, Markolf KL, Levine BD, McAllister DR, Jones KJ. Differences in the radius of curvature between femoral condyles: implications for osteochondral allograft matching. J Bone Jt Surg. 2018;100-A(15):1326–31.
12. Carpenter DP, Holmberg RR, Quartulli MJ, Barnes CL. Tibial plateau coverage in UKA: a comparison of patient specific and off-the-shelf implants. J Arthroplasty. 2014;29(9):1694–8.
13. van der Merwe J, van den Heever DJ, Erasmus PJ. Estimating regions of interest on the distal femur. Med Eng Phys. 2018;60:23–9.
14. Harrysson OLA, Hosni YA, Nayfeh JF. Custom-designed orthopedic implants evaluated using finite element analysis of patient-specific computed tomography data: femoral-component case study. BMC Musculoskelet Disord. 2007;8:91.
15. Fitz W. Unicompartmental knee arthroplasty with use of novel patient-specific resurfacing implants and personalized jigs. J Bone Jt Surg. 2009;91-A(Suppl 1):69–76.
16. Parratte S, Argenson J-NA, Pearce O, Pauly V, Auquier P, Aubaniac J-M. Medial unicompartmental knee replacement in the under-50s. J Bone Jt Surg. 2009;91-B(3):351–6.
17. Liddle AD, Pandit H, O'Brien S, Doran E, Penny ID, Hooper GJ, et al. Cementless fixation in Oxford unicompartmental knee replacement: a multicentre study of 1000 knees. Bone Jt J. 2013;95-B(2):181–7.
18. Pandit H, Liddle AD, Kendrick BJL, Jenkins C, Price AJ, Gill HS, et al. Improved fixation in cementless unicompartmental knee replacement: five-year results of a randomized controlled trial. J Bone Jt Surg. 2013;95-A(15):1365–72.
19. Chatellard R, Sauleau V, Colmar M, Robert H, Raynaud G, Brilhault J, et al. Medial unicompartmental knee arthroplasty: does tibial component position influence clinical outcomes and arthroplasty survival? Orthop Traumatol Surg Res. 2013;99(4 Suppl):S219–25.
20. Bellemans J, Colyn W, Vandenneucker H, Victor J. The Chitranjan Ranawat award: is neutral mechanical alignment normal for all patients? The concept of constitutional varus. Clin Orthop Relat Res. 2012;470(1):45–53.
21. Eckhoff DG, Bach JM, Spitzer VM, Reinig KD, Bagur MM, Baldini TH, et al. Three-dimensional mechanics, kinematics, and morphology of the knee viewed in virtual reality. J Bone Jt Surg. 2005;87-A(Suppl 2):71–80.
22. Mullaji AB, Shah S, Shetty GM. Mobile-bearing medial unicompartmental knee arthroplasty restores limb alignment comparable to that of the unaffected contralateral limb. Acta Orthop. 2017;88(1):70–4.
23. Diezi C, Wirth S, Meyer DC, Koch PP. Effect of femoral to tibial varus mismatch on the contact area of unicondylar knee prostheses. Knee. 2010;17(5):350–5.
24. Hirschmann MT, Behrend H. Functional knee phenotypes: a call for a more personalised and individualised approach to total knee arthroplasty? Knee Surg Sports Traumatol Arthrosc. 2018;26(10):2873–4.
25. Kim M-K. Unicompartmental knee arthroplasty fails to completely restore normal gait patterns during level walking. Knee Surg Sports Traumatol Arthrosc. 2018;26(11):3280–9.
26. Kozinn SC, Scott R. Unicondylar knee arthroplasty. J Bone Jt Surg. 1989;71-A(1):145–50.
27. Eriksson K, Sadr-Azodi O, Singh C, Osti L, Bartlett J. Stress radiography for osteoarthritis of the knee: a new technique. Knee Surg Sports Traumatol Arthrosc. 2010;18(10):1356–9.
28. Bergeson AG, Berend KR, Lombardi AV, Hurst JM, Morris MJ, Sneller MA. Medial mobile bearing unicompartmental knee arthroplasty: early survivorship and analysis of failures in 1000 consecutive cases. J Arthroplasty. 2013;28(9 Suppl):172–5.
29. Saragaglia D, Bevand A, International RR. Results with nine years mean follow up on one hundred and three KAPS® uni knee arthroplasties: eighty six medial and seventeen lateral. Eur J Orthop Surg Traumatol. 2018;42(5):1061–6.
30. Jones GG, Kotti M, Wiik AV, Collins R, Brevadt MJ, Strachan RK, et al. Gait comparison of unicompartmental and total knee arthroplasties with healthy controls. Bone Jt J. 2016;10(Suppl B):16–21.
31. Leenders AM. A high rate of tibial plateau fractures after early experience with patient-specific instrumentation for unicompartmental knee arthroplasties. Knee Surg Sports Traumatol Arthrosc. 2018;26(11):3491–8.
32. Ollivier M, Parratte S, Lunebourg A, Viehweger E, Argenson J-N. The John Insall award: no functional benefit after unicompartmental knee arthroplasty performed with patient-specific instrumentation: a randomized trial. Clin Orthop Relat Res. 2016;474(1):60–8.
33. Alvand A, Khan T, Jenkins C, Rees JL, Jackson WF, Dodd CAF, et al. The impact of patient-specific instrumentation on unicompartmental knee arthroplasty: a prospective randomised controlled study. Knee Surg Sports Traumatol Arthrosc. 2018;26(6):1662–70.
34. Dao Trong ML, Diezi C, Goerres G, Helmy N. Improved positioning of the tibial component in unicompartmental knee arthroplasty with patient-specific cutting blocks. Knee Surg Sports Traumatol Arthrosc. 2015;23(7):1993–8.

35. Belzile E, Rivet-Sabourin G, Bédard M, Robichaud H, Angers M, Bédard M. Évaluation de la précision d'implantation d'une prothèse unicompartimentale de genou utilisant un guide de coupe personnalisé. Orthop Traumatol Surg Res. 2017;103S:S31.
36. Vasso M, Antoniadis A, Helmy N. Update on unicompartmental knee arthroplasty: current indications and failure modes. EFORT Open Rev. 2018;3(8):442–8.
37. Liddle AD, Pandit H, Judge A, Murray DW. Effect of surgical caseload on revision rate following total and unicompartmental knee replacement. J Bone Jt Surg. 2016;98-A(1):1–8.
38. Zambianchi F, Digennaro V, Giorgini A, Grandi G, Fiacchi F, Mugnai R, et al. Surgeon's experience influences UKA survivorship: a comparative study between all-poly and metal back designs. Knee Surg Sports Traumatol Arthrosc. 2015;23(7):2074–80.
39. Jones GG, Logishetty K, Clarke S, Collins R, Jaere M, Harris S, et al. Do patient-specific instruments (PSI) for UKA allow non-expert surgeons to achieve the same saw cut accuracy as expert surgeons? Arch Orthop Trauma Surg. 2018;138(11):1601–8.
40. Schotanus MGM, Thijs E, Heijmans M, Vos R, Kort NP. Favourable alignment outcomes with MRI-based patient-specific instruments in total knee arthroplasty. Knee Surg Sports Traumatol Arthrosc. 2018;26(9):2659–68.
41. Purcell RL, Cody JP, Ammeen DJ, Goyal N, Engh GA. Elimination of preoperative flexion contracture as a contraindication for unicompartmental knee arthroplasty. J Am Acad Orthop Surg. 2018;26(7):e158–63.

20

Patellofemoral Joint Arthroplasty

Romagnoli Sergio, Petrillo Stefano, and Marullo Matteo

Key Points

- Clinical results and survivorship of PFA are improving thanks to a better understanding of the PF biomechanics, more anatomical designs and adequate surgical instrumentation.
- Onlay designs have broader indications and easier surgical technique because they completely replace the trochlea by an anterior resection. Their patella-friendly trochlea and the large amount of sizes available accommodate for patella alta or excessive TT–TG distance without the need of further surgical procedures.
- PFA in PFOA secondary to patellar instability needs a kinematic alignment in which the lateral border of the trochlea is elevated, the lateral trochlear inclination is restored, but the trochlear line remains in partial external rotation. This avoids excessive modification in retinacular ligaments tension and the need of soft tissues releases.
- PFA in primary PFOA without any trochlear dysplasia can be performed with an anatomical alignment. The anterior cut should be perpendicular to the sagittal axis of the kneevjoint and the prosthesis should replace the trochlea without modifying its anatomy and orientation. Inlay PFAs could be used.

R. Sergio (✉) · P. Stefano · M. Matteo
Joint Replacement Department, IRCCS Galeazzi Orthopaedics Institute, Milan, Italy
e-mail: Sergio.romagnoli@libero.it; s.petrillo@unicampus.it

20.1 Introduction

The first isolated patello-femoral (PF) joint arthroplasty (PFA) was a patella cap, a Vitallium shell replacing the patella and maintaining the native trochlea, proposed in 1955 by McKeever. The first PFAs replacing entire PF joint had an inlay design and came in the 1979 with the Richards and Lubinus prosthesis.

I started performing PFA in the first 1980s using inlay PFAs, the cementless Bousquet and the Cemented Cartier prosthesis. Then I have continued in the 1990s with the half-inlay Grammont and the inlay Lubinus prosthesis. However, first-generation PFAs had important limitations and poor outcomes. These PFAs were inserted in the native trochlea, replacing the articular cartilage and leaving untouched the subchondral bone, without correcting the rotational alignment of the trochlea. These unideal designs with few component sizes available, improper surgical technique, inadequate instrumentation and unfavourable indications provided poor outcomes. Indeed, good or excellent results were achieved in only 20–72% of patients at short-term and midterm follow-up, with a high incidence of early reoperations (25–35% at 5 years) due to patellar maltracking, instability, patellar clunking and soft tissue impingement [1].

In the last 20 years, I preferred the onlay PFAs, using the inlay designs only in few selected cases. Onlay prostheses completely resect the trochlea with an anterior cut similar to the one performed for total knee arthroplasty (TKA). The Avon (Stryker) and the Zimmer PFJ are examples of onlay prostheses. Second-generation PFAs allow a correction of trochlea rotation or dysplasia and are associated with good results at short-term and midterm follow-up [1]. The enhanced knowledge on PF kinematics, the higher number of component sizes available, the better surgical instrumentation and the easier surgical technique contributed to improve the results. Moreover, early complications like patellar maltracking, instability or catching and snapping of the patellar component during knee flexion were significantly reduced.

20.2 Biomechanics of the PF Joint

PF joint (PFJ), among all the knee compartments, has the most complex biomechanics. An extensive knowledge about forces acting on the PFJ as well as variables affecting them is crucial to understand the surgical technique of PFA.

Forces on the PFJ act in the sagittal, coronal and axial plane. In the sagittal plane, there is a parallelogram of forces created by the quadriceps strain force (QF) and the patellar tendon strain force (PTF). The resultant vector between these two forces is defined as the PF reaction force (PRF). It is the "pressure" on cartilage of the patella and of the trochlea. PRF increases with flexion and decreases with the anterior displacement of the tibial tuberosity (Fig. 20.1) [2].

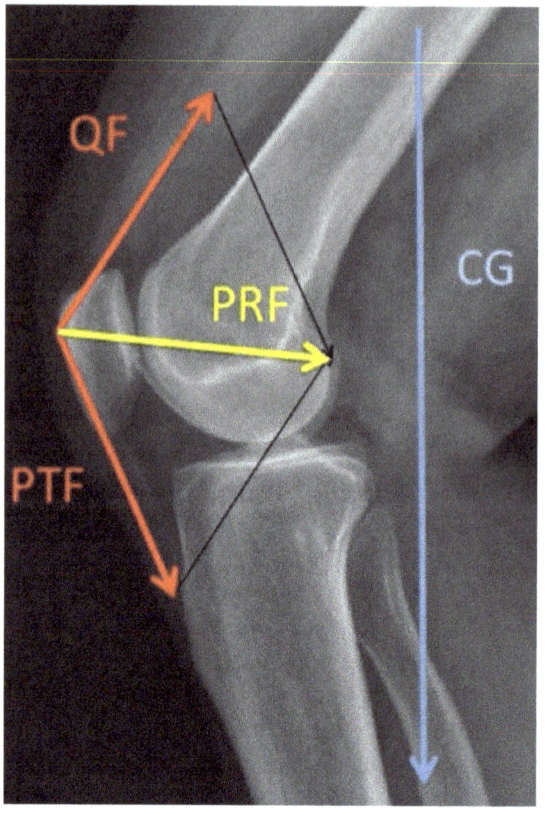

Fig. 20.1 Forces acting on the patella in the sagittal plane. The resultant vector between the quadriceps strain force (QF) and the patellar tendon strain force (PTF) is the patello-femoral reaction force (PRF). *CG* gravity centre

The moment arm acting on the PFJ depends on the distance between the vertical line created by the gravity centre and the PFJ. During stair ascending, the gravity centre comes closer to the PFJ, and the moment arm is shorter, while during stair descending, the body weight moves behind, so the distance between the gravity centre and the PFJ increases, increasing also the loadings on all knee compartments [3].

In the coronal plane, the quadriceps strain force and the patellar tendon force draw an angle, which is generally called Q angle. The Q angle determines a lateral force vector (patellar lateral force, PLF), which is maximal in complete knee extension. This is a factor contributing to lateral patellar dislocation, which is more frequent in complete knee extension (Fig. 20.2). During knee flexion, the internal rotation of the tibia neutralizes the Q angle and reduces PLF. In the coronal and axial plane, the PLF is antagonized by the reaction caused by the inclination of the lateral facet of the femoral trochlea. At 60° of knee flexion, there is a condition for patellar stability, in which the lateral trochlear inclination angle is bigger than the Q angle [4].

Even in the axial plane, there is a parallelogram of forces, in which the direction and entity of the vectors depend on knee flexion, trochlear anatomy, patellar anatomy, balance of the patello-femoral ligaments and tension/action of the quadriceps muscle.

Moreover, the mechanical axis of the lower limb influences PF biomechanics. In particular, the valgus morphotype is detrimental for

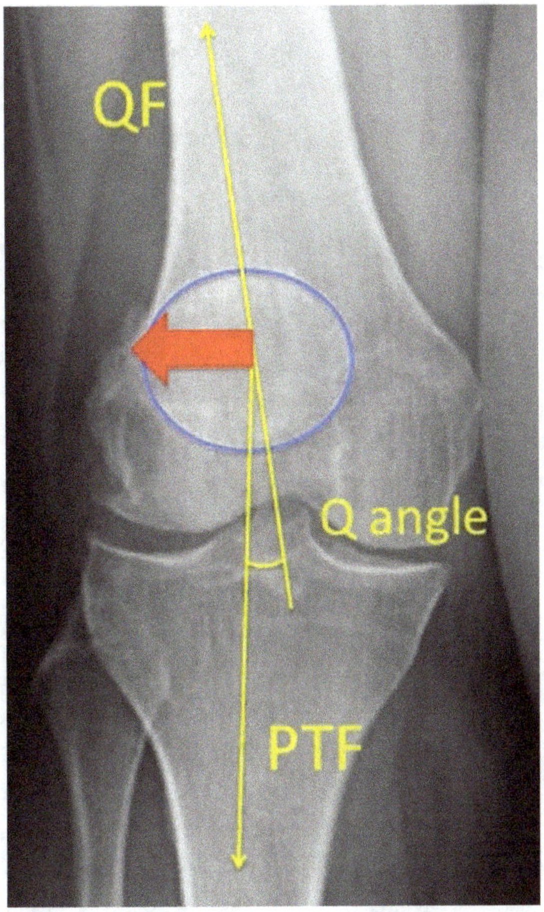

Fig. 20.2 In the coronal plane, the quadriceps strain force (QF) and the patellar tendon force (PTF) draw the Q angle. The bigger the angle, the bigger the patellar lateral force (red arrow)

a proper PF tracking; it increases the obliquity of the QF, thus increasing the Q angle and the PLF. Consequently, in high-grade valgus deformity, the patella tends to partially or completely dislocate laterally.

This condition should be considered in patients with isolated PF osteoarthritis (PFOA) and valgus deformity greater than 5°. In selected cases, it is possible to correct the coronal alignment of the knee by a femoral osteotomy (if the lateral tibiofemoral compartment is pristine) or a lateral unicompartmental knee arthroplasty (if the lateral tibiofemoral compartment is damaged, even if fairly symptomatic) and then add a PFA with easier alignment [5]. This shrewdness significantly reduces the risk of patellar dislocation and PFA failure (Fig. 20.3).

Gender has an important influence on PFJ biomechanics. It was shown that the mean Q Angle is 17° in female and 14° in male [6]. Moreover, females have a higher internal rotation of the femoral trochlea (trochlear angle) which is 2° greater in female, mainly due to a shorter medial condyle in the sagittal plane [7]. The trochlear obliquity in the coronal plane is higher in female than in male (10° vs. 7°) [8], while patellar thickness is higher in male than in female (2.57 cm vs. 2.25 cm, mean values). Moreover, males have higher medial and lateral trochlear facets and a wider trochlea. Consequently, females have smaller PFJ surface leading to load concentration, with also a higher Q angle and higher femoral internal rotation leading to patellar lateralization. Furthermore, the higher rates of trochlear dysplasia and ligament laxity in females facilitate malalignment, and all these factors explain why PFOA is significantly more frequent in female than males.

20.3 Indications

Symptomatic osteoarthritis affects the PF joint less frequently than the other compartments of the knee. Isolated PFOA has been reported in 8% of women and 2% of men over 55 years of age [9].

Three main causes determine isolated PFOA:

- Primary OA: patients with no orthopaedic antecedent and no history of patella instability. These patients are generally over 60 years old, are overweight and have a symmetrical OA of the medial and lateral patellar and trochlear facets.
- PF instability: patients with a history of objective patellar dislocation. These patients have evidence of trochlear dysplasia and/or patella alta. They are generally younger (mean age 54 years old) and often have a bilateral disease.
- Post-traumatic: patients with a history of PF fractures (young patients with a mean age at surgery of 54 years).

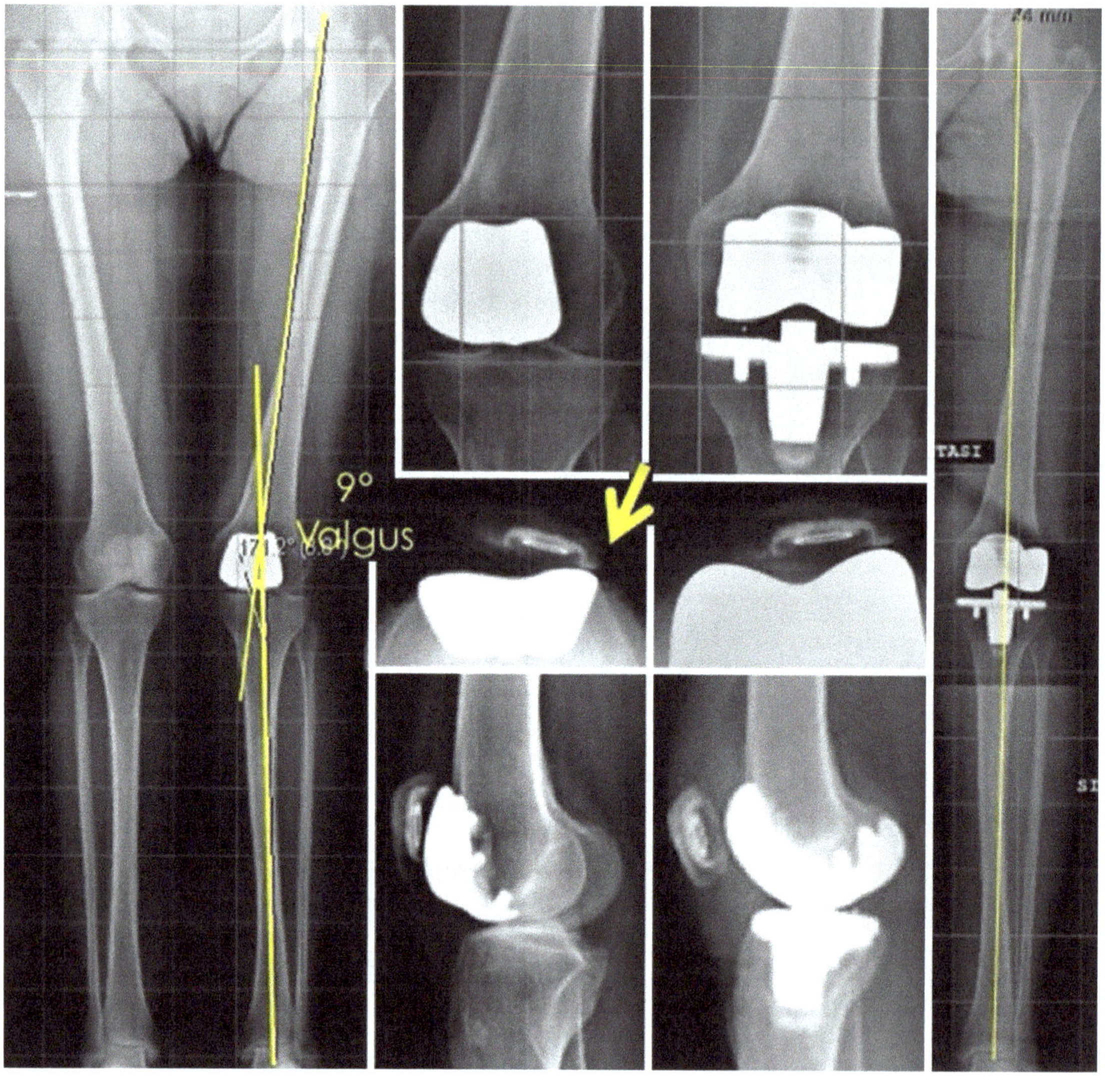

Fig. 20.3 Even if the PFA adequately replaced the native PFJ, the residual deformity (9° valgus) in the coronal plane maintained a high Q angle and consequently an excessive patellar lateral force. Clinical consequences were patellar instability and partial dislocation. The correction of mechanical axis with a TKA restored a proper PF tracking

Primary OA represents 49% of cases, while post-instability OA and post-traumatic OA account for 33% and 9% of cases, respectively [10, 11]. Trochlear dysplasia is the main factor leading to isolated PFOA. Indeed, 78% of all patients present trochlear dysplasia with crossing sign. The highest rate of dysplasia was seen in the post-instability group (66%), but even the primary OA group demonstrated a 38% of trochlear dysplasia [10, 11]. Isolated PFOA affects predominantly females (72%), with 51% of patients showing bilateral disease [10, 11].

Patients with isolated PFOA typically have significant anterior knee pain that interferes with several activities of daily living. They have difficulties in using stairs (often they need a handrail) and in getting up from a chair. They have also a limited walking capacity on flat surfaces. At clinical examination, the knee is often swollen, and typical retropatellar palpation or patellar compression evokes pain. Squatting for these patients is often impossible.

A proper radiographic evaluation of PFOA should include antero-posterior weight-bearing view, Rosenberg's view, lateral weight-bearing view and skyline view at 30° of knee flexion (Merchant's view). It is sometimes useful to take skyline views in various degrees of flexion because the pathology may be much more obvious in one position than another. Magnetic resonance imaging can be useful to assess doubtful cases or associated soft tissues lesions.

PFA preserves both cruciate ligaments and the tibiofemoral compartments, enhances stability and maintains proprioception and a more physiological tibiofemoral kinematics compared to TKA. Clinical consequences are greater comfort during daily life activities and better functional outcomes. Moreover, PFA saves more bone stock compared to a TKA, making an eventual prosthetic revision less difficult.

Indications for isolated PFA are symptomatic isolated PFOA (Iwano grade 2 or greater) and absence of tibiofemoral arthritis (Kellgren–Lawrence 2 or lower).

Contraindications are a clinically instable knee in the frontal or sagittal plane, a preoperative range of motion (ROM) less than 90°, a flexion contracture greater than 10° and inflammatory disease. The tibiofemoral cartilages should be pristine; in case one of the tibiofemoral compartments is damaged, a bicompartmental replacement (unicompartmental knee replacement, UKA and PFA) should be considered if there are no other contraindications [12].

We developed an algorithm to consider UKA in association to a PFA. There are two major criteria and two minor criteria. The two main criteria are valgus deformity greater than 5° or varus deformity greater than 4°, high adduction moment. The two secondary criteria are female sex and body mass index (BMI) >32. If two major criteria or one major + two minor criteria are present, we suggest to perform a UKA + PFA. At the same time, we developed another algorithm to recognize when performing PFA in association to UKA. Three major criteria and two minor criteria compose this algorithm. The major criteria are patello-femoral pain; patellar malalignment or lateral patello-femoral wear on X-ray axial view; and intraoperative findings of grade 3–4 patello-femoral chondral degeneration. The two minor criteria are the same of the first algorithm. If two major criteria or one major + two minor criteria are present, we suggest to add a PFA to a UKA due to high risk of PFOA progression [13].

20.4 Inlay and Onlay Designs

PFAs could be divided in two main categories: "inlay" and "onlay" prostheses. Inlay prosthesis lies inside the native trochlea, without modifying its anatomy. These are contraindicated in PFOA with high-grade trochlear dysplasia. In patella alta or in case of excessive tibial tuberosity–trochlear groove (TT–TG) distance, these inlay prostheses should be associated with other surgical procedures such as tibial tuberosity distalization or medialization.

Onlay PFA completely resects the trochlea with an anterior cut similar to the one performed for TKA. These prostheses have a bigger trochlear component compared to the inlay designs, which replaces the entire trochlea. They can be even utilized in case of high-grade trochlear dysplasia, in which the native anatomy of the trochlea is pathological and cannot be preserved, in patella alta and in cases of excessive TT–TG distance. The trochlear flange extends proximally and has a better congruency with the patella, even in case of patella alta. Increase in proximal femoropatellar contact area is of paramount importance for a proper patellar tracking in the first 30° of knee flexion, the critical range in which patellar dislocation occurs. The complete resection of the native trochlea lets to modify the position of the trochlear groove to adapt it to a lateralized tibial tuberosity, decreasing the TT–TG distance by a proximal realignment.

Onlay PFAs have broader indications without necessity of associated surgical procedures, presenting an easier surgical technique and consequently a shorter learning curve. Moreover, literature showed superior results and survivorship with onlay PFAs compared to inlay ones [13–16].

20.5 Surgical Technique

The patient is supine on the operating table. We do not use the tourniquet in any type of knee replacement for several reasons (higher risk of thromboembolic disease, slower recovery, lower range of motion, higher risk of wound complications) but principally because the tourniquet does not allow the evaluation of the balance and motion of the extensor apparatus.

PFA could be performed through any standard knee replacement incision; anyway, the most utilized surgical approach is the medial parapatellar one. Our preferred approach is mini-mid vastus. The incision should be 6–8 cm long and correspond to the proximal part of the one used for a TKA. Care must be taken to avoid damage of the meniscus or the cartilage of the tibiofemoral joint.

A lateral approach should be considered when the patella is strongly subluxated laterally or when it is planned to perform a lateral UKA. This access gives slightly less exposure of the joint, but it does not violate the quadriceps at all. Moreover, it lets to perform a fine modulation of the lateral PF and patellotibial ligaments during capsular suture after implantation.

A careful inspection of the whole joint is suggested to confirm intraoperatively the indication for PFA or to move to another surgical option.

The trochlear cut is the first bone cut to be performed, with the knee at 90° of flexion. As mentioned above, we suggest using onlay PFAs, so the trochlea should be completely resected and replaced.

In patients with primary PFOA without trochlear dysplasia, the trochlear line (TL), defined as the line connecting the anterior points of medial and lateral facets, is internally rotated relative to the posterior condylar line as the lateral facet is more prominent than the medial one and the lateral trochlear inclination (LTI) is pronounced, and the PF ligaments are balanced [17]. The PFJ works with proper biomechanics, so the PFA should not modify the native anatomy. Consequently, the prosthesis should be implanted using a kinematic or *anatomic alignment.* The anterior femoral cut should be made perpendicular to the sagittal axis of the joint. If the trochlear sulcus is still detectable, drawing Whiteside's line is helpful to identify the sagittal axis. The anterior cut should be perpendicular to the Whiteside's line and parallel to the transepicondylar axis (Fig. 20.4). Its depth should consider that the thickness of the femoral implant should replace the amount of bone and cartilage removed plus any cartilaginous wear.

In patients with PFOA secondary to trochlear dysplasia, PFJ biomechanics is completely distorted. The TL is neutral or externally rotated; the lateral trochlear facet is hypoplastic; the LTI

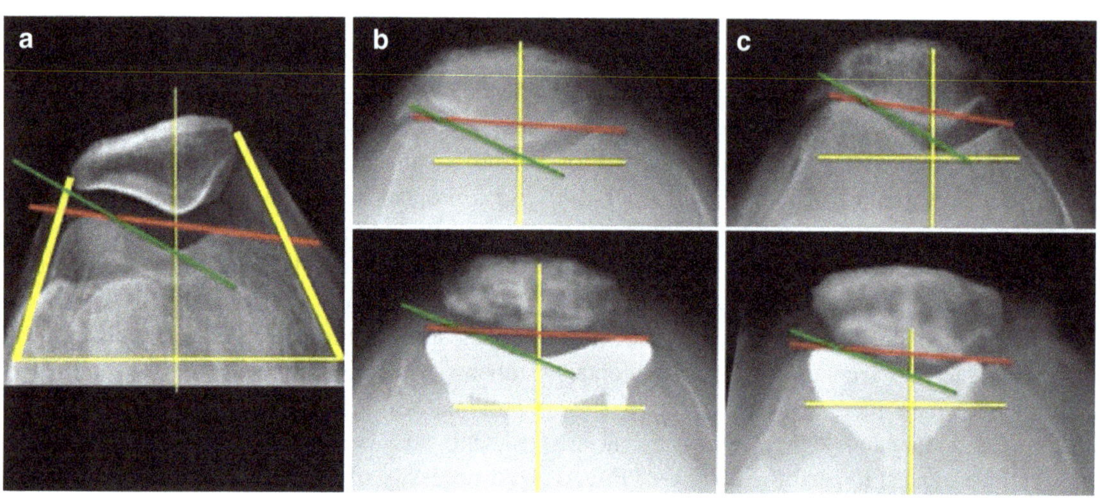

Fig. 20.4 (**a**) Anatomy of a normal PFJ. The lateral ridge is more prominent than the medial one, consequently the trochlear line (TL, red line) is internally rotated, and the lateral trochlear inclination (LTI, green line) is pronounced. In this condition, the PF ligaments are balanced (yellow lines). (**b**) Primary PFOA without trochlear dysplasia. The patella is centred. The PFJ was replaced with an onlay PFA. (**c**) Primary PFOA without trochlear dysplasia. In this case, an inlay PFA was used. In both cases, the shape and orientation of the joint were left unchanged, and the PFA has an anatomical alignment

is inadequate; the lateral patellar osteophytes are prominent; the lateral patello-femoral ligament is tensed, and the patella is displaced laterally with a load concentration on the lateral side. PFA should correct all these abnormalities, and it could be made only using an onlay design. The aim of the PFA implant is to correct the cartilage loss and deformity without stressing soft tissue structures, because PFOA is strongly related to soft tissue unbalance. For these reasons, the PFA should be performed with an anterior cut allowing a hypocorrection of the deformity, maintaining patient's morphotype. The lateral facet height must be recreated undercutting the lateral aspect of the trochlea. Anyway, in case of high-grade trochlear dysplasia, the anterior cut should maintain a slight external rotation to accommodate for the abnormally tight lateral retinaculum and abnormally lax medial retinaculum. This *adjusted kinematic alignment* will obtain a realignment with no or minimal lateral release and minimum risk of overstuffing. Kinematic alignment undercorrects the external rotation of the TL but improves the sulcus angle (SA) and the LTI. The SA depends on the prosthetic shape; the LTI depends on the shape and the rotation of the implant (Fig. 20.5). In any case, internal rotation of the trochlear component relative to the posterior condylar line should be avoided.

After the anterior cut is made, a dedicated milling guide, specific for each design of PFA, creates the allocation for the prosthetic trochlea. The correct size and placement of the trial should be chosen: the distal aspect of the implant should be flush with the articular cartilage both medially and laterally, and its mediolateral width should cover the entire trochlea, with no overstuffing. A high-velocity cutter removes a minimal amount of bone and creates the bed for the prosthesis.

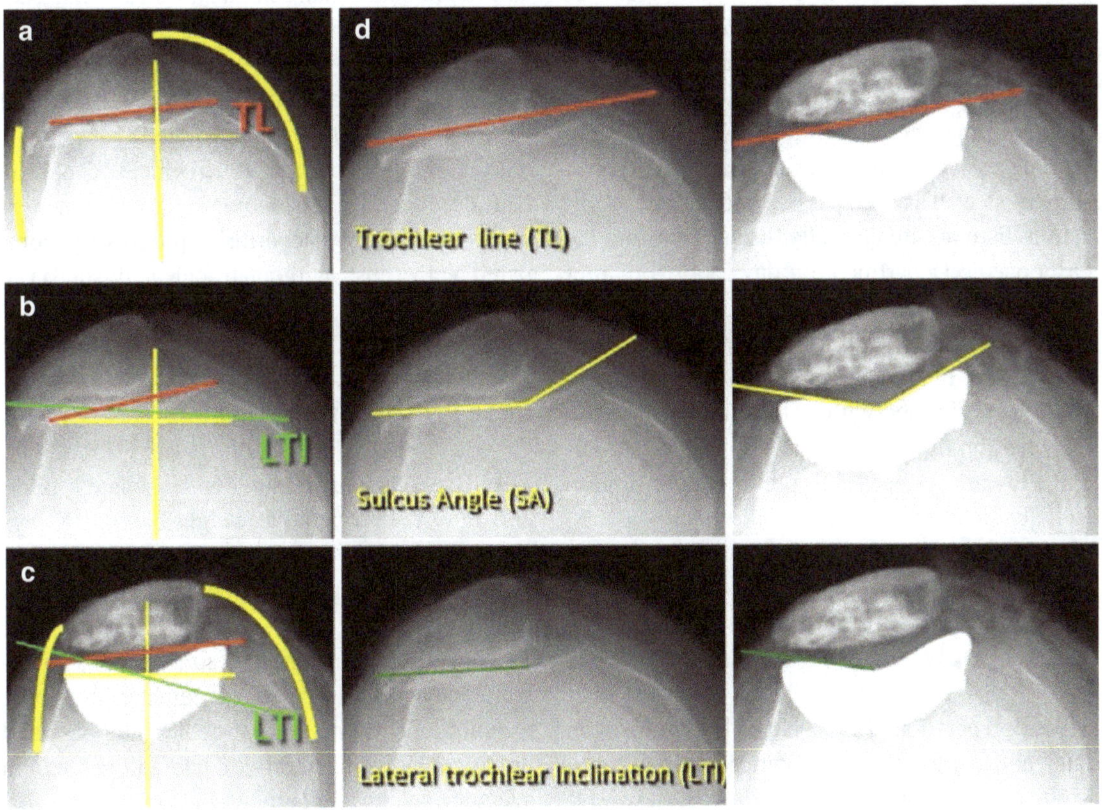

Fig. 20.5 PFOA with a dysplastic trochlea. (**a**) The lateral aspect of the trochlea is hypoplastic, and consequently the trochlear line (TL, red line) is extrarotated. The medial PF ligament is lax, and the lateral one is tight (yellow lines). (**b**) The lateral trochlear inclination (LTI, green line) is minimal. (**c**, **d**) PFA with an onlay PFA. The TL was partially corrected but remained extrarotated, the sulcus angle improved thanks to the prosthetic design, and the LTI was adequately restored. PF ligaments had only a minimal modification. PFA has a kinematic alignment

Accurate preparation of the width and depth of the bone bed is crucial to avoid any step in the cartilage-prosthesis transition zone, which could create patellar impingement and clunks.

With the knee in full extension, the patella is resurfaced. As PFOA should be considered pathology of the whole PFJ, we suggest resurfacing the patella recreating the native patellar thickness.

With the trial component in situ and after temporary closure of the capsule with 2–3 stitches or Backhaus clamps, patellar tracking should be checked. The patella should be centred into the trochlea during the whole ROM, without any impingement, clunking or subluxation. In addition, the trochlear and patellar implants should not overhang in order to prevent any soft tissue impingement and pain. When the desirable dimension of any component falls between two different sizes, we suggest choosing the smaller one. Cementing procedure starts from the trochlea and then continues with the patella. After that, PF tracking should be checked again. In PFA, capsular suture is of paramount importance, and, in particular when a lateral approach is performed, it can be modulated to adjust any minimal imperfection of the patellar tracking.

Progressive weight bearing starts the day of surgery as well as both passive and active mobilization. Patients are typically discharged from the Orthopaedic Department on day 2 post-op, after demonstrating the ability to full weight bearing with two crutches and are able to flex the knee at least 90°. In selected cases, outpatient surgery could be performed with a strict follow-up. Case Presentation figure shows an example of a bilateral PFA in a subject with pre-operative subluxated alta patellas.

20.6 Clinical Evidence of PF Replacement

Second-generation PFAs have lower revision rates and higher functional outcomes compared to first-generation inlay design prostheses [1, 14–16, 18, 19].

Recent studies reported a survivorship of 91.7% at 5 years, 83.3% at 10 years, 74.9% at 15 years and 66.6% at 20 years [1]. However, the longer follow-ups were affected by the limited results of the first-generation prostheses. When comparing more recent studies with studies published before 2010, the more recent ones reported a lower annual revision rate (1.93 vs. 2.33). The same study reported that the percentage of patients reporting good or excellent knee function varied between 86.8% and 92.5% at 5 years of follow-up. Moreover, reports from high-volume centres reported better outcomes and higher survivorship compared to data extrapolated from registries [1].

We have published our experience of 105 gender-specific PFAs at a mean follow-up of 5.5 years [12]. Sixty-four were isolated PFA, and 41 were UKA + PFA. Both groups showed a clear improvement in ROM, pain, Knee Society Score and UCLA activity score compared to preoperative values. Survivorship of these 105 implants was 95.2%. Consequently, modern PFA could be affordable both isolated than combined with a UKA, leading to excellent functional and survivorship results.

Progression of OA in the tibiofemoral components is the major long-term failure cause in PFA [1]. Dahm et al. demonstrated that patients with PFOA secondary to trochlear dysplasia had significantly less radiographic evidence of tibiofemoral joint osteoarthritis progression compared with those without trochlear dysplasia at 4 years mean follow-up [19].

Case Presentation

Fifty-five-year-old female with isolated bilateral PFOA. Preoperative weight-bearing X-rays showed pristine tibiofemoral joints and end-stage PFOA secondary to trochlear dysplasia and patella alta.

The patient underwent simultaneous bilateral PFA with an adjusted kinematic alignment technique. The prosthetic trochlea compensated the hypoplasia of lateral condyle and created an adequate sulcus angle; the trochlear line was corrected but remained externally rotated. The high-riding patella faced anyway the prosthetic trochlea without the need of further surgical procedures.

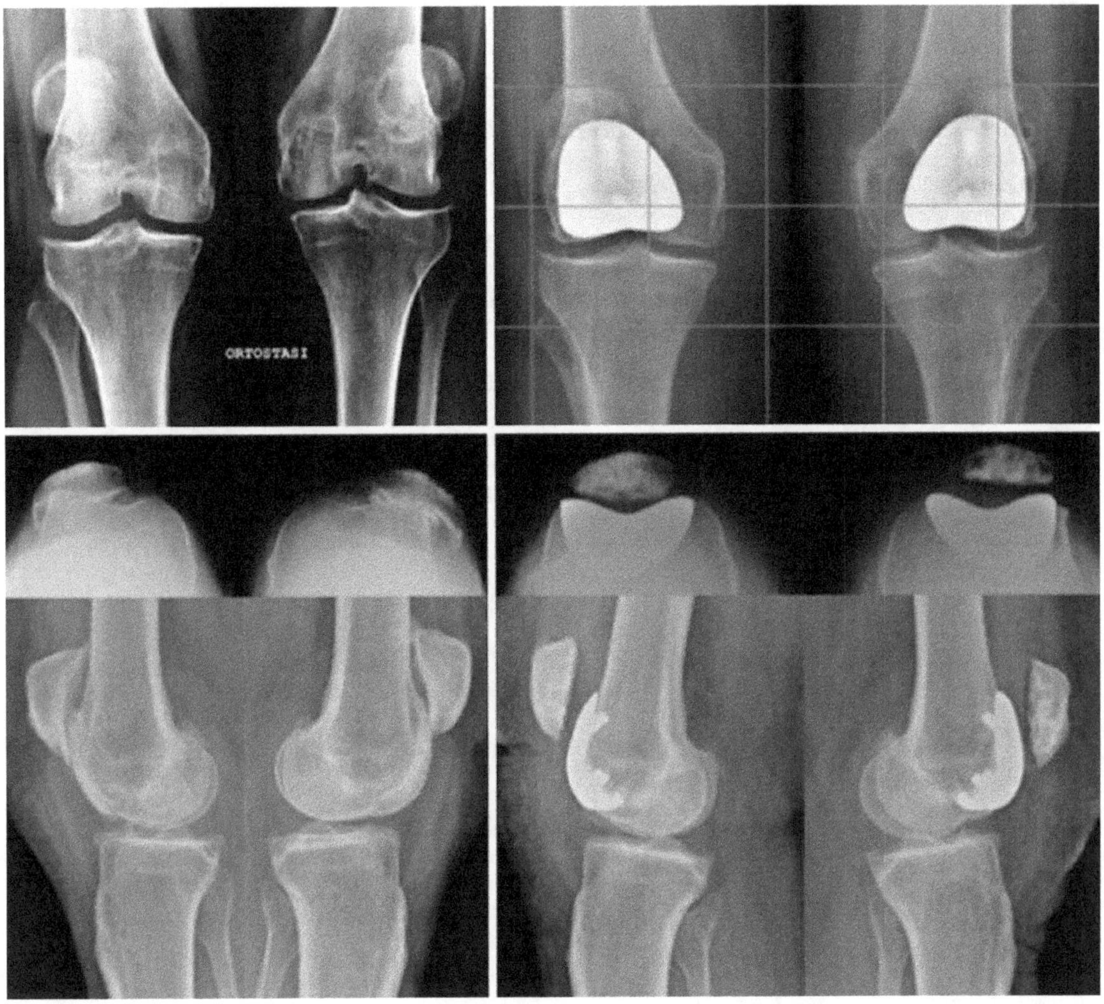

References

1. van der List JP, Chawla H, Zuiderbaan HA, Pearle AD. Survivorship and functional outcomes of patellofemoral arthroplasty: a systematic review. Knee Surg Sports Traumatol Arthrosc. 2017;25(8):2622–31. https://doi.org/10.1007/s00167-015-3878-z.
2. Scindler O, Scott N. Basic kinematics and biomechanics of the PFJ. Acta Orthop Belg. 2011;77:421–31.
3. Bandi W. Chondromalacia patellae and arthritis of the patellofemoral joint. Helv Chir Acta. 1972;11:1–70.
4. Walker PS. Contact areas and load transmission in the knee. In: American Academy of Orthopedic Surgeons: symposium on reconstructive surgery of the knee. Saint Louis: Mosby Company; 1978. p. 26–36.
5. Romagnoli S, Verde F, Zacchetti S. Bicompartmental prosthesis. In: Confalonieri N, Romagnoli S, editors. Small implants in knee reconstructions. Milan: Springer; 2013. p. 105–16.
6. Csintalan RP, Schulz MM, Woo J, McMahon PJ, Lee TQ. Gender differences in patellofemoral joint biomechanics. Clin Orthop. 2002;402:260–9.
7. Mahfouz M, Booth R Jr, Argenson J, Merkl BC, Abdel Fatah EE, Kuhn MJ. Analysis of variation of adult femora using sex -specific statistical atlases. Presented at Computer Methods in Biomechanics and Biomedical Engineering Conference; 2006.
8. Varadarajan KM, Gill TJ, Freiberg AA, Rubash HE, Li G. Gender differences in trochlear groove orientation and rotational kinematics of human knees. J Orthop Res. 2009;27:871e8. https://doi.org/10.1002/jor.20844.
9. McAlindon TE, Snow S, Cooper C, Dieppe PA. Radiographic patterns of osteoarthritis of the knee joint in the community. Ann Rheum Dis. 1992;51:844–9.
10. Dejour D, Allain J. Histoire naturelle de l'arthrose fémoro-patellaire isolée. Rev Chir Orthop. 2004;90:1S69–1S129.
11. Guilbert S, Gougeon F, Migaud H. Evolution de l'arthrose fémoro-patellaire isolée: devenir à 9 ans

de recul moyen de 80 genoux non opérés. Rev Chir Orthop. 2004;90:1S69–86.
12. Romagnoli S, Marullo M. Mid-term clinical, functional, and radiographic outcomes of 105 gender-specific patellofemoral arthroplasties, with or without the Association of Medial Unicompartmental Knee Arthroplasty. J Arthroplast. 2018;33:688–95.
13. Romagnoli S, Marullo M. What are the limits for unicompartmental knee arthroplasty? In: The young arthritic knee. Abstract book of 16èmes Journées Lyonnaises de Chirurgie du Genou 2014 Bonnin et al Editors Sauramps Medical; 2014.
14. Leadbetter WB, Ragland PS, Mont MA. The appropriate use of patellofemoral arthroplasty: an analysis of reported indications, contraindications, and failures. Clin Orthop Relat Res. 2005;436:91e9.
15. Lonner JH. Patellofemoral arthroplasty: the impact of design on outcomes. Orthop Clin North Am. 2008;39:347e54. https://doi.org/10.1016/j.ocl.2008.02.002.
16. Lonner JH, Bloomfield MR. The clinical outcome of patellofemoral arthroplasty. Orthop Clin North Am. 2013;44:271e80. https://doi.org/10.1016/j.ocl.2013.03.002.
17. Carrillon Y, Abidi H, Dejour D, et al. Patellar instability: assessment on MR images by measuring the lateral trochlear inclination-initial experience. Radiology. 2000;216:582–5.
18. Lustig S, Magnussen RA, Dahm DL, Parker D. Patellofemoral arthroplasty, where are we today? Knee Surg Sports Traumatol Arthrosc. 2012;20:1216e26. https://doi.org/10.1007/s00167-012-1948-z.
19. Dahm DL, Kalisvaart MM, Stuart MJ, Slettedahl SW. Patellofemoral arthroplasty: outcomes and factors associated with early progression of tibiofemoral arthritis. Knee Surg Sports Traumatol Arthrosc. 2014;22(10):2554–9. https://doi.org/10.1007/s00167-014-3202-3.

21

Fundamentals of CPKA

Amy Garner and Justin Cobb

Abbreviations

ACL	Anterior cruciate ligament
BCA-L	Bicompartmental knee arthroplasty (lateral)
BCA-M	Bicompartmental knee arthroplasty (medial)
Bi-UKA	Bi-unicondylar knee arthroplasty
CPKA	Combined partial knee arthroplasty
EQ-5D	EuroQol-5D Index of Quality of Life
OKS	Oxford knee score
PFA	Patellofemoral arthroplasty
PFJ	Patellofemoral joint
PKA	Partial knee arthroplasty
TCA	Tricompartmental knee arthroplasty
TKA	Total knee arthroplasty
UKA	Unicompartmental knee arthroplasty

A. Garner (✉)
MSk Lab, Imperial College London, London, UK

Health Education, Kent, Surrey and Sussex, London, UK

Royal College of Surgeons of England and Dunhill Medical Trust, London, UK
e-mail: a.garner@imperial.ac.uk

J. Cobb
MSk Lab, Imperial College London, London, UK
e-mail: j.cobb@imperial.ac.uk

Key Points

- Bone- and cruciate-preserving alternative to total knee arthroplasty.
- High-functioning arthroplasty option when the anterior cruciate ligament is intact.
- Unlinked components offer patient-specific surgery with conventional implants.
- Suitable for young, active, high-demand patients in the primary setting.
- Addition of components to existing partial knee arthroplasty offers a safer, less invasive alternative to the revision to total knee arthroplasty.

21.1 Introduction

Arthrosis commonly affects a single compartment of the knee, but may present with two or even three compartments affected. Wear to the medial tibiofemoral compartment is ten times more common than that in the lateral tibiofemoral compartment; primary patellofemoral joint (PFJ) arthrosis is least common [1, 2]. Bicompartmental disease is present in 59% of those with gonarthrosis [3]. In one study, 40% of patients over 50 years old with knee pain had radiographic evidence of combined medial compartment and PFJ wear, 24% had isolated PFJ arthrosis, whilst only 4% had isolated tibiofemoral arthrosis [4]. Degeneration of all three compartments simultaneously is rare [2]. Consequently, removal of healthy tissue in total knee arthroplasty (TKA) is common. The anterior cruciate ligament (ACL) is present in 78% of cases of patients undergoing primary knee replacement [5]. The fundamental role of the ACL in knee stability and functional gait is well described [6]; however, regardless of its functional integrity, it is resected in almost all TKAs.

TKA is associated with up to 20% patient dissatisfaction [7], significant peri-operative risk [8] and limited function when the ACL is sacrificed. However, in the absence of an effective alternative, TKA remains the standard treatment for multi-compartment arthrosis [9]. Combined partial knee arthroplasty (CPKA) is the collective term for multiple partial knee arthroplasties (PKAs) used together within the same knee, preserving healthy compartments and functional cruciate ligaments as an alternative to TKA [10]. Four combinations of CPKA exist (Fig. 21.1): Bicompartmental knee arthroplasty (BCA) refers to a patellofemoral arthroplasty (PFA) in combination with either a medial (BCA-M) or lateral (BCA-L) unicompartmental knee arthroplasty (UKA), whilst bi-unicondylar knee arthroplasty (Bi-UKA) describes an ipsilateral medial and lateral UKA [10]. All three used in combination are referred to as a tricompartmental knee arthroplasty (TCA). CPKA is not a new idea. The original Gunston knee, Charnley's 'load angle inlay' knee, the Marmor modular knee, the Cartier knee and the Oxford unicompartmental knee systems all followed a bi-unicondylar configuration.

In the presence of a functional ACL, multi-compartment arthrosis can be addressed through single-stage CPKA. Alternatively, a patient previously treated with a single PKA may be converted to a CPKA in a further operation, in the event of subsequent native compartment degeneration. The advantage of the latter, 'staged' procedure, is that the second operation may be considered a primary PKA with the benefits of a shorter hospital stay and reduced perioperative risk [8]. Advocates of CPKA argue that, in tailoring the surgery to the exact disease pattern of the patient, a second procedure may never become necessary and healthy bone and soft tissues are preserved whilst minimising the risk to the patient and optimising function and satisfaction. If a second surgery in PKA involves conversion to a standard primary TKA, this is a relatively straightforward process, especially if a kinematic technique is employed [11], which may delay or prevent the need for revision to the TKA. Opponents, however, argue that if the entire knee is replaced in the first instance, the patient may avoid the need for a second procedure altogether. Using two implants in combination, together with the potential need for additional hospital admissions, has a financial implication, though this additional cost may be offset by shorter hospital stays following both the primary and revision procedure, and fewer perioperative complications.

21.2 Case 1

A 64-year-old male presented with antero-medial right knee pain and difficulty standing up from a chair and walking up the stairs. He reported night pain, occasional giving way and now walks with a stick, but is keen to return to playing tennis. On examination, he had a moderate effusion and

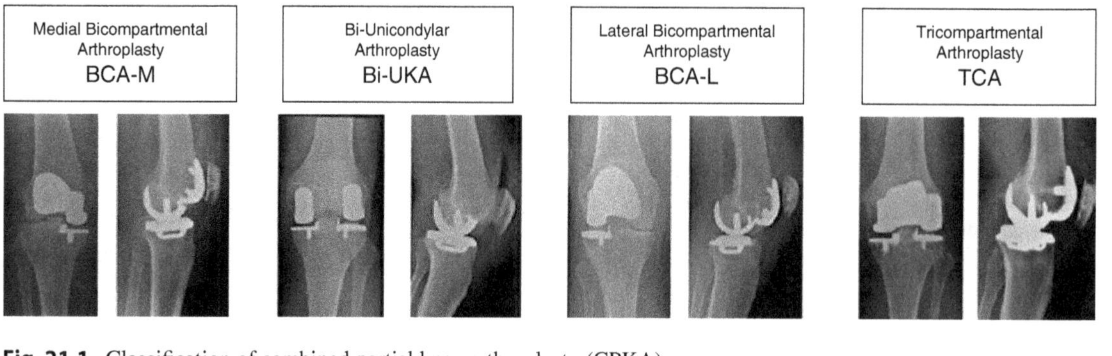

Fig. 21.1 Classification of combined partial knee arthroplasty (CPKA)

correctable varus deformity. Range of motion was 5–130°. Lachman and Anterior Drawer tests were negative. He had extrusion of the medial meniscus, but the lateral meniscus did not extrude on valgus stress. Pre-operative radiographs (Fig. 21.2) show varus alignment with significant loss of joint space in the medial compartment, osteophytes and subchondral sclerosis. There is some medial translation of the tibia on the femur. There is significant arthrosis of the lateral facet of the patellofemoral joint. The lateral compartment is well preserved with no evidence of arthrosis. On the lateral view, the ACL appears to be functional with no evidence of anterior translation of the tibia on the femur.

The patient was presented with the options for surgical management (Table 21.1) but prioritised high levels of function and opted for BCA-M. The patient was positioned supine on the operating table with a side support and foot support to hold the knee at 90° of flexion. A midline incision and medial parapatellar approach were used to access the joint. The lateral compartment was inspected and found to be disease-free. The ACL was intact. The UKA-M was undertaken first to correct the alignment and left with trial implants whilst the trochlea was prepared. The patella button was trialled to ensure it tracked smoothly over the trochlear component and

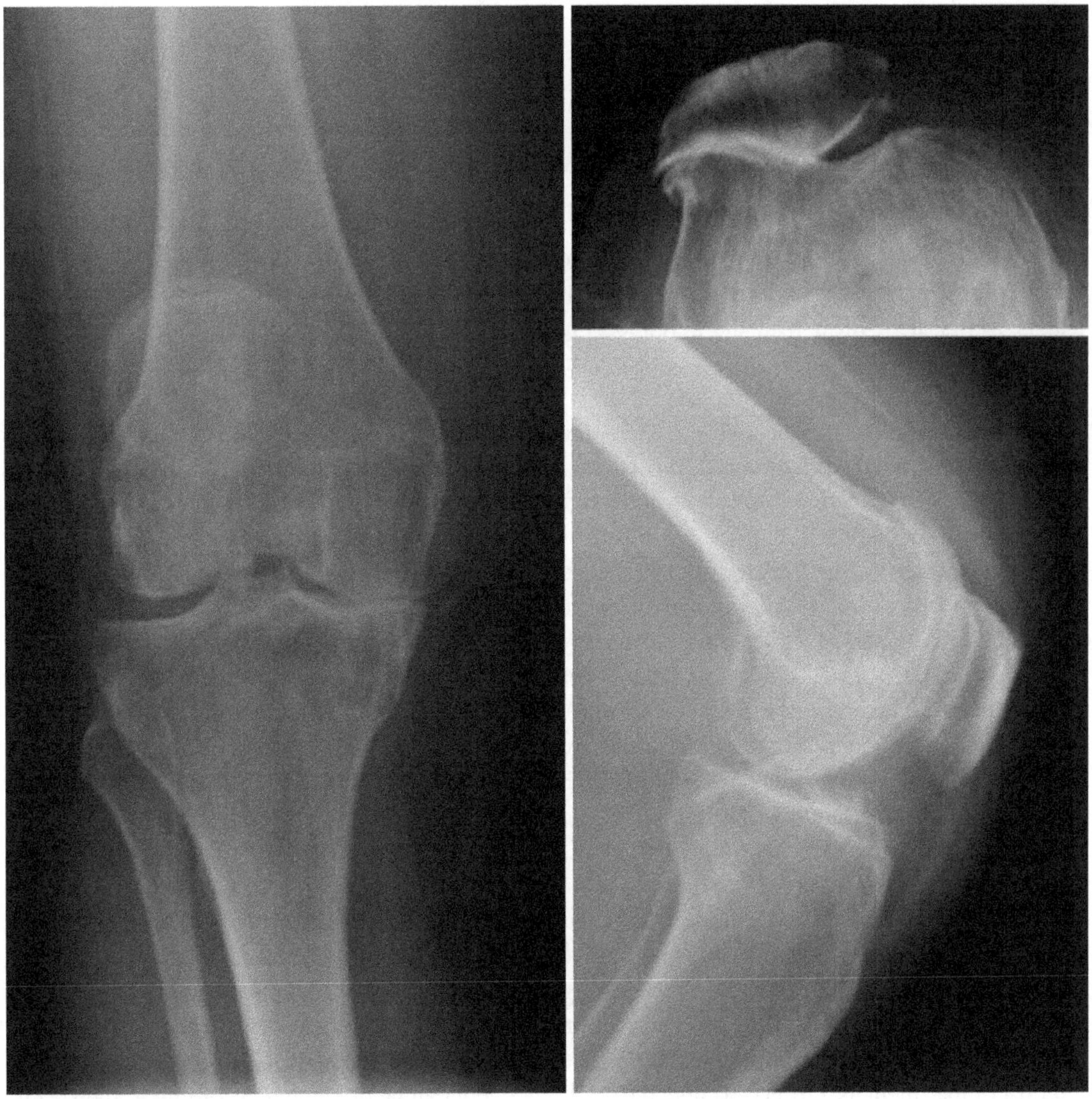

Fig. 21.2 Pre-operative radiographs, Case 1

Table 21.1 Options for surgical management of medial compartment with lateral facet patellofemoral arthrosis

Management option	Advantages	Disadvantages
TKA	Technically straightforward Widely available Lower risk for revision No risk of native compartment degeneration	ACL sacrifice—compromised function Up to 20% dissatisfaction Higher perioperative risks Longer hospital stay Removal of healthy bone (lateral compartment)
UKA-M	Bone preserving Short hospital stay Lower perioperative risks Least traumatic ACL preserving—higher function	Does not address patellofemoral arthrosis Higher revision risk Risk of further degeneration necessitating revision
PFA	Bone preserving Short hospital stay ACL preserving—higher function	Does not address medial tibiofemoral arthrosis Will not correct alignment Risk of further degeneration necessitating revision Highest revision risk (not recommended in isolation for bi-compartmental arthrosis)
BCA-M	Treats all affected compartments Bone preserving Will correct alignment ACL preserving—highest function	Risk of revision if lateral compartment fails Unknown revision rates (likely higher than TKA) Unknown perioperative risk (likely lower than TKA) Technically challenging—few surgeons perform it Higher implant costs

did not catch on the femoral component of the medial UKA. A final check to ensure the trochlear is well-seated, flush with the neighbouring cartilage, is made, to ensure the patella button transitions smoothly between implants. Care is taken not to damage the cartillage betwen the implants during bone preparation. Whilst balancing an UKA in the supine position is more difficult than in a 'dangling' support, it improves the technical ease of the PFA, so it is preferred for simultaneous BCA-M. All components were implanted simultaneously after all of the bony cuts had been performed. Tourniquet time was 64 min (surgeon average for UKA is 45 min). The patient recovered without peri-operative complication and was discharged within 48 h of surgery. Within 4 months of surgery, he had returned to full function including playing tennis twice per week. His Oxford Knee Score was 44 at 6 months, rising to 47 at 12 months and continuing at 47 6 years post-surgery. Post-operative radiographs (Fig. 21.3) show a mobile-bearing UKA-M and onlay PFA in situ, with correction of the varus deformity and tibial translation. The lateral compartment is preserved, and the ACL appears functional, and the patella button tracks adequately over the resurfaced trochlea.

21.3 Function Post-CPKA

A number of studies and expert opinions emphasise the benefits of BCA [12], including superior performance in strenuous activities such as stair climbing and jogging, compared to TKA, in part due to restored isokinetic quadriceps function [13]. High function, independent rising from a chair and reciprocal stair ascent is seen rapidly and consistently after BCA [14, 15]. Kinematics and gait patterns associated with BCA are similar to those of healthy controls [14, 16]. Compared to TKA, several studies report that patients with BCA have higher levels of satisfaction and comfort following surgery [17, 18], with good or excellent pain outcomes reported up to 12 years post-operatively in 85% of patients, 92% of whom reported satisfactory pain relief [19]. Patients experience less intra-operative blood loss [20] and greater post-operative range of movement [21] compared to matched groups undergoing TKA.

In Case 1, the femur has been addressed through two unlinked components. A significant advantage of unlinked CPKA is that each component can be orientated according to the specific anatomy of the compartment, effectively allowing the surgeon to create a custom fit, using 'off-the-

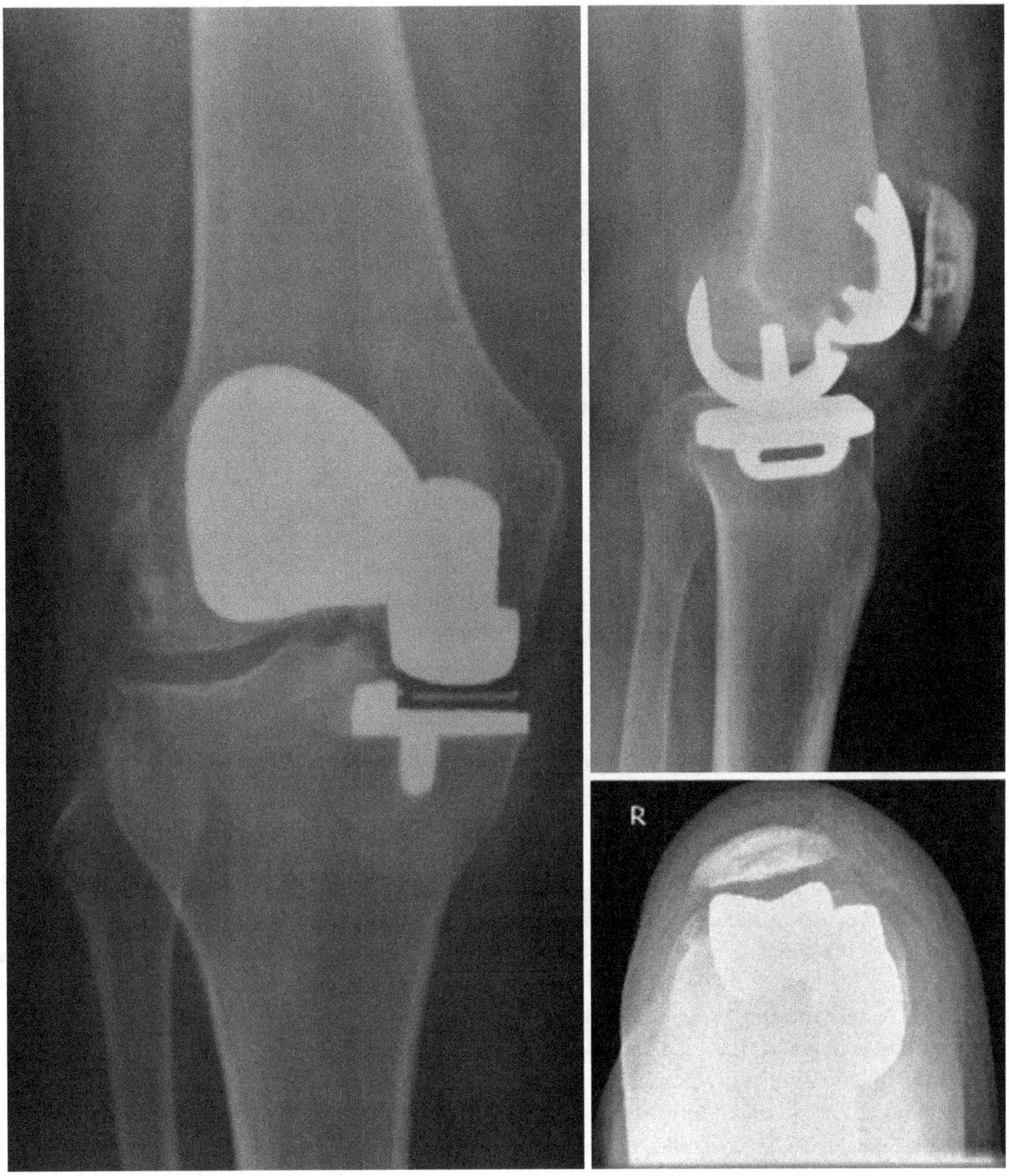

Fig. 21.3 Post-operative radiographs, Case 1, with BCA-M in situ

shelf' implants [22]. An alternative is to use a monolithic femoral component, which simultaneously resurfaces both the condyle and the trochlea. Whilst monolithic femoral components are theoretically easier to implant, early examples including the Journey Deuce (Smith and Nephew Inc., Memphis, TN, US) performed very poorly, blighted by high rates of early revision (Fig. 21.4). Malalignment, sizing difficulties, poor durability, anterior knee pain, limited range of movement and tibial component fractures were all cited as causes for early failure [13]. In one short-term study, a 12% revision rate was reported, with 25% of patients complaining of anterior knee pain [23]. In another study of 25 Journey Deuce, three were revised—two for fractured tibial trays and one for patella instability [24]. These reports, plus evidence of tibial subsidence, contributed to the US Food and Drug Administration's decision to recall the Journey Deuce prosthesis in 2010.

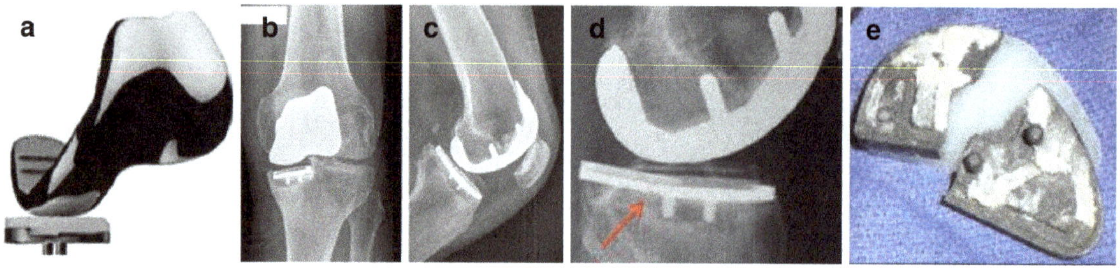

Fig. 21.4 Monolithic Journey Deuce (Smith and Nephew Inc., Memphis, TN, US) (**a**) with tibial component subsidence (**b**, **c**) and tibial baseplate fracture (**d**, **e**) [24, 25]

Contemporary monolithic designs are utilising assistive technologies including 3D-printed patient-specific instrumentation, robotics and navigation to help improve alignment accuracy and decrease the technical demands of this procedure [26] which may lead to a resurgence in interest in linked components. Modular CPKA may allow the surgeon more freedom to make subtle adjustments according to the distal femoral geometry of the femur, with promising results but a steep learning curve [21, 23, 27–29]. Some early modular BCA-M had a 46% incidence of disease progression or radiographic evidence of loosening by 17 years post-operation, likely due to poor-quality polyethylene and crude instrumentation necessitating a "free-hand" technique [30]. Aseptic loosening of the PFA implant was the main cause of failure in 20/27 revised BCA-M [30]. Experience with BCA failure, however, provided much evidence that conversion to TKA was typically straightforward, using primary TKA implants [29, 31–33]. Second-generation anterior-cut (onlay design) cemented patellofemoral components are associated with improved clinical and biochemical outcomes [34–36]. Unlinked components enable more accurate alignment [34].

21.4 Case 2

A 54-year-old male presented with lateral joint knee pain and difficulty walking on slopes. He has been a keen hill walker for many years. He reports swelling in the knee and now requires daily anti-inflammatory medications to walk short distances. On examination, he has a good range of movement but extrusion of the lateral meniscus. Lachman test was negative, and the knee felt stable, with no medial meniscal extrusion on varus stressing.

Weight-bearing radiographs (Fig. 21.5) demonstrate a valgus right knee, with Ahlback grade IV loss in the lateral compartment with some medial opening. There is severe degeneration of the lateral facet of the PFJ. The ACL appears functional on the lateral radiograph, with no evidence of anterior translation of the tibia on the femur.

This young patient prioritised high function and opted for single-stage BCA-L. A midline incision was made, followed by a lateral parapatellar arthrotomy. Additional care was taken to sublux the patella medially to enable adequate exposure. Extending the arthrotomy into the quadriceps tendon is sometimes necessary to improve the view, but may increase the associated morbidity of the procedure. The medial compartment was found to be well preserved, and the ACL was functional and intact. On the lateral side, it is particularly important to ensure the patella has a smooth transition between the femoral components of the UKA and PFA and the femoral condylar cartilage for accurate tracking. Care should be taken not to over-resect bone from the distal femur, if required, to avoid impingement of the UKA bearing in full extension. The patient experienced no peri-operative complications and returned to hill walking within 6 months. His Oxford Knee Score was 44 at 12 months post-surgery, EQ-5D 0.95/1. Post-operative radiographs (Fig. 21.6) demonstrate the BCA-L in situ and confirm that the medial compartment is preserved and alignment corrected. The patella tracks centrally across the resurfaced trochlea. In this case a mobile-bearing lateral UKA was used to prioritise high function,

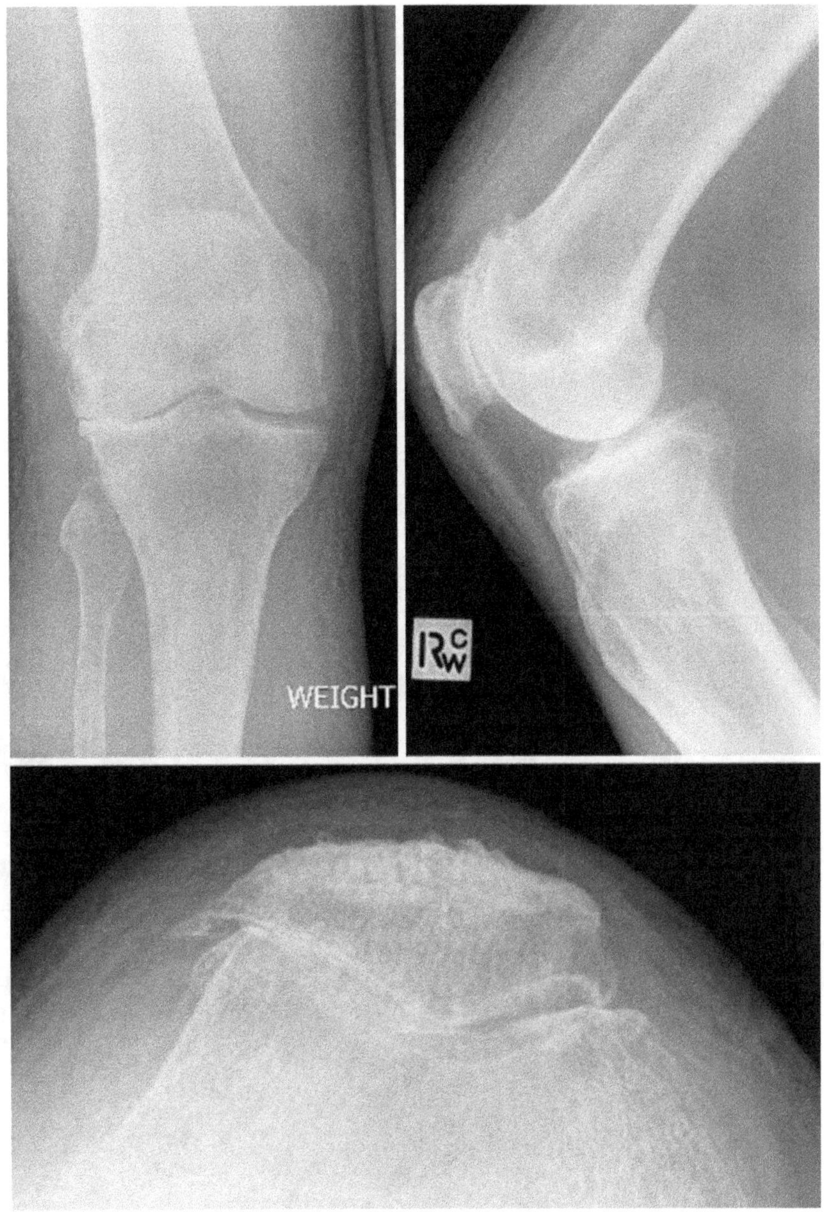

Fig. 21.5 Pre-operative radiographs, Case 2

but if concern for the risk of bearing dislocation is present, a fixed bearing device may be more appropriate.

21.5 Case 3

An 82-year-old lady presents with knee pain 14 years following a medial UKA. She now requires a walking stick but can stand from a chair and use the stairs without particular difficulty. She has diabetes mellitus type II controlled with insulin, cardiac stents and hypertension and had a transient ischaemic attack 5 years ago. On examination, she has a moderate effusion, correctable valgus deformity of <10°, 0–120 range of movement and some anterior–posterior laxity; but the medial UKA appears stable and functional. Pre-operative radiographs (Fig. 21.7) demonstrate a well-fixed medial UKA but failure of the lateral compartment. The patellofemoral compartment is relatively well preserved, and the ACL appears functional.

Progression of lateral compartment OA in patients with medial arthrosis is very rare in the absence of surgical intervention [37, 38].

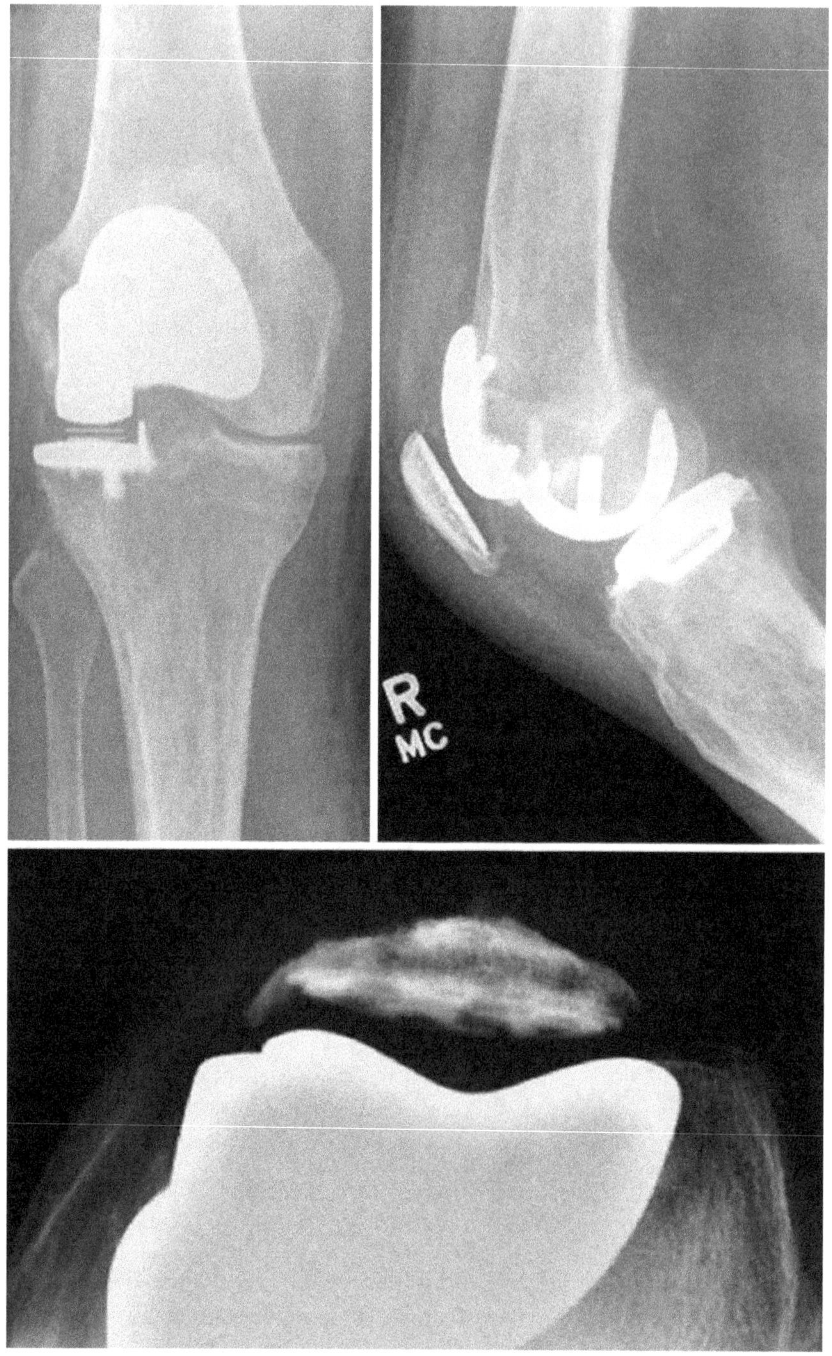

Fig. 21.6 Post-operative radiographs, Case 2, demonstrating a BCA-L in situ

After a medial UKA, lateral arthrosis is often cited as a reason for failure and revision to TKA [22]. However, multiple studies from the Oxford Group and the National Joint Registry, using data from 15- to 20-year follow-up studies, place the revision rate as between 2.3 and 2.6% [39–41], whilst our own group reported 64 knees with no polyethylene bearing dislocations [42].

The surgical options for managing Case 3's newly degenerate compartment are to remove the well-fixed, high-functioning medial UKA, sacrifice the remaining function of the ACL and patellofemoral compartment and convert to a TKA or leave the medial UKA untouched and 'convert' to a Bi-UKA through the addition of a lateral UKA [43]. Revision to TKA is commonly performed across the world, but carries

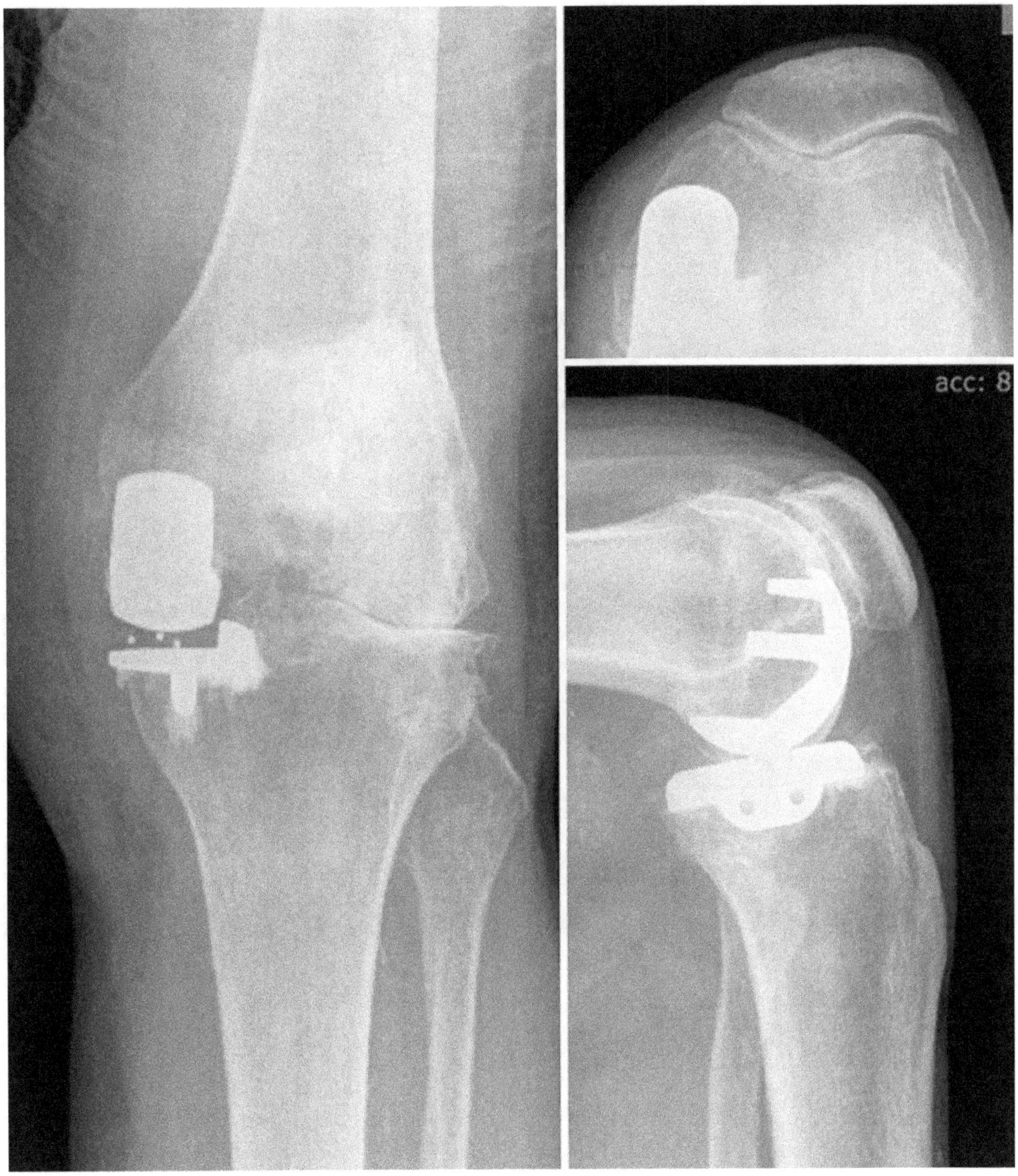

Fig. 21.7 Pre-operative radiographs, Case 3, demonstrating a UKA-M in situ

significant peri-operative risk, requiring a large surgical exposure, the risk of bone loss during implant removal and significant peri-operative risk of stroke, myocardial infarction or death [8]. Although conversion to Bi-UKA would be regarded by joint registries as a revision of the medial UKA, it is possible to perform it as though it were a primary procedure, with a small incision. Since the lateral compartment is being addressed as if a primary UKA, the procedure benefits from short tourniquet times and early hospital discharge. This patient is high risk for major surgery and opted for a smaller, safer procedure to avoid the risks associated with conversion to TKA.

It was discussed, during the consent process, that should the PFJ be worn or the ACL completely dysfunctional, the surgeon would have a low threshold for conversion to TKA. The previous UKA incision had been medial to the

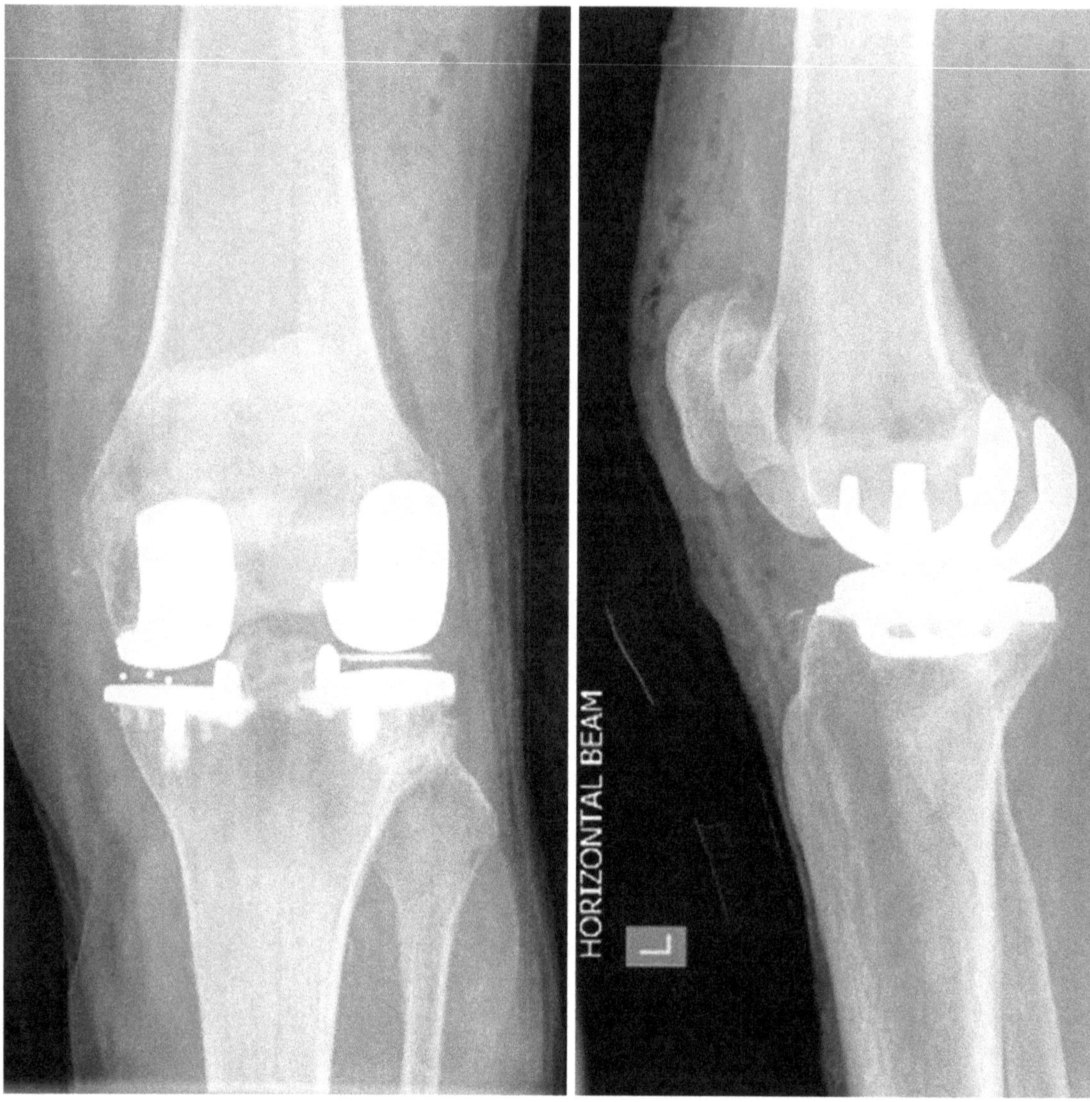

Fig. 21.8 Post-operative radiographs demonstrate conversion to Bi-UKA through the addition of a lateral UKA

midline, and therefore, a parallel lateral incision was made, leaving a 6-cm skin bridge between the wounds. Had the previous incision been more midline, it would have been re-used, but a new lateral parapatellar arthrotomy made, to access the lateral compartment. The ACL was found to be degenerate but functional, which is not considered a contra-indication in elderly low-demand patients. The medial UKA was well fixed with minimal evidence of polyethylene wear, so it was left, though in high-functioning patients the polyethylene is often exchanged if signs of wear are evident. The tourniquet time was 48 min, and the patient was discharged the following day. Post-operative radiographs (Fig. 21.8) demonstrate the Bi-UKA in situ. In this instance, a mobile bearing was used; however, due to the increased dislocation rate, a fixed bearing may be preferable in elderly, low-demand patients.

Biazzo et al. compared 19 patients undergoing single-stage Bi-UKA to a matched cohort undergoing computer-assisted TKA, showing superior outcome in terms of function and stiffness on WOMAC indexes and equivalent KSS and WOMAC Arthritis Index (pain score) [20]. Single-staged Bi-UKA is associated with shorter hospital stays than TKA [32].

21.6 Summary

CPKA is more technically demanding than TKA in theory, but is associated with excellent post-operative outcomes and superior function [18]. It is suitable both for young, high-demand patients looking for excellent function and for higher risk patients, particularly in the revision setting, providing a safer, conservative alternative to TKA.

References

1. McAlindon TE, Snow S, Cooper C, Dieppe PA. Radiographic patterns of osteoarthritis of the knee joint in the community: the importance of the patellofemoral joint. Ann Rheum Dis. 1992;51(7): 844–9.
2. Ahlbäck S. Osteoarthrosis of the knee. A radiographic investigation. Acta Radiol Diagn (Stockh). 1968;(Suppl 277):7–72.
3. Ledingham J, Regan M, Jones A, Doherty M. Radiographic patterns and associations of osteoarthritis of the knee in patients referred to hospital. Ann Rheum Dis. 1993;52(7):520–6.
4. Duncan RC, Hay EM, Saklatvala J, Croft PR. Prevalence of radiographic osteoarthritis—it all depends on your point of view. Rheumatology (Oxford). 2006;45(6):757–60.
5. Johnson AJ, Howell SM, Costa CR, Mont MA. The ACL in the arthritic knee: how often is it present and can preoperative tests predict its presence? Clin Orthop Relat Res. 2013;471(1):181–8.
6. Duthon VB, Barea C, Abrassart S, Fasel JH, Fritschy D, Menetrey J. Anatomy of the anterior cruciate ligament. Knee Surg Sports Traumatol Arthrosc. 2006;14(3):204–13.
7. Bourne RB, Chesworth BM, Davis AM, Mahomed NN, Charron KD. Patient satisfaction after total knee arthroplasty: who is satisfied and who is not? Clin Orthop Relat Res. 2010;468(1):57–63.
8. Liddle AD, Judge A, Pandit H, Murray DW. Adverse outcomes after total and unicompartmental knee replacement in 101,330 matched patients: a study of data from the National Joint Registry for England and Wales. Lancet (London, England). 2014;384(9952):1437–45.
9. Cobb J. Osteoarthritis of the knee. Precise diagnosis and treatment. BMJ. 2009;339:b3747.
10. Garner A. van Arkel RJ, Cobb J. Classification of combined partial knee arthroplasty, Bone Joint J. 2019;101-B(8):922–28.
11. Toliopoulos P, LeBlanc MA, Hutt J, Lavigne M, Desmeules F, Vendittoli PA. Anatomic versus mechanically aligned total knee arthroplasty for unicompartmental knee arthroplasty revision. Open Orthop J. 2016;10:357–63.
12. Thienpont E, Price A. Bicompartmental knee arthroplasty of the patellofemoral and medial compartments. Knee Surg Sports Traumatol Arthrosc. 2013;21(11):2523–31.
13. Palumbo BT, Henderson ER, Edwards PK, Burris RB, Gutierrez S, Raterman SJ. Initial experience of the journey-deuce bicompartmental knee prosthesis: a review of 36 cases. J Arthroplast. 2011;26(6 Suppl):40–5.
14. Wang H, Dugan E, Frame J, Rolston L. Gait analysis after bi-compartmental knee replacement. Clin Biomech (Bristol, Avon). 2009;24(9):751–4.
15. Argenson JN, Parratte S, Bertani A, Aubaniac JM, Lombardi AV Jr, Berend KR, et al. The new arthritic patient and arthroplasty treatment options. J Bone Joint Surg Am. 2009;91(Suppl 5):43–8.
16. Leffler J, Scheys L, Plante-Bordeneuve T, Callewaert B, Labey L, Bellemans J, et al. Joint kinematics following bi-compartmental knee replacement during daily life motor tasks. Gait Posture. 2012;36(3):454–60.
17. Parratte S, Ollivier M, Opsomer G, Lunebourg A, Argenson JN, Thienpont E. Is knee function better with contemporary modular bicompartmental arthroplasty compared to total knee arthroplasty? Short-term outcomes of a prospective matched study including 68 cases. Orthop Traumatol Surg Res. 2015;101(5):547–52.
18. Heyse TJ, Khefacha A, Cartier P. UKA in combination with PFR at average 12-year follow-up. Arch Orthop Trauma Surg. 2010;130(10):1227–30.
19. Cartier P, Sanouiller JL, Grelsamer R. Patellofemoral arthroplasty. 2-12-year follow-up study. J Arthroplast. 1990;5(1):49–55.
20. Biazzo A, Silvestrini F, Manzotti A, Confalonieri N. Bicompartmental (uni plus patellofemoral) versus total knee arthroplasty: a match-paired study. Musculoskelet Surg. 2019;103:63–8.
21. Tan SM, Dutton AQ, Bea KC, Kumar VP. Bicompartmental versus total knee arthroplasty for medial and patellofemoral osteoarthritis. J Orthop Surg (Hong Kong). 2013;21(3):281–4.
22. Romagnoli S, Marullo M, Massaro M, Rustemi E, D'Amario F, Corbella M. Bi-unicompartmental and combined uni plus patellofemoral replacement: indications and surgical technique. Joints. 2015;3(1):42–8.
23. Rolston L, Bresch J, Engh G, Franz A, Kreuzer S, Nadaud M, et al. Bicompartmental knee arthroplasty: a bone-sparing, ligament-sparing, and minimally invasive alternative for active patients. Orthopedics. 2007;30(8 Suppl):70–3.
24. Engh GA. A bi-compartmental solution: what the deuce? Orthopedics. 2007;30(9):770–1.
25. Stuyts B, Vandenberghe M, Bracht H, Fortems Y, Van den Eeden E, Cuypers L. Fracture of the tibial baseplate in bicompartmental knee arthroplasty. Case Rep Orthop. 2015;2015:1–5.
26. Steinert AF, Beckmann J, Holzapfel BM, Rudert M, Arnholdt J. Bicompartmental individualized knee replacement: use of patient-specific implants and instruments (iDuo). Oper Orthop Traumatol. 2017;29(1):51–8.

27. Argenson JN, Chevrol-Benkeddache Y, Aubaniac JM. Modern unicompartmental knee arthroplasty with cement: a three to ten-year follow-up study. J Bone Joint Surg Am. 2002;84(12):2235–9.
28. Wunschel M, Lo J, Dilger T, Wulker N, Muller O. Influence of bi- and tri-compartmental knee arthroplasty on the kinematics of the knee joint. BMC Musculoskelet Disord. 2011;12:29.
29. Zanasi S. Innovations in total knee replacement: new trends in operative treatment and changes in peri-operative management. Eur Orthop Traumatol. 2011;2(1–2):21–31.
30. Parratte S, Pauly V, Aubaniac JM, Argenson JN. Survival of bicompartmental knee arthroplasty at 5 to 23 years. Clin Orthop Relat Res. 2010;468(1):64–72.
31. Lonner JH. Modular bicompartmental knee arthroplasty with robotic arm assistance. Am J Orthop (Belle Mead, NJ). 2009;38(2 Suppl):28–31.
32. Confalonieri N, Manzotti A, Cerveri P, De Momi E. Bi-unicompartmental versus total knee arthroplasty: a matched paired study with early clinical results. Arch Orthop Trauma Surg. 2009;129(9):1157–63.
33. Pradhan NR, Gambhir A, Porter ML. Survivorship analysis of 3234 primary knee arthroplasties implanted over a 26-year period: a study of eight different implant designs. Knee. 2006;13(1):7–11.
34. Shah SM, Dutton AQ, Liang S, Dasde S. Bicompartmental versus total knee arthroplasty for medio-patellofemoral osteoarthritis: a comparison of early clinical and functional outcomes. J Knee Surg. 2013;26(6):411–6.
35. Pritchett JW. Anterior cruciate-retaining total knee arthroplasty. J Arthroplast. 1996;11(2):194–7.
36. Andriacchi TP, Galante JO, Fermier RW. The influence of total knee-replacement design on walking and stair-climbing. J Bone Joint Surg Am. 1982;64(9):1328–35.
37. Neogi T, Felson D, Niu J, Nevitt M, Lewis CE, Aliabadi P, et al. Association between radiographic features of knee osteoarthritis and pain: results from two cohort studies. BMJ. 2009;339:b2844.
38. Felson DT, Nevitt MC, Yang M, Clancy M, Niu J, Torner JC, et al. A new approach yields high rates of radiographic progression in knee osteoarthritis. J Rheumatol. 2008;35(10):2047–54.
39. Pandit H, Jenkins C, Gill HS, Barker K, Dodd CA, Murray DW. Minimally invasive Oxford phase 3 unicompartmental knee replacement: results of 1000 cases. J Bone Joint Surg. 2011;93(2):198–204.
40. Goodfellow J, O'Connor J, Pandit H, Dodd CA, Murray D. Unicompartmental arthroplasty with the Oxford knee. 2nd ed. Oxford: Goodfellow; 2016. p. 288.
41. Price AJ, Svard U. A second decade lifetable survival analysis of the Oxford unicompartmental knee arthroplasty. Clin Orthop Relat Res. 2011;469(1):174–9.
42. Altuntas AO, Alsop H, Cobb JP. Early results of a domed tibia, mobile bearing lateral unicompartmental knee arthroplasty from an independent centre. Knee. 2013;20(6):466–70.
43. Pandit H, Mancuso F, Jenkins C, Jackson WFM, Price AJ, Dodd CAF, et al. Lateral unicompartmental knee replacement for the treatment of arthritis progression after medial unicompartmental replacement. Knee Surg Sports Traumatol Arthrosc. 2017;25(3):669–74.

22

Custom TKA: Necessity and Surgical Technique

Elliot Sappey-Marinier, Carsten Tibesku, Tarik Ait Si Selmi, and Michel Bonnin

Key Points

1. Restore the native shape with an optimal bone implant fit.
2. Reproduce the native pre-arthritic joint line with a personalized alignment.
3. New economic system using custom single-use instruments.

As we reach the 50th anniversary of 'modern TKA', new technologies and new industrial processes render the manufacture of fully customized implants feasible. While this can be considered as a technological breakthrough, addressing several limitations of TKA, we may question whether this costly technology is worthwhile and beneficial for patients. Considering the wide range of TKA sizes now available—sometimes having millimetric-size increments—do we really need customized implants to reproduce the native anatomy?

E. Sappey-Marinier · T. A. S. Selmi · M. Bonnin (✉)
Centre Orthopédique Santy, Jean Mermoz Private Hospital, Lyon, France

C. Tibesku
KniePraxis, Straubing, Germany
e-mail: carsten@tibesku.de

22.1 Why Custom Total Knee Arthroplasty?

22.1.1 A Brief History of TKA

During the first half of the twentieth century, the pioneers of arthroplasty surgery tested surgical procedures for arthritic knees, which could be considered as 'resurfacing procedures' using soft tissue or chromium–cobalt interposition [1]. Inspired by the success of Smith-Petersen [2] with mould arthroplasty of the hip, Campbell and Boyd performed the first arthroplasty of the knee [3]. The advent of 'modern TKA' in the early 1970s introduced standardization, precision and reproducibility of surgical techniques and manufacturing processes, but abandoned the concept of personalized resurfacing. Due to the limited number of sizes available (only one femoral size existed during the first decade of total condylar knee arthroplasty) [4], optimizing a bone implant fit was challenging. During the 1980s and 1990s, the range of sizes increased, but only proportional to the original designs, assuming that all human knees had the same shape. It was only in the early 2000s that morphologic variability was investigated through the aspect ratio [5] and manufacturers developed narrow versions in their range of femurs, known as 'gender knees'.

22.1.2 The Limits of Contemporary TKA

Nowadays, surgeons can choose components from a wide range of sizes, including standard and narrow and sometimes asymmetric tibia. However, anatomic variations are not limited to large or narrow, but also include several other features, such as the trapezoidicity of the distal femur [6], the condylar radii of curvature [7], joint-line obliquity [8] and the shape of the trochlea and tibial plateaus [9]. The observed variability in morphotypes echoes the words of John Insall who warned that 'care must be taken in describing what is "normal" because of significant individual variations' and those of Werner Müller who pointed out that 'nothing is as constant as the variability of anatomy'. Therefore, the size and shape ranges used in standard TKA hardly cover the variability of the human knee, and oversizing has been reported in up to 76% on the femur and up to 90% on the tibia after TKA. It has been also demonstrated that any overhang of the implants increases the risk of residual pain and stiffness and jeopardizes functional outcomes [10–12].

Moreover, because the soft tissue envelope is non-extensible, implantation of mechanically aligned prostheses causes ligament imbalance, patellar maltracking and stiffness. These are tackled by the use of technical tricks such as ligament releases [13], external rotation of the femoral component [14] and kinematic alignment [15], all of which are 'palliative solutions' compensating for the non-anatomic shape of the implants and modification of the native alignment. It is therefore important to understand that TKA alignment and implant design are inter-related and cannot be considered separately.

22.1.3 Alignment Strategy in TKA

In the early days of TKA, the so-called *mechanical alignment (MA)* was favoured, aiming for a straight leg axis of 180° (neutral alignment), obtained via orthogonal cuts. A perfectly straight 180° leg does not mirror the average alignment, but was chosen for reasons of reproducibility and load distribution, to minimize polyethylene wear and implant loosening [16]. The mean native *joint line obliquity (JLO)* is 3°, with large inter-individual variations, comprising the mechanical lateral distal femoral angle (mLDFA), the mechanical medial proximal tibial angle (mMPTA) and the joint line convergence. The native JLO is rarely reproduced with classic orthogonal cuts, which results in asymmetric bone resections and therefore 'iatrogenic laxity'. The *anatomic alignment (AA) technique for TKA* still aims at a neutral (180°) alignment but via slightly oblique cuts (3°), which reproduces the average JLO value. The *kinematic alignment (KA) technique for TKA,* introduced later, aims to adapt the position of the implant to the soft tissue envelope, thereby restoring the native tri-dimensional alignment of the lower limb. Whatever the chosen alignment technique, a one geometrical implant design may cause bone implant mismatches when used in the wide range of human knee anatomies. So personalized implant orientation with KA may benefit to be linked to implant customization.

22.1.4 Are Patients Fully Satisfied with Standard TKA?

Despite the increasing survival of TKAs, due to innovations in biomaterials, design and surgical techniques, the satisfaction rate following TKA reported in the literature varies from 75% to 89%, with three main influencing factors: residual pain, functional outcome and preoperative expectations [17–20]. In a multicentre series of 347 non-selected TKA patients using various implants [17], we observed that only 62% of our patients were totally pain free during gait and 35% while climbing or descending stairs and 40% complained of pain while running. Only 48% of the patients declared being 'very satisfied' with the procedure, and 68% considered their operated knee to be 'normal for their age'.

22.2 The Need for Custom TKA

The Origin® custom TKA (Symbios, Yverdon-les-Bains, Switzerland) was developed between 2012 and 2017 and is CE marked since 2018. This system was conceived and designed to reproduce the native (pre-arthritic) anatomy of the knee, using a single-use custom instrumentation. The main aims are:

1. To optimize bone implant fit and avoid prosthetic overhang or under-coverage.
2. To improve ligament balancing by avoiding resection laxity due to asymmetric bone cuts.
3. To improve mid-flexion stability and kinematics by restoring the native radii of curvature.
4. To improve patellofemoral tracking by restoring the native femoral torsion and customized trochlea.
5. To facilitate restoration of the native pre-arthritic limb alignment.

Its production is based on a classic process, the chromium–cobalt femoral implant being made by standard casting, followed by machining and polishing. The tibial baseplate is made of titanium.

22.3 Design Rationale of the Origin® Implant

The Origin® prosthesis is postero-stabilized, with a proportional post-cam system that engages beyond 60° of knee flexion. The intercondylar box is proportional, in order to minimize bone sacrifice. Between 0° and 60° of knee flexion, anteroposterior stability relies on the shape of the polyethylene with a specific anterior ultracongruency. Most of the prosthetic designs retaining or sacrificing the PCL do not stabilize the femur adequately during flexion and allow a paradoxical femoral anterior sliding, which constrains the patella and reduces the quadriceps lever arm.

The femoral component reproduces the shape of the native femur, in terms of contours, radii of curvature and joint line obliquity. Because the implant and instrumentation are devised to reproduce the natural shape of the distal femur, no additional rotation is required during implantation, and the design is linked to the alignment. Therefore, no intraoperative modification of the femoral cuts or femoral rotation need be considered. The prosthetic trochlea is designed to match the shape of the native patella and to maintain its native alignment, with soft edges to avoid patellofemoral crepitus. In cases of trochlear or patellar dysplasia, the femoral trochlea implant is designed as a standard trochlea.

The tibial baseplate is asymmetric and reproduces the contours of the native plateaus, facilitating rotational positioning of the implant after bone resection. The rotation of the tibia matches the transverse tibial axis, defined by the line joining the centres of each plateau. The tibial slope is maintained in a range of 2°–5° to avoid anteroposterior instability. The tibial keel is aligned medio-laterally with the axis of the tibial metaphysis, which corresponds non-systematically to the baseplate centre. The coronal alignment of the tibial cut is maintained in ±3° range from 90°.

22.4 What Is the Process?

The design and manufacturing process of the Origin® custom TKA takes 6 weeks and requires cooperation between the surgeon and engineers. The design is based on a three-dimensional analysis of the bony anatomy of the arthritic deformities and limb alignment, based on a preoperative CT scan, using a special radiographic protocol, including the knee, hip and ankle joint. The DICOM files are collected and sent electronically to the engineering team through a secured 'Symbios box'. 3D analysis is performed with Knee-Plan® software (Symbios, Yverdon-les-Bains, Switzerland) (Fig. 22.1).

Additional clinical (range of motion of the knee, reducibility of the deformity) and radiographic information (dynamic varus–valgus XR and long leg standing XR) may also be useful. The engineering process requires several steps:

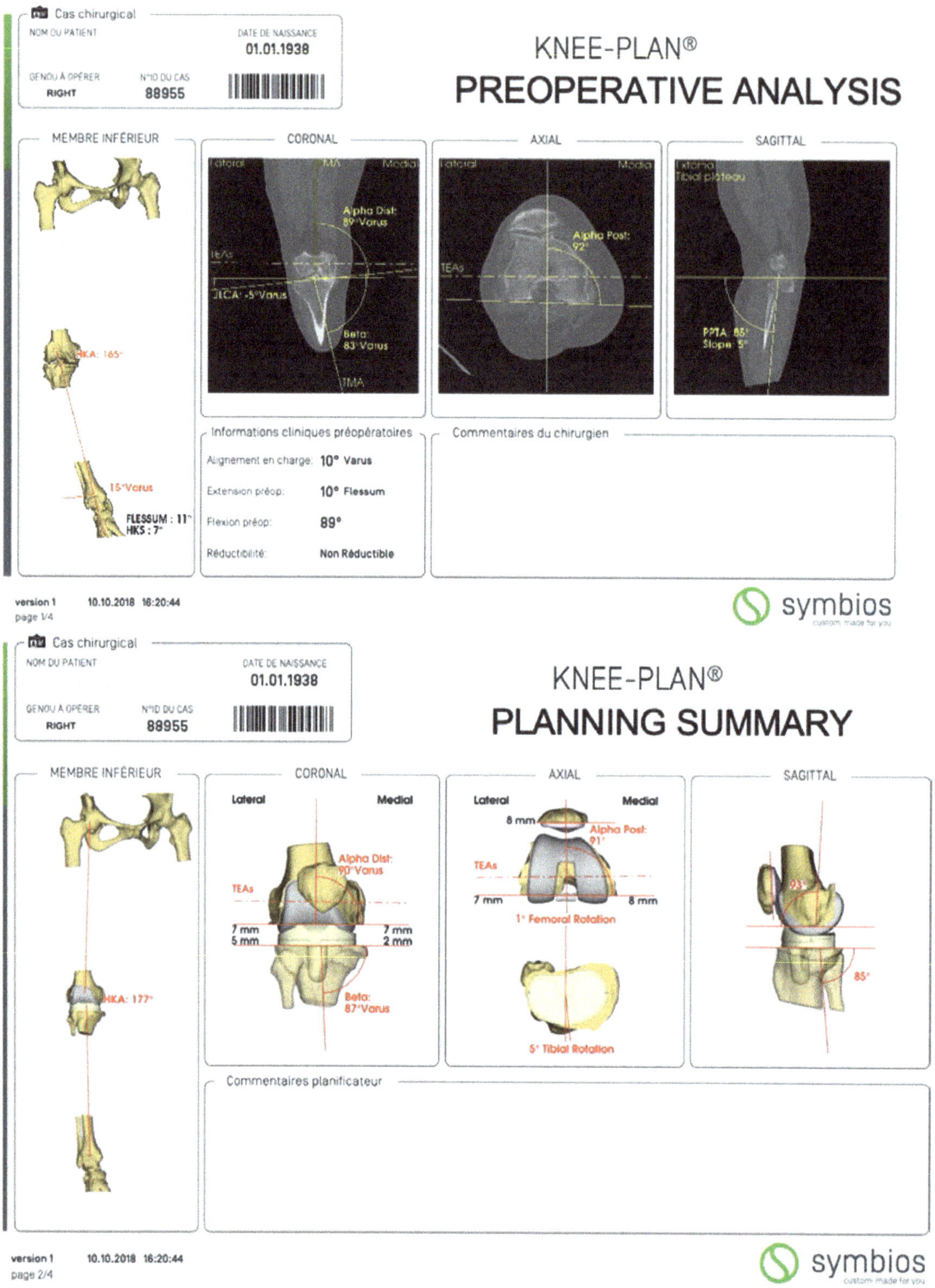

Fig. 22.1 Knee-plan pre-operative analysis

1. Semi-automated 3D reconstruction and segmentation of the distal femur, proximal tibia and patella.
2. Planning is done with Knee-Plan® software. From raw images, the alignment and bone wear are analysed, and the native (pre-arthritic) alignment is deduced. The realignment strategy is then established, including the level and orientations of the bone cuts. The aim is to reproduce the native alignment called the Origin Alignment©, in a range of ±3° from 180°, with a reproduction of the joint line obliquity in a range of ±5°, in accordance with the restricted kinematic alignment protocol from Vendittoli (Chap. 17).
3. The design of the definitive implants, trial implants and custom instruments is then finalized, using SolidWorks® software (Dassault Systèmes, Vélizy-Villacoublay, France).
4. Operative planning and the implant design are then validated online by the surgeon.
5. Manufacturing of the definitive implants is then finalized, using 'pre-shapes', previously manufactured with classic chromium–cobalt casting technology for the femur and titanium (Ta6V) for the tibial baseplate. From a wide range of 'pre-shapes', the next largest sized pre-form is chosen, and final customization is done using automated quick milling technology to reproduce the shape of the native pre-arthritic bone.
6. The custom guides are made with additive manufacturing technology using polyamide (PA2200).
7. Implants and instruments are then assembled into a single box and sent directly to the hospital.

22.5 Which Alignment Strategy?

1. The Origin® alignment aims to reproduce both native (pre-arthritic) alignment and joint line obliquity, based on the preoperative CT scan with 3D reconstruction of the hip, knee and ankle. Bone wear and arthritic deformity are assessed and corrected during 3D reconstruction. The mLDFA is recreated by reconstruction of the native femoral surface. The mMPTA is measured and recreated by a combination of bone cut adjustment (up to 3°) and an asymmetric polyethylene inlay (up to 2°), similar to the restricted kinematic alignment protocol from Vendittoli (Chap. 17).

The *native alignment*, also known as *constitutional alignment*, is determined from a combination of (1) the knee morphology obtained from a CT scan; (2) clinical data, notably the reducibility of the axis deviation and (3) the weight-bearing axis from a whole-leg standing radiograph. This Origin Alignment© does not seek to change the axis to 180°, but to restore the native alignment.

At this stage, there are certain limitations in the reconstruction of both native alignment and joint line obliquity. While it has been demonstrated that restoration of the native JLO in patients with constitutional varus decreases peak knee adduction [21], the Origin Alignment© remains within safe limits in terms of tribology, fixation with a JLO range of ±5° and a postoperative alignment—range of ±3°. Allowing for these limitations, approximately 75% of knee OA patients are suitable for Origin Alignment© [22]. The other cases are managed individually according to the surgeon's preference.

22.6 Surgical Technique

All instruments are single-use custom tools and fit in a single box weighing 3 kg.

22.6.1 Femoral Preparation

In this technique, the femoral preparation is done first (Fig. 22.2), because the femur is the driver of the knee kinematics. The first surgical step is to remove the remnants of cartilage, using electrocautery, a curette or a scalpel blade, in the areas of contact of the cutting block. The first femoral jig is secured to the bone with pins as soon

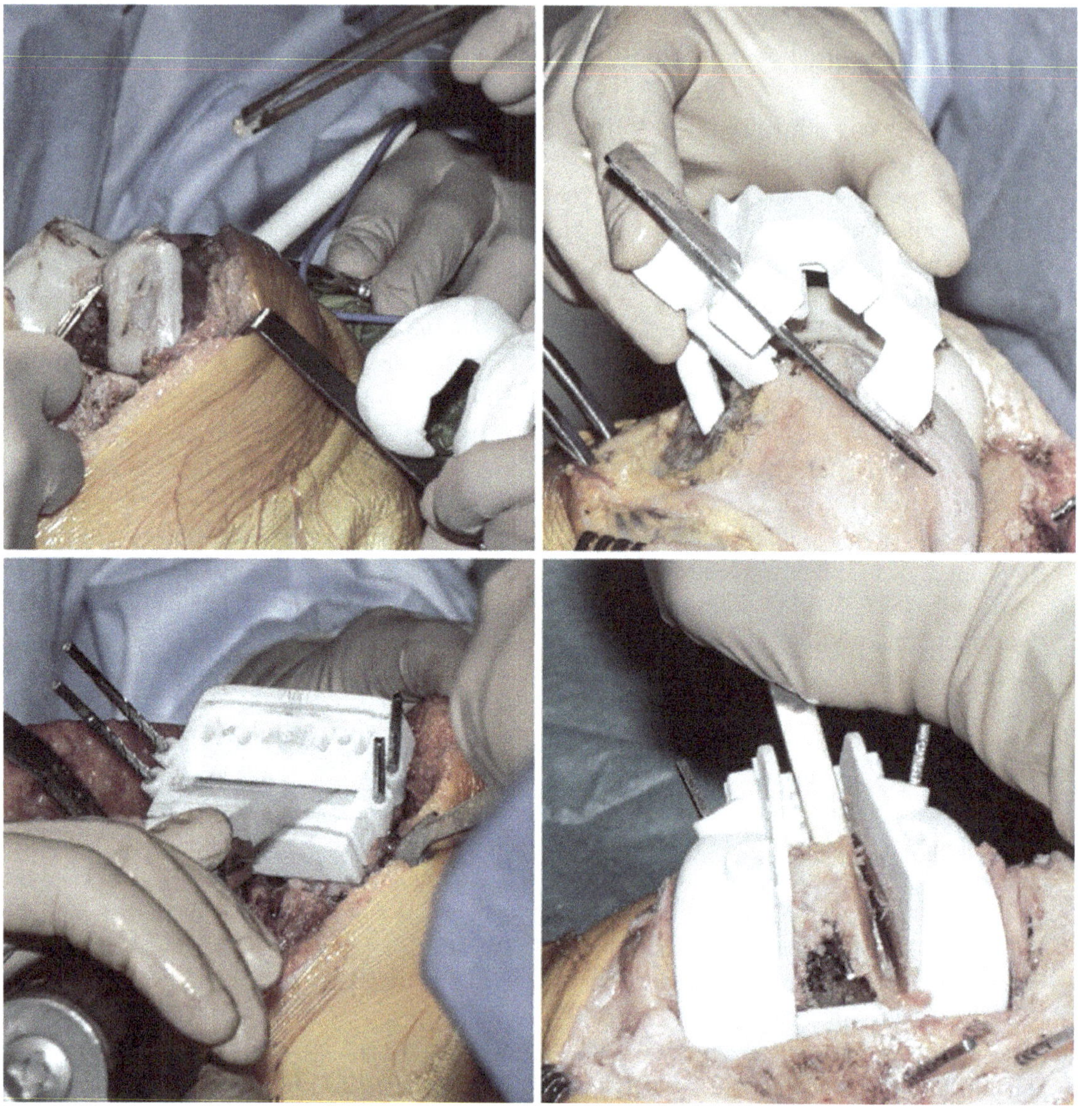

Fig. 22.2 Different steps of the femoral preparation

as a unique and stable position has been found for it, and cuts are performed with an oscillating saw. No femoral recuts are needed as the aim of the procedure is to reproduce precisely the shape of the distal condyles. The 'four in one' femoral cutting guide (second femoral jig) is positioned on the distal resected femur without any adjustment in size or rotation. The concept of femoral rotation has here no meaning because the femoral implant reproduces the shape of the distal femur and the thickness of the polyethylene reproduces the native joint line obliquity. Resection of the intercondylar femoral notch is guided by the third femoral jig. The medio-lateral contour of the bloc—specific to the patient—matches the bony contours of the femur.

The trial femoral component is positioned on the distal femur, and flexion/extension motion and valgus/varus stressing are done to assess the amount of bone wear and the level of the tibia cut.

22.6.2 Tibial Preparation

After removal of the cartilage remnants and osteophytes, the tibial jig is positioned on the

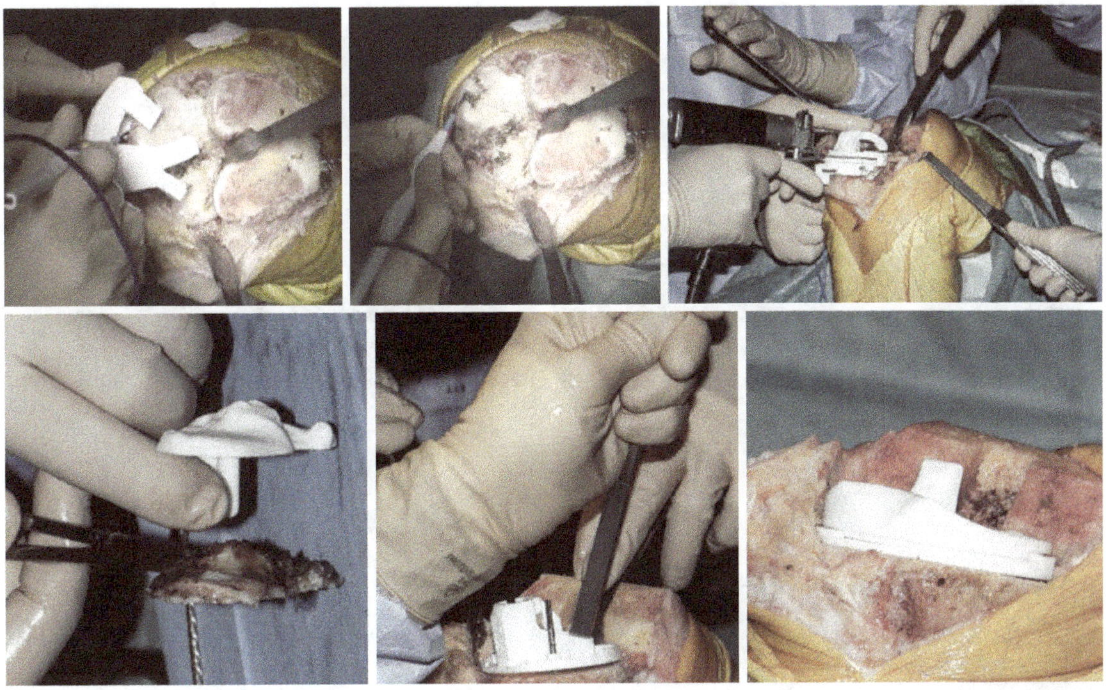

Fig. 22.3 Different steps of the tibial preparation

plateaus and secured with pins once the position is stable (Fig. 22.3). To meet the planned cut's orientation, the extramedullary alignment control rod must be centred medio-laterally to the centre of the ankle joint.

The resection provided by the tibial guide is a pre-cut of −2 mm (minus 2 mm) with respect to the planning. In most cases, a +2 mm recut must be done as a second step (corresponding to the planned resection), after checking the stability with the 'Bone Balancer' (trial femoral implants with a floating tibial component). This recut is guided by the 're-cutting guide'. In some knees with laxity, if the ligament balancing is correct after the first tibial cut (pre-cut), the additional +2 mm recut can be skipped. Conversely, in some stiff knees, an additional re-cut (+4 mm from the first cut) may be necessary, using the same 're-cutting guide'.

After obtaining a good range of motion, with a balanced knee, controlled with the 'Bone Balancer' (medio-lateral stability with a slight residual varus–valgus laxity), the definitive tibial preparation is performed. The custom tibial baseplate (keel position and contouring are patient specific) is then fixed on the resected tibia surface, and the central peg and fins are prepared.

22.6.3 Final Implantation

The trochlea of the Origin® prosthesis is designed to match the shape of the native patella (anatomic trochlea), so patellar resurfacing is not required, but is recommended in cases of severe patellar osteoarthritis.

Once all bone surfaces have been prepared, the implants are cemented, firstly with the tibia and lastly with the femoral component (Fig. 22.4). Standard closure and dressing are then performed.

22.6.4 Postoperative Care

Physiotherapy begins a few hours after surgery, with immediate full weight bearing, using crutches only for safety and without any flexion or extension restrictions. Rehabilitation is based mostly on self-rehabilitation performed under the supervision of a physiotherapist,

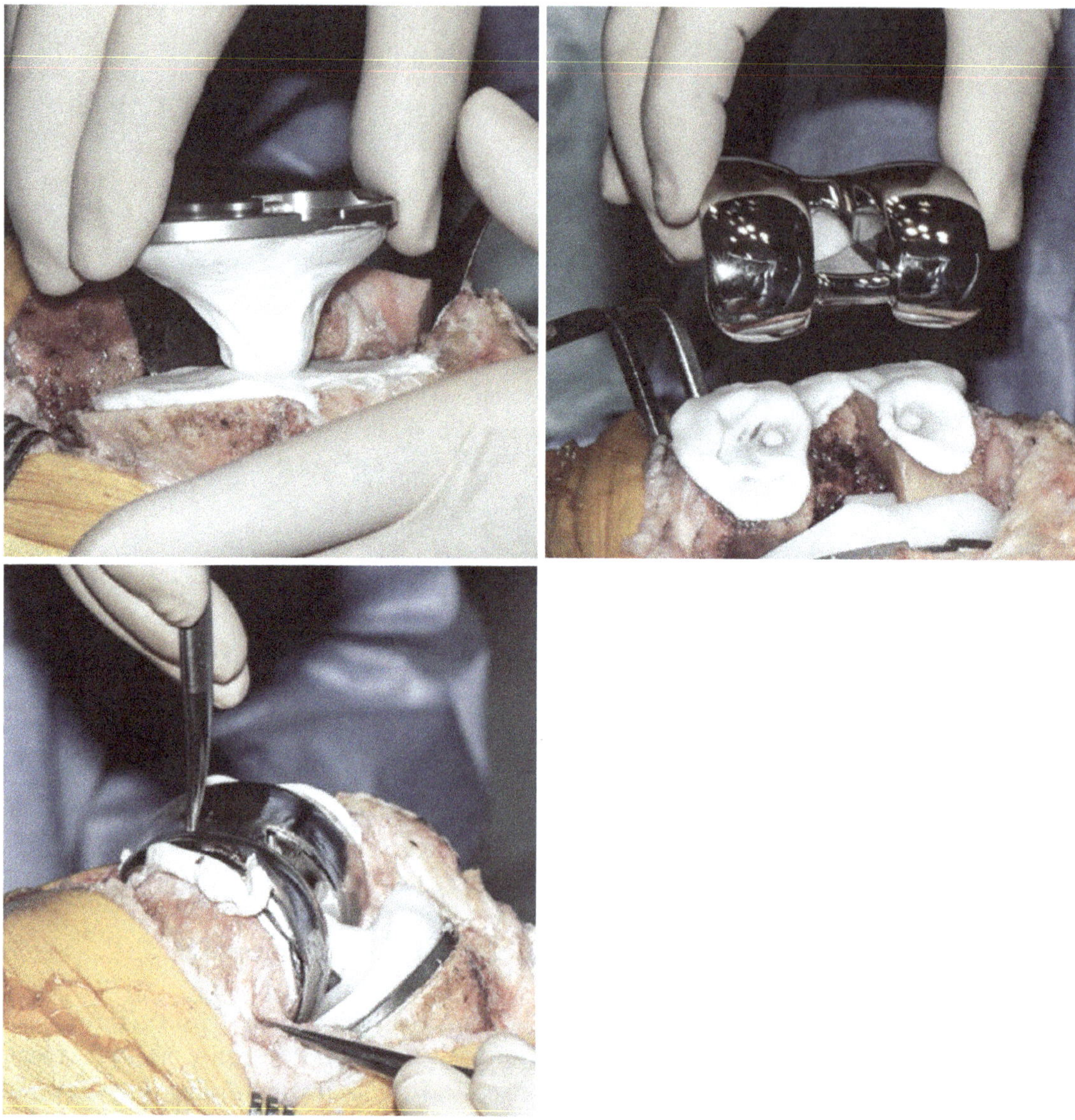

Fig. 22.4 Final cemented implantation

avoiding any active muscle strengthening earlier than 4 months postoperative.

22.7 What Are the Potential Benefits of Custom TKA?

22.7.1 Patient Benefits

This technology is based on the theory that many unsatisfactory outcomes and/or residual pain after TKA can be attributed to a lack of anatomic restoration, hardly identifiable by medical examination. Residual pain, stiffness and laxity are often secondary effects of incorrect sizing [11, 12] or malrotation [14]. Furthermore, asymmetric resections due to alignment strategy and the non-anatomic shape of the implants cause 'iatrogenic' laxities or stiffness. We therefore believe that an optimal restoration of the native anatomy—including limb alignment—may help improve functional outcomes in TKA. Also, customization of the bone cuts and implants allows engineers to minimize, as much as possible, the thickness and weight of the implants and the number of bone resections needed.

It is worth noting that custom cutting guides or navigation systems, generally used in standard implants, failed to demonstrate clear benefits in terms of outcomes and patient satisfaction. Similarly, robotic surgery might be more reliable and precise in the future, but will not solve the major difficulties due to the non-anatomic design of the implant itself. We strongly believe that TKA needs improvements to its three main pillars: (1) definition of a personalized alignment strategy; (2) improvement of surgical precision with new technology, such as robotics and (3) restoring the native knee anatomy using custom implants.

22.7.2 Benefits for the Surgeon

Customized TKA offers many advantages to the surgeon. Firstly, the surgical process is easier, because conservation or restoration of the native anatomy automatically addresses many surgical difficulties: (1) femoral and tibial rotations are adjusted during the design stage, and adjustments to component positioning are required; (2) balancing is easier, particularly at mid-flexion, due to the conservation of the condylar curvature radii and the JLO; (3) no size adjustments are needed as the bone implant fit is optimized. Secondly, planning is defined preoperatively in terms of alignment and implant positioning, which safeguards the surgeon. Thirdly, this technology may help in certain difficult cases such as (1) patients with post-traumatic extra-articular deformities where correction of the deformity is easier; (2) patients with inextractible hardware close to the joint surface, where the instruments and the implant are designed to avoid impingement; (3) patients with multioperated or previously infected bones, because no bone catheterism is required; and (4) patients with extreme anatomy, where implantation of standard TKA may be challenging.

22.7.3 Hospital Benefits

This technology is valuable for the hospital management, simplifying the process in the theatre, with a single box including the implants and instruments, all tailored for the patient. It eliminates the need for large inventories of implants and instrumentation trays. Finally, this technology dramatically decreases the need for sterilization, with a major economic impact (cost) and also ecological consequences (water used for sterilization).

References

1. Campbell W. Interposition of vitallium plates in arthroplasties of the knee. Am J Surg. 1940;47(3):639–41.
2. Smith-Petersen MN. Evolution of mould arthroplasty of the hip joint. J Bone Joint Surg Br. 1948;30B(1):59–75.
3. Jones WN. Mold arthroplasty of the knee joint. Clin Orthop Relat Res. 1969;66:82–9.
4. Insall JN, Hood RW, Flawn LB, Sullivan DJ. The total condylar knee prosthesis in gonarthrosis. A five to nine-year follow-up of the first one hundred consecutive replacements. J Bone Joint Surg Am. 1983;65(5):619–28.
5. Hitt K, Shurman JR 2nd, Greene K, McCarthy J, Moskal J, Hoeman T, Mont MA. Anthropometric measurements of the human knee: correlation to the sizing of current knee arthroplasty systems. J Bone Joint Surg Am. 2003;85-A(Suppl 4):115–22.
6. Bonnin MP, Saffarini M, Bossard N, Dantony E, Victor J. Morphometric analysis of the distal femur in total knee arthroplasty and native knees. Bone Joint J. 2016;98-B(1):49–57.
7. Howell SM, Howell SJ, Hull ML. Assessment of the radii of the medial and lateral femoral condyles in varus and valgus knees with osteoarthritis. J Bone Joint Surg Am. 2010;92(1):98–104.
8. Bellemans J, Colyn W, Vandenneucker H, Victor J. The Chitranjan Ranawat award: is neutral mechanical alignment normal for all patients? The concept of constitutional varus. Clin Orthop Relat Res. 2012;470(1):45–53.
9. Bonnin MP, Saffarini M, Mercier PE, Laurent JR, Carrillon Y. Is the anterior tibial tuberosity a reliable rotational landmark for the tibial component in total knee arthroplasty? J Arthroplasty. 2011;26(2):260.e1–7.e2.
10. Bonnin MP, Saffarini M, Shepherd D, Bossard N, Dantony E. Oversizing the tibial component in TKAs: incidence, consequences and risk factors. Knee Surg Sports Traumatol Arthrosc. 2016;24(8):2532–40.
11. Bonnin MP, Schmidt A, Basiglini L, Bossard N, Dantony E. Mediolateral oversizing influences pain, function, and flexion after TKA. Knee Surg Sports Traumatol Arthrosc. 2013;21(10):2314–24.
12. Mahoney OM, Kinsey T. Overhang of the femoral component in total knee arthroplasty: risk factors

and clinical consequences. J Bone Joint Surg Am. 2010;92(5):1115–21.
13. Insall J. Total knee replacement. In: Surgery of the knee. New York: Churchill Livingstone; 1984. p. 587–695.
14. Berger RA, Crossett LS, Jacobs JJ, Rubash HE. Malrotation causing patellofemoral complications after total knee arthroplasty. Clin Orthop Relat Res. 1998;356:144–53.
15. Howell SM, Howell SJ, Kuznik KT, Cohen J, Hull ML. Does a kinematically aligned total knee arthroplasty restore function without failure regardless of alignment category? Clin Orthop Relat Res. 2013;471(3):1000–7.
16. Parratte S, Pagnano MW, Trousdale RT, Berry DJ. Effect of postoperative mechanical axis alignment on the fifteen-year survival of modern, cemented total knee replacements. J Bone Joint Surg Am. 2010;92(12):2143–9.
17. Bonnin M, Laurent JR, Parratte S, Zadegan F, Badet R, Bissery A. Can patients really do sport after TKA? Knee Surg Sports Traumatol Arthrosc. 2010;18(7):853–62.
18. Bonnin MP, Basiglini L, Archbold HA. What are the factors of residual pain after uncomplicated TKA? Knee Surg Sports Traumatol Arthrosc. 2011;19(9):1411–7.
19. Bourne RB, Chesworth BM, Davis AM, Mahomed NN, Charron KD. Patient satisfaction after total knee arthroplasty: who is satisfied and who is not? Clin Orthop Relat Res. 2010;468(1):57–63.
20. Noble PC, Conditt MA, Cook KF, Mathis KB. The John Insall award: patient expectations affect satisfaction with total knee arthroplasty. Clin Orthop Relat Res. 2006;452:35–43.
21. Niki Y, Nagura T, Nagai K, Kobayashi S, Harato K. Kinematically aligned total knee arthroplasty reduces knee adduction moment more than mechanically aligned total knee arthroplasty. Knee Surg Sports Traumatol Arthrosc. 2018;26(6):1629–35.
22. Almaawi AM, Hutt JRB, Masse V, Lavigne M, Vendittoli P-A. The impact of mechanical and restricted kinematic alignment on knee anatomy in total knee arthroplasty. J Arthroplast. 2017;32:2133–40.

23

History, Indications and Complications of Bicruciate TKA

James W. Pritchett

Key Points

Bicruciate knee replacement is an attractive concept because it preserves rather than removes the anterior cruciate ligament and the tibial eminence. Bicruciate knee replacement is not a new procedure, but there are new bicruciate knee implant designs available. There are five key points to consider before deciding to perform a bicruciate total knee replacement:

- Preservation of both the cruciate ligaments during total knee replacement is challenging but results in excellent function and long-term survivorship.
- A total knee replacement with both cruciate ligaments intact results in more normal kinematic and clinical function compared to knee replacements with one or both ligaments resected.
- A bicruciate knee replacement requires less bone and soft tissue resection. A more normal transmission of the weight-bearing stresses is possible compared to other knee replacements.
- Preserving both cruciate ligaments mandates the correct tension on all ligaments. The joint line, knee alignment, and restoration of the surface contours are a complete match to the patient's normal (constitutional or pre-arthritic) knee.
- Paired bilateral studies have shown that patients prefer a bicruciate total knee replacement compared to other total knee replacements. Patients report more normal feel, fewer noise-related complaints, better strength and stability on stairs, and better performance in single-leg weight-bearing activities.

23.1 Introduction

Bicruciate knee replacement offers several functional benefits over other types of knee replacement. It results in a more natural feel with a greater sense of security during weight-bearing flexion, the replaced joint retains more normal biomechanical function, and the knee is stable and capable of an excellent range of motion.

Bicruciate knee replacement also offers several procedural benefits. It is more bone and soft tissue conserving, and it does not transfer weight-bearing stress into the center of the tibia through a medullary stem but loads the tibia in a more physiologic manner. The insertion technique is more demanding but less intrusive because there is no subluxation of the tibia forward on the femur during surgery.

Most surgeons prefer removing one or both cruciate ligaments, allowing the shape of the

J. W. Pritchett (✉)
Department of Orthopedic Surgery, University of Washington, Seattle, WA, USA

implants to drive the stability and motion of the knee. Also, subluxing the tibia forward is an easy and efficient way to visualize the tibia. However, with better techniques and instruments, resecting the cruciate ligaments is an unnecessary concession to convenience. Some surgeons argue that a useful anterior cruciate ligament (ACL) is not always present or that its kinematic function cannot be restored. For some patients, though, keeping their ACL is the only way to preserve their knee function. Younger and more active patients are presenting for knee replacement surgery. The ACL is intact in more than 60% of all patients presenting for total knee arthroplasty (TKA) regardless of age and stage of disease [1].

23.2 History of Bicruciate Knee Replacement

The first total condylar knee replacement was a bicruciate prosthesis. Dr. Charles O. Townley made drawings of a total knee prosthesis while a resident at Ford Hospital [2]. His design garnered an unenthusiastic reception from Sir John Charnley, a visiting professor in 1948, who claimed there would be too much metal implanted. Townley began using only the tibial component with retention of both cruciate ligaments in 1951 [2] (Fig. 23.1). Other knee implants of the 1950s and 1960s were either hinged or paired compartmental prostheses [3].

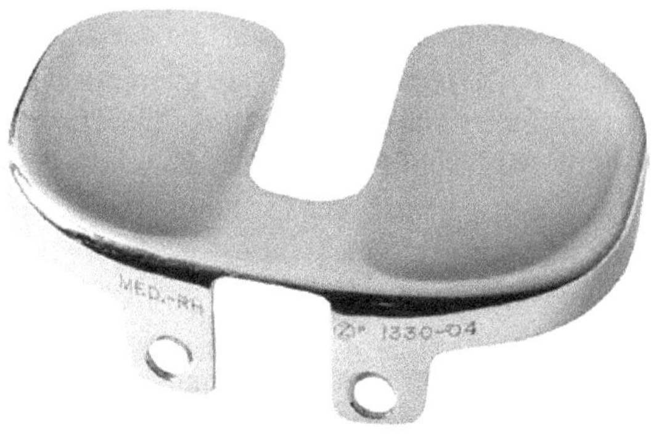

Fig. 23.1 This is a photograph of the Townley tibial articular plate used from 1951 to 1971

Seventy-five percent of Townley's articular plate patients had good clinical outcomes. In 1959, Townley added a McKeever patellar prosthesis and resurfaced the femoral condyles and trochlea with polyurethane foam (Ostamer) that had been used as a bone glue for fracture nonunions [4]. This was the first total condylar knee prosthesis (Fig. 23.2). It looked and functioned similarly to total condylar implants introduced in the 1970s [5].

Polyurethane is hydrophilic. The polyurethane Townley used ultimately softened and was absorbed and excreted through the kidneys. Polyurethane was withdrawn by the manufacturer after some reports of failures when used in fracture and arthrodesis [6]. However, none of the knee procedures failed clinically despite using a thermosetting acrylic. Bone has recuperative powers for chemical and thermal exposures. The knees functioned as a hemiarthroplasty after the polyurethane was absorbed. None required revision, and a few patients were followed for more than 30 years with functioning knees [2].

When polyethylene became available, Townley moved the metal component to the femur and used polyethylene for both the tibial and patellar components [7]. Cloutier and others later provided bicruciate knee prosthesis designs and generally with success [8]. Townley refined his bicruciate prosthesis and used it with success for the next 40 years.

23.3 Rationale for Bicruciate Knee Replacement

Normal knee function relies on smooth, uninterrupted motion that is provided by stable, well-lubricated, low-friction articular surfaces. Knee replacement involves compromises between stability and flexibility. For most surgeons, this includes removal of one or both cruciate ligaments [5]. As an alternative philosophy, a bicruciate knee replacement emphasizes minimal bone resection and limited constraint with the goal of allowing more natural movement of

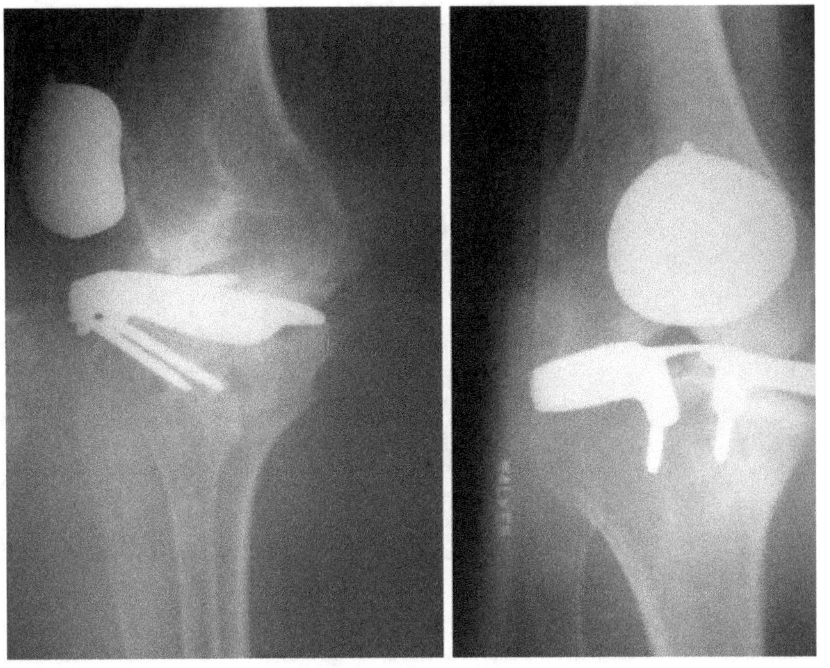

Fig. 23.2 This radiograph was taken 33 years following placement of a Townley tibial plate and McKeever patellar prosthesis. The polyurethane used to resurface the femur wore away, but the clinical function remained good

the knee compared to other prostheses [9–11]. A well-performed bicruciate total knee replacement more closely approximates the function of a normal knee. Resection of the cruciate ligaments is an unnecessary concession to custom and habit.

23.4 General Indications for Bicruciate Knee Replacement

Total knee replacement using any of the contemporary knee prostheses can be expected to improve function, reduce pain, and provide satisfactory implant survivorship. Most studies report that 20% of patients have reservations about the quality of their result even in the absence of complications.

Bicruciate total knee replacement is a demanding procedure. Precise surgical technique is necessary, as well as skill, familiarity with the technique, and the ability to work well in a confined surgical space. Bicruciate knee replacement anticipates that the ACL is functionally intact, although some ACL fibers are inevitably lost to disease. Stability as shown by the anterior drawer and Lachman maneuvers is sufficient evidence that the ACL is competent. Varus, valgus, and flexion contractures up to 15° can be accepted (Fig. 23.3). Age is not a barrier to bicruciate total knee replacement.

23.5 What Are the Best Indications?

Patients who benefit the most from bicruciate knee replacement appreciate the stability during their activities that require confidence in single-leg, weight-bearing flexion. Patients who have had their ACL reconstructed are particularly motivated to retain their ACL and understand its value (Fig. 23.3). A few patients are so committed to bicruciate replacement that they will undergo ACL reconstruction before their knee replacement.

Patients with vascular insufficiency are also motivated to undergo bicruciate knee replacement to avoid added tension on vascular structures that

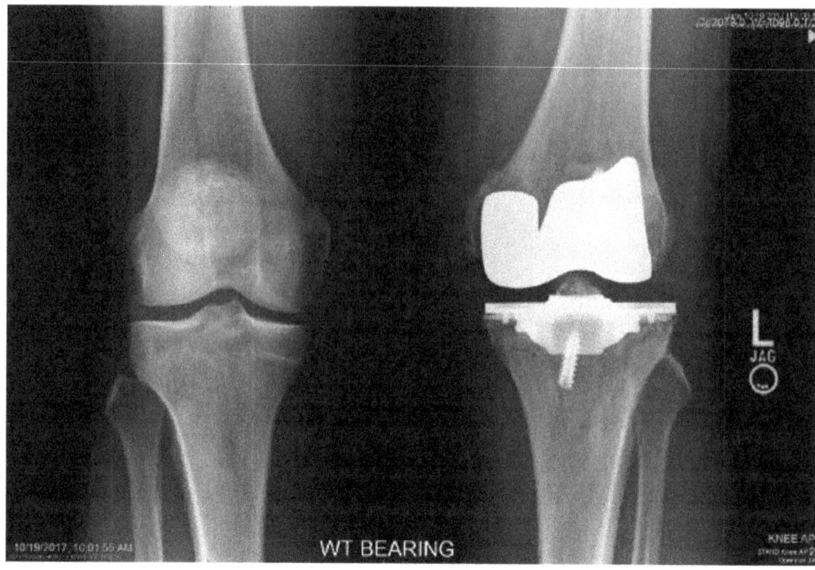

Fig. 23.3 This is a currently available bicruciate total knee prosthesis placed for severe arthritis in a patient with a prior ACL reconstruction

can result from forward subluxation of the knee. Since this is not part of a bicruciate procedure, there is a lower risk of vascular injury. Patients with a blocked medullary space of the tibia can also benefit from a bicruciate replacement since there is no medullary stem. Thus, additional procedures to remove prior fixation implants in the tibia can be avoided.

23.6 What Are the Specific Complications?

Unique complications related to bicruciate knee replacement are fracture of the tibial eminence and rupture of the ACL. Usually, these occur intraoperatively as the knee is brought from flexion into extension. If these complications occur, options are to convert to another type of prosthetic replacement or to repair/reconstruct the ACL or eminence. Screws can be used to secure an eminence fracture. A graft can be used to repair an ACL rupture, but this adds complexity to the TKA. Most commonly, if there is an ACL rupture, conversion to a medial congruent implant is recommended.

Fracture of the tibial baseplate and sometimes the polyethylene occurred in some of the older implants. The fracture has been detected on routine follow-up radiographs. It may or may not require revision based on how well the patient's knee is performing. This complication no longer occurs with forged cobalt–chromium tibial trays.

Loosening of the tibial tray occurred with one recent bicruciate prosthesis, but it was attributed to flaws in the implant design and implantation technique. This implant is no longer in common use [12].

Scar around the ACL resulting in limited motion can occur due to tensioning degenerative ACL fibers during implantation. The tension in these cases is from insufficient tibial or femoral resection or thicker than necessary tibial polyethylenes (i.e., overstuffing). A bicruciate knee should not be placed with the same ligamentous tension that might be acceptable with other designs. The intact ACL will provide all necessary stability. Restoration of motion is achieved by recessing the ACL.

23.7 Alignment Technique

Alignment is critical. Although it looks reasonable to preserve knee anatomy with the kinematic alignment, my personal experience was using an adjusted mechanical alignment technique in which I usually plan 2°–3° of varus with respect to the mechanical axis of the knee. Most commonly, the tibia is prepared with 6° posterior slope. Extramedullary guides for the tibia are preferred, as the medullary canal of the tibia is not opened in a bicruciate replacement. The medial and lateral tibial plateaus are prepared with separate sagittal and transverse cuts. Conventional instruments typically have been used; but, more recently, robotic techniques have been developed. The instruments do not need to be complex, but a careful stepwise technique is required.

23.8 Stepwise Surgical Technique

Close approximation of the anatomical contours and preservation of the strategic ligaments during implantation are the secrets of success in knee replacement. Bicruciate knee replacement requires a masterful understanding of the patient's knee. Its creativity is from mastering the simplicity of the concept. Ligamentous balancing is performed, but neither cruciate ligament is resected or recessed. Initially, alignment and balance in extension are achieved by correcting the coronal deformity with appropriate capsular and collateral ligament releases.

The femur is prepared first. A spacer is used to assure that a sufficient distal femoral cut has been made. The femoral component is an unconstrained design, and the shape of the condyles simulates a normal knee. The femur is placed in 3° of external rotation. Great care is used to place the anterior flange flush to the trochlea. The femoral component is placed directly on the posterior femoral condyle making sure any remaining cartilage or osteophytes are removed. Throughout the tibial preparation, the tibial eminence is protected by pins using a guide to assure there is no undercutting. The tibial spines and insertions of the cruciate ligaments are left in continuity with the rest of the tibia. The tibial component is placed in slight external rotation following the orientation of the ACL fibers. A spacer block is used again to assure an adequate resection of the tibia, with the goal of using the thinnest tibial inserts of 8 mm. If there are insufficient distal femoral or proximal tibial cuts or inadequate ligament balancing, the tibial eminence can fracture, and/or the ACL can rupture as the knee is moved from flexion into extension.

It is important to have the correct ligament tension at the conclusion of the procedure. The knee should have a smooth, uninterrupted, full range of motion at the end of the procedure. There should be no need to stretch out any remaining contractures.

Preparation for the keel of the tibial prosthesis is made anteriorly. The tibial implant is placed first followed by the femoral component. The patella is prepared to receive a dome-shaped prosthesis. Patellar tracking is verified. Since the joint line has not been elevated and the knee is well balanced, lateral retinacular release is not necessary.

23.9 Clinical Evidence Supporting Bicruciate Total Knee Replacement

Bicruciate total knee replacement has been performed since 1971. There have been improvements in the quality of the polyethylene, the metallurgy of the tibial tray, and instrumentation. Townley first reported the results of 80 bicruciate TKAs in 1973 with good or excellent results in 84% at 2 years [7]. In 1985, he reported on 532 procedures, and 89% had good or excellent outcomes at 1.5–11 years [13]. Tibial loosening occurred in 2%. In 1988, Townley presented his results as his Presidential Address to the American Knee Society [14]. He also introduced porous-coated fixation. The implant survivorship at 16 years post-TKA in 1700 patients was 92%, and 90% of his patients had good or excellent outcomes [2, 7, 13].

The Hermes AC total knee replacement was designed by Cloutier in 1977 [8]. At 22 years of follow-up, the survival rate was 82%, 12% were revised for polyethylene wear, and 4.3% were revised for aseptic loosening. Overall, 87% of patients had good or excellent results. The mean AP laxity was 1 mm [8]. Buechel and Pappas [15] reported that 91% of meniscal-bearing TKAs with bicruciate preservation survived 20 years.

The author [15] conducted a competing-risks survivorship analysis of 537 TKA procedures at 23 years follow-up and found that survivorship was 94%; 5.6% were revised, most commonly because of polyethylene wear. Late ACL ruptures occurred in two patients. The mean AP laxity at 23 years post-TKA was 2 mm with two revisions for instability.

23.9.1 Patient Satisfaction

Implant survivorship is not a synonym for satisfaction. The generally accepted patient-reported outcome measures may not be accurate. Therefore, for the 23-year review mentioned previously [16], I asked five questions (Table 23.1). In response, 96% of patients had their pain relief expectations met, 95% of patients returned to their regular activities, 69% had their expectations about sports participation met, 90% were overall satisfied, and 75% would recommend the surgery to another individual [16].

23.9.2 Patient Preference

Determining a patient's preference is an alternative method to traditional patient-reported outcomes. It offers another way to understand the relative importance of attributes from the patient's point of view. Patient preference studies are concerned with measuring patient values. Patient preferences come directly from the patient without interpretation. Patient preferences are the best way to determine benefit when no option is clearly superior to another and when patients' views vary considerably or are different from the views of the healthcare providers. It is a very powerful tool in assessing outcomes of knee replacement surgery because surgeons have strong preferences about both technique and implants. Surgeons' preferences may not reflect their patients' values.

Comparing patients and procedures is difficult regardless of how carefully the study is designed and executed. Twins, but not clones, have been studied to determine similarities and differences for some medical conditions. In bilateral knee replacement studies, patients serve as their own controls, thus eliminating the effects of personality, age, gender, diagnosis, bone quality, and activity level. If the same surgeon using the same technique, indications, and treatment methods performs the care, then a high level of confidence in the data is warranted [17–19].

The author performed a patient preference study starting in 1987 [19]. There were 640

Table 23.1 Results of patient satisfaction questionnaire [16]

Questions	Met completely (%)	Met (%)	Neutral (%)	Probably not (%)	Not met (%)
1. Were your expectations regarding pain relief met?	78	18	1	1	2
2. Were your expectations regarding return to regular activity met?	53	43	2	1	1
3. Were your expectations regarding return to sports and recreational activity met?	49	20	15	8	8
4. Were you satisfied with your knee replacement?	71	19	8	1	1
5. Would you recommend this surgery to a friend?	75	21	2	1	1

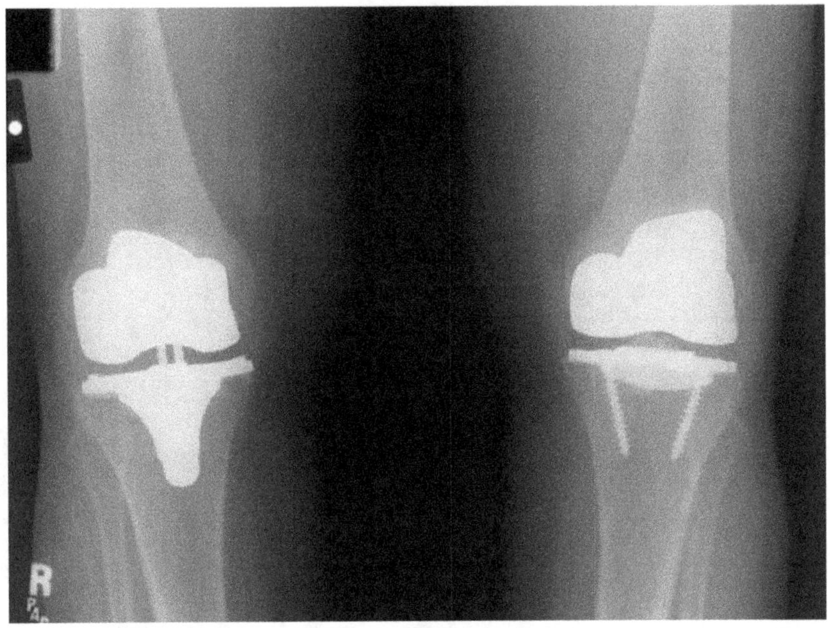

Fig. 23.4 This is a patient with a bicruciate total knee replacement on one side and a contralateral posterior stabilized prosthesis

patients (1280 knees) enrolled prospectively to evaluate patient preferences in total knee prostheses. Staged bilateral TKA was performed using a different randomly selected prosthesis on each knee (Fig. 23.4). Five different prostheses were used: bicruciate (ACL-PCL), medial pivot (MP), posterior stabilized (PS), posterior cruciate retaining (PCL), and mobile bearing (MB). Each procedure was performed using the same technique with only slight variation as needed to accommodate the different implants. Fair and poor results were excluded to provide a valid comparison, and a minimum of 4 years of follow-up was required. There were 551 patients (1102 knees) who met the inclusion criteria [17–19]. The noise patients experienced after their knee replacement was also evaluated [19]. Using a temperature probe, the temperature of the synovial fluid was measured in 50 patients to assess the amount of heat generated by the implant [20].

Range of motion, pain relief, alignment, and stability did not vary by prosthesis type. The bicruciate prosthesis generated the least amount of heat and least noise. The PS knee had the most noise, generated the second highest amount of heat, and was the least preferred knee. The MP was equal to the ACL–PCL as most preferred and had the second fewest noise concerns. Patients gave the following reasons for their knee preference: feels more normal; stronger on stairs; superior single-leg weight bearing; flexion stability; fewer clunks, pops, and clicks; and don't know. Overall, 89% of patients preferred the ACL–PCL knee over the PS, 76% preferred the MP to the PS and PCL, and 61% preferred MP to the MB [17–19, 21].

23.10 Bicruciate Implant Design Features

Successful bicruciate total knee replacement is most dependent on the correct design of the tibial component. The thinnest possible component is desirable, and strength is important, as early tibial implant designs were known to fracture. A supportive keel is placed on the undersurface of the tibial component. Fixation pegs or holes for screws are necessary for firm fixation of the tibia. The reduced contact area of the bicruciate tibial

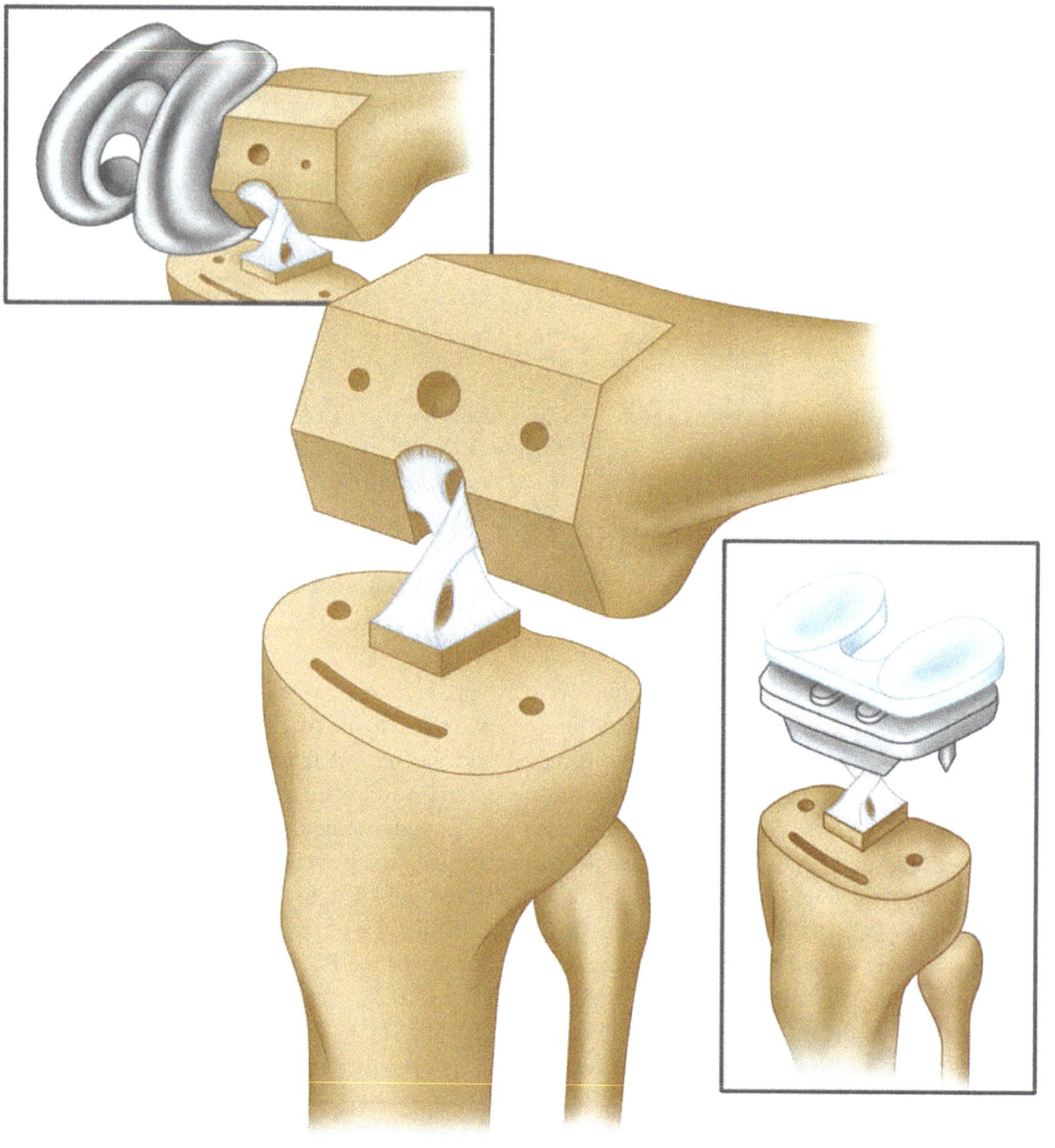

Fig. 23.5 This is a drawing of a Townley bicruciate total knee prosthesis

component to the proximal tibia compared to other total knee designs mandates precise insertion technique. Both cemented and cementless fixations have been used with equal results.

An all-polyethylene tibial implant was used in the 1970s. Metal backing was added to allow for modularity. Wear of conventional polyethylene was a concern, and it was the most common failure mode. Improvements in polyethylene and polyethylene sterilization methods have greatly reduced wear. The shape of the tibial polyethylene component is very important. Flat-shaped tibial polyethylenes were used for many years, but the femoral rollback in the lateral component was insufficient, leading to less flexion than is now desired (Fig. 23.5). A posterior bevel for the lateral tibial polyethylene insert allows much improved rollback and greater knee flexion [22]. There is a slight concavity to the medial tibial insert. The medial and lateral inserts may be 1 or 2 mm different in thickness. The tibial tray is anatomically rather than symmetrically shaped.

The bicruciate femoral component is subtlety distinct from most other posterior cruciate-retaining total knee designs. The radius of curvature of the medial femoral condyle is slightly larger than the lateral. The trochlear groove is anatomically shaped rather than deepened. Right and left femoral components are necessary. The femoral component is available in both cobalt–chromium and oxidized zirconium, and fully ceramic models are being investigated (Fig. 23.3) [23].

Predicate bicruciate knee replacements suffered from design flaws. The BP, Geomedic, and Cloutier were used in the 1970s and 1980s [3, 8, 15]. The femur was multiradius with a nonanatomic trochlea. The tibia was symmetric with symmetric polyethylene inserts. The implants were placed with mechanical alignment which made the ACL and PCL difficult to balance. The future of bicruciate knee replacement may include patient-specific implants, kinematic alignment and precision bone preparation, and ligament balancing.

23.11 Why Do I Recommend Bicruciate Total Knee Replacement?

I recommend bicruciate total knee replacement to patients with intact cruciate ligaments who need the highest functional outcomes. Bicruciate TKA is a demanding procedure to perform; however, it is possible to master the procedure. It is as reproducible as other methods once experience is gained. Not subluxing the knee reduces trauma. It is a benefit not to elevate the joint line and to leave the operating room with all four ligaments with the correct tension. It is also more reliable to depend on the knee's natural kinematic balance for knee stability rather on than the shape of metal and polyethylene.

Patients whose activities require a stable single-leg stance benefit from bicruciate total knee replacement. The recovery from surgery is rapid, and recovery is to a higher level of function. Tibiofemoral instability requiring revision virtually does not occur with bicruciate knee replacement. The patellofemoral joint tracking benefits as well. Patients report a more normal feeling knee; fewer complaints of noise such as clunking, popping, and clicking; better strength and stability on stairs; and better performance in single-leg weight-bearing activities. Most importantly, in paired bilateral studies, patients prefer bicruciate total knee replacement to their other implant choices. As with any TKA, proper patient selection is necessary to assure a successful clinical outcome and a satisfied patient.

Clinical Case

A 49-year-old professional golfer presented after experiencing several years of progressive knee pain. He had been treated with nonsteroidal anti-inflammatory drugs (NSAIDs), an unloader brace, and injections with steroids. He could no longer compete professionally in golf due to his knee pain.

His physical examination showed a flexion contracture with a range of motion of 10°–110°. The motion was stable. There was no forward subluxation of the tibia on the femur with either the anterior drawer or Lachman maneuvers. Radiographic examination showed bone-on-bone contact with a severe varus wear pattern (Fig. 23.6). The patient requested TKA. In golf, balance is critically important. Stability in single-knee weight-bearing flexion is necessary to properly execute a golf shot at the professional level.

The patient elected to undergo a bicruciate total knee replacement, which was performed without complication. The postoperative stability was complete, the range of motion improved to 0°–140°, and the patient was pain free. He returned to professional competition and won a tournament at the highest possible level at age 52. He continues to play golf at age 68. His knee implant remains in place and without any sign of wear or other complications (Fig. 23.6b).

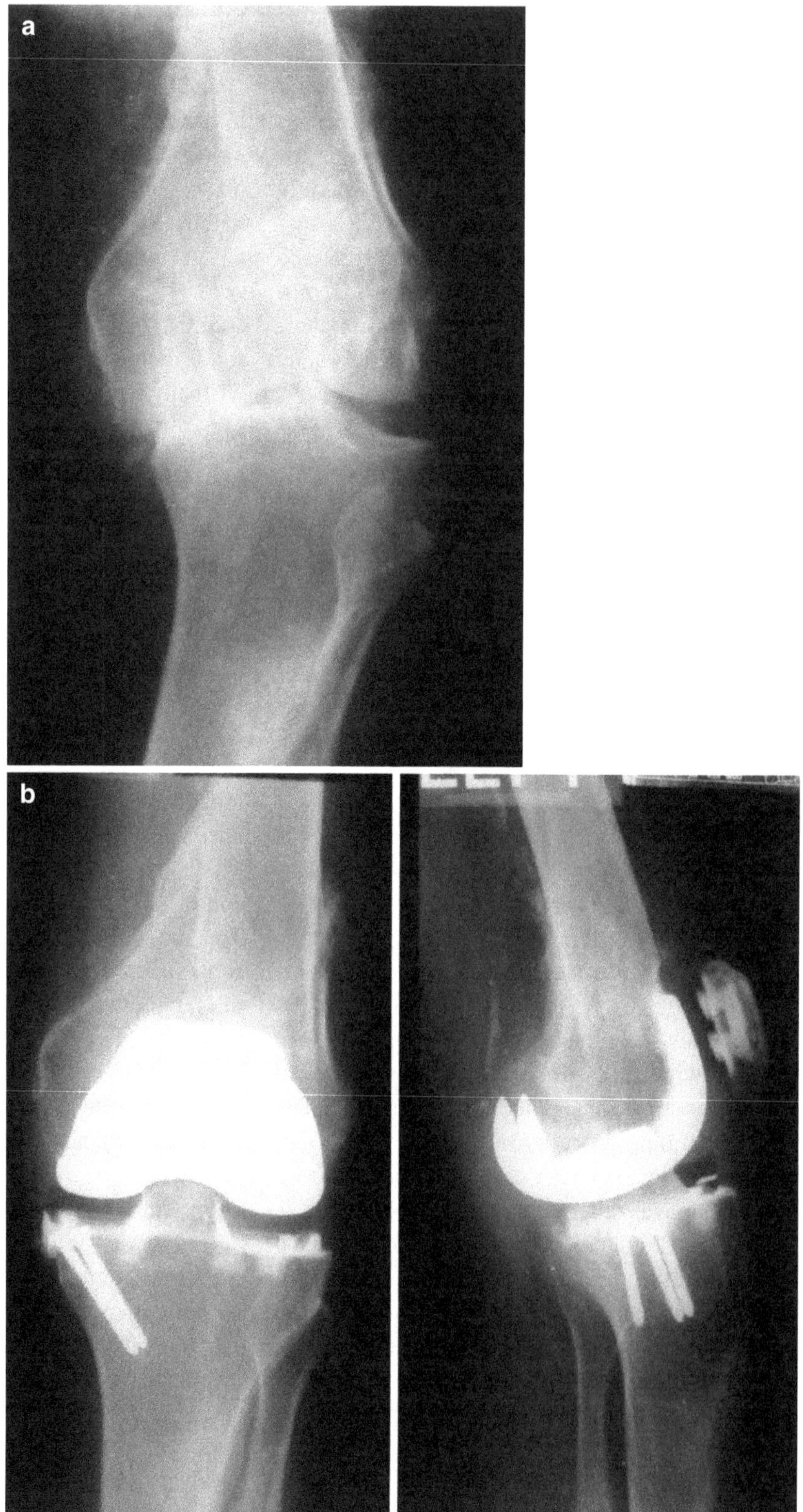

Fig. 23.6 (**a**) The 49-year-old golf professional was seen in 1976 for severe arthritis with a varus deformity. (**b**) The result of his Townley anatomic knee remained good 24 years later

References

1. Cushner FD, La Rosa DF, Vigorita VJ, Scuderi GR, Scott WN, Insall JN. A quantitative histologic comparison: ACL degeneration in the osteoarthritic knee. J Arthroplast. 2003;18:687–92.
2. Townley CO. Articular-plate replacement arthroplasty for the knee joint. 1964. Clin Orthop Relat Res. 1988;236:3–7.
3. Robinson RP. The early innovators of today's resurfacing condylar knees. J Arthroplast. 2005;20(1):2–26.
4. Pritchett JW. Total articular knee replacement using polyurethane. J Knee Surg. 2019;32(3):101–6.
5. Insall JN. Presidential address to the Knee Society. Choices and compromises in total knee arthroplasty. Clin Orthop Relat Res. 1988;226:43–8.
6. Redler I. Polymer osteosynthesis. A clinical trial of Ostamer in forty-two patients. J Bone Joint Surg Am. 1962;44:1621–52.
7. Townley CO. Knee joint arthroplasty: long-term results of the tibial articular replacement plate and its current use in an anatomic total knee arthroplasty. Clin Orthop Relat Res. 1973;94:311–2.
8. Sabouret P, Lavoie F, Cloutier JM. Total knee replacement with retention of both cruciate ligaments: a 22-year follow-up study. Bone Joint J. 2013;95-B:917–22.
9. Fuchs S, Tibescu CO, Genkinger M, Laass H, Rosenbaum D. Proprioception with bicondylar sledge design prostheses retaining cruciate ligaments. Clin Orthop Relat Res. 2003;406:148–54.
10. Komistek RD, Allain J, Anderson DT, Dennis DA, Goutallier D. In vivo kinematics for subjects with and without an anterior cruciate ligament. Clin Orthop Relat Res. 2002;404:315–25.
11. Stiehl JB, Komistek RD, Cloutier JM, Dennis DA. The cruciate ligaments in total knee arthroplasty: a kinematic analysis of 2 total knee arthroplasties. J Arthroplast. 2000;15:545–50.
12. Christensen JC, Brothers J, Stoddard GJ, et al. Higher frequency of reoperation with a new bicruciate-retaining total knee arthroplasty. Clin Orthop Relat Res. 2017;475:62–9.
13. Townley CO. The anatomic total knee resurfacing arthroplasty. Clin Orthop Relat Res. 1985;192:82–96.
14. Townley CO. Total knee arthroplasty. A personal retrospective and prospective review. Clin Orthop Relat Res. 1988;236:8–22.
15. Buechel FF, Pappas MJ. Long-term survivorship analysis of cruciate-sparing versus cruciate-sacrificing knee prostheses using meniscal bearings. Clin Orthop Relat Res. 1990;260:162–9.
16. Pritchett JW. Bicruciate-retaining total knee replacement provides satisfactory function and implant survivorship at 23 years. Clin Orthop Relat Res. 2015;473:2327–33.
17. Pritchett JW. Anterior cruciate-retaining total knee arthroplasty. J Arthroplast. 1996;11:194–7.
18. Pritchett JW. Patient preferences in knee prostheses. J Bone Joint Surg Br. 2004;86:979–82.
19. Pritchett JW. Patients prefer a bicruciate-retaining or the medial pivot total knee prosthesis. J Arthroplast. 2011;26:224–8.
20. Pritchett JW. Heat generated by knee prostheses. Clin Orthop Relat Res. 2006;442:195–8.
21. Pritchett JW. A comparison of the noise generated from different types of knee prostheses. J Knee Surg. 2013;26:101–4.
22. Pinskerova V, Johal P, Nakagawa S, et al. Does the femur roll-back with flexion? J Bone Joint Surg Br. 2004;86:925–31.
23. Tria AJ Jr. A contemporary bicruciate total knee arthroplasty. Semin Arthroplast. 2017;28:65–70.

Part VII

Achieving Implants Position through Tools in Personalized Knee Arthroplasty

24

Calipered KA and the Surgical Techniques

Alexander J. Nedopil, Stephen M. Howell, and Maury L. Hull

24.1 Overview

This chapter presents the philosophy of kinematic alignment (KA) and the surgical technique for setting the positions of the components using ten calipered measurements, manual instruments, and nine verification checks. The adoption of kinematic alignment is increasing. Four meta-analyses, three randomized trials, and a national multicenter study showed that patients treated with KA total knee arthroplasty (TKA) reported significantly better pain relief, function, and flexion and a more normal feeling knee than patients treated with mechanically aligned (MA) TKA [1–8]. Two randomized trials that limited the severity of the preoperative knee deformities showed similar clinical outcomes [9, 10]. KA co-aligns the axes of the femoral and tibial components with the three axes of the native knee without restrictions on the level of preoperative deformities [11]. The surgical goal of restoring the native alignments of the limb, Q-angle, and joint lines unique to each patient depends on accurately setting the components coincident to the native joint lines, which co-aligns the axes. The surgical goal of restoring the laxities, tibial compartment forces, knee adduction moment, and gait to those of the native knee without ligament release balances the TKA and promotes long-term implant survival [12–19]. A description of the calipered technique of KA with manual instruments, the sequence for measuring bone positions and resection thicknesses, the intraoperative recording of these measurements on the verification worksheet (Fig. 24.1), and the use of decision trees for balancing the TKA with the medial pivot CS and CR inserts are shown (Figs. 24.2 and 24.3). Calipered measurements of the thicknesses of the femoral and tibial bone resections restore the native joint lines with high reproducibility when they are adjusted within ±0.5 mm of the femoral and tibial components after compensating for cartilage and bone wear and the 1 mm kerf from the saw cut [20–22]. Because calipered measurements are a basic surgical skill, inexpensive, and highly reliable, they should be a required verification check when performing kinematic alignment with manual instruments, patient-specific guides, navigation,

A. J. Nedopil · S. M. Howell (✉) · M. L. Hull
Department of Orthopedic Surgery, Orthopedic Surgeon Adventist Health Lodi Memorial, Lodi, CA, USA
e-mail: mlhull@ucdavis.edu

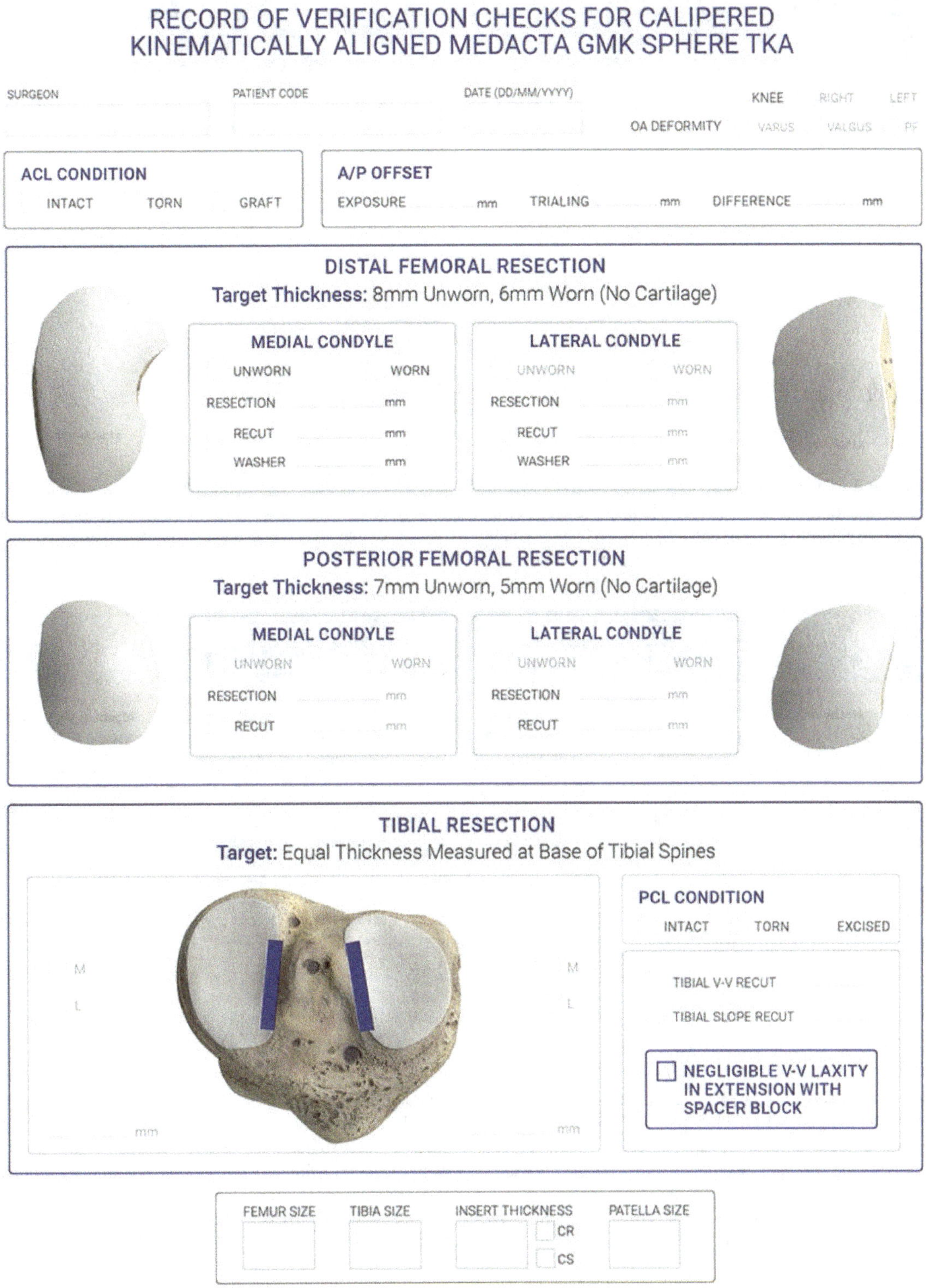

RECORD OF VERIFICATION CHECKS FOR CALIPERED KINEMATICALLY ALIGNED MEDACTA GMK SPHERE TKA

SURGEON
PATIENT CODE
DATE (DD/MM/YYYY)
KNEE RIGHT LEFT
OA DEFORMITY VARUS VALGUS PF

ACL CONDITION
INTACT TORN GRAFT

A/P OFFSET
EXPOSURE mm TRIALING mm DIFFERENCE mm

DISTAL FEMORAL RESECTION
Target Thickness: 8mm Unworn, 6mm Worn (No Cartilage)

MEDIAL CONDYLE
UNWORN WORN
RESECTION mm
RECUT mm
WASHER mm

LATERAL CONDYLE
UNWORN WORN
RESECTION mm
RECUT mm
WASHER mm

POSTERIOR FEMORAL RESECTION
Target Thickness: 7mm Unworn, 5mm Worn (No Cartilage)

MEDIAL CONDYLE
UNWORN WORN
RESECTION mm
RECUT mm

LATERAL CONDYLE
UNWORN WORN
RESECTION mm
RECUT mm

TIBIAL RESECTION
Target: Equal Thickness Measured at Base of Tibial Spines

M
L
mm
M
L
mm

PCL CONDITION
INTACT TORN EXCISED

TIBIAL V-V RECUT
TIBIAL SLOPE RECUT

NEGLIGIBLE V-V LAXITY IN EXTENSION WITH SPACER BLOCK

FEMUR SIZE
TIBIA SIZE
INSERT THICKNESS CR CS
PATELLA SIZE

Fig. 24.1 Verification checks consisting of serial calipered measurements of bone positions and resection thicknesses within ±0.5 mm of target are recorded intraoperatively on a worksheet. Recording these steps validates that the femoral and tibial components are kinematically aligned coincident to the native femoral and tibial joint lines before cementation

DECISION-TREE FOR BALANCING A CALIPERED KINEMATICALLY ALIGNED MEDACTA **GMK SPHERE CR** TKA					
Tight in Flexion & Extension	**Tight in Flexion Well-Balanced in Extension**	**Tight in Extension Well-Balanced in Flexion**	**Well-Balanced in Extension and Loose in Flexion**	**Tight Medial & Loose Lateral in Extension**	**Tight Lateral and Loose Medial in Extension**
Recut tibia and remove 1-2mm more bone.	Increase posterior slope until exposure A-P offset is restored at 900 of flexion.	Remove posterior osteophytes. Strip posterior capsule. Insert trial components & gently manipulate knee into extension.	Add thicker insert and recheck knee extends fully. When knee does not fully extend check PCL tension. When PCL is incompetent use **GMK Sphere CS** Insert.	Remove medial osteophytes. Reassess. Recut tibia in 1-2° more varus. Insert 1 mm thicker insert.	Remove lateral osteophytes. Reassess. Recut tibia in 1-2° more valgus. Insert 1 mm thicker insert.

Fig. 24.2 The decision tree lists six corrective measures for balancing the KA TKA with a posterior cruciate ligament-retaining (CR) sphere insert. The balancing steps adjust the proximal–distal level and varus–valgus and slope orientations of the tibial resection and insert thickness without recutting the femur or releasing the collateral, retinacular, and posterior cruciate ligaments

DECISION-TREE FOR BALANCING A CALIPERED KINEMATICALLY ALIGNED MEDACTA **GMK SPHERE CS** TKA					
Tight in Flexion & Extension	**Tight in Flexion Well-Balanced in Extension**	**Tight in Extension Well-Balanced in Flexion**	**Well-Balanced in Extension and Loose in Flexion**	**Tight Medial & Loose Lateral in Extension**	**Tight Lateral and Loose Medial in Extension**
Recut tibia and remove 1-2mm more bone.	Confirm complete resection of the PCL. Increase posterior slope until natural A-P offset is restored at 90° of flexion.	Remove posterior osteophytes. Strip posterior capsule. Insert trial components & gently manipulate knee into extension.	Add thicker insert and recheck knee extends fully. If still loose in flexion, then reduce slope or resect 1-2 mm bone from distal femur and add thicker **GMK Sphere CS** insert.	Remove medial osteophytes. Reassess. Recut tibia in 1-2° more varus. Insert 1 mm thicker insert.	Remove lateral osteophytes. Reassess. Recut tibia in 1-2° more valgus. Insert 1 mm thicker insert.

Fig. 24.3 The decision tree lists six corrective measures for balancing the KA TKA with a posterior cruciate ligament-substituting (CS) sphere insert. The balancing steps adjust the proximal–distal level and varus–valgus and slope orientations of the tibial resection and insert thickness without releasing collateral, retinacular, and posterior cruciate ligaments. When the posterior cruciate ligament is unintentionally transected with the saw or detached from the tibia the flexion space increases whereas the extension space does not. Bone grafting the posterior 1/3 rd of the tibial resection, recutting the tibia in less slope, and resecting 2 mm of bone from the distal femur and using a thicker insert are strategies for compensating for the increase in flexion space laxity

and robotics. Examples of treatment of patients with severe varus and valgus deformities and flexion contractures treated with KA TKA without ligament release are shown. Finally, the reasons for the low risk of tibial component failure, low risk of patellofemoral instability, and high implant survival at 10 years after KA TKA are explained [11, 23, 24].

24.2 Co-aligning the Axes of the Femoral and Tibial Components with the Three Axes of the Native Knee Is the Philosophy of Kinematic Alignment

The term "kinematic alignment" indicates the surgeon follows the philosophy of co-aligning the axes of the femoral and tibial components with the three axes of the native knee without ligament release and without restrictions on the degree of preoperative varus, valgus, flexion, and extension deformities [3, 21, 25–27]. Calipered measurements of femoral and tibial bone resections verify the alignment of the components coincident to the native joint lines and co-alignment of the axes of the components with the three "kinematic" axes of the native knee (Fig. 24.4) [22]. The first axis is in the native femur and connects the center of the best-fit circles to the posterior femoral condyles from 20° to 120° like an axle passing through two wheels. This axis controls the arc of flexion and extension of the tibia with respect to the femur [26, 28–31]. The second axis is in the native femur and lies parallel and averages 10 mm anterior and 12 mm proximal to the first axis. This axis controls the arc of flexion and extension of the patella with respect to the femur [25, 27]. The flexion–extension plane lies perpendicular to the two femoral axes in the extended knee [32, 33]. The third axis is in the native tibia and lies perpendicular to the two femoral axes and native joint lines of the femur and tibia. This axis controls internal–external rotation of the tibia with respect to the femur [25, 26]. Because the orientations of three kinematic axes are closely parallel or perpendicular to the native joint lines, setting the femoral and tibial components coincident to the native joint lines after compensating for cartilage wear and the kerf of the saw cut closely co-aligns the axes of the components with those of the native knee, which preserves the native resting lengths of the collateral, posterior cruciate, and retinacular ligaments [21, 22, 34].

24.3 First Surgical Goal: Restore the Native Joint Lines, Q-Angle, and Limb Alignments Unique to Each Patient

Restoring the native joint lines, Q-angle, and limb alignments unique to each patient is the first surgical goal of calipered KA TKA [3, 21, 35].

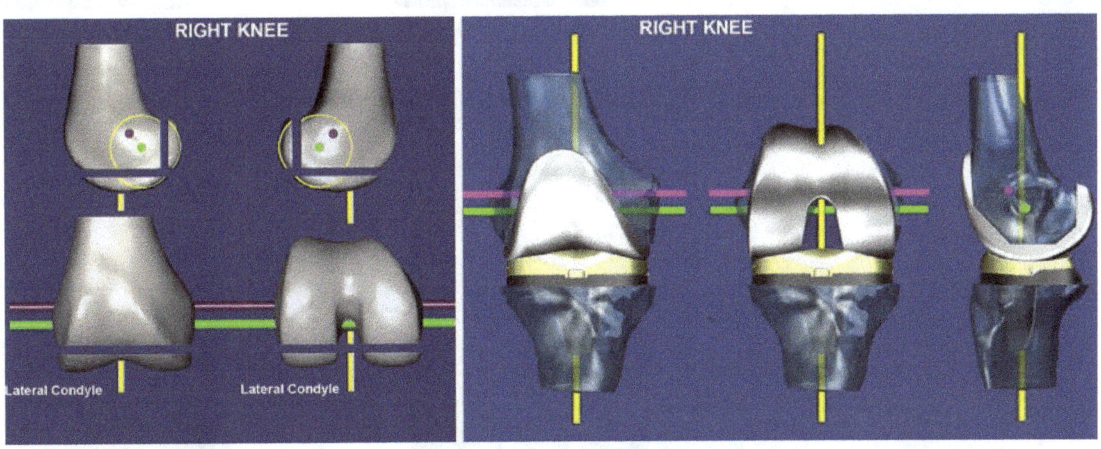

Fig. 24.4 Projections of the right distal femur (left) and KA TKA (right) show the parallel and perpendicular relationships between the three "kinematic" axes of the native knee show the anatomic basis of the philosophy of co-aligning the axes of the components with those of the native knee [48]. The flexion–extension axis of the tibia is the green line, the flexion–extension axis of the patella is the magenta line, and the internal–external axis of the tibia is the yellow line. All three axes are closely parallel or perpendicular to the joint lines of the native knee. Resecting bone from the distal and posterior femur condyles equal in thickness to the condyles of the femoral component after compensating for 2 mm of cartilage wear and 1 mm kerf of the saw cut sets the femoral component coincident to the native joint lines and co-aligns the axes

There is a growing body of evidence that a substantial number of native limbs do not have a neutral or 0° hip–knee–ankle (HKA) angle prior to the onset of osteoarthritis [12, 31, 35–38]. The maximum range reported for the HKA angle is 7°–12° for constitutional varus and −4° to −16° for constitutional valgus for people in the United States, Korea, India, and Belgium [31, 36–38]. Hence, when mechanical alignment changes constitutional varus and valgus alignment to a 0° HKA angle, the native joint lines and Q-angle are changed. Changing the native joint lines overly tensions or slackens the collateral, retinacular, and posterior cruciate ligaments and frequently creates an extension–flexion imbalance in a compartment that is uncorrectable with a soft tissue release [18, 19, 35, 36, 39–42] (Figs. 24.5 and 24.6). The technique of kinematic alignment using ten calipered measurements is highly reproducible as the left to right symmetry of the distal lateral femoral angle (DLFA), proximal medial tibial angle (PMTA), Q-angle, and HKA angle is restored to that of the native limb in >95% of patients with negligible risk of varus

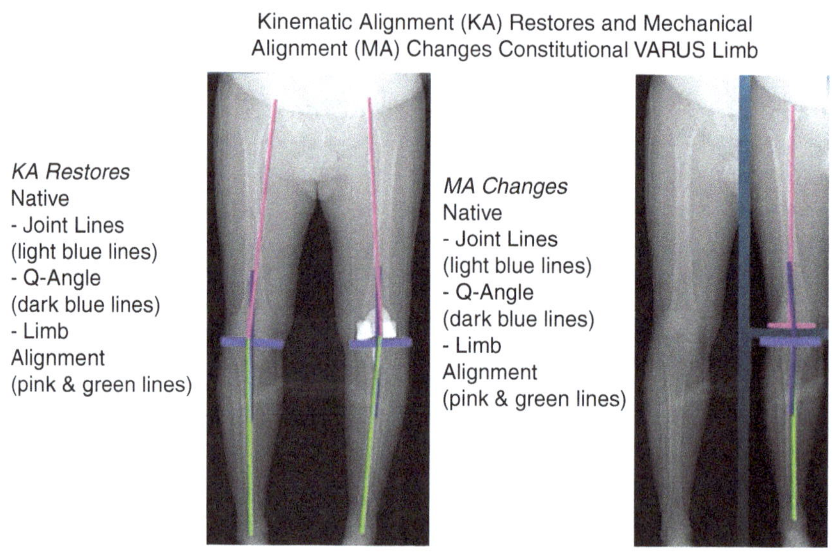

Fig. 24.5 Composite of a patient with a constitutional varus limb (left) shows calipered KA restored the native joint lines (light blue lines), Q-angle (dark blue lines), distal lateral femoral angle (pink lines), and proximal medial tibial angle (green lines) in the limb with the TKA without ligament release (right)

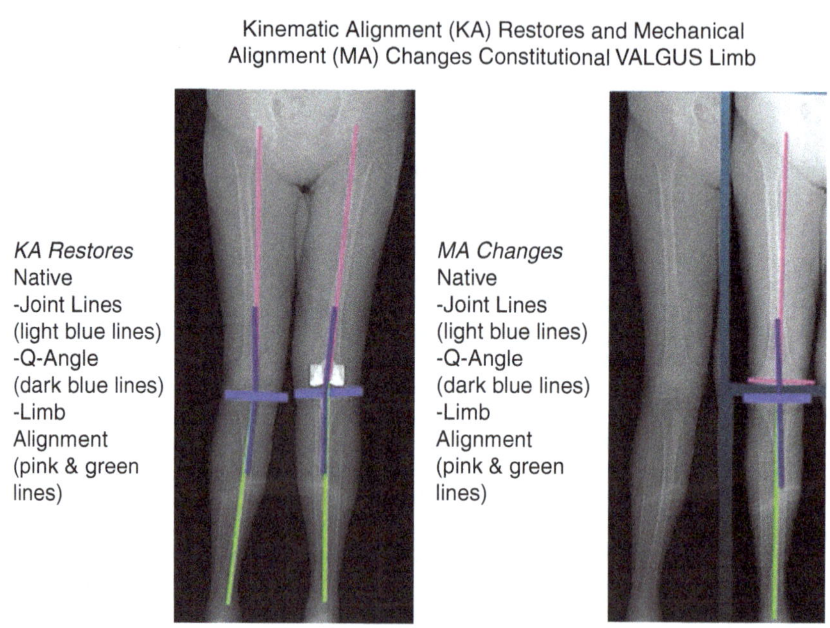

Fig. 24.6 Composite of a patient with a constitutional valgus limb (left) shows calipered KA restored the native joint lines (light blue lines), Q-angle (dark blue lines), distal lateral femoral angle (pink lines), and proximal medial tibial angle (green lines) in the limb with the TKA without ligament release (right)

alignment of the tibial component with respect to the native tibial joint line [20, 21].

24.4 Second Surgical Goal: Restore Laxities, Tibial Compartment Forces, and Knee Adduction Moment of the Native Knee Without Ligament Release

Restoring the native laxities, tibial compartment forces, knee adduction moment, and gait without ligament release is the second surgical goal of calipered KA TKA [12, 13, 16–19, 43]. The varus–valgus and internal–external rotation laxities of the native knee are looser at 45° and 90° of flexion than at 0° (Fig. 24.7). The penalty for performing gap-balancing TKA, which tightens the native laxities at 45° and 90° to match those at 0° of flexion, is overly tight ligaments relative to those of the native knee that patients might perceive as pain, stiffness, and limited extension and flexion [14, 19].

Most TKA techniques resect the ACL and replace the articular cartilage and menisci with implants of graduated sizes with conformities and stiffnesses different from the native knee. A study in cadaveric knees showed that kinematic alignment with a posterior cruciate ligament-retaining implant restored 35 of 40 measures of laxity (8 laxities × 5 flexion angles) to those of the native knee. The restoration of most of the native laxities suggests that femoral and tibial components aligned with KA compensate for the articular cartilage, menisci, and ACL [16].

KA without ligament release limits high compartment forces by restoring those of the native knee [17–19, 43]. There is no evidence of medial or lateral compartment overload even in the subset of patients with alignment of the tibial joint line and limb in a varus or valgus outlier range according to MA criteria [19]. In contrast, the medial and lateral tibial compartment forces after mechanical alignment and ligament release to a 0° hip–knee–ankle with measured resection and gap-balancing techniques are three to six times higher than those of the native knee at 0°, 45°, and 90° of flexion [17, 19, 42, 44]. Hence, KA without ligament release restores native medial and lateral tibial compartment forces, whereas MA with ligament release does not [17–19].

KA restores the native joint line obliquity [7, 12, 45], which reduces the peak knee adduction moment during gait and better restores normal gait when compared to MA TKA [12, 13]. A low knee adduction moment is one explanation for the negligible risk of varus failure of the tibial component 2–10 years after KA TKA [11, 23]. Hence, KA is a promising option in limbs with constitutional varus alignment and large coronal bowing of the tibial shaft as the low knee adduction moment and more normal gait lowers the risk of medial compartment overload [12].

24.5 Calipered Technique for Setting the Femoral Component Coincident to the Native Femoral Joint Line with Verification Checks

The following sequence of surgical steps, calipered measurements, and adjustments and the intraoperative recording of these measurements on a verification worksheet set the proximal–distal position and varus–valgus orientation of the femoral component coincident to the native distal joint line at 0° and the anterior–posterior position and internal–external orientation of the femoral component coincident to the native posterior joint line at 90° with high reproducibility (Fig. 24.4) [21, 24, 32]. The femoral mechanical axis, trans-epicondylar axis, and anterior–posterior axis (Whiteside's line) are not of interest or use when kinematically aligning the femoral component [26, 31, 39, 40, 46, 47].

Flex the knee to 90°. Expose the knee using a medial approach. Position the short arm of the offset caliper against the distal medial femoral condyle and the long arm against the anterior tibia (Fig. 24.8). Orient the long arm

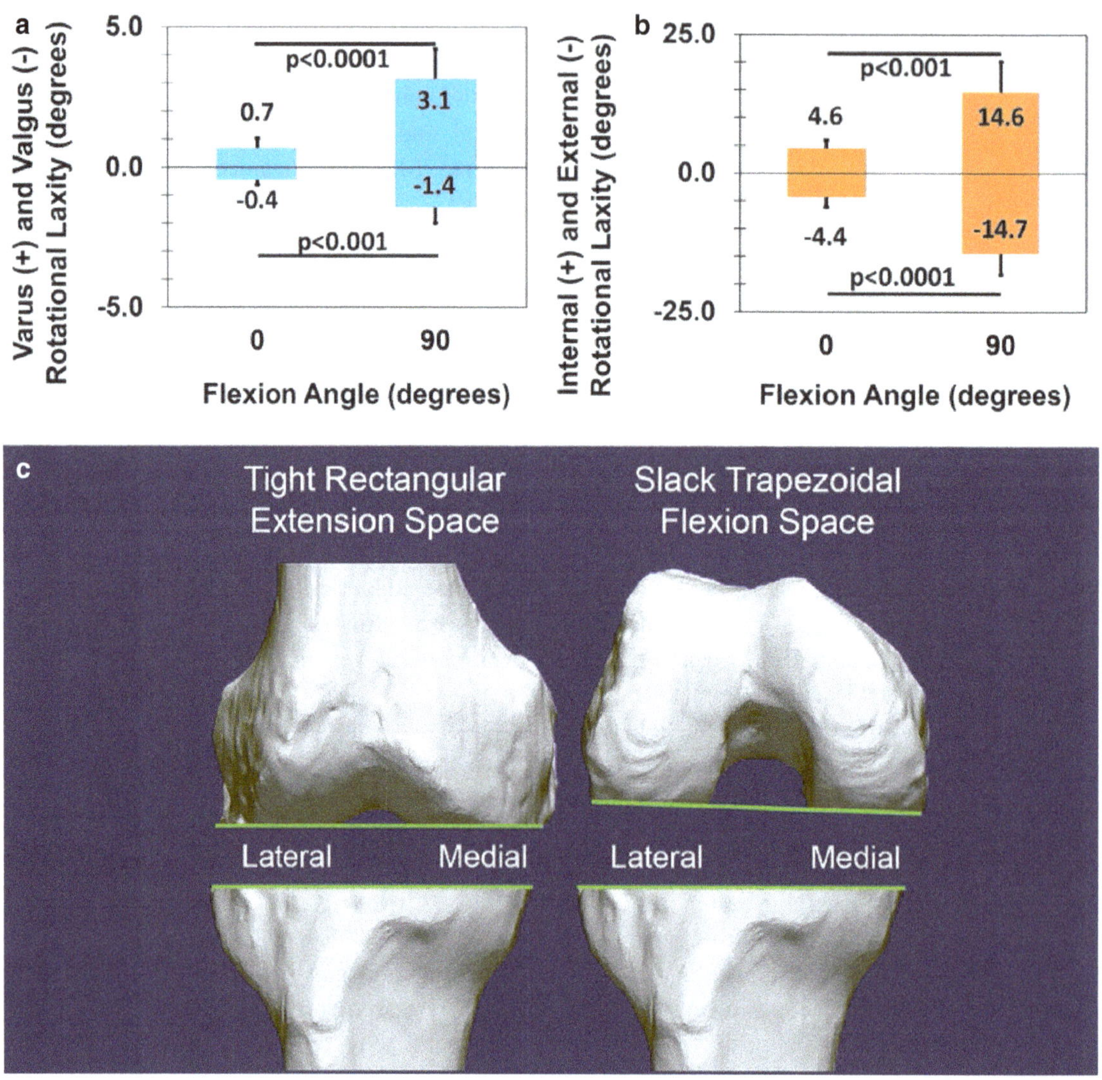

Fig. 24.7 Column graphs show the varus–valgus and internal–external rotational laxities of the native knee are greater at 90° than at 0° of flexion (**a**, **b**) [14, 15]. During knee arthroscopy, the surgeon notices these relative differences in laxity as a tight rectangular space when the knee is in extension and a slack trapezoidal space with more laxity laterally than medially when the knee is in flexion. The schematic shows that the resections of the femur and tibia with calipered KA restore the tight rectangular extension space and slack trapezoidal flexion space of the native knee (**c**). Hence, calipered KA restores 35 of 40 measures of laxity of the native knee [16], whereas the MA concept of gap balancing overtightens the flexion space that patients may perceive as pain, stiffness, and limited flexion [14]

parallel to the patellar tendon. Measure the distance of the offset. Subtract 2 mm when cartilage is worn to bone on the medial femoral condyle [48].

Verification Check 1: Record the offset measurement on an electronic or paper version of the verification worksheet (Fig. 24.1). During final balancing before cementation of the components, adjustments are made to the slope of the tibial resection and insert thickness until the offset is matched within 0 ± 1 mm, which restores the native laxities and tibial compartment forces of the flexion space (Fig. 24.7) [15, 16, 48].

Expose the knee fully and assess the locations of cartilage wear on the distal femur. Remove any partially worn cartilage to bone with a ring curette. Set the flexion–extension orientation of the femoral component by starting the diameter hole for the positioning rod midway between the top of the intercondylar notch and the anterior

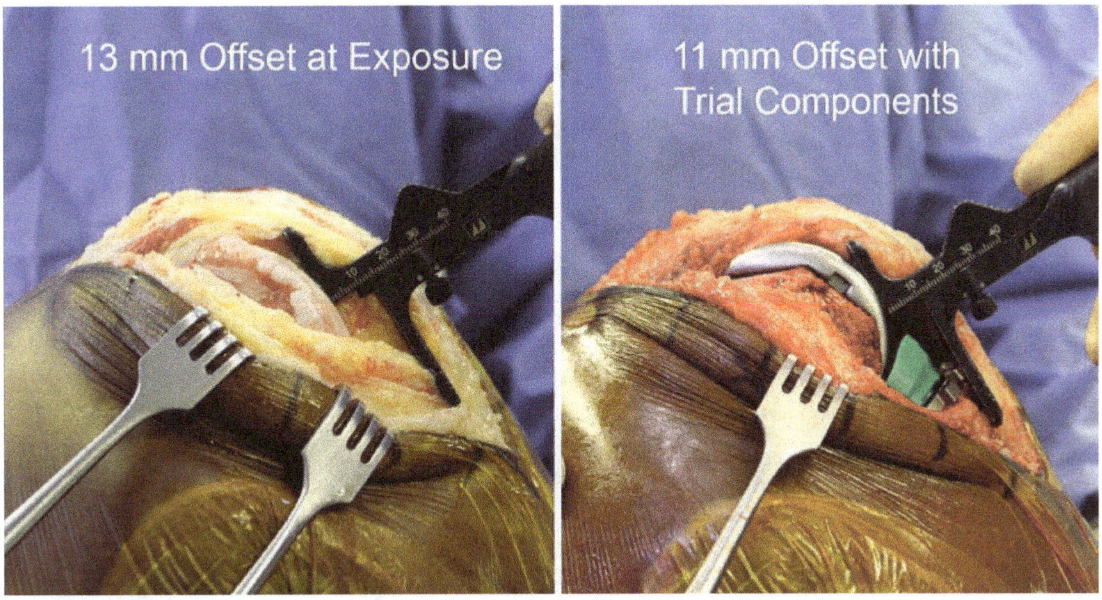

Fig. 24.8 Intraoperative photographs of a right knee in 90° of flexion show the caliper measurement of the "offset" of 13 mm between the distal medial femur and the anterior tibia at the time of exposure with the longer arm of the caliper-oriented parallel to the patellar tendon in the sagittal plane (left). When cartilage is worn to bone, subtract 2 mm from the measurement. During final balancing before cementation of the components, the slope of the tibial resection and insert thickness are adjusted until the offset with trial components matches the corrected offset of the knee at the time of exposure of 11 mm and passive internal–external rotation of the tibia ~±14° like the native knee (right) (Fig. 24.7) [14]. A 2° increase in the posterior slope and a 2 mm decrease in the insert thickness translates the tibia ~3 mm posterior [17, 53]

cortex (Fig. 24.9). Keep a 5–10 mm bridge of bone between the posterior rim of the drill hole and the top of the intercondylar notch. Orient the drill perpendicular to a plane coincident to the distal surface of the femur and parallel with the anterior cortex of the femur. Drill and then insert a positioning rod 8–10 cm.

Verification Check 2: Keeping a 5–10 mm bridge of bone between the posterior rim of the drill hole and the top of the intercondylar notch limits flexion of the femoral component to within 1° ± 2° with respect to the anatomic axis of the distal femur resulting in a negligible risk of patellofemoral instability [49–51].

Set the proximal–distal position and varus–valgus orientation of the femoral component by using an offset distal referencing guide (Fig. 24.10). Select the offset of the guide so that a compensation of 2 mm is added to the distal femoral condyle(s) with cartilage wear. Do not correct for distal femoral bone wear as it is negligible even in the most arthritic knees [34, 48]. Slide the selected offset distal referencing guide over the intramedullary rod. Confirm the offset surface of the guide contacts both distal femoral condyles. Pin the guide and resect the distal femur. Measure the thicknesses of the distal medial and lateral bone resections with a caliper. Adjust the resections of the distal femur until their thicknesses match the distal condyles of the femoral component within ±0.5 mm after compensating for 2 mm of cartilage wear and a 1 mm kerf from the saw cut.

- Correct a 1 or 2 mm underresection of the distal femoral condyles by removing more bone from the distal femur with use of a 1 mm distal recut guide or by repositioning the distal femoral resection guide 2 mm more proximal.
- Correct a 1 or 2 mm overresection of a distal femoral condyle by filling the gap by placing a 1 or 2 mm-thick washer on the corresponding fixation peg of the 4-in-1 block.

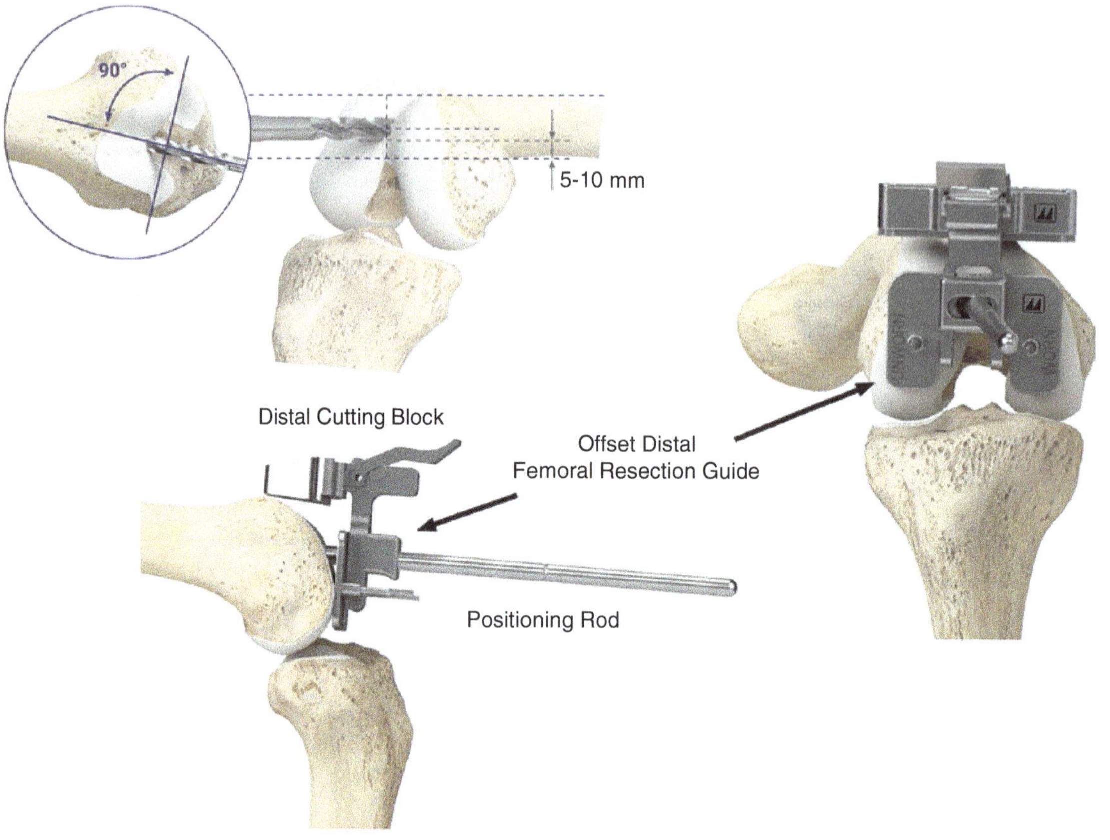

Fig. 24.9 Schematic shows the method for limiting flexion of the femoral component, which results in a negligible risk of patellofemoral instability [49–51]. Start the drill hole midway between the anterior limit of the notch and the anterior cortex of the femur (short blue-dotted line). Orient the drill perpendicular to a plane coincident to the distal surface of the femur and parallel with the anterior cortex of the femur. A starting point that keeps a 5–10 mm bone bridge between the posterior rim of the drill hole and the top of the intercondylar notch limits flexion of the femoral component to within 1° ± 2° with respect to the anatomic axis of the distal femur [50]

Verification Check 3: Record the calipered measurements on the verification worksheet (Fig. 24.1). The calipered measurements restore the varus–valgus orientation of the femoral component to the contralateral native limb in 97% of subjects [21].

Set the anterior–posterior position and internal–external orientation of the femoral component by selecting a posterior referencing guide set in 0° rotation and positioning the feet of the guide in contact with the posterior femoral condyles (Fig. 24.11). In the most varus osteoarthritic knee, the use of the 0° posterior referencing guide is correct because complete cartilage wear is rare on the posterior medial femoral condyles. In the most severe valgus osteoarthritic knee, the 0° posterior referencing guide occasionally requires rotation of the foot of the guide 1–2 mm posterior from the worn posterior lateral femoral condyle. Do not correct for posterior femoral bone wear as it is negligible even in the most arthritic knees [34, 48].

Size the femoral component by positioning the stylus on the anterior femur. Drill the holes for the 4-in-1 chamfer block. Insert the 4-in-1 chamfer block remembering to place a 1 or 2 mm-thick washer on the corresponding fixation peg to correct for a 1 or 2 mm overresection of a distal femoral condyle. Make the posterior resections before making the anterior and chamfer cuts. Measure the thicknesses of the distal medial and lateral bone resections with a caliper. Adjust the resections of the posterior femur until their

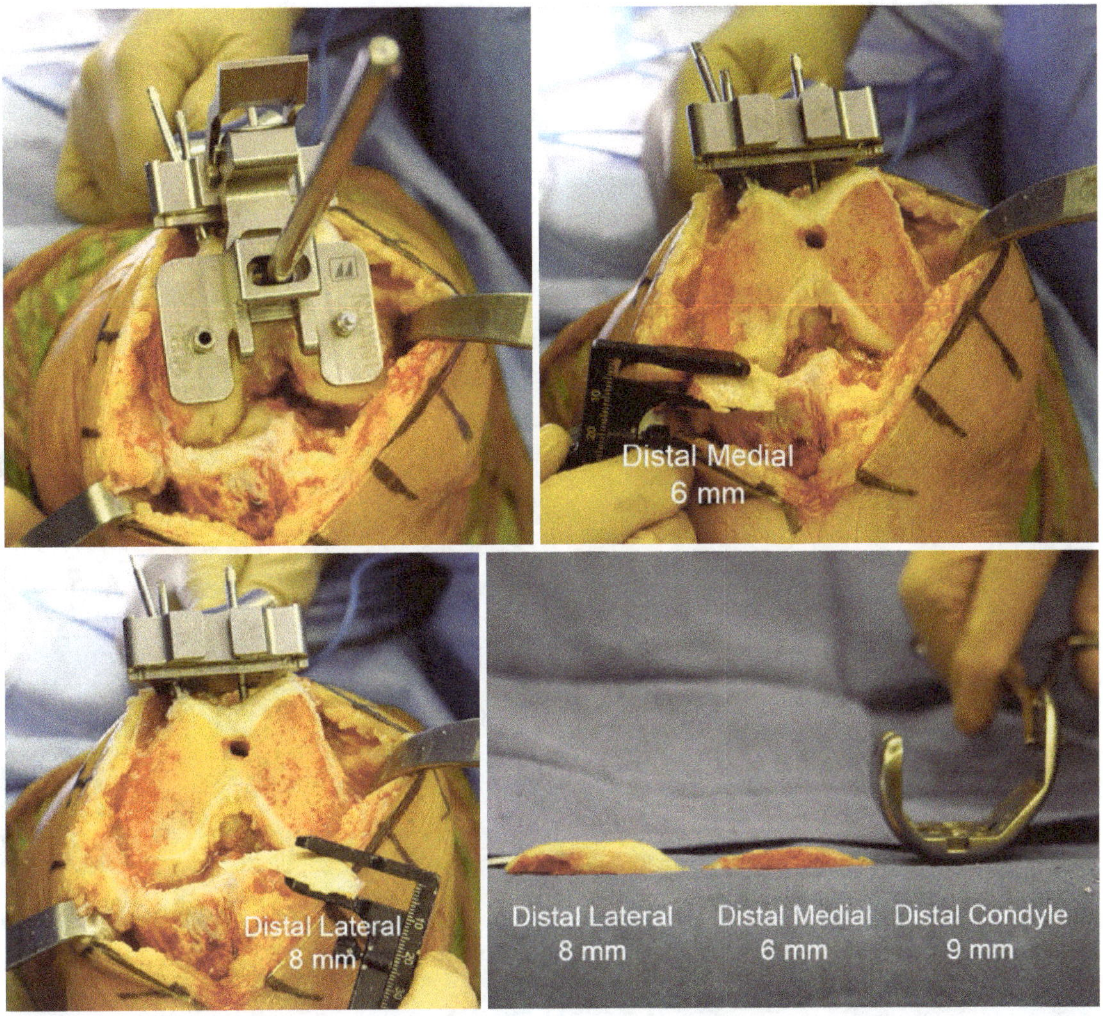

Fig. 24.10 Composite of a left varus osteoarthritic knee shows the steps for kinematically aligning the femoral component coincident to the distal joint line of the native femur. Pin the offset distal femoral resection guide with the "WORN" mark overlying the medial femoral condyle and the "UNWORN" mark overlying the lateral femoral condyle (upper left). Measure the distal medial resection with a caliper (upper right). Measure the distal lateral resection with a caliper (lower left). The distal condyles of the femoral component are 9 mm thick (lower right). Hence, the distal medial and lateral femoral resections should be 6 and 8 mm thick, which compensate for the 1 mm of kerf of the saw and the 2 mm of cartilage wear on the distal medial femoral condyle. Recording these calipered measurements verifies the varus–valgus orientation of the femoral component is coincident to the native joint line and matches the contralateral native limb in 97% of the subjects [21]

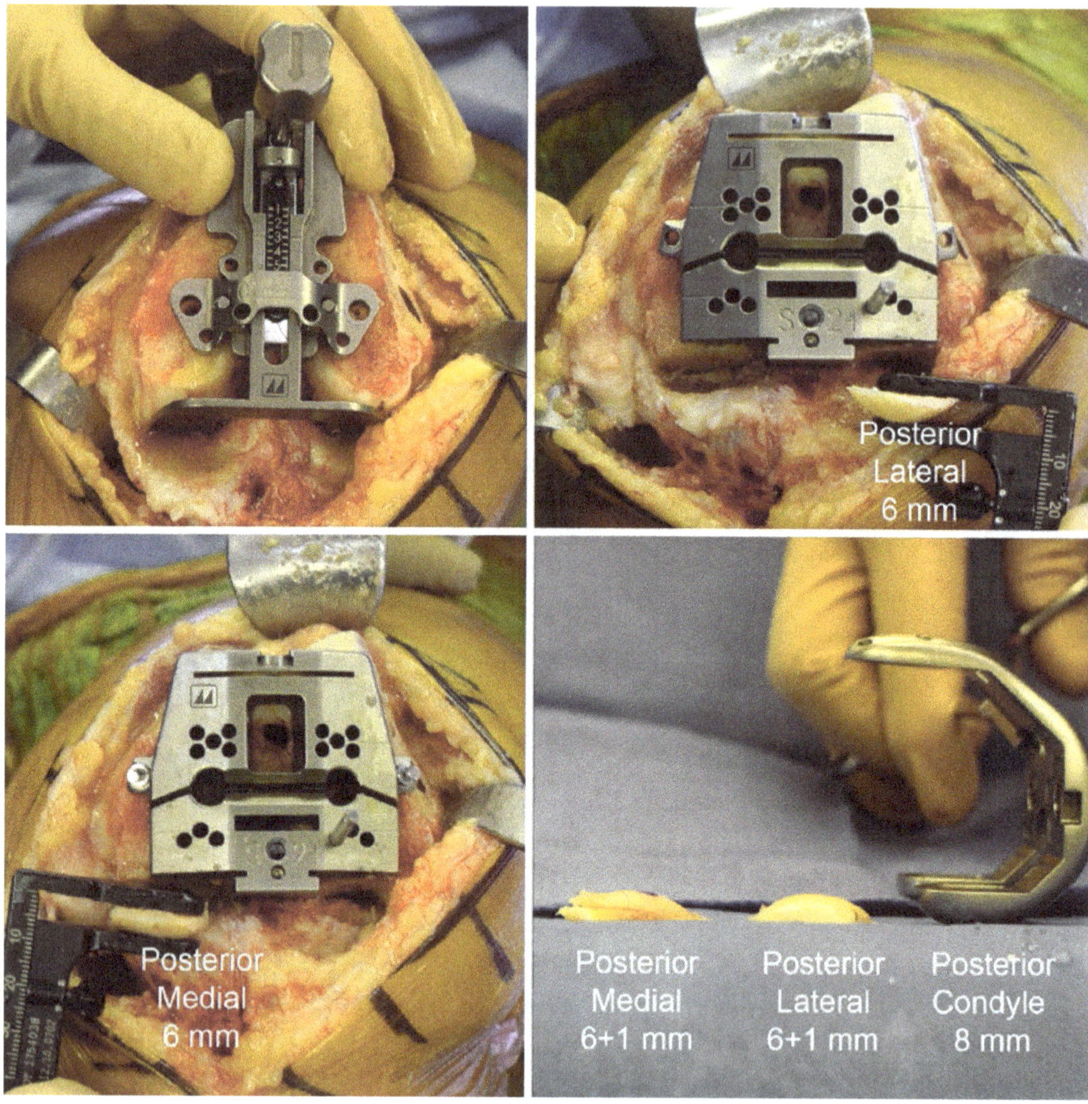

Fig. 24.11 Composite of a left varus osteoarthritic knee shows the steps for kinematically aligning the femoral component coincident to the posterior joint line of the native femur. Insert a posterior referencing guide set at 0° rotation and drill holes for the 4-in-1 chamfer block (upper left). Measure the posterior lateral resection with a caliper (upper right). Measure the posterior medial resection with a caliper (lower left). Hence, the posterior medial and lateral resections should be 7 mm thick, which compensates for the 1 mm kerf of the saw (lower right). The +1 indicates 1 mm of additional bone was resected to correct a saw blade that skived during the initial posterior resection. Recording these calipered measurements verifies the internal–external orientation of the femoral component is coincident to the posterior joint line of the native knee within 0° ± 1.1 [32]

thicknesses match the posterior condyles of the femoral component within ±0.5 mm after compensating for 2 mm of cartilage wear when present and a 1 mm kerf from the saw cut. When a posterior femoral resection is 1–2 mm too thick or too thin, elongate the pin hole in the direction of the correction and translate the 4-in-1 chamfer block as needed. Insert the oblique compression screws and secure the reposition of the chamfer block. Make the anterior and chamfer femoral resections.

Verification Check 4: Record the calipered measurements on the verification worksheet (Fig. 24.1).The calipered measurements reproducibly restore the internal–external orientation of the femoral component within 0° ± 1.1° of the posterior joint line and the flexion–extension plane of the native knee [32].

24.6 Calipered Technique for Setting the Tibial Component Coincident to the Native Tibial Joint Line with Verification Checks

The following sequence of surgical steps, calipered measurements, and adjustments verify the proximal–distal position and the varus–valgus, flexion–extension, and internal–external orientations of the tibial component are coincident to the native tibial joint line. The tibial mechanical axis, intramedullary canal, and tibial tubercle are not of interest or use when KA the tibial component [11, 21, 40, 47, 52].

Use an extramedullary tibial guide as a support for positioning the tibial resection guide and not as a method for referencing the ankle (Fig. 24.12). Set

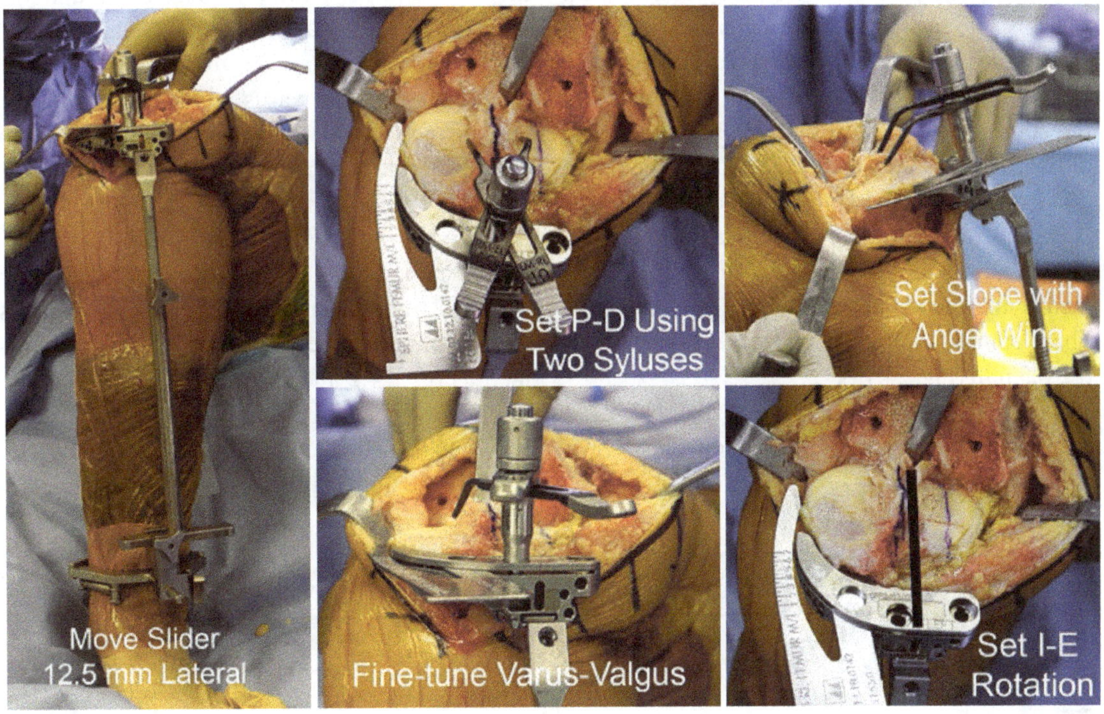

Fig. 24.12 Composite of a right knee shows the steps for KA the tibial component. Set the varus–valgus position of the tibial resection by applying a conventional extramedullary tibial resection guide to the ankle and moving the slider 12.5 mm lateral from the 0 mm position (left). Set the proximal–distal position by registering the tips of the two styluses at the base of each tibial spine in an area with intact cartilage (upper middle). Set the slope by adjusting the anterior–posterior slider at the ankle until the plane of the angel wing parallels the medial tibial joint line after compensating for cartilage and bone wear (upper right). Fine-tune the varus–valgus and slope orientation of the tibial resection guide to compensate for cartilage and bone wear (lower middle). Set internal–external orientation by rotating the tibial cutting guide until the line on the top of the guide is parallel to a line drawn between the tibial spines (black line) and a line representing the major axis of the elliptical-shaped lateral tibial condyle (faint blue line) (lower right)

the varus–valgus orientation of the tibial resection guide parallel to the articular surface of the native tibia by translating the medial–lateral slider at the ankle 12.5 mm lateral, which achieves an anatomic or ~2–3° varus orientation to the tibial mechanical axis in most patients [3, 10]. Set a conservative proximal–distal position for the tibial resection by positioning the tips of the two styluses with the 8 mm offset at the base of each tibial spine in an area with intact cartilage. Insert an angel wing on the medial side of the tibial cutting guide. Set the slope of the resection of the medial tibial plateau by adjusting the anterior-posterior slider at the ankle until the plane of the angel wing parallels the medial tibial joint line after compensating for cartilage and bone wear. Set internal–external orientation by rotating the tibial cutting guide until the line on the top is parallel to a line drawn between the tibial spines and a line representing the major axis of the elliptical-shaped lateral tibial condyle [32]. Visually fine-tune the varus–valgus and slope orientation of the tibial resection guide to compensate for cartilage and bone wear. Pin the guide and resect the proximal tibia. Examine the medial edge of the tibial resection and confirm the plane of the tibial resection parallels the plane of the articular surface of the tibia after compensating for wear. Use a caliper and measure the thickness of the medial and lateral tibial condyles at the base of the tibial spines, which should be similar within 0 ± 0.5 mm (Fig. 24.13).

Verification Check 5: Record the calipered measurements on the verification worksheet (Fig. 24.1).

Flex the knee to 90°. Insert the tightest-fitting spacer block (choose from 10, 11, 12, 13, and 14 mm) between the femur and tibia. Recut the tibia using the 2 mm recut guide when the flexion space is too tight for a 10 mm spacer.

Verification Check 6: With the knee in 90° of flexion, internally and externally rotate the spacer and assess the relative tightness between the medial and lateral compartments. Confirm the spacer fits tighter in the medial compartment, fits looser in the lateral compartment, and pivots about the medial compartment, which restores a trapezoidal flexion space like the native knee (Fig. 24.7) [14].

Place the knee in full extension. Reinsert the spacer. Retract the soft tissues and visually examine the varus–valgus laxity between the femoral resection and spacer block and between the spacer block and tibial resection. Confirm the varus–valgus laxity is negligible and the difference in the gaps between the medial and lateral compartments is within 0 ± 0.5 mm, which restores the varus–valgus laxity of the native knee in full extension and native limb and joint line alignments with high reproducibility [14, 21]. Remember to account for over-resections of the distal femoral condyle. Perform one of the corrective steps listed in the decision trees when the varus–valgus laxity is greater in either the medial or lateral compartment (Figs. 24.2 and 24.3).

- When the lateral compartment is 2 mm tighter, recut the tibia using the 2° valgus recut guide.

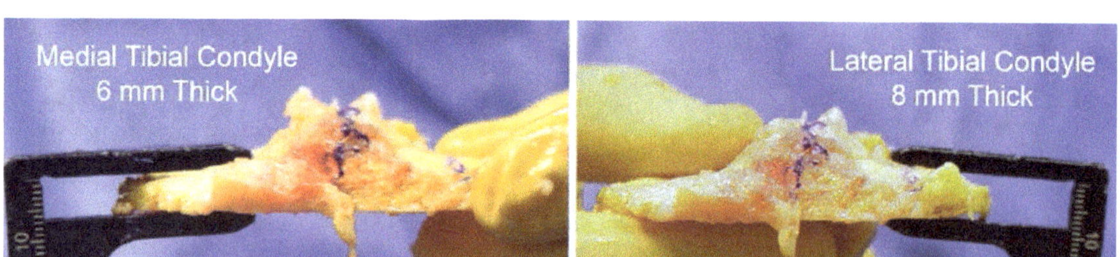

Fig. 24.13 Composite of a right knee shows a caliper measuring a 6 mm-thick medial tibial condyle and an 8 mm-thick lateral tibial condyle at the base of the tibial spines. Expect the medial side to be tight and the lateral side loose when visually examining the varus–valgus laxity between the femoral resection, spacer block, and tibial resection with the knee in full extension. In this case, the use of a 2° varus recut guide removed 2 mm of bone from the medial tibial condyle and restored the negligible varus–valgus laxity and tight rectangular space of the native knee in extension (Fig. 24.7) [13, 15]. The negligible varus–valgus laxity verifies the orientation of the tibial component matches the contralateral native limb in 97% of subjects [14, 16, 21]

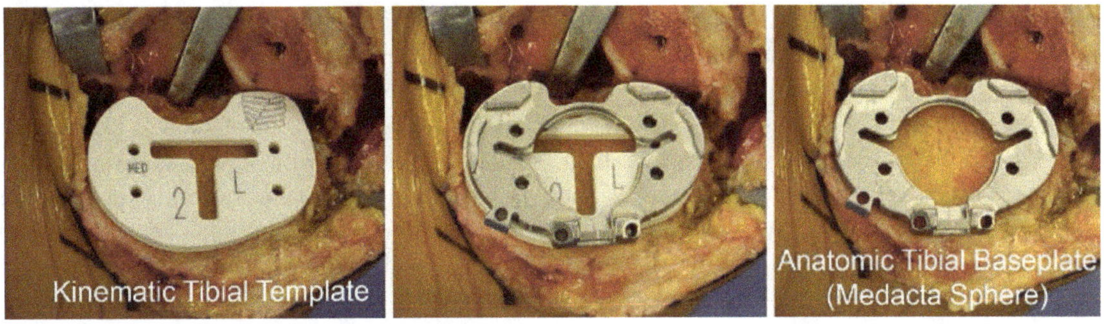

Fig. 24.14 Composite of a right knee shows the steps for KA internal–external rotation of the tibial component. Best-fitting the largest kinematic tibial template within the cortical boundary of the tibial resection assists the surgeon in accurately setting the I–E rotation of the tibial component parallel to the F–E plane of the knee when performing KA TKA (left) [33]. The anatomic shape of the trial tibial baseplate (Medacta) matches the kinematic tibial template (middle). Best fitting the largest trial tibial baseplate within the cortical boundary of the tibial resection verifies the internal–external rotation of the tibial component is within 0° ± 4° of the flexion–extension plane of the knee, which restores high-level knee function (right) [32, 33]

- When the medial compartment is 2 mm tighter, recut the tibia using the 2° varus recut guide.
- When a 1 mm correction is required, place the ~1 mm-thick angle wing between the recut guide and the tibia resection and make a 1° recut.

Verification Check 7: Negligible varus–valgus laxity restores the native rectangular space in full extension with a negligible mean varus–valgus laxity of <±1° and tibial joint line, knee, and limb alignment (Fig. 24.7) [14, 20, 21, 32, 43].

View the entire surface of the proximal tibial resection to size and position the anatomic tibial baseplate (Medacta) (Fig. 24.14). The anatomic shapes of the six trial tibial baseplates match closely those of seven kinematic tibial templates, which reproducibly set internal–external rotation of the tibial component within 0° ± 4° of the flexion–extension plane of the native knee [33]. Select the largest trial tibial baseplate that fits within the cortical boundary of the tibial resection. Rotate the trial tibial baseplate until the edge is parallel with the cortex. Pin the trial tibial baseplate and create the slot for the stem.

Verification Check 8: Setting the internal–external orientation of the anatomic tibial baseplate to within 0° ± 4° of the flexion–extension plane of the knee restores high-level knee function [32, 33]. Because the mediolateral location of the tibial tubercle varies, the medial border and medial one-third of the tibial tubercle are unreliable landmarks for setting the rotation of the tibial component on the tibia [52].

Finally, insert trial components and assess the varus–valgus laxities with the knee in full extension and 15–20° of flexion and the anterior offset of the tibia on the medial femur, internal–external rotation, and posterior and distraction translation of the tibia with the knee in 90° of flexion while referring to the corrective measures in the Sphere CR and Sphere CS decision trees (Figs. 24.2 and 24.3). The common principle of these decision trees is that fine-tuning the proximal–distal position and the varus–valgus and flexion–extension (slope) orientations of the tibial resection balances the knee. Balancing is accomplished without ligament release.

24.6.1 Final Verification with Trial Components Check 9

- *Place the knee in full extension:* Retract the soft tissues and visually examine the varus–valgus laxity between the femoral component and tibial insert, which should be negligible like the native knee (Fig. 24.7) [14, 15].
  - Correct a 1° varus or 1° valgus instability because this degree of laxity is greater than the native knee and is associated with instability in extension [14].

- *Place the knee in 15–20° of flexion:* Check varus–valgus laxity. The medial side should open ~1 mm and the lateral side ~2–3 mm and be looser than in full extension (Fig. 24.7).
  - When the lateral side opens more than ~3–4 mm, verify the tibial resection is not in excessive valgus by remeasuring the tibial resection at the base of the tibial spines.
- *Place the knee in 90° of flexion:*
  - When the posterior cruciate ligament is intact and the CR insert is used, adjust the slope of the tibial resection and thickness of the insert until the anterior offset of the tibia from the distal medial femoral condyle matches the knee at the time of exposure. A 2° increase in the posterior slope and a 2 mm decrease in the insert thickness translates the tibia ~3 mm posterior [17, 53]. Confirm the tibia internally and externally rotates ~±14° like the native knee (Figs. 24.2 and 24.7) [14, 48].
  - When the posterior cruciate ligament is resected and the sphere CS insert for a medial ball and socket implant is used, check the posterior drawer and distract the tibia. When the insert rides too posterior on the femoral component and the flexion space is slack, use a thicker insert and tighten the flexion space. When the thicker insert limits knee extension, recut 1–2 mm more bone from the distal femur. Refer to the corrective steps in the fourth column of the Sphere CS decision tree (Fig. 24.3).

24.7 Kinematic Alignment Corrects Severe Varus Deformities Without Ligament Release

Since 2006, all patients suitable for a primary total knee replacement were treated following the principles of kinematic alignment which are to co-align the axes and joint lines of the components with the three "kinematic" axes and joint lines of the pre-arthritic or native knee without placing restrictions on the preoperative deformity, and postoperative correction and without ligament release. During these 13 years, there were over 5000 primary KA TKAs from which all patients with severe deformities secondary to post-traumatic arthritis, progressive osteoarthritis post high tibial osteotomy, and patients with multiple-level deformity were included.

Surprisingly, intrinsic contracture and stretching of the collateral and posterior cruciate ligaments were exceedingly uncommon. Preoperatively, the AP radiographs of chronic varus or valgus deformities often showed a joint space larger than typical suggesting intrinsic stretching or laxity of the lateral or medial collateral ligament, whereas intraoperatively these ligaments were not lax. The AP radiograph of a knee with a fixed flexion contracture explains the inconsistency. The lateral and medial laxity of a flexed knee is several millimeters more than the extended knee, which is why flexion is the preferred position for performing an arthroscopic meniscectomy. When treating a patient with extrinsic laxity of a collateral or posterior cruciate ligament secondary to trauma, components are still aligned coincident with the native joint lines with use of the kinematic principles, and added constraint with use of implants that offer a box in the femoral component and a post on the tibial insert compensates for the extrinsic laxity. The use of cones and short stem extensions enables positioning of components coincident with the native joint line with a low risk of stem impingement of the femoral and tibial cortex.

24.7.1 Case Example, History

A 58-year-old male tore his ACL and PCL in his right knee in a motorcycle injury at age 24 and had an open medial meniscectomy. Preoperatively, the knee had advanced post-traumatic, postsurgical osteoarthritis with a 20° varus deformity and 15° fixed flexion contracture and limited range of motion from 15° to 90° of flexion (Fig. 24.15). Varus–valgus

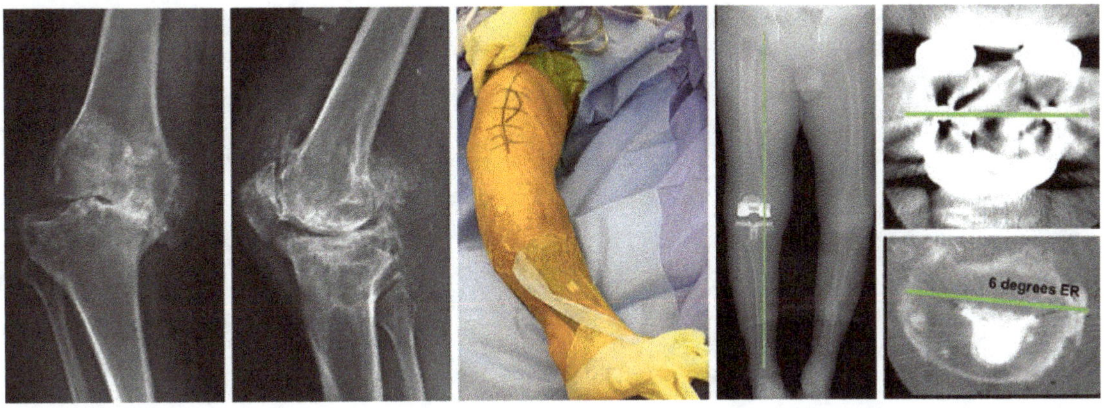

Fig. 24.15 Composite shows the preoperative radiographs of a post-traumatic knee with a severe varus deformity, flexion contracture, and chronic posterior cruciate ligament insufficiency; an intraoperative photograph of the varus deformity; and a postoperative computer tomographic scanogram of the limb and axial views of the femoral and tibial components. The AP radiograph shows a lateral joint space larger than typical suggesting intrinsic laxity of the lateral collateral ligament. Intraoperatively, the lateral collateral ligament was not lax. The AP radiograph of a knee with a fixed flexion contracture explains the inconsistency. The lateral laxity of a flexed knee is several millimeters more than the extended knee, which is why flexion is the preferred position for performing an arthroscopic lateral meniscectomy. Following the principles of kinematic alignment, the TKA restored the native alignment and laxities of the knee without a release of the medial collateral ligament and was performed with the posterior cruciate ligament substituting implants because of the torn posterior cruciate ligament

laxity testing at 0° and 30° indicated an intact MCL and LCL. Lachman and posterior drawer tests indicated chronic ACL and PCL insufficiency. His Oxford Knee Score was 11 points (48 best, 0 worst), Knee Society Score was 31 points, and Knee Society Function Score was 40 points.

24.7.2 Postoperative Result

KA with use of a posterior cruciate ligament substituting implant because of the torn PCL corrected this severe varus deformity of 20° and flexion contracture of 15° without ligament release. Postoperatively, the patient had a 6° varus hip–knee–ankle angle. The 6° angle between the transverse axes of the components was less than 106°, which is compatible with high function [24, 32]. At 2 years, the patient ambulated without difficulty or pain, range of motion improved to 0°–115°, and the Oxford Knee Score increased from 11 to 45 points, the Knee Society Score increased from 31 to 98 points, and Knee Society Function Score increased from 40 to 70 points.

24.8 Kinematic Alignment Corrects Severe Valgus Deformities Without Ligament Release

24.8.1 Case Example, History

A 68-year-old female with a prior arthroscopic meniscectomy developed osteoarthritis of the knee with a 25° valgus deformity, 17° fixed flexion contracture, and limited range of motion from 20° to 105° of flexion (Fig. 24.16). Varus–valgus laxity testing at 0° and 30° indicated an intact MCL and LCL. Lachman and posterior drawer tests indicated an intact ACL and PCL. Her Oxford Knee Score was 13 points (0 worst, 48 best), Knee Society Score was 24 points, and Knee Society Function Score was 30 points.

24.8.2 Postoperative Result

KA with use of a posterior cruciate ligament retaining implant corrected this severe valgus deformity and flexion contracture without ligament release. Postoperatively, the patient had a 3°

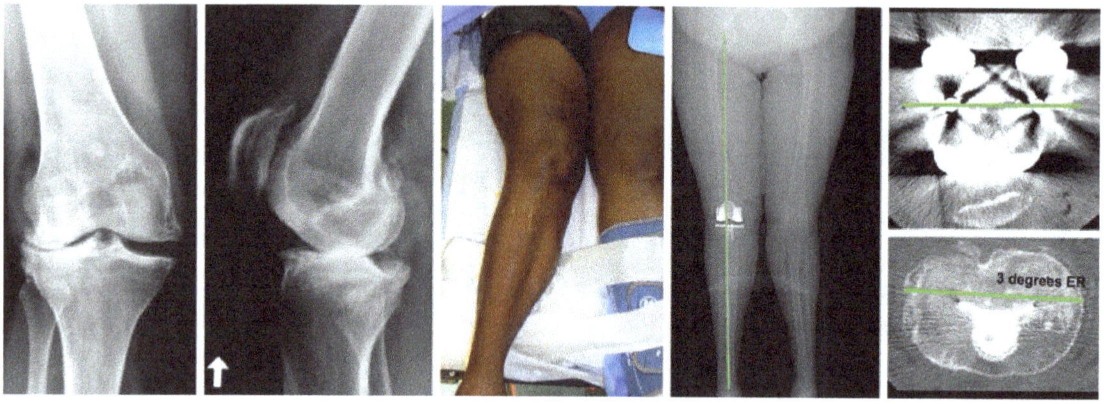

Fig. 24.16 Composite shows the preoperative radiographs of the knee with severe valgus deformity, intraoperative photograph of the severe valgus deformity, postoperative computer tomographic scanogram of the limb, and axial views of the femoral and tibial components. The AP radiograph shows a medial joint space larger than typical suggesting intrinsic laxity of the medial collateral ligament. Intraoperatively, the medial collateral ligament was not lax. The AP radiograph of a knee with a fixed flexion contracture explains the inconsistency. The medial laxity of a flexed knee is several millimeters more than the extended knee, which is why flexion is the preferred position for performing an arthroscopic medial meniscectomy. Following the principles of kinematic alignment, the TKA restored the alignments of the tibial joint line, knee, Q-angle, and limb close to those of the contralateral or native limb without release of the lateral collateral or lateral retinacular ligament in this patient with an intact posterior cruciate ligament

valgus hip–knee–ankle angle. The transverse axes of the femoral and tibial components were within 3° of parallel, which is compatible with high function [24, 32]. At 2 years, the patient ambulated without difficulty or pain, range of motion improved to 0°–119°, and the Oxford Knee Score increased from 13 to 44 points, Knee Society Score increased from 41 to 98 points, and Knee Society Function Score increased from 30 to 70 points.

24.9 Kinematic Alignment Has a Low Risk of Tibial Component Failure, Low Risk of Patellar Instability, and High Implant Survival at 10 Years

Accurately setting the slope of the tibial component in the sagittal plane results in negligible failure of the tibial component after KA [11, 23, 54, 55]. At 2–9 years of follow-up, the 0.3% incidence of tibial component failure (8 of 2725 prostheses) of patients treated with KA TKA was comparable if not lower than the 1.0% (54 of 5342 prostheses) incidence of failure from aseptic loosening of the femoral and/or tibial component for patients treated with MA TKA (Fig. 24.17) [56]. In kinematic alignment, posterior subsidence or posterior edge wear is the mechanism of tibial component failure, which is caused by resecting the tibia in 7° greater slope than the native [23]. In MA, varus or medial overload is the mechanism of tibial component failure, which is caused by uncorrectable instability in a compartment from changing the constitutional limb alignment to neutral and a high knee adduction moment during gait [12, 35, 39, 40]. Hence, restoring the slope of the native tibial joint line lowers the risk of posterior subsidence and posterior edge wear of the tibial component when performing KA TKA [11, 23].

Three biomechanical advantages explain the negligible risk of varus tibial loosening after kinematically aligned TKA. First, KA provides more physiological strains in the collateral ligaments than MA TKA by restoring the native joint lines and constitutional alignment without releasing ligaments [41]. Second, KA provides medial and lateral tibial compartment forces comparable to those of the native knee with no evidence of

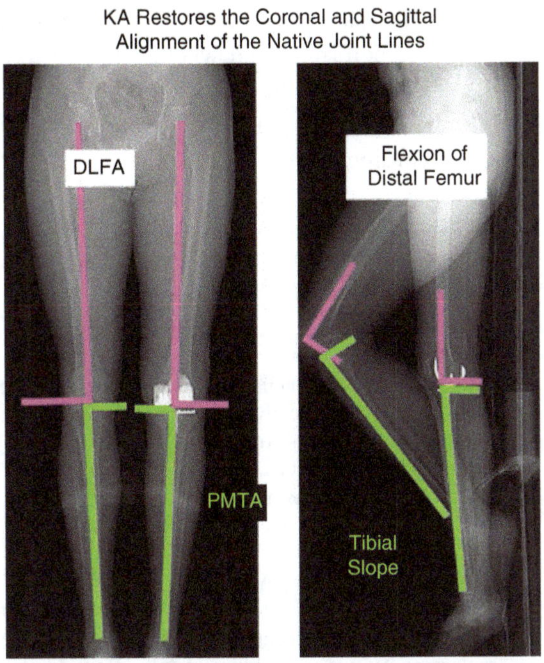

Fig. 24.17 Composite shows calipered KA restored the distal lateral femoral angle (DLFA) and proximal medial tibial angle (PMTA) of the TKA to those of the native knee in the sagittal plane (left) and the flexion–extension orientation of the distal femoral joint line and proximal tibial joint line of the TKA to those of the native knee in the coronal plane (right)

tibial compartment overload even when the postoperative alignments of the limb, knee, and tibial component are within the varus or valgus outlier range according to mechanical alignment criteria [17–19]. Third, KA is an especially promising option for patients with large varus coronal bowing of the tibia because the knee adduction moment and risk of varus overload are lower than after MA TKA [12].

Accurately setting the flexion of the femoral component in the sagittal plane results in negligible patellofemoral instability after KA [49–51]. At 1–10 years of follow-up, there is a 0.4% incidence of patellofemoral instability (13 of 3212 prostheses) in patients treated with kinematically aligned TKA. In KA, flexion of the femoral component greater than 10° with respect to the anatomic axis of the distal femur increased the risk of patellofemoral instability by downsizing the femoral component ~1–2 sizes, reducing the cross-sectional area of the trochlea, reducing the proximal reach of the flange by ~8 mm, and delaying the engagement of the patella during early flexion [49, 51]. A change in the native Q-angle does not cause patellofemoral instability as KA restores the native Q-angle, whereas mechanical alignment increases or decreases the native Q-angle in limbs with varus or valgus constitutional alignment, respectively (Figs. 24.5 and 24.6) [35]. The design of the femoral component does not cause patellofemoral instability as KA more closely restores the groove location and the sulcus angle of the native trochlea and trochlea morphology without overstuffing than mechanical alignment [57, 58]. Internal rotation about the center of the femoral component of ~3 relative to mechanical alignment does not cause patellofemoral instability as the ~1.5 mm increase in the distance between the lateral prosthetic trochlea and lateral femur is negligible [49]. The use of a distal referencing guide attached to an intraosseous positioning rod limits flexion of the femoral component to 1 ± 2° with respect to the femoral anatomic axis, which is 9° less than patients with patellofemoral instability (Fig. 24.9) [50]. Hence, limiting flexion of the femoral component lowers the risk of patellofemoral instability when performing kinematically aligned TKA [51].

The 10-year implant survivorship of a single-surgeon series of KA TKAs performed without restricting the degree of preoperative varus–valgus and flexion deformity is comparable if not higher than two single-surgeon series of MA TKAs. Using aseptic revision at 10 years as the end point, the 98.5% implant survival after 220 KA TKAs was 5.5% higher than the ~93% implant survival after 398 MA TKAs in the United States [59] and 4.5% higher than the ~94% implant survival after 270 MA TKAs in the United Kingdom [60]. The estimated number of revisions for 1000 patients is 15 for KA TKA and 70 and 60, respectively, for the US and UK studies of MA TKA. In the study of KA, four of seven revisions were associated with excessive flexion of the femoral component ($N = 3$) and reverse slope of the tibial component ($N = 1$) in the sagittal plane. Limiting flexion of the femoral component and restoring the slope of the native tibia could have lowered the incidence of these revisions [23,

49–51]. The postoperative alignment of the tibial component, knee, and limb in varus and valgus outlier ranges according to mechanical alignment criteria does not adversely affect the 10-year implant survival, yearly revision rate, and level of function as measured by the Oxford Knee and WOMAC scores [11]. Hence, restoring the native joint lines, Q-angle, and limb alignments unique to each patient results in high long-term implant survival regardless of the degree of preoperative varus-valgus and flexion deformity and postoperative alignment.

24.10 Summary

This chapter presented the philosophy of calipered KA and the surgical technique for setting components coincident to the native joint lines using ten calipered measurements, manual instruments, and nine verification checks. KA co-aligns the axes of the femoral and tibial components with the three axes of the native knee without ligament releases and without restricting the level of preoperative deformities and postoperative correction. The surgical goals are (1) restoration of the native alignments of the limb, Q-angle, and joint lines unique to each patient and (2) restoration of the laxities, tibial compartment forces, knee adduction moment, and gait of the native knee without ligament release. Measurement of the thicknesses of the femoral and tibial bone resections with a caliper and adjustment of the resections until they match those of the components after compensating for cartilage and bone wear and the 1 mm kerf from the saw cut restores the native joint lines with high reproducibility. These measurements are recorded intraoperatively on a worksheet, which verifies kinematic positioning of the components before cementation. Decision trees for balancing the TKA with CR and CS medial pivot tibial inserts balance the knee by adjusting the varus–valgus and slope of the tibial resection and not by releasing ligaments. Finally, the restoration of native alignment and tibial compartment forces lowers the risks of tibial component failure and patellofemoral instability and results in high implant survival at 10 years regardless of the level of preoperative deformity and whether the postoperative alignments of the tibial component, knee, and limb are within varus and valgus outlier ranges according to MA criteria.

References

1. Calliess T, Bauer K, Stukenborg-Colsman C, Windhagen H, Budde S, Ettinger M. PSI kinematic versus non-PSI mechanical alignment in total knee arthroplasty: a prospective, randomized study. Knee Surg Sports Traumatol Arthrosc. 2017;25(6):1743.
2. Courtney PM, Lee GC. Early outcomes of kinematic alignment in primary total knee arthroplasty: a meta-analysis of the literature. J Arthroplast. 2017;32(6):2028.
3. Dossett HG, Estrada NA, Swartz GJ, LeFevre GW, Kwasman BG. A randomised controlled trial of kinematically and mechanically aligned total knee replacements: two-year clinical results. Bone Joint J. 2014;96-B(7):907.
4. Lee YS, Howell SM, Won YY, Lee OS, Lee SH, Vahedi H, Teo SH. Kinematic alignment is a possible alternative to mechanical alignment in total knee arthroplasty. Knee Surg Sports Traumatol Arthrosc. 2017;25(11):3467.
5. Nam D, Nunley RM, Barrack RL. Patient dissatisfaction following total knee replacement: a growing concern? Bone Joint J. 2014;96-B(11 Supple A):96.
6. Li Y, Wang S, Wang Y, Yang M. Does kinematic alignment improve short-term functional outcomes after total knee arthroplasty compared with mechanical alignment? A systematic review and meta-analysis. J Knee Surg. 2018;31(1):78.
7. Matsumoto T, Takayama K, Ishida K, Hayashi S, Hashimoto S, Kuroda R. Radiological and clinical comparison of kinematically versus mechanically aligned total knee arthroplasty. Bone Joint J. 2017;99-B(5):640.
8. Nakamura S, Tian Y, Tanaka Y, Kuriyama S, Ito H, Furu M, Matsuda S. The effects of kinematically aligned total knee arthroplasty on stress at the medial tibia: a case study for varus knee. Bone Joint Res. 2017;6(1):43.
9. Waterson HB, Clement ND, Eyres KS, Mandalia VI, Toms AD. The early outcome of kinematic versus mechanical alignment in total knee arthroplasty: a prospective randomised control trial. Bone Joint J. 2016;98-B(10):1360.
10. Young SW, Walker ML, Bayan A, Briant-Evans T, Pavlou P, Farrington B. The Chitranjan S. Ranawat award: no difference in 2-year functional outcomes using kinematic versus mechanical alignment in TKA: a randomized controlled clinical trial. Clin Orthop Relat Res. 2017;475(1):9.

11. Howell SM, Shelton TJ, Hull ML. Implant survival and function ten years after kinematically aligned total knee arthroplasty. J Arthroplast. 2018;33:3678.
12. Niki Y, Nagura T, Nagai K, Kobayashi S, Harato K. Kinematically aligned total knee arthroplasty reduces knee adduction moment more than mechanically aligned total knee arthroplasty. Knee Surg Sports Traumatol Arthrosc. 2018;26(6):1629.
13. Blakeney W, Clément J, Ing M, Desmeules F, Hagemeister N, Rivière C, Vendittoli P. Kinematic alignment in total knee arthroplasty better reproduces normal gait than mechanical alignment. Knee Surg Sports Traumatol Arthrosc. 2019;27:1410–7.
14. Roth JD, Howell SM, Hull ML. Native knee laxities at 0 degrees, 45 degrees, and 90 degrees of flexion and their relationship to the goal of the gap-balancing alignment method of total knee arthroplasty. J Bone Joint Surg Am. 2015;97(20):1678.
15. Roth JD, Hull ML, Howell SM. The limits of passive motion are variable between and unrelated within normal tibiofemoral joints. J Orthop Res. 2015;33(11):1594.
16. Roth JD, Hull ML, Howell SM. Analysis of differences in laxities andneutral positions from native after kinematically aligned TKA using cruciate retaining implants. J Orthop Res. 2019;37:358–69.
17. Shelton TJ, Howell SM, Hull ML. A total knee arthroplasty is stiffer when the intraoperative tibial force is greater than the native knee. J Knee Surg. 2019;32:1008–14.
18. Shelton TJ, Howell SM, Hull ML. Is there a force target that predicts early patient-reported outcomes after kinematically aligned TKA? Clin Orthop Relat Res. 2019;477:1200–7.
19. Shelton TJ, Nedopil AJ, Howell SM, Hull ML. Do varus or valgus outliers have higher forces in the medial or lateral compartments than those which are in-range after a kinematically aligned total knee arthroplasty? Limb and joint line alignment after kinematically aligned total knee arthroplasty. Bone Joint J. 2017;99-B(10):1319.
20. Johnson JM, Mahfouz MR, Midillioglu MR, Nedopil AJ, Howell SM. Three-dimensional analysis of the tibial resection plane relative to the arthritic tibial plateau in total knee arthroplasty. J Exp Orthop. 2017;4(1):27.
21. Nedopil AJ, Singh AK, Howell SM, Hull ML. Does calipered kinematically aligned TKA restore native left to right symmetry of the lower limb and improve function? J Arthroplast. 2018;33(2):398.
22. Riviere C, Iranpour F, Harris S, Auvinet E, Aframian A, Chabrand P, Cobb J. The kinematic alignment technique for TKA reliably aligns the femoral component with the cylindrical axis. Orthop Traumatol Surg Res. 2017;103(7):1069.
23. Nedopil AJ, Howell SM, Hull ML. What mechanisms are associated with tibial component failure after kinematically-aligned total knee arthroplasty? Int Orthop. 2017;41(8):1561.
24. Nedopil AJ, Howell SM, Rudert M, Roth J, Hull ML. How frequent is rotational mismatch within 0 degrees +/−10 degrees in kinematically aligned total knee arthroplasty? Orthopedics. 2013;36(12):e1515.
25. Coughlin KM, Incavo SJ, Churchill DL, Beynnon BD. Tibial axis and patellar position relative to the femoral epicondylar axis during squatting. J Arthroplast. 2003;18(8):1048.
26. Hollister AM, Jatana S, Singh AK, Sullivan WW, Lupichuk AG. The axes of rotation of the knee. Clin Orthop Relat Res. 1993;(290):259.
27. Iranpour F, Merican AM, Baena FR, Cobb JP, Amis AA. Patellofemoral joint kinematics: the circular path of the patella around the trochlear axis. J Orthop Res. 2010;28(5):589.
28. Pinskerova V, Iwaki H, Freeman MA. The shapes and relative movements of the femur and tibia at the knee. Der Orthopade. 2000;29(Suppl 1):S3.
29. Iwaki H, Pinskerova V, Freeman MA. Tibiofemoral movement 1: the shapes and relative movements of the femur and tibia in the unloaded cadaver knee. J Bone Joint Surg Br. 2000;82(8):1189.
30. Weber WE, Weber EFM. Mechanik der menschlichen Gehwerkzeuge. Göttingen: Verlag der Dietrichschen Buchhandlung; 1836.
31. Eckhoff DG, Bach JM, Spitzer VM, Reinig KD, Bagur MM, Baldini TH, Flannery NM. Three-dimensional mechanics, kinematics, and morphology of the knee viewed in virtual reality. J Bone Joint Surg Am. 2005;87(Suppl 2):71.
32. Nedopil AJ, Howell SM, Hull ML. Does malrotation of the tibial and femoral components compromise function in kinematically aligned total knee arthroplasty? Orthop Clin North Am. 2016;47(1):41.
33. Paschos NK, Howell SM, Johnson JM, Mahfouz MR. Can kinematic tibial templates assist the surgeon locating the flexion and extension plane of the knee? Knee. 2017;24(5):1006.
34. Nam D, Lin KM, Howell SM, Hull ML. Femoral bone and cartilage wear is predictable at 0 degrees and 90 degrees in the osteoarthritic knee treated with total knee arthroplasty. Knee Surg Sports Traumatol Arthrosc. 2014;22(12):2975.
35. Singh AK, Nedopil AJ, Howell SM, Hull ML. Does alignment of the limb and tibial width determine relative narrowing between compartments when planning mechanically aligned TKA? Arch Orthop Trauma Surg. 2017;138(1):91.
36. Bellemans J, Colyn W, Vandenneucker H, Victor J. The Chitranjan Ranawat award: is neutral mechanical alignment normal for all patients? The concept of constitutional varus. Clin Orthop Relat Res. 2012;470(1):45.
37. Shetty GM, Mullaji A, Bhayde S, Nha KW, Oh HK. Factors contributing to inherent varus alignment of lower limb in normal Asian adults: role of tibial plateau inclination. Knee. 2014;21(2):544.
38. Song MH, Yoo SH, Kang SW, Kim YJ, Park GT, Pyeun YS. Coronal alignment of the lower limb and

the incidence of constitutional varus knee in Korean females. Knee Surg Relat Res. 2015;27(1):49.
39. Gu Y, Howell SM, Hull ML. Simulation of total knee arthroplasty in 5 degrees or 7 degrees valgus: a study of gap imbalances and changes in limb and knee alignments from native. J Orthop Res. 2017;35(9):2031.
40. Gu Y, Roth JD, Howell SM, Hull ML. How frequently do four methods for mechanically aligning a total knee arthroplasty cause collateral ligament imbalance and change alignment from normal in white patients? J Bone Joint Surg. 2014;96(12):e101.
41. Delport H, Labey L, Innocenti B, De Corte R, Vander Sloten J, Bellemans J. Restoration of constitutional alignment in TKA leads to more physiological strains in the collateral ligaments. Knee Surg Sports Traumatol Arthrosc. 2015;23(8):2159.
42. Meneghini RM, Ziemba-Davis MM, Lovro LR, Ireland PH, Damer BM. Can intraoperative sensors determine the "target" ligament balance? Early outcomes in total knee arthroplasty. J Arthroplast. 2016;31(10):2181.
43. Roth JD, Howell SM, Hull ML. Kinematically aligned total knee arthroplasty limits high tibial forces, differences in tibial forces between compartments, and abnormal tibial contact kinematics during passive flexion. Knee Surg Sports Traumatol Arthrosc. 2018;26(6):1589.
44. Verstraete MA, Meere PA, Salvadore G, Victor J, Walker PS. Contact forces in the tibiofemoral joint from soft tissue tensions: implications to soft tissue balancing in total knee arthroplasty. J Biomech. 2017;58:195.
45. Ji HM, Han J, Jin DS, Seo H, Won YY. Kinematically aligned TKA can align knee joint line to horizontal. Knee Surg Sports Traumatol Arthrosc. 2016;24(8):2436.
46. Eckhoff D, Hogan C, DiMatteo L, Robinson M, Bach J. Difference between the epicondylar and cylindrical axis of the knee. Clin Orthop Relat Res. 2007;461:238.
47. Howell SM, Kuznik K, Hull ML, Siston RA. Longitudinal shapes of the tibia and femur are unrelated and variable. Clin Orthop Relat Res. 2010;468(4):1142.
48. Howell SM, Papadopoulos S, Kuznik KT, Hull ML. Accurate alignment and high function after kinematically aligned TKA performed with generic instruments. Knee Surg Sports Traumatol Arthrosc. 2013;21(10):2271.
49. Brar AS, Howell SM, Hull ML, Mahfouz MR. Does kinematic alignment and flexion of a femoral component designed for mechanical alignment reduce the proximal and lateral reach of the trochlea? J Arthroplast. 2016;31(8):1808.
50. Ettinger M, Calliess T, Howell SM. Does a positioning rod or a patient-specific guide result in more natural femoral flexion in the concept of kinematically aligned total knee arthroplasty? Arch Orthop Trauma Surg. 2017;137(1):105.
51. Nedopil AJ, Howell SM, Hull ML. What clinical characteristics and radiographic parameters are associated with patellofemoral instability after kinematically aligned total knee arthroplasty? Int Orthop. 2017;41(2):283.
52. Howell SM, Chen J, Hull ML. Variability of the location of the tibial tubercle affects the rotational alignment of the tibial component in kinematically aligned total knee arthroplasty. Knee Surg Sports Traumatol Arthrosc. 2013;21(10):2288.
53. Christen B, Heesterbeek P, Wymenga A, Wehrli U. Posterior cruciate ligament balancing in total knee replacement: the quantitative relationship between tightness of the flexion gap and tibial translation. J Bone Joint Surg Br. 2007;89(8):1046.
54. Howell SM, Howell SJ, Kuznik KT, Cohen J, Hull ML. Does a kinematically aligned total knee arthroplasty restore function without failure regardless of alignment category? Clin Orthop Relat Res. 2013;471(3):1000.
55. Howell SM, Papadopoulos S, Kuznik K, Ghaly LR, Hull ML. Does varus alignment adversely affect implant survival and function six years after kinematically aligned total knee arthroplasty? Int Orthop. 2015;39(11):2117–24.
56. Ritter MA, Davis KE, Meding JB, Pierson JL, Berend ME, Malinzak RA. The effect of alignment and BMI on failure of total knee replacement. J Bone Joint Surg Am. 2011;93(17):1588.
57. Lozano R, Campanelli V, Howell S, Hull M. Kinematic alignment more closely restores the groove location and the sulcus angle of the native trochlea than mechanical alignment: implications for prosthetic design. Knee Surg Sports Traumatol Arthrosc. 2019;27:1504–13.
58. Riviere C, Iranpour F, Harris S, Auvinet E, Aframian A, Parratte S, Cobb J. Differences in trochlear parameters between native and prosthetic kinematically or mechanically aligned knees. Orthop Traumatol Surg Res. 2018;104(2):165.
59. Parratte S, Pagnano MW, Trousdale RT, Berry DJ. Effect of postoperative mechanical axis alignment on the fifteen-year survival of modern, cemented total knee replacements. J Bone Joint Surg Am. 2010;92(12):2143.
60. Bonner TJ, Eardley WG, Patterson P, Gregg PJ. The effect of post-operative mechanical axis alignment on the survival of primary total knee replacements after a follow-up of 15 years. J Bone Joint Surg Br. 2011;93(9):1217.

25

Utilization of Personalized Instruments for KA TKA

William G. Blakeney and Pascal-André Vendittoli

Key Points

- Performing a kinematically aligned (KA) TKA requires accurate planning of resections and precise tools to achieve the set goals.
- CT-based patient-specific instrumentation (PSI) is our preferred method for performing KA TKA implantation.
- The restricted kinematic alignment protocol (rKA) has been developed as an alternative solution to the "true" KA technique in situations of patients with atypical knee anatomy.
- The rKA protocol limits the femoral and tibial prosthesis coronal alignment to within ±5° of neutral, with the overall combined lower limb coronal orientation within ±3° of neutral.
- PSI allows for pre-operative planning and fine-tuning adjustments.
- Compared to standard instruments, computer navigation or robotic surgery, PSI results in a shorter operating time and decreased instrumentation.
- PSI is a simple, standardised solution for a patient-specific rKA protocol in TKA, with many benefits to the surgeon and patient.

W. G. Blakeney
Department of Surgery, CIUSSS-de-L'Est-de-L'Ile-de-Montréal, Hôpital Maisonneuve Rosemont, Montréal, QC, Canada

Department of Surgery, Albany Health Campus, Albany, WA, Australia

P.-A. Vendittoli (✉)
Department of Surgery, CIUSSS-de-L'Est-de-L'Ile-de-Montréal, Hôpital Maisonneuve Rosemont, Montréal, QC, Canada

Department of Surgery, Université de Montréal, Montréal, QC, Canada

25.1 Personalized Instrumentation to Reproduce Patients' Specific Anatomy

There is a very wide variation in patients' knee anatomy. The precise restoration of this anatomy during total knee arthroplasty (TKA) may improve knee balance, clinical function and patient satisfaction. In the early ages of TKA, implant sizes and surgical precision were limited. The amount of deviation from a patient's anatomy that may impact on clinical results is not clear. However, in the era of personalized joint replacement, we believe that a precision of within 2 mm or 2° should be the goal. Performing a kinematically aligned (KA) TKA requires accurate planning of resections and precise tools to achieve the set goals. Patient-specific instrumentation is a very attractive solution. These patient-specific instruments (PSI) are constructed based upon preoperative planning using either tomographic or magnetic resonance imaging. 3D models of the patient's knee, hip and ankle are reconstructed and anatomical landmarks are identified to set the parameters of tibia and femur resections according to the surgeon's preferences. Intraoperatively, the custom guides or PSI is applied to the bone surfaces to guide resections. The PSI defines both the implant orientation and size.

Generally, CT-based imaging is preferred for KA TKA, as measurement of the patient's bony anatomy is required to measure the constitutional knee alignment of the patient. The majority of patients undergoing TKA have minimal bone loss with most of the articular surface wear being cartilaginous. Aligning the resections to the bony anatomy of the femur and tibia, accounting for an equal cartilage layer medial and lateral, allows restoration of the native joint line and alignment. When bone loss is present, however, this should be considered when planning resection planes. A meta-analysis compared the accuracy of MRI- and CT-based systems for PSI [1]. They reported the incidence of outliers greater than 3° was 12.5% for CT-based systems vs. 16.9% for MRI-based systems, though this difference was not statistically significant.

The accuracy of PSI has been assessed by numerous studies and meta-analyses [2–10]. Three meta-analyses reported improved coronal femoral alignment with PSI compared to conventional instrumentation [6–8]. However, four other meta-analyses failed to detect a significant difference [2–5]. The tibial coronal alignment was demonstrated to favour conventional instrumentation over PSI in four meta-analyses [2, 4, 5, 8], whereas three did not detect any significant differences [3, 6, 7]. No significant difference was detected in femoral sagittal alignment in any of the meta-analyses. Four studies found an increased risk of tibial sagittal plane malalignment with PSI [2, 4, 5, 8]. One study found improved rotational alignment with PSI [10]. These studies all looked at the accuracy of a mechanical alignment (MA) protocol. The accuracy of PSI for a KA technique is likely to replicate these results.

25.2 Restricted Kinematic Alignment Protocol and Personalized Instrumentation

We developed and have used clinically, since 2011, a restricted KA protocol (rKA, see Chap. 17) [11]. The PSI method described (MyKnee®, Medacta International SA, Castel San Pietro, Switzerland) is our preferred method for performing rKA TKA implantation. Pre-operative CT scans according to the standardised MyKnee® protocol are taken. Cutting blocks and 3D bone models of the knee are then produced according to the preferences of the surgeon. The rKA protocol aims to reproduce the patient's constitutional knee anatomy within a defined safe range [11, 12]. The rKA technique limits the femoral and tibial prosthesis coronal alignment to within ±5° of neutral, with the overall combined lower limb coronal orientation within ±3° of neutral. As discussed previously (see rKA, Chap. 17), in more complex cases requiring modification of the anatomy of both tibia and femur to stay within these limits, our practice is to preserve femoral anatomy as closely as possible and perform greater modifications on the tibial side. We believe that the femoral flexion axis plays the more significant role in knee kinematics. Femoral rotation is set at 0° of rotation to the posterior condyles. The femoral size is matched to the best fit of the distal femoral anatomy, and sagittal orientation is set to avoid notching, usually at 2–4° of flexion with respect to the mechanical axis of the femur. The tibial posterior slope is set at 3° as recommended by the manufacturer. Application of the rKA protocol is performed by an experienced MyKnee® engineer at Medacta International. Then, the pre-operative plan is sent to the surgeon according to these specifications for approval (Fig. 25.1). Images of the cuts and implants are simulated and provided (Fig. 25.2). The surgeon can modify the pre-operative plan if desired.

At the time of surgery, sterilised 3D bone models are provided with the PSI cutting guides (Fig. 25.3). Femoral and tibial cutting guides can be tested on the 3D bone models to assess the optimal fit (Fig. 25.4). As we use a CT-based

MyKnee | CT BASED | REV.0 - 28.nov.2018

MyKnee Surgical Planning Report

CASE CODE	[redacted]
SURGEON	Pascal-André Vendittoli
SURGERY DATE	2018-12-22
SURGICAL APPROACH	Medial
PRODUCT	GMK-Sphere
BLOCKS	STD+MIS

LEFT TOTAL KNEE	PRE-OP	POST-OP
HKA	175.5	180.0
Femoral Valgus (from bone)	2.0	2.0
Tibial Varus (from bone)	2.0	2.0
Tibia Posterior Slope	13.0	2.0
Epicondyles vs Post. Cond.	2.0	

IMPLANTS	DEFAULT	CHANGED
Femoral Implant Size	3+	
Tibial Implant Size	3	

PRE-OP LONG AXIS

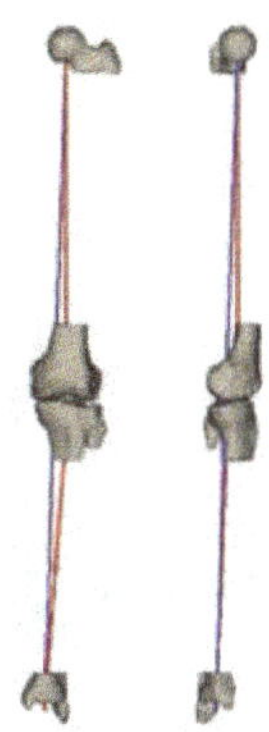

CAUTION

This case is based on CT data:

REMOVE FROM THE BONE THE CARTILAGE AND SOFT TISSUES COVERING THE CUTTING BLOCK CONTACT AREAS.

All measurements shown are from the bone and do not include the thickness of the cartilage.

FEMUR

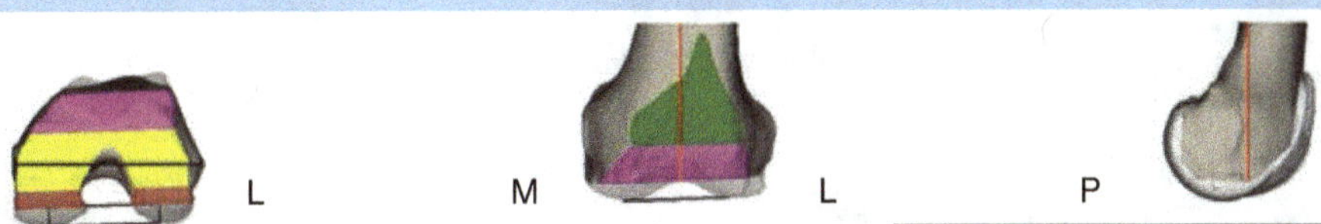

	DEFAULT	CHANGED
FEMORAL RESECTIONS [mm]		
Lateral Posterior Cut	8	
Medial Posterior Cut	8	
Lateral Distal Cut	8	
Medial Distal Cut	8	
FEMORAL ANGLES [deg]		
Valgus	2	
Flexum	3	
ROTATION [deg]		
External Rotation vs. Post. Condyles	0	

CAUTION

Accurately clear the posterior condyles from any osteophytes and overhanging bone.

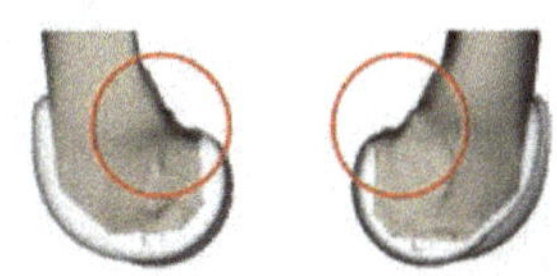

TIBIA

	DEFAULT	CHANGED
TIBIAL RESECTIONS [mm]		
Lateral Tibial Cut	9	
Medial Tibial Cut	9	
TIBIAL ANGLES [deg]		
Varus	2	
Posterior Slope	2	

COMMENTS

Biomechanical and Radiostereometric Analysis of the GMK Sphere Primary Total Knee Replacement.
A Randomized, Double Blind Comparison of Anatomical Versus Mechanical Alignment in Total Knee Replacement.

Medacta | **CONFIDENTIAL** | myknee@medacta.ch | M08.59 rev.7

Fig. 25.1 Preoperative plan for rKA alignment

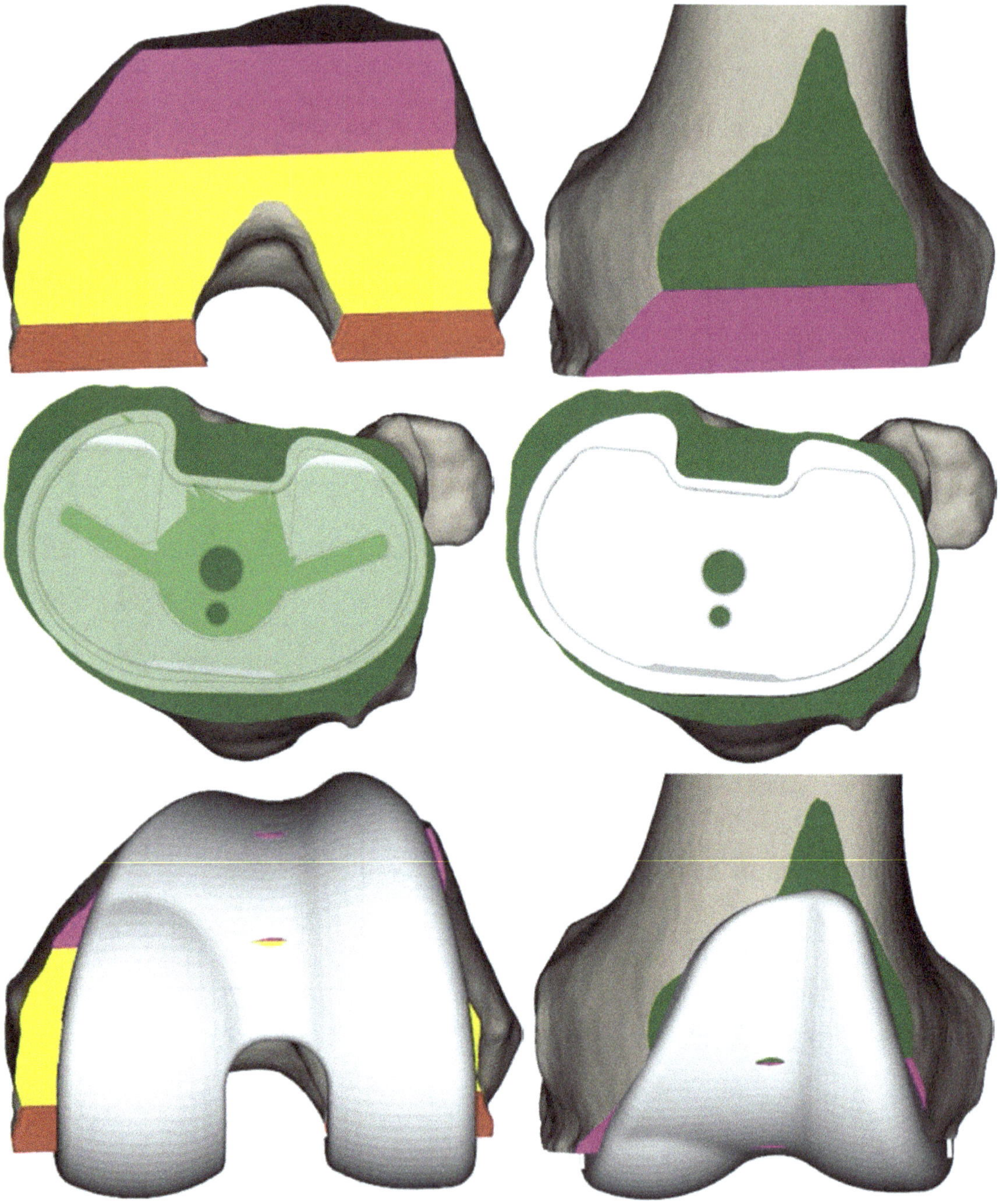

Fig. 25.2 Images of the resulting bone cuts with and without the implant are provided

protocol, the cartilage and soft tissues covering the cutting block contact areas must be removed from the bone with the help of a diathermy blade. The contact areas can be identified on the bone model (Fig. 25.2). The femoral cutting block is then placed manually on the distal femur, in the position of maximum stability (Fig. 25.5). Once the positioning is deemed satisfactory, the cutting block is fixed with pins. As well as positioning the guide for distal femoral resection, these pins set the rotation of the 4-in-1 cutting guide and hence femoral rotation.

For the tibial resection, the process is repeated with the tibial guide and bone model. To ensure

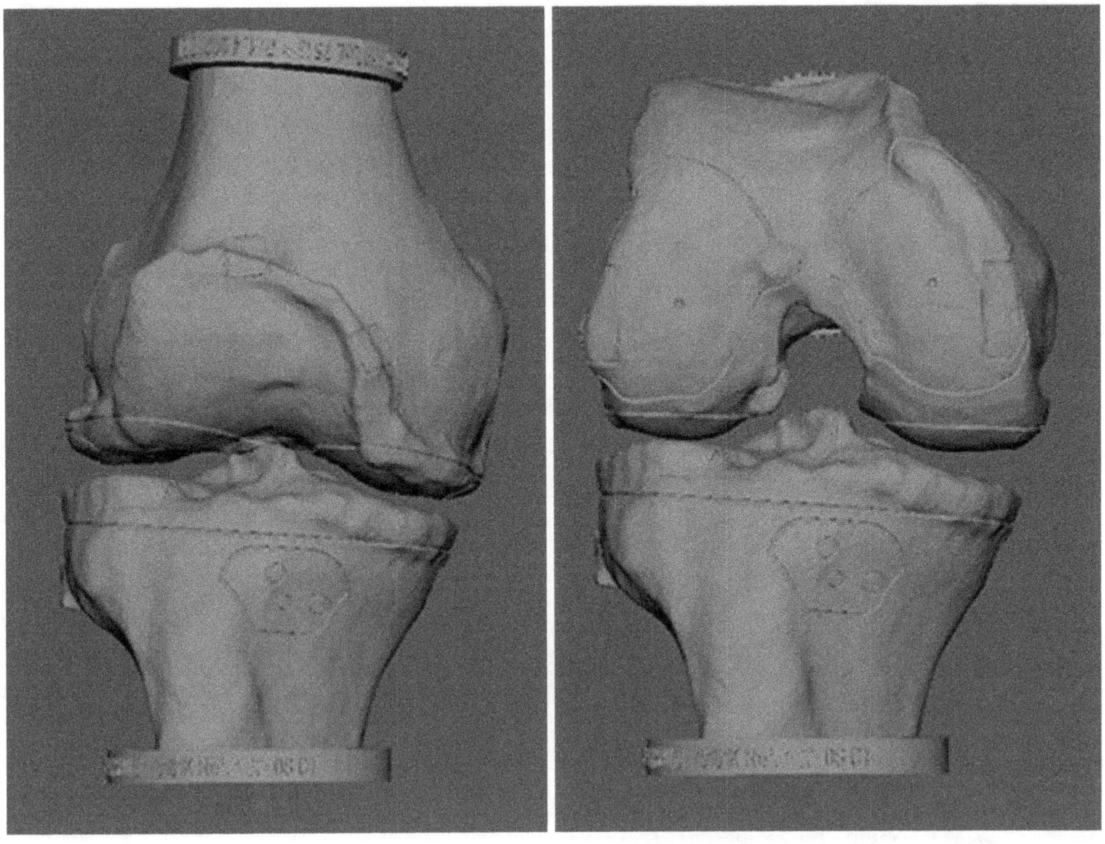

Fig. 25.3 3D bone models for an rKA case showing the equal medial and lateral cut thicknesses and the resulting joint line

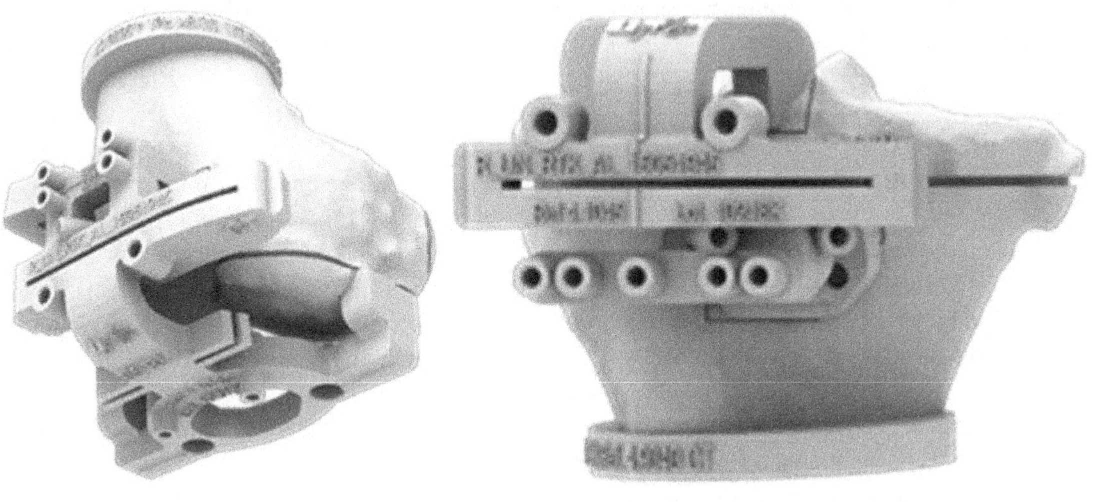

Fig. 25.4 Cutting blocks assembled on the 3D bone models to assess the optimal fit

maximum stability of the guide, the surgeon should verify that the points of contact between the tibial cutting block and the tibial bone correspond with the bone model (Fig. 25.4). Once the cutting guide has been properly positioned on the tibia, cut parameters are automatically set for the knee according to the preoperative plan (Fig. 25.6). With implant trials in place,

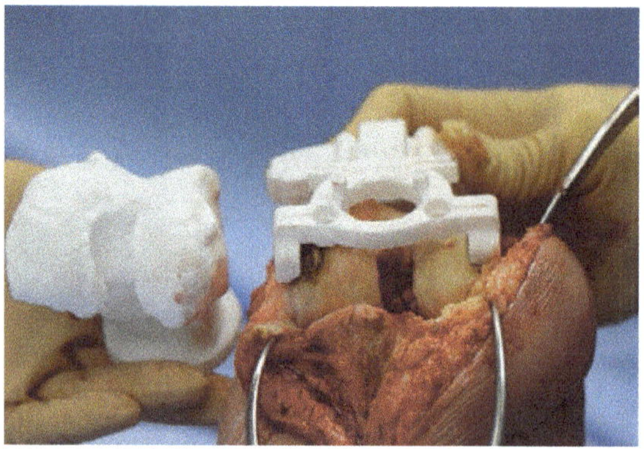

Fig. 25.5 Femoral block on the femur

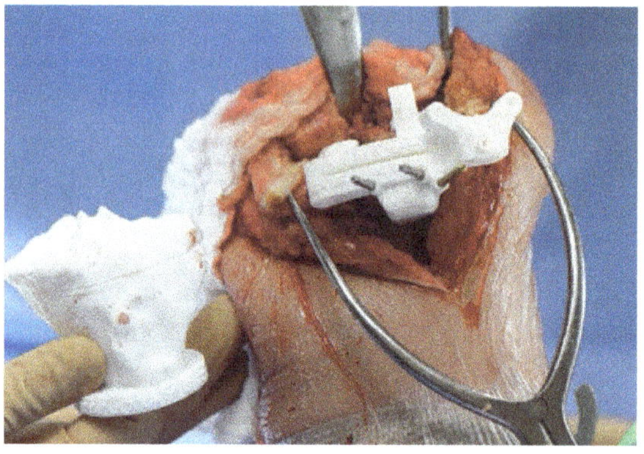

Fig. 25.6 Tibial block on bone

we adjust tibial rotation manually to match the femur in flexion and extension.

25.3 Benefits of Patient-Specific Instruments

The PSI method used by the authors (MyKnee®, Medacta International SA, Castel San Pietro, Switzerland) has demonstrated accuracy of implant positioning in a number of studies [13–16]. A study of 50 consecutive TKAs performed using the MyKnee® PSI reported 98% were within 3° of the planned HKA angle [13]. Predicted coronal plane orientation of the tibial and femoral components was achieved in 100% and 96% of patients, respectively. The sagittal orientation of the femoral and tibial components was achieved in 98% and in 92% of patients, respectively. Accurate femoral rotation within 3° of planned was accomplished in 90% of patients.

The majority of studies assessing PSI have demonstrated improved positioning of the femoral component compared to the tibia. It is the authors' experience that the femoral cutting guide is easier to position accurately due to the conforming anatomy of the distal femur. We would recommend that when positioning the tibia, the surgeon spends extra time to confirm accurate placement. Secondary checks may be performed with the alignment guides and following resection with callipers. In most cases of rKA TKA, no ligament imbalance is created. Using PSI for rKA thus simplifies the TKA procedure to a precise application of the cutting block on the patient's bone and avoidance of cut deviation using the oscillating saw. We prefer to use the Precision saw blade (Stryker, USA) for these procedures. This saw blade has an oscillating tip, but the core of the blade stays still. It eliminates blade vibration in the PSI cutting slot which avoids creation of plastic wear/debris.

Another benefit of PSI is standardisation of the procedure with all the planning done preoperatively, compared to computer navigation [11] or robotic surgery where it is done at the time of surgery. It is also rare to require recutting, in contrast to the calliper technique with conventional instrumentation (see Chap. 24). This may result in a shorter operating time. A meta-analysis demonstrated minor reductions in total operative time (−4.4 min, $p = 0.002$) and blood loss (−37.9 mL, $p = 0.015$) for PSI compared to conventional instrumentation [17]. The included studies all used mechanical alignment technique for implanting TKA. The time saved may be greater with a patient-specific alignment technique, where bespoke planning is required.

Other potential benefits include decreased instrumentation with less tray processing requirements and improved accuracy for the novice or low-volume surgeon (Fig. 25.7). A trial comparing PSI with conventional instrumentation demonstrates a 90-min reduction in instrument processing time [18]. With savings

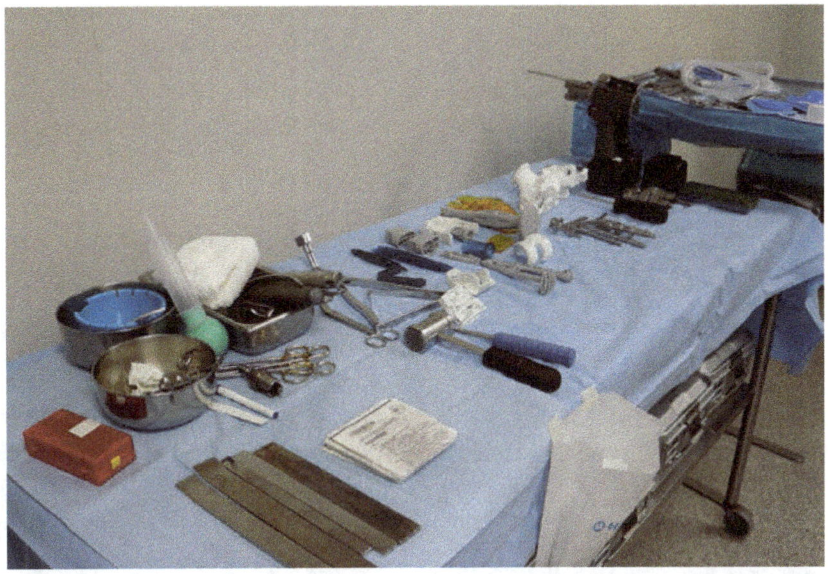

Fig. 25.7 Minimal instrumentation to perform TKA

in labour, instrumentation and surgical time, this equated to a total savings of $628 per case. They did note, however, that this was offset by the high cost of pre-operative imaging and fabrication of the PSI. These costs, however, are likely to be much less than those associated with robotic surgery, particularly in low-volume centres. Experienced surgeons are more accurate in their bone cuts using standard TKA instrumentation compared to surgeons with less experience [19]. Patient-specific instrumentation has been shown to improve accuracy of inexperienced surgeons to the equivalent of expert surgeons, in a study using sawbone knee models [20]. Most of the clinical studies comparing the accuracy of PSI with conventional instrumentation are conducted in high-volume centres with experienced arthroplasty surgeons [8] and may be subject to expert bias.

PSI is a simple, standardised solution for a patient-specific rKA protocol in TKA, with many benefits to the surgeon and patient.

25.4 Case Example

An active 58-year-old female, with advanced knee osteoarthritis, presents for consideration of TKA, after failure of conservative treatment. Six years ago, she had a right TKA in another institution with unsatisfying clinical results (pain and stiffness). Two years ago, she underwent a right TKA revision (by the initial surgeon) which did not improve her right knee function. She is severely disabled by her left knee OA but very hesitant to accept another TKA after the disappointing right knee results (Fig. 25.8). We offered her a left knee rKA TKA with PSI. A pre-operative planning CT scan demonstrates pre-operative femoral valgus of 2° and tibial varus of 2° (Figs. 25.1 and 25.2). The pre-operative HKA was 4.5° varus, as a result of cartilage wear on the medial side of the tibia. The patient elected to undergo TKA using the rKA protocol. As is the case with ~50% of cases, no modifications were required from her pre-operative constitutional alignment to stay within the safe range defined in our protocol, allowing a pure KA implantation. Frontal alignment was therefore 2° valgus for the femoral component and 2° varus for the tibial component, with an overall postoperative HKA of 0°. The patient underwent an uneventful post-operative recovery (Fig. 25.8b). At 4 months post-surgery, her prosthetic knee felt natural without restrictions. She is now requesting us to perform a second revision of her right knee to correct the implant orientations.

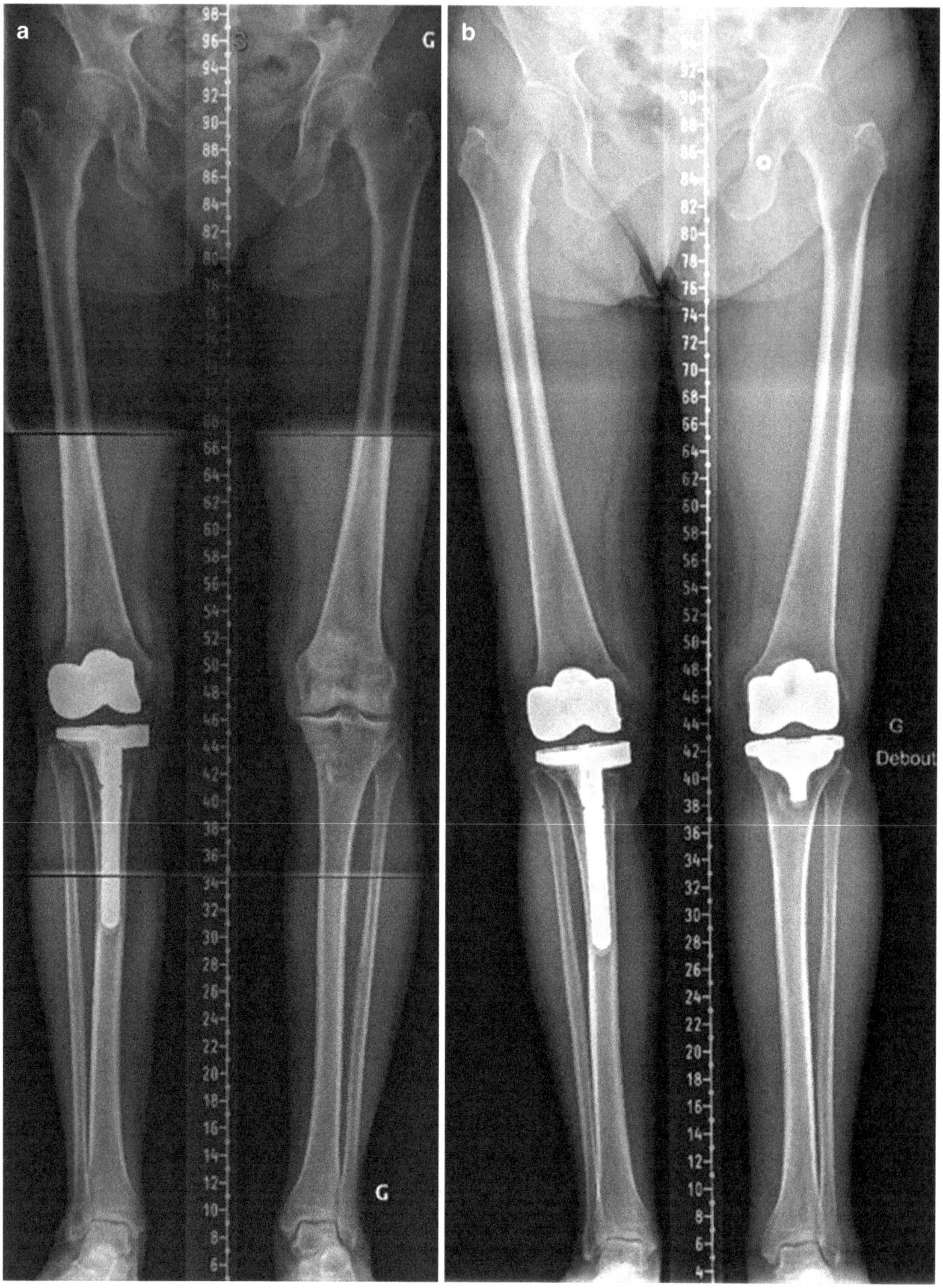

Fig. 25.8 Preoperative (**a**) and post-operative (**b**) standing long radiographs of the left knee rKA TKA with PSI. Patient unsatisfied with her right revision TKA (performed elsewhere) requested to be revised a second time

References

1. Stirling P, Valsalan Mannambeth R, Soler A, Batta V, Malhotra RK, Kalairajah Y. Computerised tomography vs magnetic resonance imaging for modeling of patient-specific instrumentation in total knee arthroplasty. World J Orthop. 2015;6(2):290–7. Epub 2015/03/21
2. Fu H, Wang J, Zhou S, Cheng T, Zhang W, Wang Q, et al. No difference in mechanical alignment and femoral component placement between patient-specific instrumentation and conventional instrumentation in TKA. Knee Surg Sports Traumatol Arthrosc. 2015;23(11):3288–95. Epub 17 Jul 2014
3. Jiang J, Kang X, Lin Q, Teng Y, An L, Ma J, et al. Accuracy of patient-specific instrumentation compared with conventional instrumentation in total knee arthroplasty. Orthopedics. 2015;38(4):e305–13. Epub 23 Apr 2015
4. Shen C, Tang ZH, Hu JZ, Zou GY, Xiao RC, Yan DX. Patient-specific instrumentation does not improve accuracy in total knee arthroplasty. Orthopedics. 2015;38(3):e178–88. Epub 12 Mar 2015
5. Zhang QM, Chen JY, Li H, Chai W, Ni M, Zhang ZD, et al. No evidence of superiority in reducing outliers of component alignment for patient-specific instrumentation for total knee arthroplasty: a systematic review. Orthop Surg. 2015;7(1):19–25. Epub 25 Feb 2015
6. Sharareh B, Schwarzkopf R. Review article: patient-specific versus standard instrumentation for total knee arthroplasty. J Orthop Surg (Hong Kong). 2015;23(1):100–6. Epub 30 Apr 2015
7. Cavaignac E, Pailhe R, Laumond G, Murgier J, Reina N, Laffosse JM, et al. Evaluation of the accuracy of patient-specific cutting blocks for total knee arthroplasty: a meta-analysis. Int Orthop. 2015;39(8):1541–52. Epub 11 Oct 2014
8. Thienpont E, Schwab PE, Fennema P. A systematic review and meta-analysis of patient-specific instrumentation for improving alignment of the components in total knee replacement. Bone Joint J. 2014;96-B(8):1052–61. Epub 3 Aug 2014
9. Ageberg E, Björkman A, Rosén B, Roos EM. Principles of brain plasticity in improving sensorimotor function of the knee and leg in patients with anterior cruciate ligament injury: a double-blind randomized exploratory trial. BMC Musculoskelet Disord. 2012; 13:68.
10. Mannan A, Akinyooye D, Hossain F. A meta-analysis of functional outcomes in patient-specific instrumented knee arthroplasty. J Knee Surg. 2017;30(7):668–74. Epub 3 Dec 2016
11. Hutt JRB, LeBlanc MA, Massé V, Lavigne M, Vendittoli PA. Kinematic TKA using navigation: surgical technique and initial results. Orthop Traumatol Surg Res. 2016;102(1):99–104.
12. Almaawi AM, Hutt JRB, Masse V, Lavigne M, Vendittoli P-A. The impact of mechanical and restricted kinematic alignment on knee anatomy in total knee arthroplasty. J Arthroplast. 2017;32(7):2133–40.
13. Nabavi A, Olwill CM, Do M, Wanasawage T, Harris IA. Patient-specific instrumentation for total knee arthroplasty. J Orthop Surg (Hong Kong). 2017;25(1):2309499016684754. Epub 1 Feb 2017
14. Lyras DN, Greenhow R, Loucks C. Restoration of the mechanical axis in total knee artrhoplasty using patient-matched technology cutting blocks. A retrospective study of 132 cases. Arch Bone Joint Surg. 2017;5(5):283–9. Epub 12 Dec 2017
15. Koch PP, Muller D, Pisan M, Fucentese SF. Radiographic accuracy in TKA with a CT-based patient-specific cutting block technique. Knee Surg Sports Traumatol Arthrosc. 2013;21(10):2200–5. Epub 15 Aug 2013
16. Anderl W, Pauzenberger L, Kolblinger R, Kiesselbach G, Brandl G, Laky B, et al. Patient-specific instrumentation improved mechanical alignment, while early clinical outcome was comparable to conventional instrumentation in TKA. Knee Surg Sports Traumatol Arthrosc. 2016;24(1):102–11. Epub 20 Oct 2014
17. Thienpont E, Schwab PE, Fennema P. Efficacy of patient-specific instruments in total knee arthroplasty: a systematic review and meta-analysis. J Bone Joint Surg Am. 2017;99(6):521–30. Epuв 16 Mar 2017
18. Barrack RL, Ruh EL, Williams BM, Ford AD, Foreman K, Nunley RM. Patient specific cutting blocks are currently of no proven value. J Bone Joint Surg Br. 2012;94(11 Suppl A):95–9. Epub 9 Nov 2012
19. Plaskos C, Hodgson AJ, Inkpen K, McGraw RW. Bone cutting errors in total knee arthroplasty. J Arthroplast. 2002;17(6):698–705. Epub 7 Sept 2002
20. Jones GG, Logishetty K, Clarke S, Collins R, Jaere M, Harris S, et al. Do patient-specific instruments (PSI) for UKA allow non-expert surgeons to achieve the same saw cut accuracy as expert surgeons? Arch Orthop Trauma Surg. 2018;138:1601–8. Epub 5 Sept 2018

26

Technical Aspects and Tips to Perform Computer-assisted Surgery and Robotic Surgery

M. Cievet-Bonfils, C. Batailler, T. Lording,
E. Servien, and S. Lustig

26.1 Introduction

Computer-assisted surgery (CAS) and robotic surgery have shown promise for joint replacement by improving surgical precision regarding bone resections and ligament balance [1]. The objective is not to substitute the surgeon, but rather to assist the surgeon with the goal to perform a more precise implantation.

Data suggest that systems involving 3D preoperative planning and custom guides are being employed more frequently and benefit the precision of the implantation. The inconveniences of these systems are the need for pre-operative computed tomography (CT) scan with specific protocol and the cost for manufacturing the custom guides.

An evolution of robotic surgery has been developed and relies on a bone morphing step during surgery, such as with the NAVIO system (Smith Nephew®) [2, 3]. Preoperative CT imaging is therefore no longer necessary. These systems have the potential to improve the surgical accuracy for knee arthroplasty. Nevertheless, the surgical steps and the potential difficulties must be understood. This chapter presents the technical aspects of this evolution, current and future applications, and surgical tips to perform robotic or computer-assisted surgery easily.

26.2 Computer-Assisted Surgery and Robotics

CAS and robotic surgery permit intra-operative definition of distal femoral and proximal tibial bone anatomy through the bone morphing process, as well as determination of mechanical axes (femoral, tibial and limb) and knee range of motion.

Robotic surgery permits dynamic acquisition of ligament laxity during the planning phase, assists placement of cutting guides and finally allows the evaluation of residual ligament laxities.

Implants positioning is performed accurately with the robotic system and 3D planning during surgery. With the system BlueBelt (Smith and Nephew®), bone resection is done by the surgeon who manipulates the handpiece, while the computer retracts the burr when the handpiece moves outside the planned bone resection zone. This specific system needs minimal preoperative imaging. We do not perform any pre-operative 3D imaging but only a standard radiographic assessment.

M. Cievet-Bonfils · C. Batailler · E. Servien
S. Lustig (✉)
Orthopaedic Department, Lyon North University Hospital, Lyon, France
e-mail: maxime.cievet-bonfils@chu-lyon.fr; cecile.batailler@chu-lyon.fr; elvire.servien@chu-lyon.fr

T. Lording
Melbourne Orthopaedic Group, Windsor, VIC, Australia

26.3 Unicompartmental Knee Arthroplasty

Implanting femoro-tibial or patello-femoral UKAs is technically demanding, and its success depends on the quality of the indication and its implantation. This makes these procedures ideal for use of robotic technology.

26.3.1 Medial UKA Surgical Technique

26.3.1.1 Installation

The patient is placed in a supine position, with a lateral support and a foot wedge to maintain the knee at 90° of flexion. A tourniquet can be used according to surgeon preference.

The NAVIO PFS console consists of three elements:

- An infrared camera (as in a conventional surgical navigation system) that must be installed about 1 m from the surgical field, facing the operator, so as to permanently visualize the femoral and tibial sensors.
- A touch screen covered with a sterile drape. It is located within reach of the operator, most often at the level of the contralateral hip.
- A console controlling the robotic burr and irrigation during resection. The handpiece can be held in one hand and is connected to the console by a cable and the irrigation tubing.

The first step is positioning of the femoral and tibial sensors, most often in a percutaneous fashion to the tibia and with a minimal subvastus approach to the femur so as not to pass through the quadriceps. These sensors must be visible throughout the procedure and throughout the range of motion of the knee. The incision is parapatellar (medial or lateral), typically from the patellar superior pole to about 1 cm below the joint line, over a length of about 10 cm. It is important that osteophytes are removed before any registration by the ligament balancing system.

26.3.1.2 Point of Interest Acquisition

This stage of the procedure used to be long and tedious with older CAS systems, but advances in computing and technology have made it possible to optimize it. To ensure that the sensors are stable throughout the procedure, a reference point is identified at the tibia and femur, allowing the surgeon to check with the probe that the sensors have not moved.

The hip centre is acquired by repeated circumduction movements of the leg with a maximum permissible error of 0.9 mm. The internal and external malleoli are acquired at the ankle directly with the probe. The full range of motion of the knee is then recorded, thanks to a complete flexion–extension movement without constraint in varus nor valgus. The same extension–flexion movement is then performed with a stress in valgus (or varus in the case of lateral unicompartmental) in order to record the reducibility of the deformation throughout the range of motion. This dynamic acquisition is essential because it allows the system to consider ligament laxity during the planning phase.

Points of interest are then acquired on the femur with the probe: the centre of the knee (at the top of the notch), the most distal, most posterior and the most anterior points of the medial condyle (which corresponds to the contact between the most anterior point of the tibial plateau and the femoral condyle in complete extension of the knee). The femoral acquisition continues with a bone morphing phase of the surface of the condyle using the probe (Fig. 26.1).

The same sequence is then repeated for the tibia: the centre of the tibia, the most distal point of the tibial cup, the most posterior point (for which access is made difficult by the intact femoral condyle), the most medial point and the most anterior point. The anteroposterior axis of the tibia is also recorded, before finishing the tibial acquisition with a phase of surface bone morphing.

26.3.1.3 Planning

This is one of the essential steps of the robotic system because it allows real-time dynamic planning, taking into account the reducibility of the deformation.

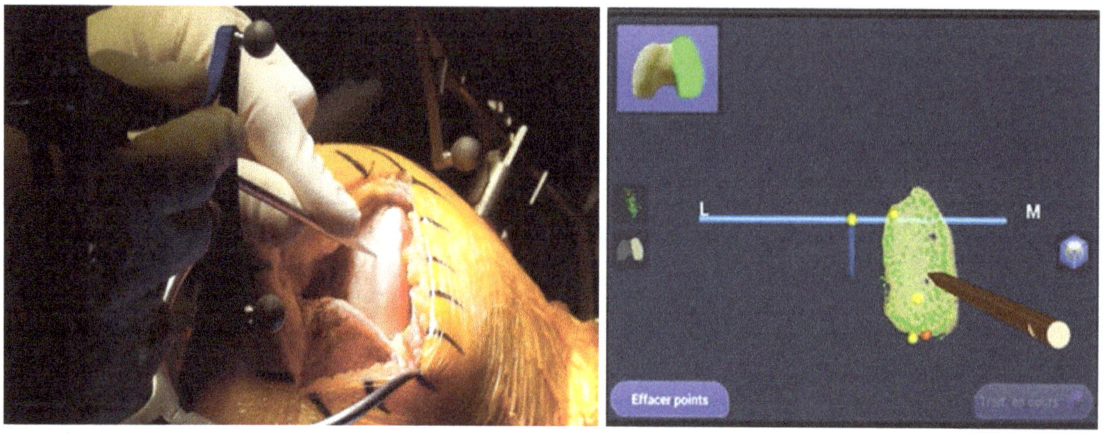

Fig. 26.1 Femoral condyle bone morphing

The first step is to choose the size of the femoral implant, which can be modified at any time during the surgery. Then we choose the position of the femoral component, within the three planes of space. A separate screen split into four parts demonstrates the exact position of the implant in relation to the shape of the femoral condyle. The touch screen allows manipulation of a 3D view of the femoral condyle with the implant planned, in order to precisely visualize the final position. The angular values of this femoral implant are visible at any time: varus/valgus, flexion and rotation.

The objective is to obtain maximal coverage of the bone surfaces, maintaining the joint line height and avoiding impingement with the massive tibial spines.

The same steps are then performed for the tibial component. We first decide the size of the implant and the thickness of the polyethylene. Then we choose the varus/valgus, rotation, tibial slope and positioning of the implant in relation to the tibial spines. The touch screen also allows rotation of 3D images to accurately visualize the positioning of the implant in the three planes of space. As always for a unicompartmental prosthesis, tibial bone resection should be minimized.

The next step is to visualize the consequences of our planning in terms of the angular correction (preoperative vs. postoperative) between 0° and 120° of flexion. At this stage, we can change the position of the tibial implant (varus/valgus, slope, rotation, resection depth) and femoral implant (varus/valgus, flexion, rotation, resection height) and visualize the consequences on the final angular correction. These parameters not only take into account static acquisitions but also the initial dynamic acquisitions, and therefore the reducibility of the deformation at each flexion angle (Fig. 26.2).

The final stage of planning is to visualize contact points between the components during flexion, which allows lateralization or medialization if necessary of either component to better centre this point of contact. You can freely navigate between the different planning screens. Once the desired result is obtained, the final choice is validated.

26.3.1.4 Preparation of Bone Surfaces

Once the planning is validated, we can prepare the bone surfaces. The assembly of the robotic burr with the irrigation system and the calibration phase takes a few seconds. A final control step allows you to visualize the area to be drilled. We check that it corresponds visually to the area where you want to position the implant.

We usually start with the femur which is more easily accessible. It is also possible to start with the tibia if desired. An automatic feedback system only burrs the planned area. If you leave this area, the burr is retracted, making it impossible to resect bone in an undesired area by mistake. The remaining bone depth to be removed is continuously displayed on the screen in a colour-coded fashion, which makes it possible to orient the

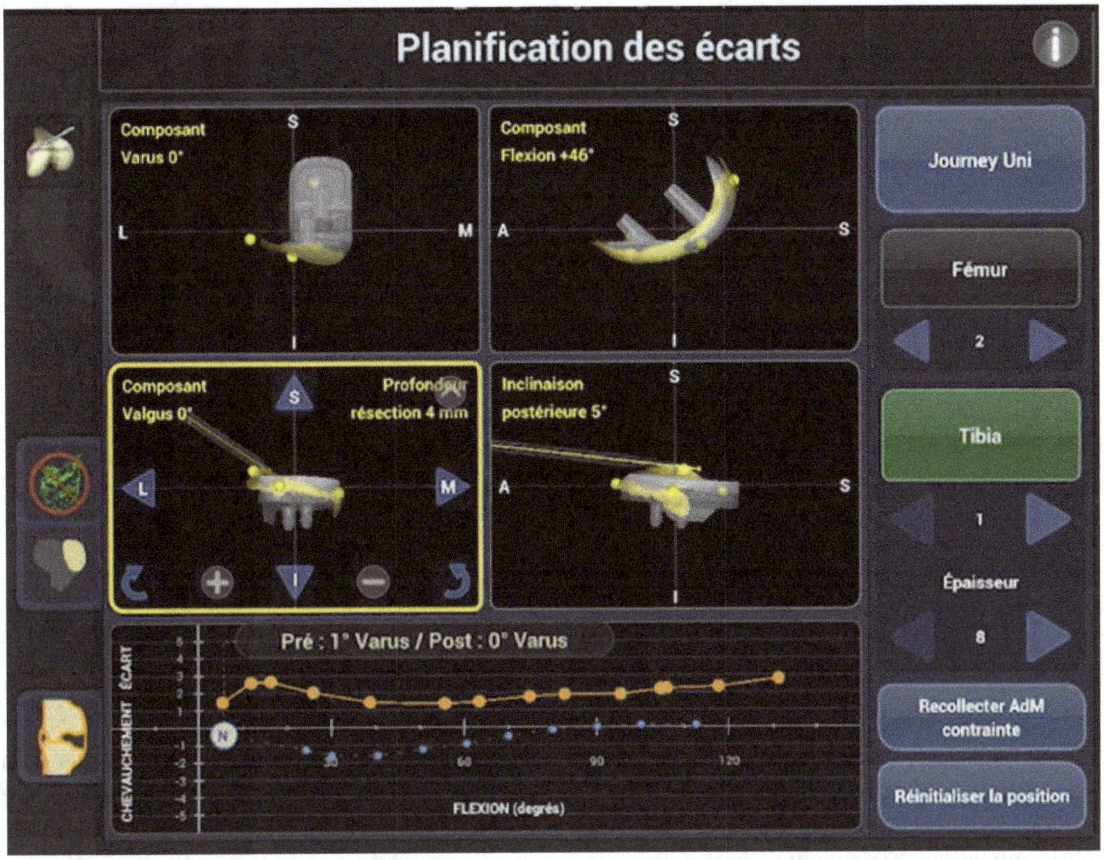

Fig. 26.2 Global knee balance planning according to the positioning of femoral and tibial implants

burr in an efficient way. The surgeon has complete freedom of movement; the robotic system only retracts the burr when it is moved outside the planned area. We gradually mobilize the knee in hyperflexion to reach the posterior femoral region. It is sometimes necessary to burr the tibia before being able to access the most posterior part of the femoral condyle.

Once the femur is prepared, we move on to the tibia with the same visual control. We begin on the most anterior part of the tibia, gradually extending to the entire planned surface. It is possible to use the most anterior part of the bone resection as a guide for a saw, and to saw the posterior part, in order to save a few minutes of operative time. A rasp is then used to file down any irregularities in the bone resections once burring is finished. The meniscus, easily accessible at this stage, is then removed. The last step consists of drilling for the anchoring lugs of the femoral implant under visual control.

26.3.1.5 Trial and Final Implants

We can then place the trial implants and display on screen the correction angle obtained as well as the ligament balance throughout the range of motion. Cementation and fixation of final implants are done according to surgeon preference. We can once again check the angular correction and balancing of the knee with the final implants in situ.

26.3.1.6 Results

In our experience with the NAVIO system, the results and particularly the positioning of the implants have been significantly improved. One of the essential parameters for the success of a knee joint prosthesis is to reproduce the joint line level [4]. Our results published on unicompartmental prostheses have shown that this parameter was very well controlled with this robotic system while giving favourable clinical results in the short and medium term since 2013 [5]. Hopefully, longer term results will confirm these encouraging initial radiological and clinical findings. In literature, the mean implant positioning is not significantly improved with robotic-assisted UKA. By contrast, the reduction of outliers is significant [6] and thus very relevant to reduction of failure. Ponzio and Lonner have reported that aggressive tibial resection is less frequent during robotic-assisted UKA [3].

Studies on robotic-assisted UKA report satisfying short- and medium-term survival rates [7]. Nevertheless, no comparative study has demonstrated a better survival rate for robotic-assisted UKA, compared to conventional UKA. Published rates of revision after robotic-assisted UKA vary from 3% to 10% at midterm [8–10].

26.4 Patello-Femoral Knee Arthroplasty

Patello-femoral prosthesis involves different difficulties. However, it is probably one of the best indications for robotic surgery, as ideal positioning requires a precise understanding of the three-dimensional anatomy of the distal femur. The bone preparation requires the use of a burr, even with conventional instrumentation. 3D planning is made easy by the acquisition phase of the NAVIO system, which produces a 3D model of the trochlea and records the reference axes (bi-epicondylar, Whiteside, femoral mechanical). It is thus possible to visualize the desired 3D positioning of the trochlear implant and to ensure a perfect transition of the femoral implant with the cartilage of the femoral condyles, before the bone resection. The preparation phase is facilitated by the controlled burring system with the robotic handpiece that burrs the cartilage and the subchondral bone according to the planning, in a more reproducible fashion than with standard instrumentation. Very few studies described results of robotic-assisted patella-femoral prosthesis, and these studies are not comparative. The first series reported satisfying functional scores and a good implant positioning [11].

26.5 Total Knee Arthroplasty

26.5.1 Computer-Assisted Surgery

Computer-assisted surgery was pioneered in the early 1990s, with the first total knee replacement performed in 1997. Computer navigation offers intra-operative dynamic assessment of alignment, balance and kinematics.

The computer-assisted system is composed of two elements:

- An infrared camera that must be installed about 1 m from the surgical field, facing the operator, so as to permanently visualize the sensors during all the surgery.
- A touch screen.

The surgery starts by placing sensors on the femur and the tibia. We then acquire the different mechanical angles and the hip centre with the use of the handpiece. A standard approach is then used to access the bone surfaces. The handpiece is used to perform bone morphing of the femoral condyles and the tibial plateau. We then place the bone cutting guide on the femur to perform the distal cut.

The bone cutting guides can be controlled in varus/valgus, flexion/extension and internal/external rotation for both the femur and the tibia. They have sensors that allow the computer system to calculate the angles of bone cutting. When adjusting the cutting guides, the operator can see on the screen the effect it will have on the bone cut. The operator can then make the cuts following the planning on the screen. After the cuts are performed, the surgery is the same as for a traditional total knee replacement.

26.5.2 Robotic

Computer-assisted surgery systems help place cutting guides using anatomical and ligament balance data. The NAVIO system is an evolution using more detailed anatomical data, especially regarding the soft tissues (Fig. 26.3). In fact, acquisitions are made throughout the range of

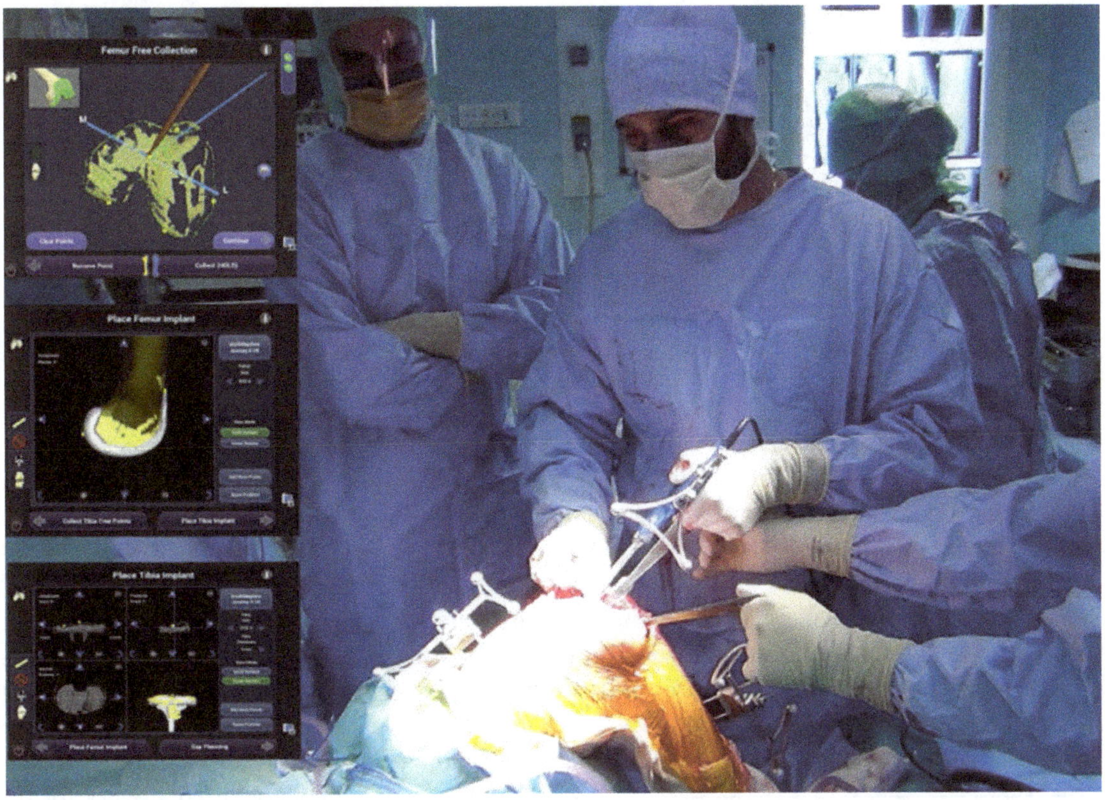

Fig. 26.3 Total knee arthroplasty with NAVIO system

motion in order to place the femoral and tibial components to optimize stability throughout the full range of motion, not only at 0° and 90° of flexion.

Balancing and soft tissue release can be checked and improved during the data collection phase. The alignment and the possible ligament contractions or laxities will be collected through all the range of motion.

Sizing and positioning of the components are done before any bone cutting. Virtual planning allows sizing and positioning of implants corresponding to anatomy and ligament balance. Once the planning is validated, the surgeon uses the robotic burr to make four holes in the distal femur and two to four holes in the proximal tibia. The cutting guides are placed using these holes as guides and then fixed on the bone (Fig. 26.4). Virtual cuts can be visualized on the screen before making them by placing a tool in the cutting slot. These cuts can also be checked after completion with the same tool.

The trial implants are then placed, and examination of the ligament balance through the full range of motion can be compared to the initial plan, before cementation of the final implants.

This type of programming is particularly interesting when using implants reproducing the kinematics of the knee. Indeed, they require taking into account not only the bone references but also the soft tissues in order to reproduce ideal articular kinematics. The robotic assistance allows finalizing this reflection by realizing the gesture with a suitable precision.

26.5.3 Literature

In a study comparing conventional versus computer-assisted surgery for TKA with 5-year follow-up, Cip et al. did not show any difference in implant survival rate, but poorer accuracy for mechanical axis and tibial slope in the conventional group. Clinical examination

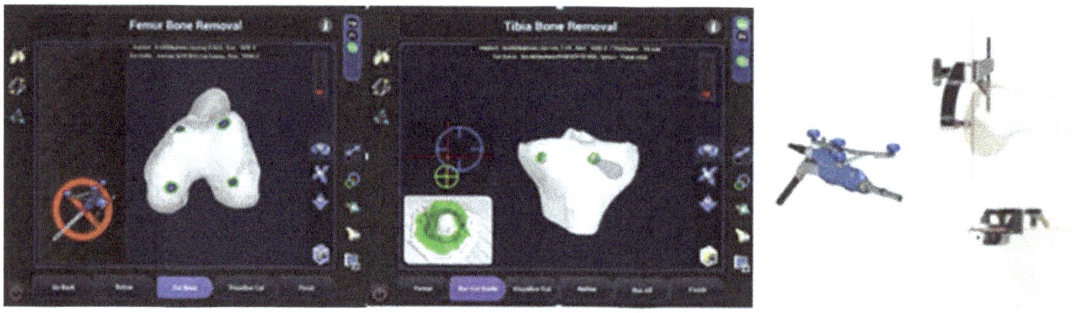

Fig. 26.4 Preparation of the femoral and tibial cutting guides' position with the robotic handpiece

showed no difference between the two groups; however, the Knee Society Score was better in the navigated group [12]. There are very few studies on robotic-assisted TKA. These studies are essentially preliminary studies without comparative group or long-term follow-up. A long-term follow-up and a randomized study are necessary to reliably assess the benefit of robotic-assisted TKA.

26.6 What's Next?

The success of robotic surgery systems suggests that their place in operating theatres will become more and more important. It may provide significant support for the placement of bi-cruciate-retaining knee replacement prostheses, which require a thorough understanding of the different characteristics of the medial and lateral compartments, as well as precise bone preparation. The protection of the tibial spine should also be simpler with the use of a burr guided by a robotic handpiece.

Currently, a recent concept is developed for the lower limb alignment during TKA. The kinematic alignment (KA) of TKA allows to conserve a part of the knee constitutional deformity and to obtain a more physiological knee with easy ligament balancing. Several studies have reported better functional outcomes after a kinematic alignment with a better restoration of a normal gait [13, 14]. Very few TKA ancillaries exist to perform accurately a KA. Some studies have assessed the efficiency of a robotic surgery system to obtain a satisfying KA and to compare outcomes with mechanical alignment [15–17]. In a randomized study, Yeo et al. compared the outcomes and gait analysis after robotic-assisted TKA with either a KA or a mechanical alignment [15]. After a follow-up of 8 years, they find the same results between both groups. The robotic-assisted surgery could be very interesting to perform an accurate kinematic alignment during TKA. This use is still uncommon with few studies. More studies are needed to assess the potential of robotic-assisted surgery for the KA.

The field of knee prosthesis revision, exponentially growing, should also benefit from robotic surgery. The preparation of areas of bone loss will allow precise adjustment for wedges or cones, combined with careful planning of the revision prosthesis taking into account the ligament balance prior to removal of the implants to be revised.

26.7 Case Example

A patient of 40 years consults for painful unstable patella. She had history of recurrent patellar dislocation, which was partially improved by distalization of the anterior tibial tuberosity. The patient presented with a knee being valgus aligned but without any stiffness, a patellar maltracking and a J sign. The X-rays showed patellofemoral osteoarthritis and trochlear dysplasia type D (Dejour classification) and normal patellar height (Fig. 26.5). The tibial tuberosity–trochlear groove (TT–TG) distance, as measured on CT scan, was 35 mm.

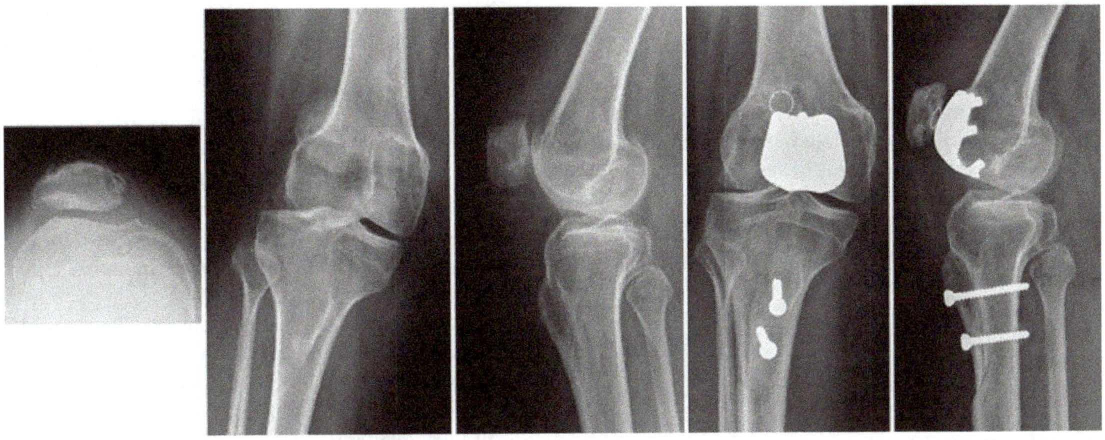

Fig. 26.5 Pre- and post-operative knee radiographs

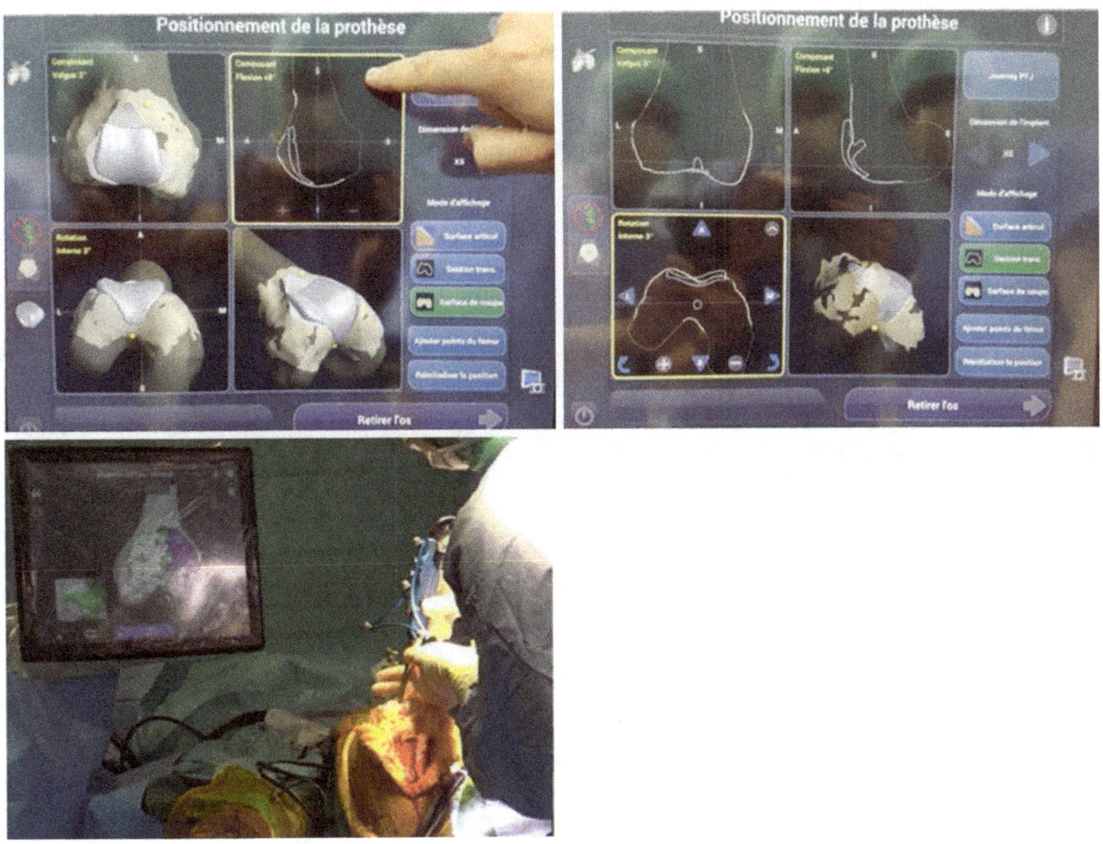

Fig. 26.6 Implant positioning with the robotic assistance before bone removal with the retro-controlled burr

She undertook a bilateral patello-femoral prosthesis associated with medialization of the anterior tibial tuberosity. The robotic assistance allowed precise implantation of the trochlea component in the three dimensions to obtain a good patellar tracking without impingement. In this indication, it is sound to lateralize a little the trochlea in order to improve the tracking and to drill sufficiently in order to avoid the increase of the constraints in the anterior compartment (Fig. 26.6).

References

1. van der List JP, Chawla H, Joskowicz L, Pearle AD. Current state of computer navigation and robotics in unicompartmental and total knee arthroplasty: a systematic review with meta-analysis. Knee Surg Sports Traumatol Arthrosc. 2016;24:3482–95.
2. Lonner JH, Moretti VM. The evolution of image-free robotic assistance in unicompartmental knee arthroplasty. Am J Orthop (Belle Mead NJ). 2016;45: 249–54.
3. Ponzio DY, Lonner JH. Robotic technology produces more conservative tibial resection than conventional techniques in UKA. Am J Orthop (Belle Mead NJ). 2016;45:E465–8.
4. Weber P, Schroder C, Laubender RP, et al. Joint line reconstruction in medial unicompartmental knee arthroplasty: development and validation of a measurement method. Knee Surg Sports Traumatol Arthrosc. 2013;21:2468–73.
5. Herry Y, Batailler C, Lording T, Servien E, Neyret P, Lustig S. Improved joint-line restitution in unicompartmental knee arthroplasty using a robotic-assisted surgical technique. Int Orthop. 2017;41:2265–71.
6. Bell SW, Anthony I, Jones B, MacLean A, Rowe P, Blyth M. Improved accuracy of component positioning with robotic-assisted unicompartmental knee arthroplasty: data from a prospective, randomized controlled study. J Bone Joint Surg Am. 2016;98: 627–35.
7. Marcovigi A, Zambianchi F, Sandoni D, Rivi E, Catani F. Robotic-arm assisted partial knee arthroplasty: a single centre experience. Acta Biomed. 2017;88: 54–9.
8. Pearle AD, van der List JP, Lee L, Coon TM, Borus TA, Roche MW. Survivorship and patient satisfaction of robotic-assisted medial unicompartmental knee arthroplasty at a minimum two-year follow-up. Knee. 2017;24:419–28.
9. Plate JF, Augart MA, Seyler TM, et al. Obesity has no effect on outcomes following unicompartmental knee arthroplasty. Knee Surg Sports Traumatol Arthrosc. 2017;25:645–51.
10. Gladnick BP, Nam D, Khamaisy S, Paul S, Pearle AD. Onlay tibial implants appear to provide superior clinical results in robotic unicompartmental knee arthroplasty. HSS J. 2015;11:43–9.
11. Turktas U, Piskin A, Poehling GG. Short-term outcomes of robotically assisted patello-femoral arthroplasty. Int Orthop. 2016;40:919–24.
12. Cip J, Widemschek M, Luegmair M, Sheinkop MB, Benesch T, Martin A. Conventional versus computer-assisted technique for total knee arthroplasty: a minimum of 5-year follow-up of 200 patients in a prospective randomized comparative trial. J Arthroplast. 2014;29:1795–802.
13. Blakeney W, Clement J, Desmeules F, Hagemeister N, Riviere C, Vendittoli PA. Kinematic alignment in total knee arthroplasty better reproduces normal gait than mechanical alignment. Knee Surg Sports Traumatol Arthrosc. 2019;27:1410–7.
14. Courtney PM, Lee GC. Early outcomes of kinematic alignment in primary total knee arthroplasty: a meta-analysis of the literature. J Arthroplast. 2017;32:2028–2032.e2021.
15. Yeo JH, Seon JK, Lee DH, Song EK. No difference in outcomes and gait analysis between mechanical and kinematic knee alignment methods using robotic total knee arthroplasty. Knee Surg Sports Traumatol Arthrosc. 2019;27:2385.
16. Calliess T, Ettinger M, Savov P, Karkosch R, Windhagen H. Individualized alignment in total knee arthroplasty using image-based robotic assistance: video article. Orthopade. 2018;47:871–9.
17. Urish KL, Conditt M, Roche M, Rubash HE. Robotic total knee arthroplasty: surgical assistant for a customized normal kinematic knee. Orthopedics. 2016;39:e822–7.

27

An Augmented Reality Platform for Patient-Specific Hip and Knee Joint Arthroplasties

Edouard Auvinet, Cedric Maillot, and Chukwudi Uzoho

- Augmented reality is a new navigation that allows the superposition of clinical information in the sight of the surgeon.
- The planning and performing of patient-specific joint replacement techniques, but also the training for orthopaedic surgeries will benefit from the augmented reality systems.
- Augmented reality platform availability is related to improvement in computing power capacity, tracking system precision and environment understanding algorithm development.

This chapter aims to introduce some elements of reflection regarding the use of an augmented reality platform for patient-specific hip and knee joint arthroplasties. The chapter is composed of three main parts. The first part proposes a brief presentation of the 'reality concept' and the recent technological progresses that have made this new technology ready for use in the OR. The second part describes the augmented reality process and addresses the technological bottlenecks, which still need to be addressed. The last part provides several case examples, using such technology in the OR.

E. Auvinet (✉) · C. Maillot
Orthopaedic and Trauma Surgery Department, UZ Gent, Ghent, Belgium

Health Innovation and Research Institute, UZ Gent, Ghent, Belgium

MSK Lab, Imperial College, London, UK
e-mail: e.auvinet@imperial.ac.uk

C. Uzoho
MSK Lab, Imperial College, London, UK
e-mail: chukwudi.uzoho16@imperial.ac.uk

27.1 From Reality to Augmented Reality

Surgeons are used to interacting with their surgical environment. During the procedure, surgeons use all their senses to perform complex tasks at an optimal standard. However, visual, touch and sound sensation are the ones most readily relied on during their practice. Their aptitude to assess the situation with their senses have been learned and refined through their medical training, and also with the experience acquired during clinical practice.

In recent decades, digital technologies used in augmented reality have been developed in order to interact with the human senses. These technologies enable user projection into a reality described through a digital memory. This "digital" reality is then rendered to human sense through a digital interface. The interface mediums include an image for the eyes, a sound for the ears and pressure for the touch. When the digital system is able to measure the action of the user, it can then alter the digital reality and represent its new version to the user.

Except for the touch sense, these technologies have been widely used for computer games particularly with "First-Person Shooter" games where the picture is rendered on a screen. This case uses non-immersive virtual reality as the user is still connected with part of their reality. The recent development of immersive helmets allows one to cut the user from their reality and expose the user to a stereoscopic display. In this case, each eye has its own display, and the computer renders a picture from a different position for each eye. The stereoscopic perception of the user allows a full 3D immersion in the virtual environment. Further to this, the augmented reality headset uses stereoscopic projection of virtual objects on the real environment of the user.

Since their inception, digital technologies used in augmented reality have aimed to alter the user's senses. Indeed, digital systems are able to handle information representing an object, a scene or some information about the scene, which creates a sort of reality. Several products have been developed that allow such interfaces to deliver virtual information to the user's senses. The major senses that have been targeted are that of vision and sound. Screens and audio devices were the first to help the digital system in better presenting virtual information to the user. Touch sense has also been addressed through the development of haptic devices. But this sense is particularly difficult as it involves delivery of mechanical forces which are difficult to produce with wearable devices. The augmented reality concept, which aims at projecting information from a virtual reality into the user's reality, needs to understand the user reality and to render the virtual objects properly.

Information usability is intimately related to the quality of the information and its presentation. For example, it would be difficult to prepare a plan on a low-quality image display and with a low precision bone surface. This has been a technological bottleneck for several years. In the last decades, the digital world has improved in both technology and availability. Indeed, technological progress introduces higher computing power, better output interface and smaller devices. The computing power increased in an exponential way. The last super computer Tianhe-2 is 2.73×10^{12} times more powerful than the IBM 704 released in 1954.

Following the increase in computing power, availability improved as well. For example, the Cray-2 released in 1985 and the iPhone 6 have similar computing power. As shown in Table 27.1, the technological advances allow us nowadays to transport and easily use the device. The device has also become more available, with less than a hundred of Cray-2 sold, whilst over 220 million iPhone 6 devices have been delivered. The level of expertise is also an important factor as to the use of Cray-2 device, requires a computer scientist or an engineer, whilst almost anyone can operate an iPhone 6. A second key factor is also cost. The Cray-2 price was US$32 million versus the US$649 for the iPhone 6. Improvements in display devices and computing power for image rendering have driven further advancements in picture quality and better bridged the fidelity to the reality (Fig. 27.1).

Table 27.1 Difference of power consumption, weight and price for the Cray 2 and the iPhone 6

	Cray 2	iPhone 6
Power consumption	195,000 W	~1 W
Weight	2500 kg	0.129 kg
Cost	US$32 million	US$649

This table shows the difference of power consumption, weight and cost for the Cray 2 and the iPhone 6 which have an equivalent computing power

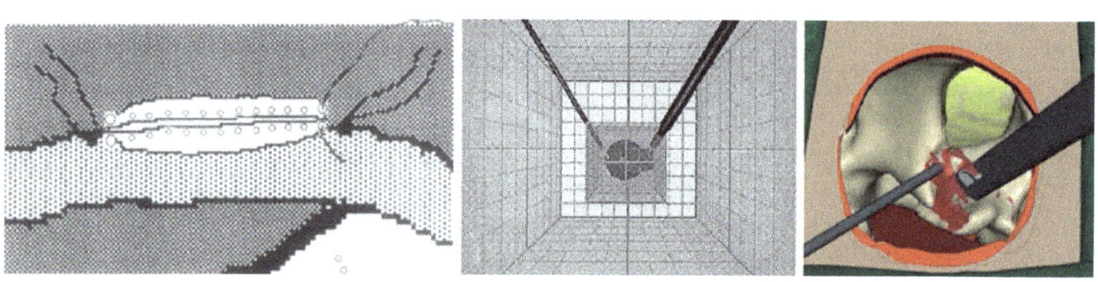

Fig. 27.1 The tryptic of images produced by virtual reality platforms show the evolution of the rendering quality along the years, which increase the realism perception level by the user. Image 1994, image 2002, image 2019 (images, adapted from [9–11])

The haptic feeling is a particular part which is associated with the robotic domain.

This short comparison helps to figure out the important improvement of the digital technologies, which propelled the recent development of augmented reality into the clinical domain. Surgical outcomes can be improved with better planning and the availability of implant positioning parameters that are visible in real time. Augmented reality is one potential technology that could allow one to present additional information to the clinician in order to assist during the surgery.

27.2 How Does Augmented Reality Works?

Augmented reality technologies aim to introduce virtual elements into the user's environment. The information used needs to be related with the reality, meaning that the system will need to measure and understand the user reality, process it to compute the information required, and then render it to project this information to the user in correlation with the reality. For that purpose, patient position as well as the relative positions of equipment like tools and display devices is a crucial element to measure and it is mandatory in order to compute feedback information.

27.2.1 Tracking

To measure and track the objects position, several technologies have been proposed. This could be done with three classes of measuring methods: with contact, semi-contact, and contactless. This depends on link between the object and the measuring equipment.

With the contact system, there is a mechanical link between the measuring system and the object. For example, the Acrobot uses a digitizer arm to locate the position and orientation of the objects. The arm is anchored into the bone and each articulation of the arm measures all the spatial parameters with the length and the angular values between each arm's segments.

The semi-contact system relies on a contact link between the anatomy and the marker and a contactless link between the markers and the cameras. The marker's 3D positions are computed from a triangulation of marker's 2D position in each camera of the optical system. Thanks to a unique spatial configuration of each markers attached to the object, the system is able to recognize the object. This method is actually used by the majority of navigation systems.

The contactless system is more recent and still a concept in development. In this case, there is nothing in contact with the patient's anatomy. The tracking is done without the need to attach any markers on the patient. It has been possible with the apparition of depth cameras as shown by Liu et al. [1]. The depth camera is an active sensor that projects a structured light pattern onto the scene. Thanks to this projected pattern, the depth camera can reconstruct the 3D surface of the scene. In this case, the anatomy of the object becomes its own marker. The tracking is done by identifying and following the surfaces along the time. However, this method is at its early stages with only a proof of concept having been proposed in the literature. This method is very promising as it could track not only bone position but also bone shape modification. For the contact and semi-contact method, the user needs to take samples of the bone surface with a dedicated tool in order to register the bone surface with the tracking device, rather than the contactless system, which already delivers a sample of the 3D surface of the object. This bone surface sample will be used in the computing stage for bone registration.

For the augmented reality system, the semi-contact and contactless tracking system will be the most suitable. Figure 27.2 shows an example of a hybrid solution of semi-contact and contactless tracking, while the drill is tracked with an attached marker, the femoral head is tracked with the depth camera.

The bottleneck for the contact and semi-contact tracking system is the need of a bone shape digitizing stage at the beginning of the procedure and for each bone modification control, which requires some time to be performed. However, they are robust to the bone shape modification because they

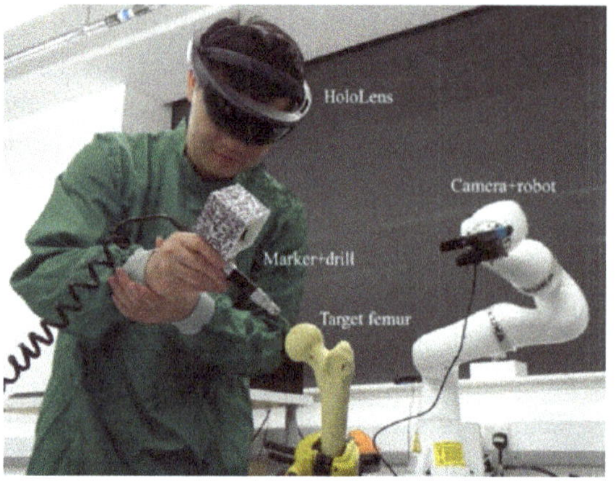

Fig. 27.2 The setup for a proof of concept of an intraoperative augmented reality assistance system. This system introduces the use of a contactless tracking system for the femoral part and a visual feedback for the user in the augmented reality headset. A particularity of this setup is the automatic positioning of the depth camera by the robot arm which insures the visibility of the femoral part when an occlusion occurs. The tool is still tracked with a classical semi-contact tracking method with an attached marker (Adapted from [1])

rely on the markers to perform the tracking. For the contactless, the bottleneck relates to the depth sensor precision and the scene understanding of the 3D shape measured to separate and identify the different objects in the scene.

27.2.2 Computing

The computing part of the process consists in two operations. The first operation is the registration of the anatomical parts tracked with the preoperative images. The second operation is to compute clinical index from raw information, which, for example, compare the actual situation with the preoperative plan. The registration operation is required due to the different positions adopted by the patient during their preoperative imaging and the actual position of the patient in the OR. This operation needs to identify the corresponding elements from the preoperative information and the intraoperative one in order to compute the spatial transformation between them. In orthopaedic surgery, this operation is made easier because of the solid nature of the bone in contrast to solely soft tissue procedures. For the contact and semi-contact tracking method, this operation is already robust and used in most navigation systems. It usually uses a fiducial-based registration method. In this case, anatomical fiducials are annotated in the preoperative images and then the surgeon identifies them intraoperatively. It strives to find the spatial transformation, which will make the bone sample points fit with the preoperative surface of the bone. In this case, identification of the bone surface has been done by the surgeon, who themselves have recognized and sampled them. This registration is commonly done by applying an iterative closest point method between the surface issued from the computer tomography scan and intraoperative sample points. With the contactless method, this operation is more difficult because the depth camera records the environment, bones, soft tissues and the background. The first step of the analysis is to distinguish the nature of the tissues. Once this is complete, the bone surface measured could then be compared with the related bone surface measured in the preoperative medical imaging. The second computing operation focuses on the processing of positional information previously obtained for both the patient anatomy and the equipment in order to deliver clinically relevant information. For instance, this will compare the actual intraoperation situation with the preoperative or intraoperative planning. To this end, for each particular operation step, the relevant information will be compared. For example, during the TKA femoral extremity bone cut, the position of the oscillating saw will be compared with the femur position. This will allow the system to compute the relative position of the actual cutting plane with the preoperative plan. Then two valuable pieces of clinical information could be extracted, including the angular error between the normal planes and the error distance to the correct entry point in the bone.

27.2.3 Visualization

Visualization will produce the image that will be presented to the user. In the case of augmented reality, this image representing the digital reality must be aligned with surgeons' reality. To this end, the tracking information of the objects and the headset allows then to define the viewpoint in the reality and render the virtual object at the correct location. Figures 27.3 and 27.4 show examples of visual feedback where clinical information is presented in the sight of the surgeon. In Fig. 27.4, this information is overlaid on the real object as opposed to what is shown in Fig. 27.3 where the information is placed outside the scene object as a virtual dashboard. The actual bottleneck is the time taken by the system to adapt to a change of situation, for example, in cases of fast motion, when the position of the viewpoint might be different between the moment when tracking information is measured, the moment when the image rendering is finished and finally the moment when the picture is displayed. This would create some inconsistency in the visual feedback. This problem might be resolved, by reducing the tracking and rendering delay, which could happen with improvement of the technological performance.

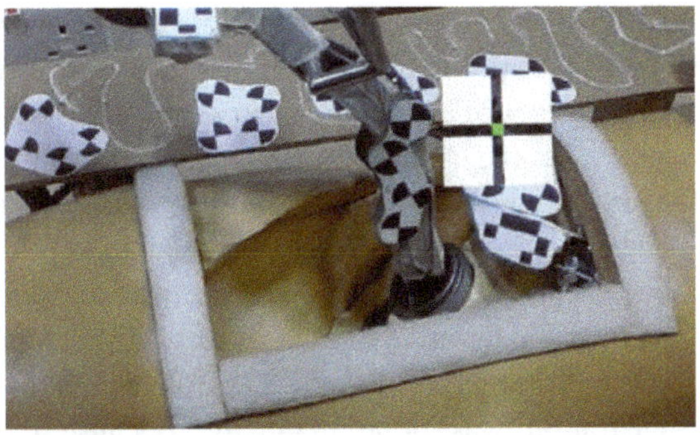

Fig. 27.3 This image represents the view of the student through the AR headset. The green dot on the crossbar represents the distance to the target, vertically for the inclination angle and horizontally for the anteversion angle. This dot remains red until the error is less than 1° for both angles. (Adapted from [8])

27.3 How Augmented Reality Could Support Surgery?

The success of the total hip and knee replacements is related with the correct positioning of the implant. Precise implantation is of upmost

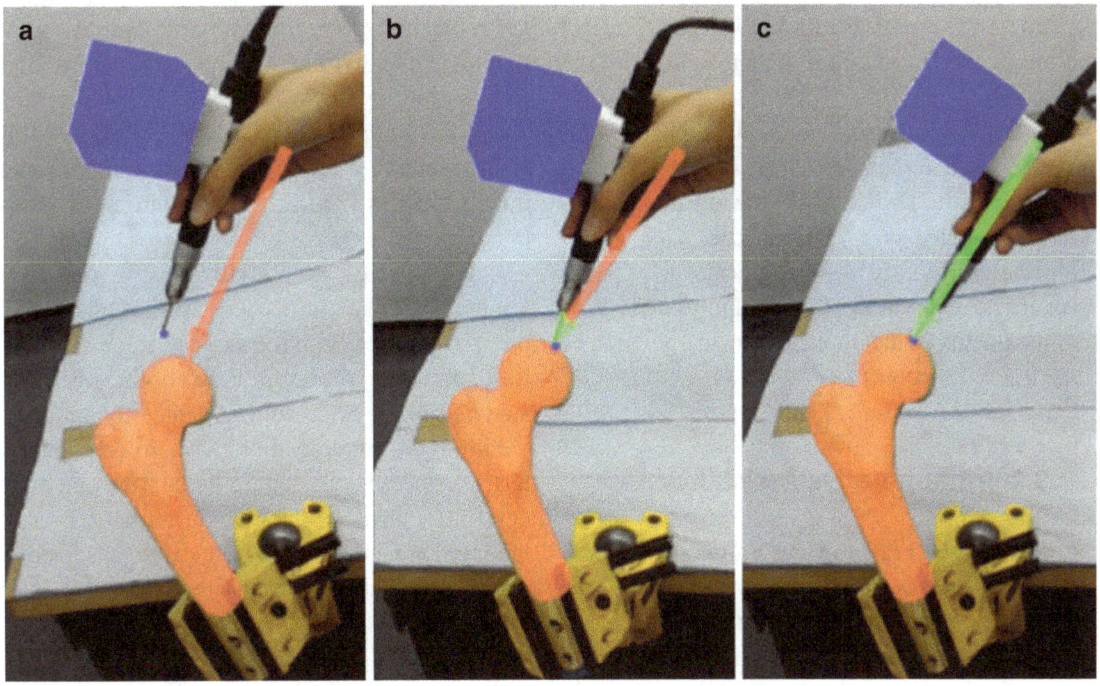

Fig. 27.4 This image shows the visual feedback seen by the user for the femoral head drilling component in hip resurfacing. The arrow indicates the entry point and orientation target. (**a**) The arrow is fully red because neither the orientation nor the entry point errors are, respectively, inferior to 1° and 1 mm. (**b**) The entry point error is lower than 1 mm, indicated by the green arrow tip. (**c**) The orientation error is less than 1°, indicated by the green complete green arrow (Adapted from [1])

importance when the implantation is personalized by considering the individual joint's anatomy and kinematics. Namely, following a precise patient-specific planning, implantation has to be as much precise and a real-time feedback of this precision is needed, to ensure the final outcome is what the surgeon had planned. Augmented reality will soon integrate itself within different activities of orthopaedic practice. Indeed, several steps of the surgery may benefit a 3D representation of information. Several of the improvements would occur during preoperative and intraoperative planning, intraoperative assistance and training of the surgeon.

27.3.1 Preoperative and Intraoperative Planning

To prepare the surgery, the practitioner takes into account numerous facets of information. However, the shape of the anatomy is often presented with 2D information such as radiographs or CT scan layers or even 3D surface but presented as 2D representation on screens. The 3D nature of this information is then limited by the presentation interface. Thanks to the new augmented reality headset, which allow each eye to have its own screen, the planning can be now executed with 3D information being more accurately presented in a 3D interface. This would help the clinician to fully appreciate the spatial properties, depth perception, and ultimately benefit the quality of the implantation and potentially the clinical outcomes.

27.3.2 Intraoperative Assistance

Nowadays, several devices already provide intraoperative assistance, such as navigation or robotics systems. However, the main interface used to display the feedback information is a screen sitting aside the operating zone. This means that the surgeon must split their attention between the operating field and the screen. Augmented reality technology helps the surgeon to focus his attention on the patient, by overlaying feedback information directly into the field of view. This enhances the theatre ergonomics. The surgeon is able to appreciate information feedback from the navigation system whilst keeping the visual clues required for precise motor control of their gesture. A first step in this direction has been investigated by Pr Rodriguez who uses a projection of the navigation screen into the sight of the surgeon. This first simplified step avoids the need of precise positioning of the headset and the issue of real-time constraint needed for image processing, to ensure the reliability of the superposition of the feedback information directly onto the patient. In shoulder surgery, Pr Gregory [2] used the Hololens where registration was done manually. Because the Hololens localize itself in the room referential, as soon as the positioning error of the Hololens (±5 mm [3]) or the patient moves, the registration is no longer valid and needs to be corrected. This highlights the importance of the tracking stage in augmented reality technology.

Finally, personalized kinematic techniques for replacing hip and knee joints aim at reproducing the individual's joint anatomy in addition to considering kinematics joint parameters. AR technology may improve precision in restoring the native anatomy and also enable better quality control after implantation of final components.

Soon, the technology will be ready to overlay all the information needed by the surgeon in order to proceed with the surgery. Such information might be used through all the operative steps, from the bone cutting plane orientation to the implant's final position. Also, in certain conditions, once the procedure has started and bone cuts have been made, the position of several landmarks needed to mark the implant position might have been altered. These marks may no longer be reliable, jeopardizing the final implant position.

Some preclinical application tests have already been investigated for hip and knee surgeries. For hip arthroplasty surgery, Fotouhi et al. [4] used a real-time RGBD data overlay on

C-arm data to help cup positioning in total hip arthroplasty, achieving a low error level for translation, anteversion, and abduction of 1.98 mm, 1.10°, and 0.53°, respectively. Liu et al. [1] used depth data with robotic assistance for hip resurfacing guide-hole drilling. The position and orientation of the drilled holes were compared with the preoperative plan and the mean errors were found to be approximately 2 mm and 2°. Van Duren et al. [5] used digital fluoroscopic imaging simulator using orthogonal cameras to track coloured markers attached to the guide-wire for the insertion of a dynamic hip screw. The accuracy of the algorithm was shown to increase with the number of iterations up to 20 beyond which the error asymptotically converged to an error of 2 mm. Hiranaka et al. [6] showed that using an augmented reality to project the fluoroscope monitor in the sight of the surgeon during a femoral head nail insertion helped in improving accuracies as well as radiation exposure and insertion time. In knee surgery, Dario et al. [7] used an augmented reality mechatronic tool for arthroscopy, which had an overall system error of 3–4 mm.

These preliminary results show that augmented reality could help the surgeon to gain in efficiency and safety during TKA and THA procedures, particularly in the context of personalized implant positioning.

27.3.3 Training

Augmented reality will soon have a major role to play in various aspects of medical practice. For example, augmented reality has been used in a training platform to provide feedback on the acetabular cup orientation relative to the target. By such means, the trainee could enhance their precision in placing the acetabular cup with optimal inclination and version with real-time feedback from the AR headset. This method might help to avoid any break in the visual feedback and refined motor control training. For example, an augmented reality training platform for acetabular cup positioning had nearly the same performance in training a medical student [8] as for conventional training with expert feedback. The visual feedback from the platform shown in Fig. 27.3 was comparable to expert feedback in training for this critical part of the THA.

27.4 Conclusion

Augmented reality technology will undoubtedly soon play an important role in assisting joint replacement surgery. Unlike computer-navigation system and robotics, it is likely that AR may similarly contribute to improving the precision of implantation with better intraoperative ergonomics and workflow, without adding significant extra-cost to the procedure. Some technological bottlenecks have to be solved before AR technology can be fully integrated in daily clinical practice.

References

1. Liu H, Auvinet E, Giles J, Rodriguez F. Augmented reality based navigation for computer assisted hip resurfacing: a proof of concept study. Ann Biomed Eng. 2018;46(10):1595–605.
2. Gregory T, Gregory J, Sledge J, Allard R, Mir O. Surgery guided by mixed reality: presentation of a proof of concept. Acta Orthop. 2018;89(5):480–3.
3. Auvinet E, Galna B, Aframian A, Cobb J. O100: validation of the precision of the Microsoft HoloLens augmented reality headset head and hand motion measurement. Gait Posture. 2017;57(1):175–6.
4. Fotouhi J, Alexander CP, Unberath M, Taylor G, Lee SC, Fuerst B, et al. Plan in 2D, execute in 3D: an augmented reality solution for cup placement in total hip arthroplasty. J Med Imaging. 2018;5(02):1.
5. van Duren BH, Sugand K, Wescott R, Carrington R, Hart A. Augmented reality fluoroscopy simulation of the guide-wire insertion in DHS surgery: a proof of concept study. Med Eng Phys. 2018;55:52–9.
6. Hiranaka T, Fujishiro T, Hida Y, Shibata Y, Tsubosaka M, Nakanishi Y, et al. Augmented reality: the use of the PicoLinker smart glasses improves wire insertion under fluoroscopy. World J Orthop. 2017;8(12):891–4.
7. Dario P, Tonet O, Megali G. A novel mechatronic tool for computer-assisted arthroscopy. IEEE Trans Inf Technol Biomed. 2000;4(1):15.
8. Logishetty K, Western L, Morgan R, Iranpour F, Cobb JP, Auvinet E. Can an augmented reality headset improve accuracy of acetabular cup orientation

in simulated THA? A randomized trial. Clin Orthop Relat Res. 2019;477:1190–9.
9. Ota D, Loftin B, Saito T, Lea R, Keller J. Virtual reality in surgical education. Comput Biol Med. 1995;25(2):127–37.
10. Seymour NE, Gallagher AG, Roman SA, O'Brien MK, Bansal VK, Andersen DK, Satava RM. Virtual reality training improves operating room performance results of a randomized, double-blinded study. Ann Surg. 2002;236(4):458–64.
11. De Luca G, Choudhury N, Pagiatakis C, Laroche D. A multi-procedural virtual reality simulator for orthopaedic training. Virtual, augmented and mixed reality. Applications and case studies. HCII 2019. Lect Notes Comput Sci. 2019;11575:256–71.

28

Kinematically Aligned (KA) Knee Components and Total Knee Arthroplasty

Raj R. Thakrar and Sam Oussedik

Key Points

- Kinematically aligned (KA) knee components are implanted using the patient's joint surfaces and ligament tensions for reference rather than mechanical axes.
- This alternative alignment requires alternative assessment of post-operative radiographs.
- Implant positioning must be measured against the patient's own anatomy and as such is likely to result in valgus femoral positioning, varus tibial positioning and a resultant oblique joint line in the majority of patients.
- Evaluating three-dimensional images allows assessment in all three planes and will provide more accurate information regarding rotational alignment.

28.1 Introduction

Radiological assessment following knee arthroplasty surgery remains an essential aspect of routine post-operative care. Although outcomes after total knee arthroplasty (TKA) are increasingly focused on functional outcome scores, conventional radiographs still have a major role in the diagnosis and management of complications following surgery. In particular, component alignment in the coronal plane has been highlighted as playing an important role in implant survivorship of mechanically aligned (MA) TKA [1–4].

The Knee Society Total Knee Arthroplasty Roentgenograpic Evaluation and Scoring System published originally in 1989 [5, 6] is based on the anatomical axis, and allows for a systematic approach to the reporting of radiographs following TKA, providing a universally common method. However, the assessment and, more importantly, interpretation of post-operative TKA alignment may be influenced by the surgical philosophy adopted.

In this chapter, we aim to discuss how kinematic alignment (KA) in TKA may influence this interpretation of post-operative radiographs. Furthermore, we question whether conventional methods of short limb anteroposterior and lateral radiographs alone are sufficient in assessing the KA TKA.

28.2 What Is Kinematic Alignment?

Movement of the knee joint is achieved through the biomechanical interaction of the soft tissue component (ligaments and menisci) together with femoral and tibial articulating surfaces. Mean femoral joint angle (FJA) is approximately

R. R. Thakrar
Department of Orthopaedics, East and North Hertfordshire NHS Trust, Hertfordshire, UK

S. Oussedik (✉)
Department of Orthopaedics, University College London Hospital NHS Trust, London, UK

3° valgus and tibial joint angle (TJA) measures 3° varus to their respective mechanical axes [7]. Consequently, mean constitutional knee joint alignment is 3° varus to the mechanical axis of the lower limb.

First described by Freeman et al., the MA approach to TKA remains the gold standard. The technique aims to create a neutral lower limb alignment. This is achieved through preparing the distal femoral and proximal tibial cuts perpendicular to their respective mechanical axes. In addition, the posterior femoral condyle is cut in 3° external rotation. The net effect is thought to be equal load distribution through a newly orientated joint line with favourable survivorship outcomes reported when this is achieved [3, 8, 9].

More recently, however, work by Stephen Howell and colleagues has suggested an alternative approach to alignment in TKA, formally referred to as KA. Much of the work on KA has been driven by high patient dissatisfaction rates following the MA TKAs [10] bringing into question this surgical philosophy. KA works on the principle of correcting the arthritic deformity to restore the patient's own constitutional joint orientation, delivering a more "personalized" joint replacement. Considering the amount of bone and cartilage loss, resurfacing of the joint is achieved by adapting the bone resection thickness to match the implant thickness.

Appreciation of the KA approach requires an understanding of the kinematic axis of the knee joint. Much of the biomechanical rationale behind KA was introduced by Hollister et al. in the early 1990s [11] and more recently by the work of Eckhoff et al. [12]. Whilst the mechanical axis of the knee is based on a 2D schema of the joint (coronal and sagittal planes), the kinematic axis refers to its 3D orientation. By definition, the three kinematic axes include:

- Primary transverse axis (or cylindrical or transcondylar axis):

  This passes through the centre of a circle fit to the articular surface of the medial and lateral femoral condyles and represents the axis about which the tibia flexes on the femur from 10° to 120°.
- Secondary transverse axis:

  This axis is parallel and proximal to the primary axis and is the transverse axis about which the patella flexes and extends on the femur.
- Longitudinal axis:

  This is represented by the longitudinal axis of the tibia about which the tibia internally and externally rotates on the femur. The longitudinal axis is perpendicular to the primary and secondary axes.

The key operative goal of KA is to co-align the transverse axis of an appropriately sized femoral component to the primary transverse axis of the femur with the aim of restoring the normal interrelationships amongst the three axes.

28.3 How Does Implant Position Vary Between MA and KA?

To date, much of the literature evaluating postoperative alignment in TKA is based on the mechanically aligned knee using the aforementioned standardised radiographic views. The radiographic assessment of the MA knee will often demonstrate the joint to be in 4–6° of valgus (tibiofemoral anatomic angle) with optimal range reported as 2–7° by Fang et al. [8]. The alignment of the femoral component usually lies in 5–9° of valgus relative to the long axis of the femur [13]. The tibial component is placed perpendicular to the long axis of the tibia. Ritter et al. reported in their series of 6070 TKAs with a minimum follow-up of 2 years that implant failure was most likely to occur if placed <90° relative to the tibial axis (i.e. valgus) and the femoral component >8° valgus.

In contrast, component alignment in a KA prosthetic knee is somewhat more variable. A study by Dossett et al. [14] reported their short-term radiological results of an RCT comparing kinematically and mechanically aligned knee joints. They noted a tendency of placing the femoral component in a greater degree of valgus and tibial component in varus in the KA group. Importantly, they reported that the overall lower limb mechanical alignment was similar amongst the two groups with an average hip–knee–ankle angle of 0.3° varus in the KA group compared to 0° in the MA group. They concluded that the native joint line obliquity (best appreciated on weight-bearing long leg alignment views) was more closely restored in the KA group in comparison to the MA joints.

The results of this study have been echoed in a recent systematic review by Lee et al. [15] comparing KA and MA TKA. They concluded that whilst overall knee and limb alignments are similar amongst the two groups, the individual component alignment tends to be positioned in a greater degree valgus and varus in the femur and tibia, respectively, in the KA group. They also went on to conclude that the joint line obliquity in the KA group resembled that of the normal knee joint, something MA TKA fails to achieve.

28.4 Approach to Radiological Assessment of the KA TKA

Conventional weight-bearing anteroposterior and lateral radiographs are routinely used to assess the quality of implant positioning. Unlike in MA TKAs, with KA the ipsilateral pre-operative radiographs or the normal contralateral side knee is used as a reference for comparison.

Using these radiographs, component alignment in the coronal plane can be evaluated as the angle created between the anatomical axis of the bone and a line tangential to the articulating surface of the respective components with the aim of matching these angles pre- and post-operatively (Fig. 28.1). Furthermore, the coronal plane also allows assessment of the joint line obliquity (Fig. 28.2) on weight-bearing views.

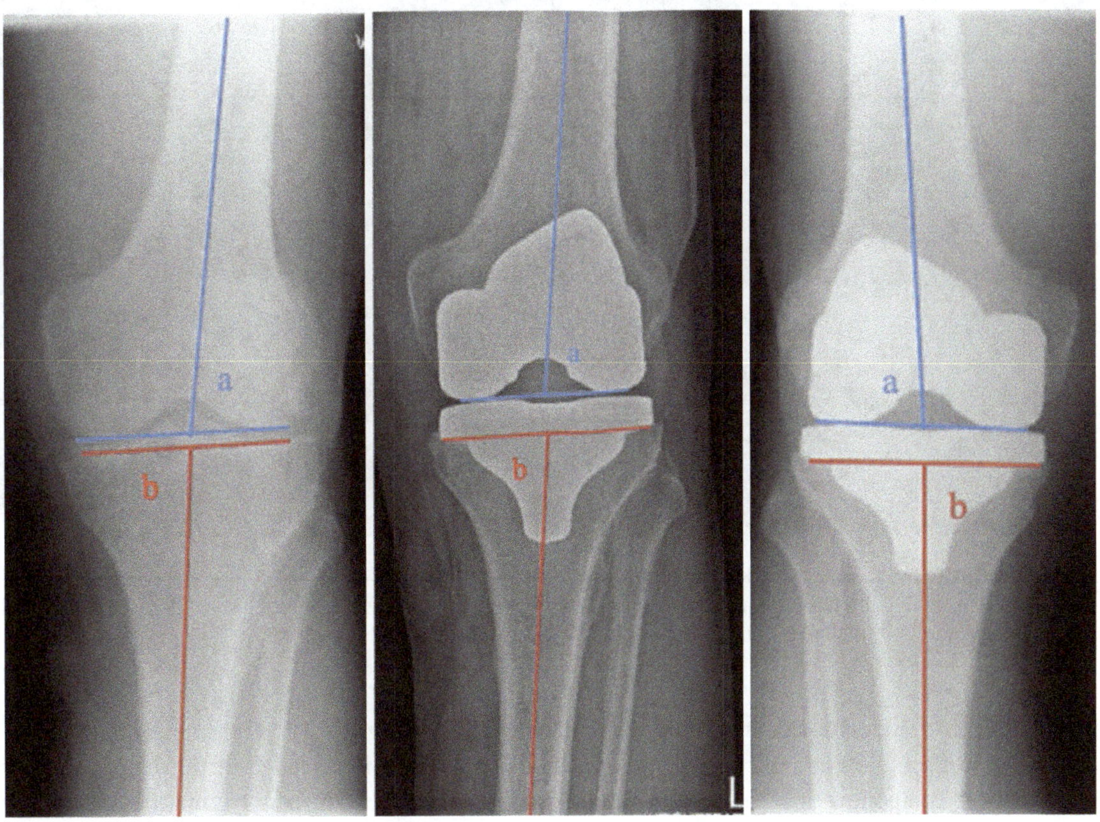

Fig. 28.1 Evaluation of component position using the anatomical axis. Comparison of pre-operative and post-operative angles demonstrates restoration of LDFA (**a**) and MPTA (**b**) angles following KA TKA (central image). In contrast, a change in these angles is noted on the contralateral knee where MA approach was utilised (right image)

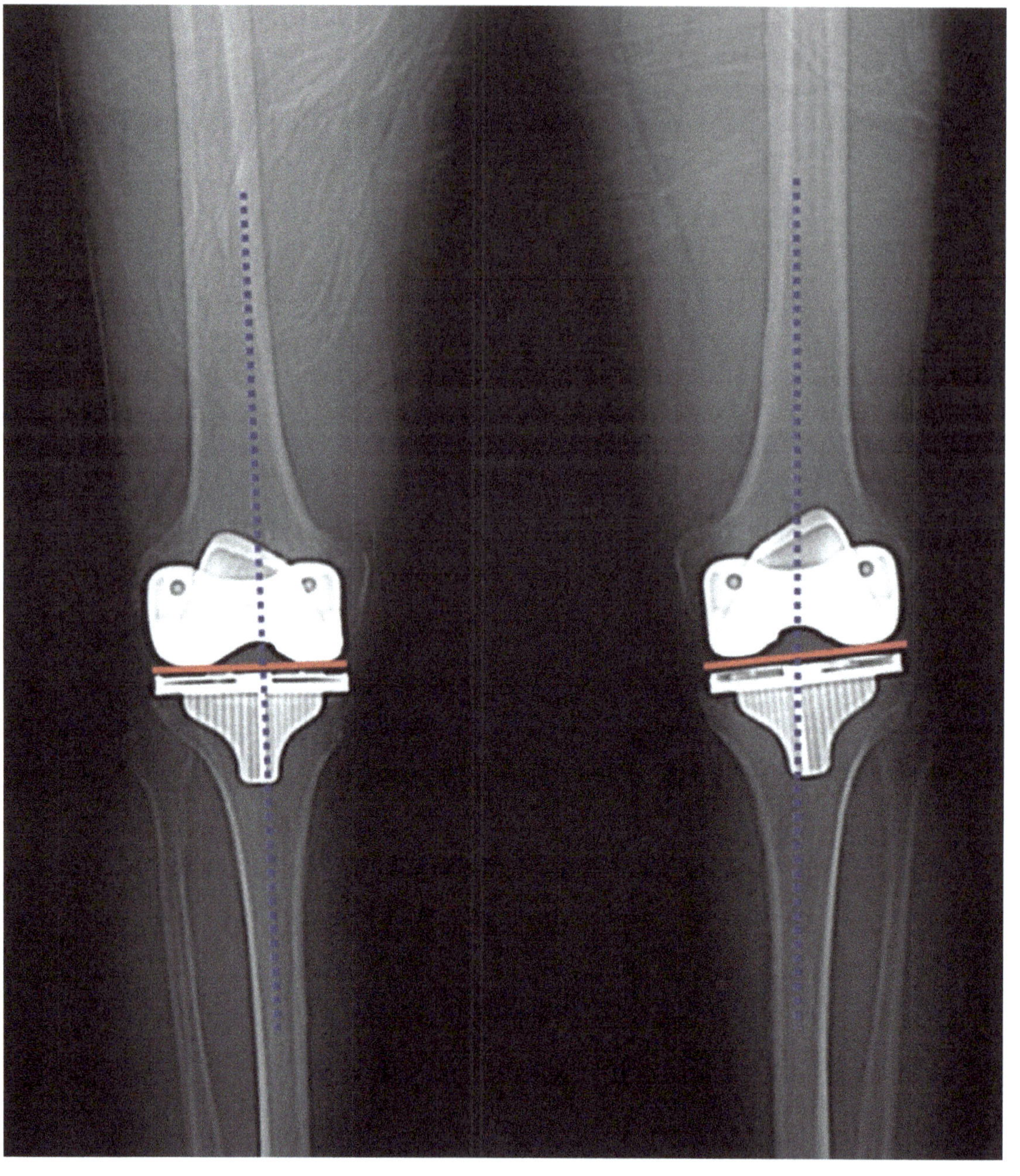

Fig. 28.2 Composite shows (1) the KA TKA (left knee) restores the natural joint line obliquity (red line) and maintains natural limb alignment (blue line) despite the appearance of a varus tibial component anatomical alignment; (2) the MA TKA (right knee) changes the natural joint line obliquity (red line)

On lateral view, assessment of the femoral component offset gives an indication of whether the femoral component has been over-/undersized or excessively anteriorised. The posterior condylar offset is defined as the maximum thickness of the posterior condyle projected posteriorly to a line tangential to the posterior cortex of the femur (Fig. 28.3). Decreasing offset potentially restricts knee range of movement secondary to impingement of the tibial component on the posterior femoral shaft. Equally, excessive anteriorisation of the femoral component can lead to overstuffing of the patellofemoral compartment leading to poor outcomes. Assessment

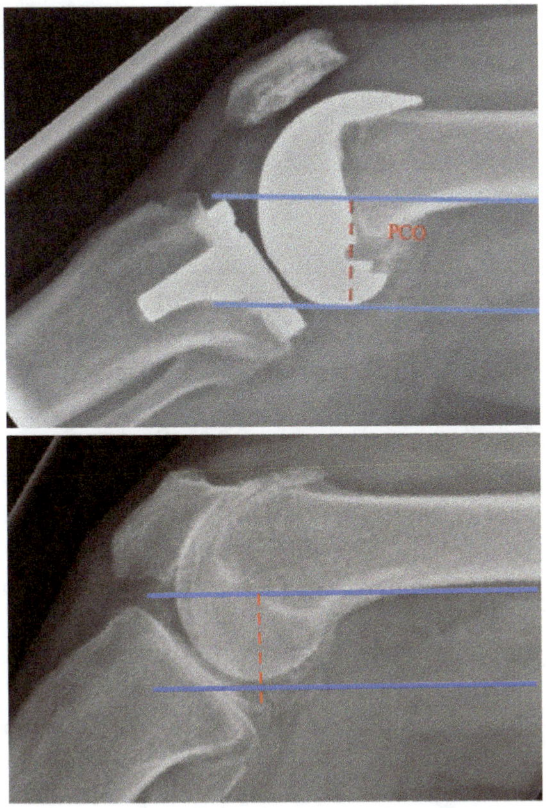

Fig. 28.3 Measurement of posterior condylar offset (PCO) pre- and post-op. Identified as the perpendicular distance between two parallel lines representing posterior cortex of femur and posterior femoral condyle

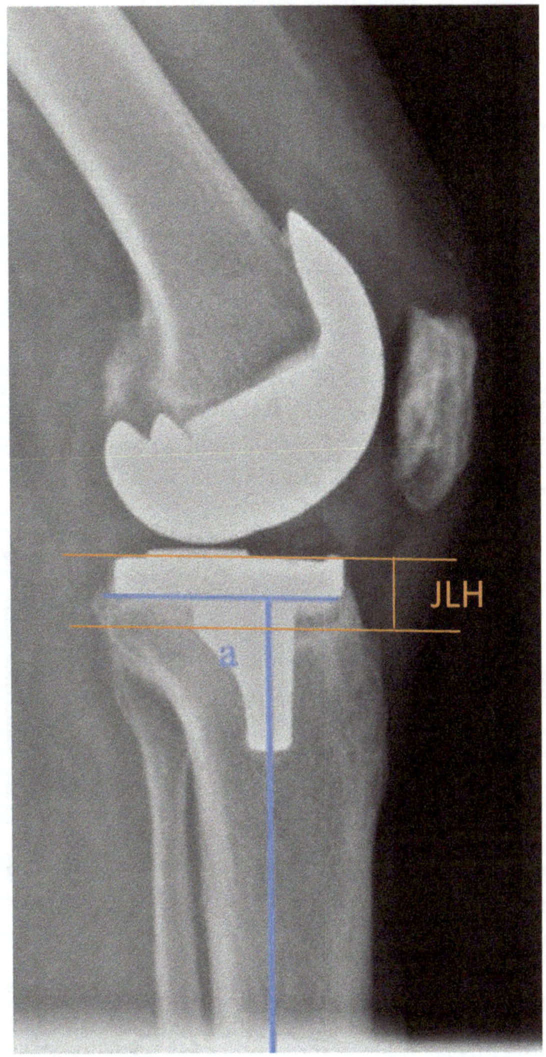

Fig. 28.4 Assessment of tibial slope (**a**) and joint line height (JLH)

of the posterior condyle contour matching that of the femoral component is also a useful method of assessing femoral sizing in the sagittal plane.

The tibial component is typically positioned where it can provide maximal bone coverage whilst optimising patellar tracking. Restoration of tibial slope ensures joint stability in the AP plain whilst allowing for deep flexion of the knee and maintaining knee kinematics. The posterior tibial slope is obtained from the intersection of a line drawn through the mid-shaft of the tibia and a line tangential to the tibial component (Fig. 28.4).

Maintenance of joint line height also plays an important role in knee kinematics, influencing knee range of movement and patellar femoral joint contact forces [16]. This is likely through its effect on the functionality of the posterior cruciate ligament. Assessment of joint line height can be made on lateral view radiographs. Typically, it is measured as the perpendicular distance between superior margin of the tibial tubercle and the weight-bearing parallel surface of the tibial component (Fig. 28.4).

Post-operative patella baja can negatively influence the outcomes for TKA through patellar maltracking and furthermore restricting range of movement. It is defined as a decrease in length of the patellar tendon by 10% of its preoperative value. Surgical techniques such as excessive Hoffa's fat pad excision resulting in tendon ischaemia are common causes for patella baja post-TKA [17–19]. Equally, it is important to note that factors such as implant design and elevation of the joint line can also influence patellar height measurement with bi-cruciate-substituting knees demonstrating a more similar pattern of patellar tendon shortening during flexion to the native knee joint as compared with cruciate-retaining knee designs [20]. Whilst there are a number of recognised techniques for measurement of patellar height, the Insall–Salvati ratio has a number of theoretical advantages in that it is not influenced by the position of the joint line, size of the knee, position of the knee or radiographic magnification. The measurement was first described in 1971 [21]. It is calculated as the ratio of the length of the patellar tendon to the diagonal length of the patella (Fig. 28.5). A later modification of this measurement by Grelsamer and Meadows was introduced in 1992 to compensate for the ambiguity of identifying the true patella and patellar tendon lengths [22]. This modified value may be used as an adjunct to the Insall–Salvati ratio.

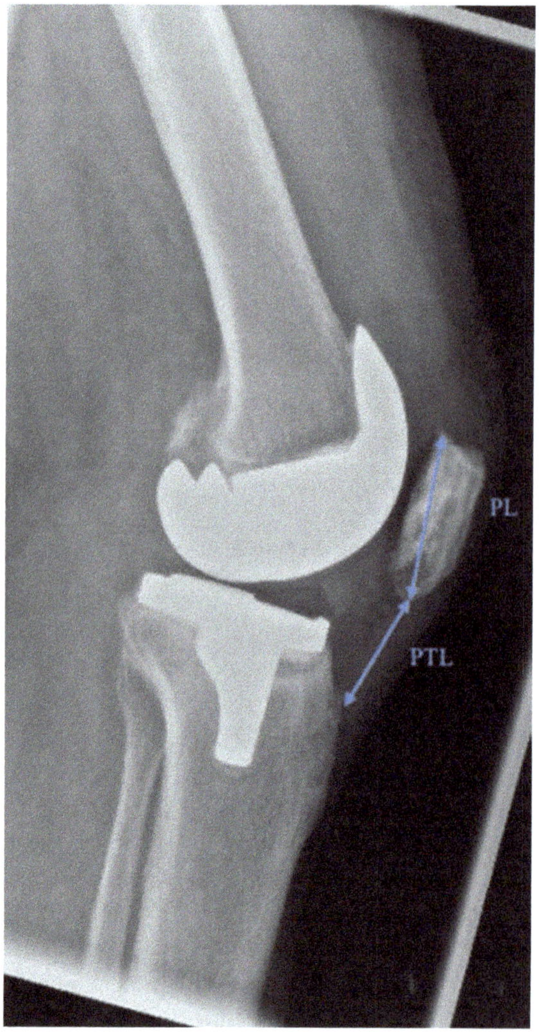

Fig. 28.5 Assessment of patellar height. Original description of the Insall–Salvati ratio expressed as a ratio of the patellar tendon length (PTL) over the patellar length (PL)

28.5 Is Traditional Short Leg Radiographic Assessment of Kinematic TKA Sufficient?

It is traditional practise that assessment of component position and overall tibiofemoral alignment post-TKA be made on short leg radiographs. In the outpatient setting, these are easier to perform and limit the degree of radiation exposure to the patient.

Whilst there is sufficient evidence to support that this method delivers an adequate degree of clinical information [23], a number of more recent studies have questioned accuracy of short leg views when compared to hip–knee–ankle standing long leg views for evaluation of coronal alignment [24, 25]. Furthermore, whilst non-weight-bearing radiographs provide information on component alignment relative to the anatomical axis of the femur and tibia, they fail to demonstrate exactly how the knee prosthesis is functionally loaded, assessment of which is relevant in both MA and KA philosophy. A study by Hutt et al. [26] highlighted the importance of this. They evaluated post-op radiographs of 50 KA TKAs. Their results reported that when looking at the tibial component relative to the mechanical axis of the tibia (as one would do on a short leg film assessment), a misleading, excessive degree of varus malalignment was noted (66% outliers to the safe zone of >3° varus); however, when assessing the joint line angle on weight-bearing long leg views, this outlier group was significantly smaller (12%). Hutt concluded that KA TKA often produces a joint line angle in varus relative to the mechanical axis of the tibia; when weight bearing, however, the actual joint line orientation becomes more acceptable, and this may explain promising early results in terms of survivorship of the KA knee joint despite X-ray appearances.

Despite this, however, it is generally considered that weight-bearing long leg views are more relevant in the assessment of the MA TKA or in the research setting. For KA TKA, the traditional short leg views provide sufficient information to allow comparison of component position to pre-operative distal femoral and proximal tibial alignment in both coronal and surgical planes as described earlier.

28.6 Role of CT Evaluation

Thus far, this chapter has described the approach to 2D coronal and sagittal plane assessment of implant position following KA TKA. Currently, there is no literature to support the superiority of a 3D imaging modality such as 3D computer tomography (3D-CT) over 2D radiographs in assessing the KA TKA. We attribute this to the fact that KA is a relatively new concept with much of the current literature being focused on the assessment of patient outcomes and implant survivorship. What is evident, however, is that whilst the standard views discussed thus far allow for varus/valgus and AP positioning of the components to be assessed, they are of limited value on assessment of axial rotational alignment [27–29]. Furthermore, a number of studies have identified challenges relating to the accurate assessment of subtle malposition on plain radiographs owing to variations in limb position and magnification [30, 31]. Early described methods of assessment of rotation are limited to implant design and [32, 33]; hence, the current gold standard for assessment of rotation involves cross-sectional imaging in the form of CT scan [34], which is the case irrespective of whether an MA or KA philosophy has been adopted.

With regard to the KA knee, as discussed earlier, this philosophy is focused on a 3D model of the knee joint. In this scenario, CT may play a role in assessing, in particular, the position of the femoral component in the axial plane. A study by Hirschmann et al. compared the accuracy of conventional radiographs, transverse 2D-CT and 3D-CT reconstruction in assessing the position and orientation of TKA components. They concluded that their protocol of 3D-CT reconstruction for the assessment of rotational, sagittal and coronal orientation of the components reduced measurement errors as evident through less variability in inter- and intra-observer error. A limitation of CT, however, remains the inability to routinely perform weight-bearing imaging, which as mentioned earlier plays an important role when it comes to understanding functional loading of the joint. Hence, until such imaging becomes routinely available, it would have to be proposed that weight-bearing radiographs remain a useful alternative.

Equally, it is also important at this point to consider the clinical relevance of routine assessment of the axial orientation in KA TKA. Based on the surgical strategy of a measured resection tool adopted in this technique, the likelihood of failing to perform a cut parallel to the posterior femoral condyles is theoretically low. This, combined with a larger tolerance for axial orientation of the tibial component (in the order of 30–40°), may suggest that the overall axial orientation of the KA TKA (contrary to MA TKA), is unlikely to become a significant cause of clinical issues and therefore has little merit in being assessed.

28.7 Summary

KA TKA is becoming an increasingly popular philosophy with promising early reports on functional outcome and patient satisfaction. Assessment of the functionally loaded joint appears to be a key component in evaluation of the KA TKA. Conventional methods of short limb X-rays with anatomical assessment of component position provide sufficient information, especially when used in the context of referencing off pre-operative or contralateral normal limb radiographs. There is, however, some suggestion in the literature that short leg views may be misinterpreted as showing component malposition with excessive varus/valgus component alignment as compared to the acceptable safe zones when adopting the KA strategy. Equally the role of post-operative CT scan remains inconclusive in routine assessment of implant position.

Pearls and Pitfalls

1. KA in TKA has promising early clinical results.
2. Current approach to short leg views in post-operative assessment is adequate in assessing the KA joint.
3. Comparison of post-operative radiographs to either ipsilateral pre-operative or contralateral side normal radiographs is important as part of the evaluation process for assessment of accuracy of component positioning.
4. CT imaging in addition to long leg views plays a more important role in the evaluation of the MA TKA or in the context of research. Their role in routine assessment of the KA TKA remains inconclusive.

Clinical Case

A 62-year-old gentleman with bilateral knee osteoarthritis presented with severe mechanical pain in his left knee (Figs. 28.6 and 28.7). The limb was significantly varus aligned, but correctable. The patient was implanted with a KA medial pivot TKA design, using manual instrumentation and a callipered technique (Fig. 28.8). When planning and performing this case, the difficulty was in estimating the bone loss in the medial compartment. On comparison with the

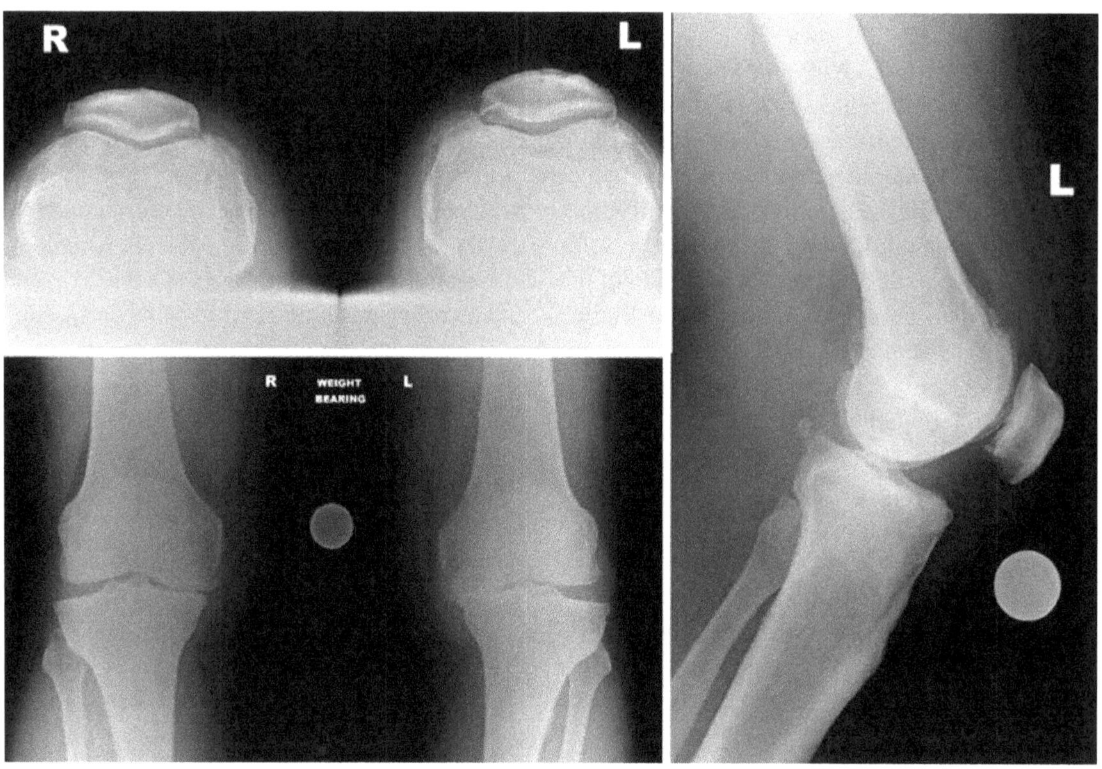

Fig. 28.6 Bilateral knee osteoarthritis primarily affecting the medial knee compartment, being more severe on the left knee

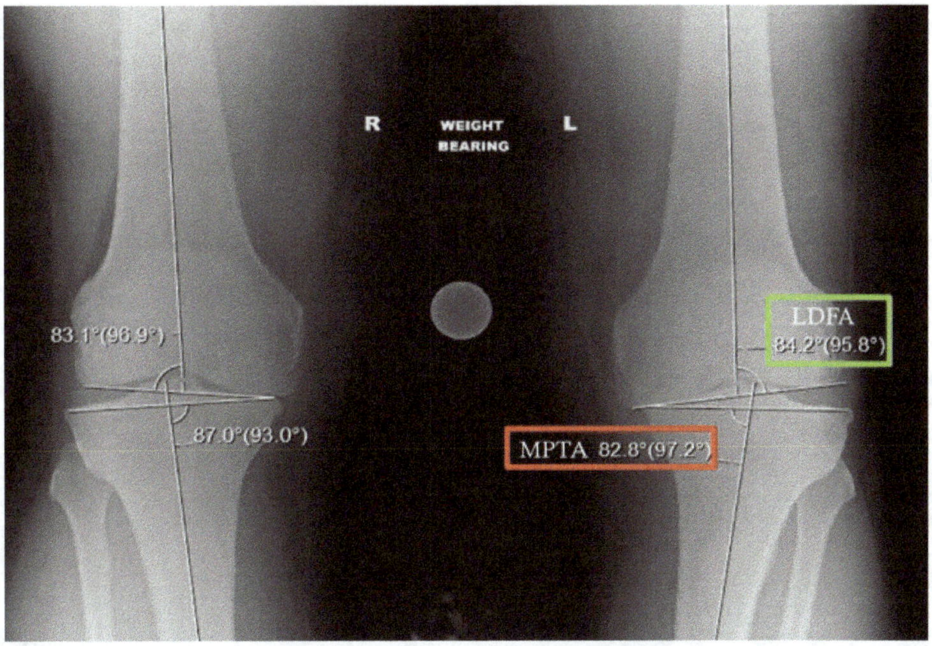

Fig. 28.7 Measurement of anatomical lateral distal femoral (LDFA) and medial proximal tibial (MPTA) angles on short film. The right knee is likely to have negligible bone loss and therefore may serve to estimate the pre-arthritic orientation of the femoral and tibial joint lines. The bone loss was estimated to be 1 mm on the distal femoral condyle (84.2°– 83.1° = 1.1°) and 4 mm on the medial tibial plateau (82.8°– 87° = 4.2°), as 1° of additional knee deformity approximately corresponds to 1 mm of articular surface bone loss

right knee, which shows negligible bone loss, a 4 mm and a 1 mm loss of bone were estimated on the tibial and femoral sides, respectively.

The quality control for kinematic positioning of knee implants can be done intraoperatively, rather than on the post-operative radiograph alone. This is achieved through calliper measurement of the width of each bone cut, compensating for cartilage and bone loss, with the aim of matching the component thickness. As calliper measurements are precise, this method is indisputably the best way to guarantee correct kinematic positioning. Post-operatively, assessment of the quality of a kinematic implantation is possible by comparing radiographic orientation of artificial and native joint lines (distal femur and proximal tibia). For comparison, it is possible to use either the contralateral knee (ideally on post-operative frontal radiograph capturing both knees) or the preoperative images of the operated knee. In this specific case with significant bone loss, it is sensible to use the contralateral knee for the post-operative radiographic quality control (Figs. 28.7 and 28.9). While short films are sufficient for assessing the quality of a kinematic implantation, long films are also valuable and inform on the prosthetic limb alignment (hip–knee–ankle [HKA] angle).

While 2D images are subject to imprecisions in measurements (2D rendering of a 3D volume, high influence on frontal measures of knee rotation in axial and sagittal planes), 3D images enable more accurate assessment and should therefore become the standard.

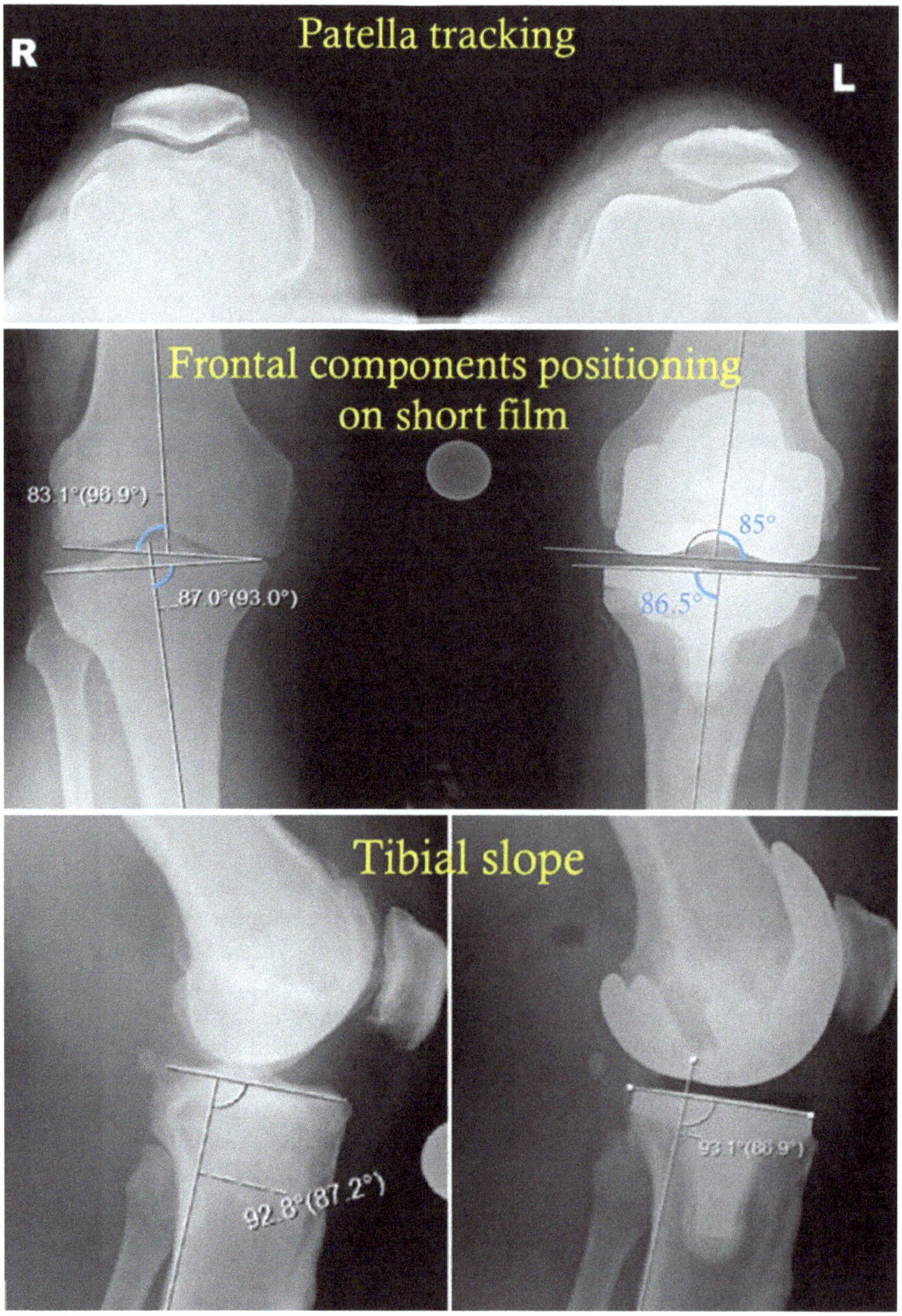

Fig. 28.8 Short film knee radiographs (skyline, frontal and lateral) enable assessment of the quality of a kinematic implantation by comparing the orientation of the joint lines between the right (native) and left (prosthetic) knees. The patellar tracking was considered excellent intraoperatively with the 'no thumb technique'; however, the patella was unexpectedly laterally shifted on the skyline view; its significance is unknown, and the patient had no complaints at her 1-year follow-up. Regarding frontal figures, it is likely that angular differences between knees are mainly the consequence of measurement imprecisions (2D radiograph), as the intraoperative calliper checks indicated accurate bone cuts, therefore guaranteeing correct restoration of the pre-arthritic distal femoral joint line orientation

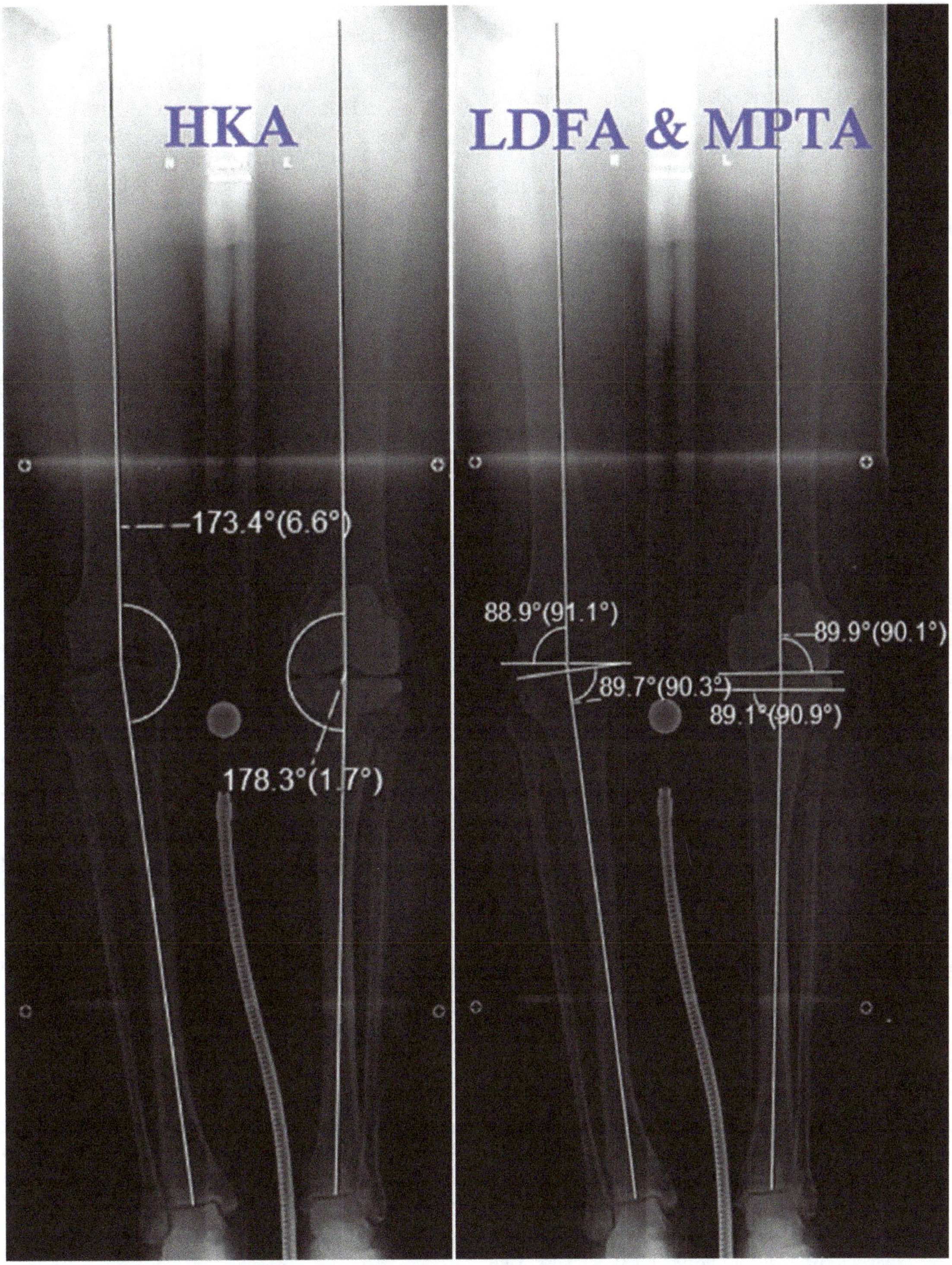

Fig. 28.9 Long films also enable assessment of the quality of the frontal component positioning (mechanical LDFA and MPTA angles), in addition to indicating the post-operative limb alignment by measurement of the hip–knee–ankle (HKA) angle. In this case, the frontal kinematic positioning of components resembles that of a mechanical implantation; nevertheless, the axial and sagittal positioning of components would still differ between techniques of alignment

References

1. Longstaff LM, Sloan K, Stamp N, Scaddan M, Beaver R. Good alignment after total knee arthroplasty leads to faster rehabilitation and better function. J Arthroplast. 2009;24(4):570–8. [cited 2018 Jul 30]. http://www.ncbi.nlm.nih.gov/pubmed/18534396
2. Choong PF, Dowsey MM, Stoney JD. Does accurate anatomical alignment result in better function and quality of life? Comparing conventional and computer-assisted total knee arthroplasty. J Arthroplast. 2009;24(4):560–9. [cited 2018 Jul 30]. http://www.ncbi.nlm.nih.gov/pubmed/18534397
3. Ritter MA, Davis KE, Meding JB, Pierson JL, Berend ME, Malinzak RA. The effect of alignment and BMI on failure of total knee replacement. J Bone Joint Surg Am. 2011;93(17):1588–96. [cited 2018 Jul 30]. http://www.ncbi.nlm.nih.gov/pubmed/21915573
4. Benjamin J. Component alignment in total knee arthroplasty. Instr Course Lect. 2006;55:405–12. [cited 2018 Jul 31] http://www.ncbi.nlm.nih.gov/pubmed/16958475
5. Ewald FC. The Knee Society total knee arthroplasty roentgenographic evaluation and scoring system. Clin Orthop Relat Res. 1989;248:9–12. [cited 2018 Aug 12]. http://www.ncbi.nlm.nih.gov/pubmed/2805502
6. Scuderi GR, Bourne RB, Noble PC, Benjamin JB, Lonner JH, Scott WN. The new knee society knee scoring system. Clin Orthop Relat Res. 2012;470(1):3–19. https://doi.org/10.1007/s11999-011-2135-0. [cited 2018 Jul 30]. http://link.springer.com/
7. Moreland JR, Bassett LW, Hanker GJ. Radiographic analysis of the axial alignment of the lower extremity. J Bone Joint Surg Am. 1987;69(5):745–9. [cited 2018 Aug 11]. http://www.ncbi.nlm.nih.gov/pubmed/3597474
8. Fang DM, Ritter MA, Davis KE. Coronal alignment in total knee arthroplasty. J Arthroplast. 2009;24(6):39–43. [cited 2018 Aug 11]. http://www.ncbi.nlm.nih.gov/pubmed/19553073
9. Jeffery RS, Morris RW, Denham RA. Coronal alignment after total knee replacement. J Bone Joint Surg Br. 1991;73(5):709–14. [cited 2018 Aug 9]. http://www.ncbi.nlm.nih.gov/pubmed/1894655
10. Bourne RB, Chesworth BM, Davis AM, Mahomed NN, Charron KDJ. Patient satisfaction after total knee arthroplasty: who is satisfied and who is not? Clin Orthop Relat Res. 2010;468(1):57–63. [cited 2018 Jun 3]. http://www.ncbi.nlm.nih.gov/pubmed/19844772
11. Hollister AM, Jatana S, Singh AK, Sullivan WW, Lupichuk AG. The axes of rotation of the knee. Clin Orthop Relat Res. 1993;290:259–68. [cited 2018 Jun 3]. http://www.ncbi.nlm.nih.gov/pubmed/8472457
12. Eckhoff DG. Three-dimensional mechanics, kinematics, and morphology of the knee viewed in virtual reality. J Bone Joint Surg. 2005;87(suppl_2):71. https://doi.org/10.2106/JBJS.E.00440. [cited 2018 Aug 12]. http://jbjs.org/cgi/doi/
13. Allen AM, Ward WG, Pope TL. Imaging of the total knee arthroplasty. Radiol Clin North Am. 1995;33(2):289–303. [cited 2018 Aug 12]. http://www.ncbi.nlm.nih.gov/pubmed/7871170
14. Dossett HG, Swartz GJ, Estrada NA, LeFevre GW, Kwasman BG. Kinematically versus mechanically aligned total knee arthroplasty. Orthopedics. 2012;35(2):e160–9. [cited 2018 Aug 11]. http://www.ncbi.nlm.nih.gov/pubmed/22310400
15. Lee YS, Howell SM, Won Y-Y, Lee O-S, Lee SH, Vahedi H, et al. Kinematic alignment is a possible alternative to mechanical alignment in total knee arthroplasty. Knee Surg Sports Traumatol Arthrosc. 2017;25(11):3467–79. [cited 2018 Sep 30]. http://www.ncbi.nlm.nih.gov/pubmed/28439636
16. Figgie HE, Goldberg VM, Heiple KG, Moller HS, Gordon NH. The influence of tibial-patellofemoral location on function of the knee in patients with the posterior stabilized condylar knee prosthesis. J Bone Joint Surg Am. 1986;68(7):1035–40. [cited 2019 Mar 24]. http://www.ncbi.nlm.nih.gov/pubmed/3745240
17. Kayler DE, Lyttle D. Surgical interruption of patellar blood supply by total knee arthroplasty. Clin Orthop Relat Res. 1988;229:221–7. [cited 2019 Mar 24]. http://www.ncbi.nlm.nih.gov/pubmed/3349681
18. Weale AE, Murray DW, Newman JH, Ackroyd CE. The length of the patellar tendon after unicompartmental and total knee replacement. J Bone Joint Surg Br. 1999;81(5):790–5. [cited 2019 Mar 24]. http://www.ncbi.nlm.nih.gov/pubmed/10530838
19. Lee G-C, Cushner FD, Scuderi GR, Insall JN. Optimizing patellofemoral tracking during total knee arthroplasty. J Knee Surg. 2004;17(3):144–9; discussion 149–50. [cited 2019 Mar 24]. http://www.ncbi.nlm.nih.gov/pubmed/15366269
20. Brilhault J, Ries MD. Measuring patellar height using the lateral active flexion radiograph: effect of total knee implant design. Knee. 2010;17(2):148–51. [cited 2019 Mar 24]. http://www.ncbi.nlm.nih.gov/pubmed/19720535
21. Insall J, Salvati E. Patella position in the normal knee joint. Radiology. 1971;101(1):101–4. [cited 2019 Mar 24]. http://www.ncbi.nlm.nih.gov/pubmed/5111961
22. Grelsamer RP, Meadows S. The modified Insall-Salvati ratio for assessment of patellar height. Clin Orthop Relat Res. 1992;282:170–6. [cited 2019 Mar 24]. http://www.ncbi.nlm.nih.gov/pubmed/1516309
23. Patel DV, Ferris BD, Aichroth PM. Radiological study of alignment after total knee replacement. Int Orthop. 1991;15(3):209–10. https://doi.org/10.1007/BF00192296. [cited 2018 Aug 12]. http://link.springer.com/
24. Park A, Stambough JB, Nunley RM, Barrack RL, Nam D. The inadequacy of short knee radiographs in evaluating coronal alignment after total knee arthroplasty. J Arthroplast. 2016;31(4):878–82. [cited 2018 Sep 12]. http://www.ncbi.nlm.nih.gov/pubmed/26410551
25. Abu-Rajab RB, Deakin AH, Kandasami M, McGlynn J, Picard F, Kinninmonth AWG. Hip–knee–ankle radiographs are more appropriate for assessment of

post-operative mechanical alignment of total knee arthroplasties than standard AP knee radiographs. J Arthroplast. 2015;30(4):695–700. [cited 2018 Aug 12]. http://www.ncbi.nlm.nih.gov/pubmed/25702592
26. Hutt J, Massé V, Lavigne M, Vendittoli P-A. Functional joint line obliquity after kinematic total knee arthroplasty. Int Orthop. 2016;40(1):29–34. [cited 2018 Aug 12]. http://www.ncbi.nlm.nih.gov/pubmed/25795248
27. Dennis DA. Evaluation of painful total knee arthroplasty. J Arthroplasty. 2004;19(4 Suppl 1):35–40. [cited 2018 Sep 30]. http://www.ncbi.nlm.nih.gov/pubmed/15190547
28. Mandalia V, Eyres K, Schranz P, Toms AD. Evaluation of patients with a painful total knee replacement. J Bone Joint Surg Br. 2008;90(3):265–71. [cited 2018 Sep 30]. http://www.ncbi.nlm.nih.gov/pubmed/18310744
29. Toms AD, Mandalia V, Haigh R, Hopwood B. The management of patients with painful total knee replacement. J Bone Joint Surg Br. 2009;91(2):143–50. https://doi.org/10.1302/0301-620X.91B2.20995. [cited 2018 Sep 30]. http://online.boneandjoint.org.uk.
30. Bäthis H, Perlick L, Tingart M, Lüring C, Zurakowski D, Grifka J. Alignment in total knee arthroplasty. A comparison of computer-assisted surgery with the conventional technique. J Bone Joint Surg Br. 2004;86(5):682–7. [cited 2018 Sep 30]. http://www.ncbi.nlm.nih.gov/pubmed/15274263
31. Skyttä ET, Lohman M, Tallroth K, Remes V. Comparison of standard anteroposterior knee and hip-to-ankle radiographs in determining the lower limb and implant alignment after total knee arthroplasty. Scand J Surg. 2009;98(4):250–3. [cited 2018 Sep 30]. http://www.ncbi.nlm.nih.gov/pubmed/20218424
32. Takai S, Yoshino N, Isshiki T, Hirasawa Y. Kneeling view: a new roentgenographic technique to assess rotational deformity and alignment of the distal femur. J Arthroplasty. 2003;18(4):478–83. [cited 2018 Aug 12]. http://www.ncbi.nlm.nih.gov/pubmed/12820092
33. Eckhoff DG, Piatt BE, Gnadinger CA, Blaschke RC. Assessing rotational alignment in total knee arthroplasty. Clin Orthop Relat Res. 1995;((318)):176–81. [cited 2018 Aug 12]. http://www.ncbi.nlm.nih.gov/pubmed/7671514
34. Jazrawi LM, Birdzell L, Kummer FJ, Di Cesare PE. The accuracy of computed tomography for determining femoral and tibial total knee arthroplasty component rotation. J Arthroplast. 2000;15(6):761–6. [cited 2018 Aug 12]. http://www.ncbi.nlm.nih.gov/pubmed/11021452

29

Concept of 'À La Carte' Joint Replacement

Charles Rivière, Ciara Harman,
and Kartik Logishetty

Key Points

- The goal of arthroplasty is to replace arthrosis with high-performance prosthetic joints which accommodate the high expectations and increased life expectancy of modern patients.
- A dogmatic, one-size-fits-all approach to treating arthrosis is unlikely to deliver reproducible, optimal clinical outcomes.
- Decisions regarding choice of approach, implant design, configuration and component orientation should be individualised depending on each patient's anatomy and biomechanics, and should be a shared process between the patient and surgeon.
- Surgeons should aim to reproduce normal function through personalized kinematically aligned, conservative (soft tissue and bone) joint replacement techniques.
- This 'à la carte' approach to joint replacement challenges current trends. It is technically challenging, but represents the state of the art for arthroplasty. Thus, it targets sub-specialised, high-volume, expert surgeons.

C. Rivière (✉)
The MSK Lab, Imperial College London,
White City Campus, London, UK

South West London Elective Orthopaedic Centre,
Epsom, UK

C. Harman
South West London Elective Orthopaedic Centre,
Epsom, UK

K. Logishetty
The MSK Lab, Imperial College London,
White City Campus, London, UK
e-mail: k.logishetty@imperial.ac.uk

29.1 The 'À La Carte' Joint Replacement Philosophy (Fig. 29.1)

Hip and knee arthroplasties are life-changing procedures, reducing pain and restoring function after end-stage arthrosis. Almost 90% of patients who have undergone hip arthroplasty, and 82% after knee arthroplasty, report improvement in quality of life after surgery [1]; this leaves a significant number of dissatisfied patients. The modern surgeon can make decisions regarding surgical approach, implant design and component orientation. However, it is challenging to gain proficiency in a wide variety of surgical configurations. A smaller repertoire is technically and economically more feasible, and thus a one-size-fits-all approach is commonplace. Hip and knee arthroplasties are forgiving procedures, most frequently performed in older patients without high functional demands. The future arthroplasty surgeon is faced with new challenges—patients with higher demand, expectations and longer life expectancy, in addition to an increasing burden of revision surgery. Here, we discuss 'a la carte' joint replacement (Fig. 29.1), which is both patient specific and bone/soft tissue conservative. It may improve overall satisfaction while conserving bone stock in the event of future revision surgery.

This concept is borne of the observation that each patient is unique, so a dogmatic approach to managing joint degeneration cannot consistently deliver reproducible, optimal clinical outcomes. Bone quality, joint anatomy, biomechanics and kinematics vary widely between patients. 'À la carte' joint replacement aims to tailor each surgical decision based on these factors and patient expectations. Where feasible, conservative surgery performed through smaller incisions or using bone-preserving implant designs, such as compartmental knee arthroplasty and hip-resurfacing arthroplasty, should be favoured to ease and secure potential future revision procedures. Decisions regarding choice of approach, implant design, fixation and configuration and component orientation are therefore made with a patient-specific philosophy. The goal is to replace joints with high-performance prostheses, which respect and restore native biology.

Kinematic alignment (KA) in hip [2, 3] *and knee* [4, 5] *arthroplasty* aims to restore function by placing components in positions and orientations which work in harmony with native joint biomechanics. The KA technique aims to restore the native joint anatomy, plus or minus adjusting the component position to adapt to the individual spine–hip relationship (hip replacement) or knee biomechanics (knee replacement) [6, 7]. These techniques are described in detail in Chaps. 11, 16, 17, 24 and 25. In summary, hip KA is a departure from traditional 'safe zones' for implant orientation. It focuses on achieving a centre of rotation, acetabular inclination and combined femoral and acetabular version which confers a stable and impingement-free range of motion. This dynamic concept is of particular relevance in patients with altered relationships between the hip, pelvis and spine, most commonly seen in the elderly, or after spinal arthrodesis. Knee KA focuses on restoring the native, pre-arthritic flexion of the tibia and patella around two transverse femoral axes (cylindical and patella axis, respectively) and rotation of the tibia around a longitudinal axis. This aims to restore the native joint line's height and orientation to balance the

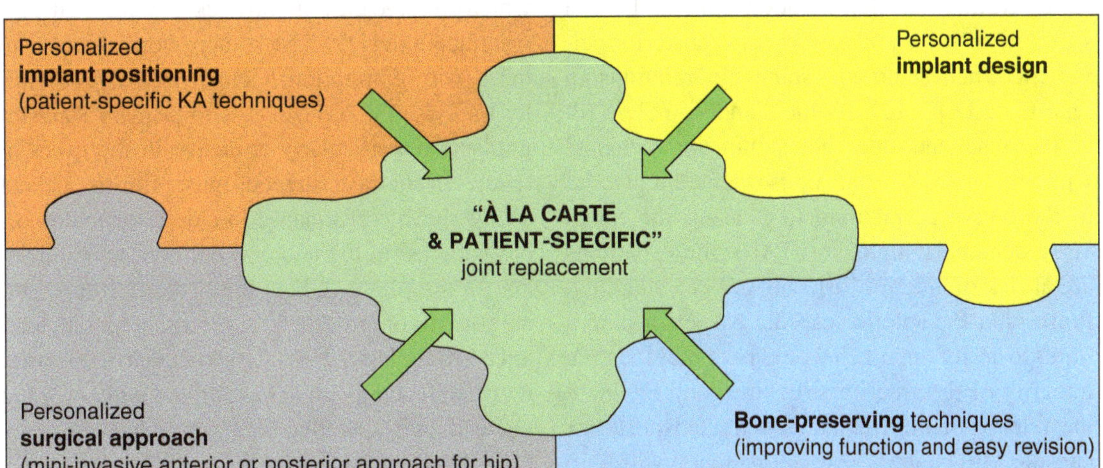

Fig. 29.1 The concept of 'a la carte and patient-specific joint replacement' consists of personalizing every aspect of the surgery. The decisions regarding choice of approach, implant design and components' orientation are made on a patient-specific basis. The goals are to replicate the constitutional joint anatomy unless severely abnormal, adjust component orientation to compensate for poor joint biomechanics and preserve as much as possible the bone stock and the integrity of the peri-articular soft tissue environment

collateral ligaments and restore patellofemoral and tibiofemoral kinematics. Hip and knee KAs take into account the patient's unique joint anatomy, peri-articular soft tissue balance and joint kinematics to produce a biomechanically friendly prosthetic joint. This may improve components' life span through improving prosthetic joint biomechanics (reducing risks of prosthetic impingement and edge loading) whilst improving patient function and satisfaction [8, 9].

The *choice of surgical approach* is of particular interest in hip arthroplasty, where it can have a significant impact on early recovery and longer term clinical outcomes. The most commonly debated approaches to the hip are the posterior (Moore) approach and the direct anterior (Hueter) approach (DAA). The posterior approach offers excellent exposure and is considered the most versatile for revision hip surgery. The anterior approach is intermuscular, internervous, and technically more demanding, but facilitates early rehabilitation and can be performed through an aesthetic 'bikini' incision. When choosing between them, surgeons should consider the age and functional demands of the patient, the presence of anterior or posterior soft tissue contractures, the technical demand of the procedure and probably the individual spine–hip relationship in addition (Fig. 29.2) [2]. Elderly patients who suffer from spine degeneration tend to have a stiff lumbar spine and an increased posterior pelvic tilt when standing—spine–hip relationship type C or D [2, 10]. As the standing pelvic tilt of these patients does not significantly change with arthroplasty, if the cup is orientated parallel to the native acetabulum (e.g. using the transverse acetabular ligament, TAL), these patients are at risk of anterior dislocation when standing. Preserving the anterior capsule by performing a mini-posterior approach would both maintain the integrity of the anterior structures, and facilitate the release of the frequently retracted posterior capsule. In contrast, young patients with hip osteoarthritis secondary to pincer-type femoroacetabular impingement disease are likely to display spine–hip relationship type B [2]. The pelvis has insufficient posterior tilt when moving from standing to sitting positions [11]. Thus, after THR, patients are at risk of posterior dislocation. Preserving the integrity of posterior soft tissue structures is sound, and an anterior approach with the cup device sufficiently anteverted is therefore more likely to restore stable range of motion. When the spine–hip relationship is normal (type 2A) [2], either approach is appropriate, although the authors favour the DAA as it does not require post-operative 'hip precautions' and is associated with an earlier return to function [12].

The *selection of the optimal implant design* depends on multiple patient-specific factors, including the patient's functional demands, bone quality (bone density and bone stock), joint morphology, the likelihood of revision surgery (which is mainly influenced by the patient's age at the time of surgery) and the risk of prosthetic instability. Younger patients may benefit from implant designs that are hard wearing and only require conservative bone resection. These properties facilitate high performance and longevity and the potential for easier revision. Compartmental knee arthroplasty (using unicondylar and/or patellofemoral implants), performed on patients without tricompartmental arthrosis, ligamentous instability and significant flexion contracture, is a safer and higher functioning alternative to total knee arthroplasty [13]. Hip-resurfacing and neck-sparing total hip arthroplasties are also conservative options which preserve the femoral neck. Patients with hip-resurfacing devices have a more normal gait than those with conventional length stems. The ability to revise these prostheses to primary standard implants is particularly attractive in the event of failure. In contrast, surgeons must prioritise patient safety above performance in elderly or multimorbid patients. In the authors' opinion, unicondylar knee arthroplasty (UKA) is suitable for appropriate patients of any age. When compared with total knee arthroplasty, UKA is associated with faster return to function, higher functional outcomes and reduced peri-operative morbidity and mortality [14, 15], even in those aged over 75 years [16]. With regards to hip arthroplasty, the use of collared stems, large-diameter heads and dual-mobility implants should be promoted, as they reduce the risks of subsidence and peri-operative femoral fracture [14] and instability [10], respectively.

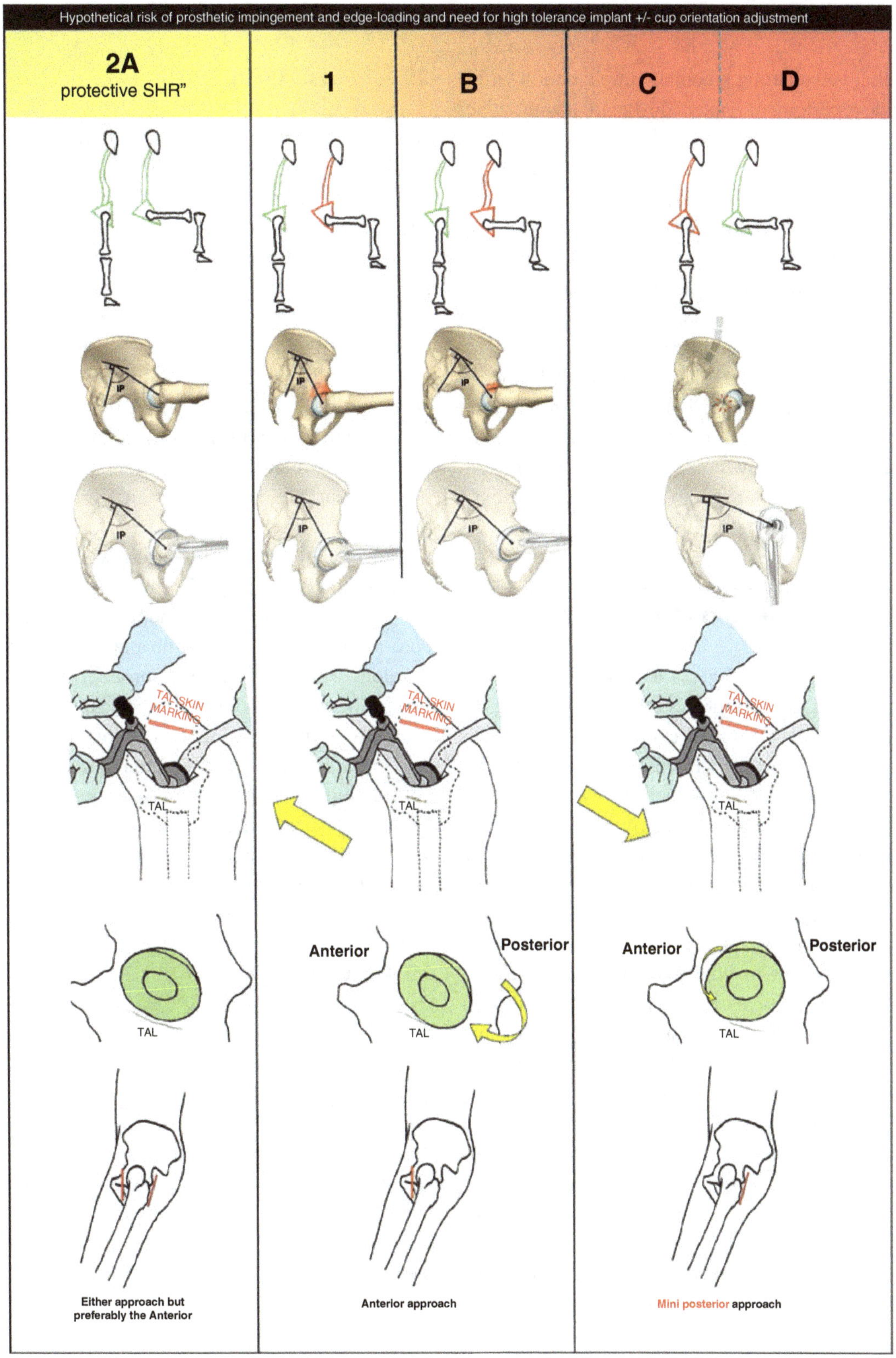

Fig. 29.2 This figure illustrates how the definition of an individual spine-hip relationship influences the personalization of the implantation of THR components. Defining a patient's spine–hip relationship (SHR) subsequently guides the surgical plan, with regards to the choice of surgical approach, implant design and orientation

29.2 Can It Be Done?

Reliably executing kinematic implantation with a wide repertoire of implant designs and approaches necessitates a high level of expertise. The 'a la carte' concept represents the state of the art for implanting joint components and targets highly specialised, high-volume, expert joint replacement surgeons who have received training in each technique. The use of technological assistance such as navigation, patient-specific cutting guides or custom implants may be helpful for reaching higher surgical reliability. Ultimately, delivering personalized and conservative joint replacement depends on the individual surgeon's ability to flexibly consider and then perform procedures tailored to a given patient's requirements.

29.3 Challenging the Status Quo

The concept of 'a la carte' joint replacement challenges the current trend for rationalising the procedures and implants available in a surgeon's armamentarium. Cost-effective arthroplasty is a worthy social goal—reducing unwanted variation in a healthcare system by using affordable implants in technically forgiving procedures. On average, satisfactory function after arthroplasty is more likely if a procedure is capably and frequently performed by most surgeons. Surgeons are less likely to challenge the status quo by offering innovative or creative personalized solutions that are less frequently performed or more technically difficult, such as bicompartmental knee arthroplasty and neck-sparing or resurfacing hip arthroplasty. Open reporting of individual surgeon outcomes has instead encouraged surgeons to perform procedures that are difficult to revise and produce generally good outcomes [17]. The 'a la carte' approach is an evidence-based philosophy but demands an additional level of expertise. Delivering kinematic alignment, compartmental knee arthroplasty and conservative hip arthroplasty requires experience beyond current basic training, but may produce outstanding short- and longer term outcomes when executed by expert surgeons.

29.4 Case Illustrations

29.4.1 Case 1 (Fig. 29.3)

A sagittally balanced 80-year-old patient with right hip osteoarthritis (inserts b, c) and a degenerative, stiff spine responsible for a mixed-type spine–hip relationship type B/C (normal pelvic incidence ≈ 55° and low-standing lumbar lordosis ≈ 21° for a 24° mismatch, low delta sacral slope ≈ 10°) (insert a). The patient had a 10° excessive pelvic retroversion when standing, causing a compensated sagittal spinal imbalance, and a 10° lack of pelvic retroversion when sitting. Anatomically aligning total hip arthroplasty components in this patient would result in unfavourable kinematics and impingement during standing (from posterior edge-loading and instability) and sitting (from anterior edge-loading and instability). To prevent these risks, the patient received a kinematically aligned dual-mobility total hip arthroplasty performed through a mini-posterior approach. This preserved the integrity of the anterior capsule, while anatomical implantation (no adjustment) of a dual-mobility cup increases the range of motion before impingement and instability (inserts e, f). To reduce the risk of intra-operative femoral fracture or subsidence, a dual taper-collared cementless stem was implanted.

29.4.2 Case 2 (Fig. 29.4)

A 62-year-old highly active patient with a right osteoarthritic hip (inserts 4b, c) and spine–hip relation type B (normal pelvic incidence ≈ 60°, normal standing lumbar lordosis ≈ 52°, low delta sacral slope ≈ 6°) (insert 4a). Anatomically aligning total hip arthroplasty components would result in unfavourable kinematics and impingement when sitting (posterior edge-loading) and posterior instability. To reduce these risks, the patient received a kinematically aligned total hip arthroplasty performed through a minimally invasive direct anterior approach, preserving the integrity of the posterior capsule and external rotator muscles. The stem was anatomically implanted, maintaining native

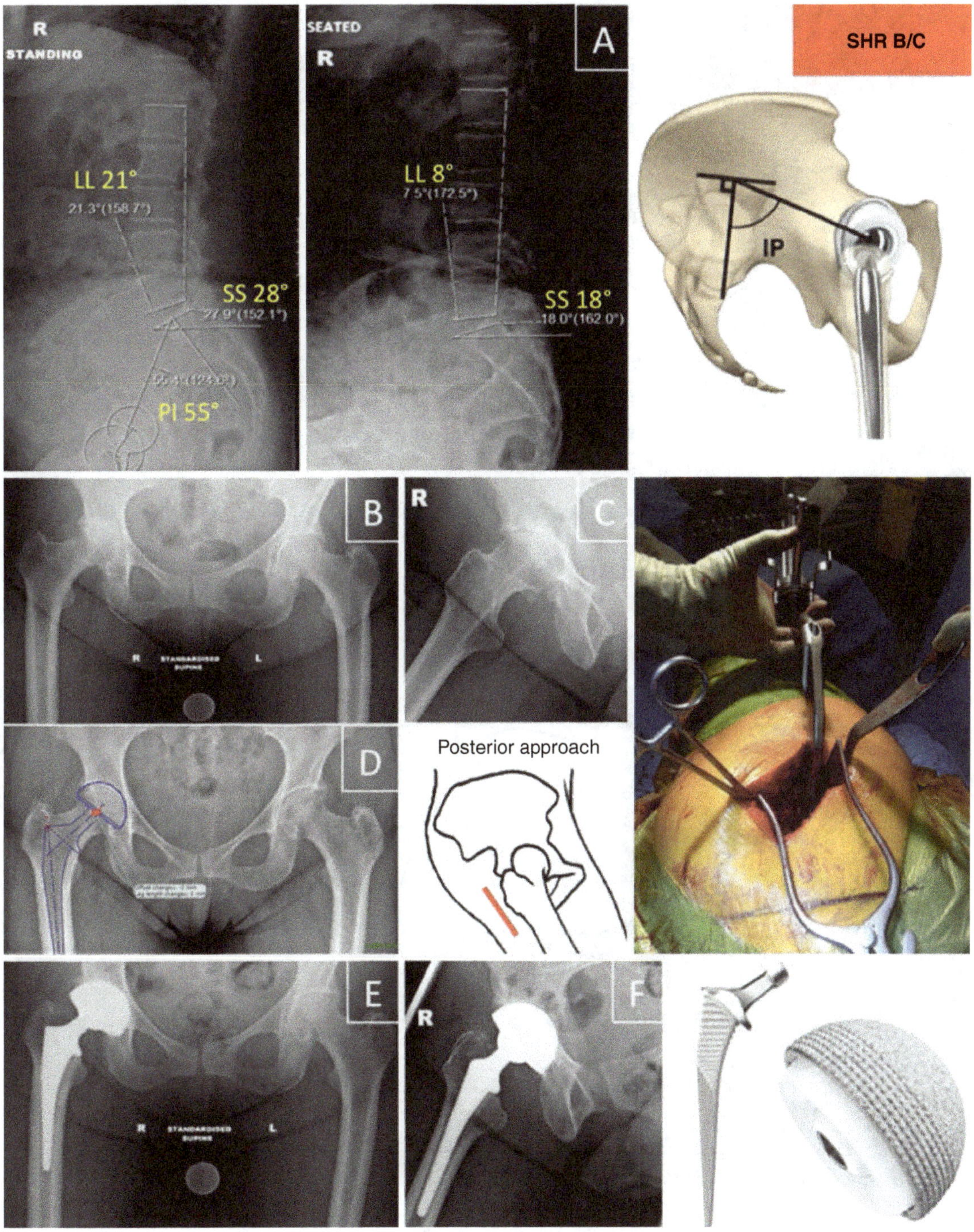

Fig. 29.3 Case 1: Right hip osteoarthritis in an elderly patient with good bone quality and spine–hip relationship type B/C. This was managed with kinematically aligned THR using a cementless collared stem and dual-mobility cup, performed through the posterior approach. Pre-operative lateral lumbo-pelvic radiographs (**a**) in standing (left) and sitting (right) positions. Pre-operative antero-posterior standing pelvic (**b**) and lateral right hip (**c**) radiographs. Digital KA-THA templating (**d**). Post-operative antero-posterior supine pelvic (**e**) and lateral right prosthetic hip (**f**) radiographs

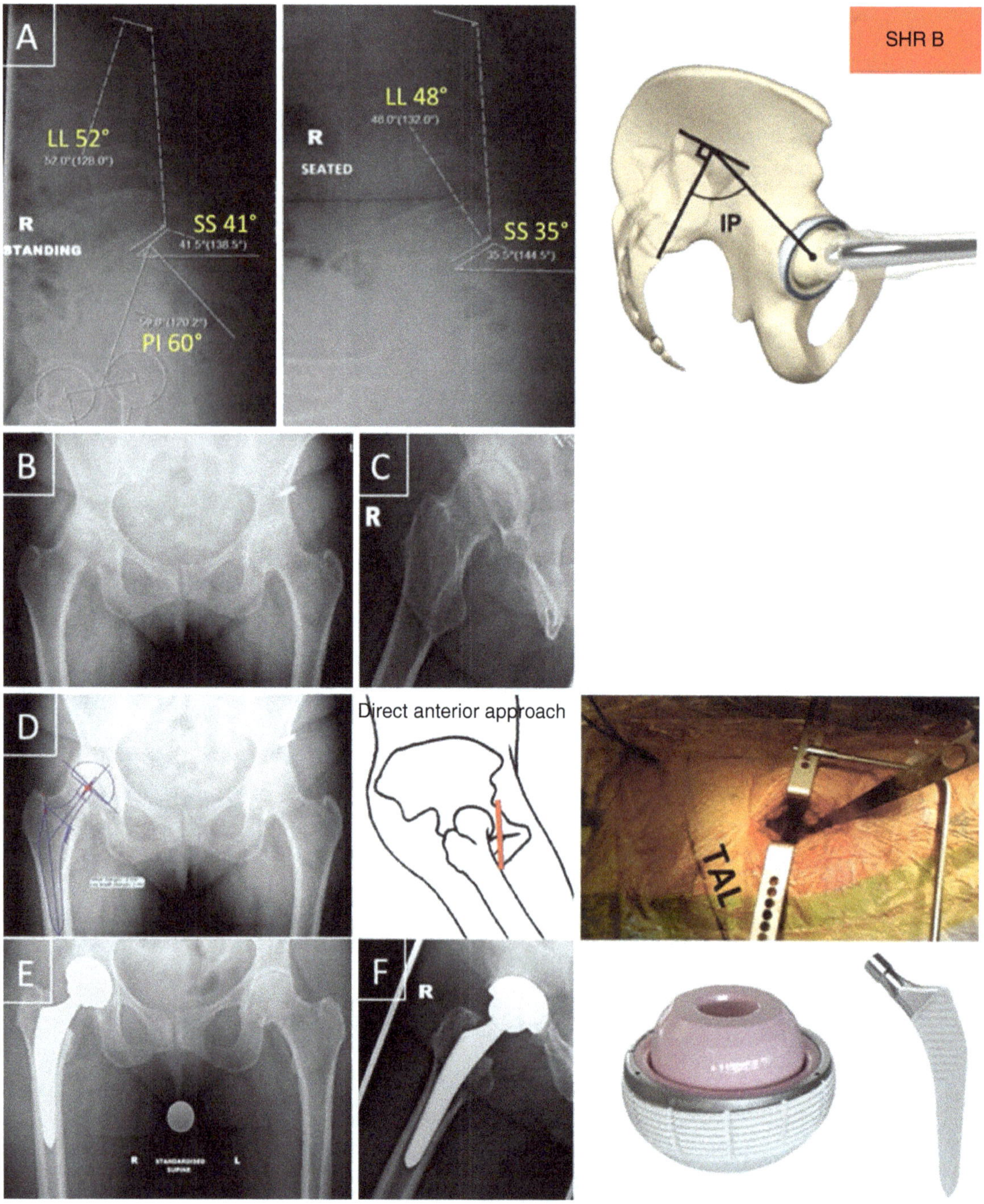

Fig. 29.4 Case 2: A highly active patient with right hip osteoarthritis and spine–hip relation type B. This was managed with kinematically aligned THR using a cementless collarless stem and a large ceramic-on-ceramic bearing, performed through the anterior approach. Pre-operative lateral lumbo-pelvic radiographs (**a**) in standing (left) and sitting (right) positions. Pre-operative antero-posterior standing pelvic (**b**) and lateral right hip (**c**) radiographs. Digital KA-THA templating (**d**). Post-operative antero-posterior supine pelvic (**e**) and lateral right prosthetic hip (**f**) radiographs

femoral version; the cup orientation was slightly adjusted with an additional 5° of anteversion relative to the transverse acetabular ligament (TAL) skin mark; a 36 mm ceramic-on-ceramic bearing was chosen for stability and durability (inserts 4e, f).

References

1. Provisional Quarterly Patient Reported Outcome Measures (PROMs) in England—Data Quality Note April 2017 to March 2018.
2. Rivière C, Lazennec J-Y, Van Der Straeten C, Auvinet E, Cobb J, Muirhead-Allwood S. The influence of spine-hip relations on total hip replacement: a systematic review. Orthop Traumatol Surg Res. 2017;103(4):559–68.
3. Riviere C. Kinematic versus conventional alignment techniques for total hip arthroplasty: a retrospective case control study. Orthop Traumatol Surg Res. 2019;105:895–905.
4. Howell SM, Papadopoulos S, Kuznik KT, Hull ML. Accurate alignment and high function after kinematically aligned TKA performed with generic instruments. Knee Surg Sports Traumatol Arthrosc. 2013;21(10):2271–80.
5. Rivière C, Iranpour F, Auvinet E, Howell S, Vendittoli P-A, Cobb J, et al. Alignment options for total knee arthroplasty: a systematic review. Orthop Traumatol Surg Res. 2017;103(7):1047–56.
6. Almaawi AM, Hutt JRB, Masse V, Lavigne M, Vendittoli P-A. The impact of mechanical and restricted kinematic alignment on knee anatomy in total knee arthroplasty. J Arthroplast. 2017;32(7): 2133–40.
7. Hutt JRB, LeBlanc M-A, Massé V, Lavigne M, Vendittoli P-A. Kinematic TKA using navigation: surgical technique and initial results. Orthop Traumatol Surg Res. 2016;102(1):99–104.
8. Price AJ, Alvand A, Troelsen A, Katz JN, Hooper G, Gray A, et al. Knee replacement. Lancet. 2018;392(10158):1672–82.
9. Takahashi T, Ansari J, Pandit H. Kinematically aligned total knee arthroplasty or mechanically aligned total knee arthroplasty. J Knee Surg. 2018;31(10): 999–1006.
10. Dagneaux L, Marouby S, Lazic S, Canovas F, Riviere C. Dual mobility device reduces the risk of prosthetic hip instability for patients with degenerated spine: a case-control study. Orthop Traumatol Surg Res. 2019;105:461–6.
11. Grammatopoulos G, Speirs AD, Ng KCG, Riviere C, Rakhra KS, Lamontagne M, et al. Acetabular and spino-pelvic morphologies are different in subjects with symptomatic cam femoro-acetabular impingement: acetabular and spinopelvic morphology in FAI. J Orthop Res. 2018;36(7):1840–8.
12. Taunton MJ, Trousdale RT, Sierra RJ, Kaufman K, Pagnano MW. John Charnley Award: randomized clinical trial of direct anterior and miniposterior approach THA. Clin Orthop. 2018;476(2):216–29.
13. Burn E, Liddle AD, Hamilton TW, Judge A, Pandit HG, Murray DW, et al. Cost-effectiveness of unicompartmental compared with total knee replacement: a population-based study using data from the National Joint Registry for England and Wales. BMJ Open. 2018;8(4):e020977.
14. Commitee NS. National Joint Registry for England, Wales, Northern Ireland and the Isle of Man: 15th annual report, 2017. National Joint Registry Centre. 2018.
15. Arirachakaran A, Choowit P, Putananon C, Muangsiri S, Kongtharvonskul J. Is unicompartmental knee arthroplasty (UKA) superior to total knee arthroplasty (TKA)? A systematic review and meta-analysis of randomized controlled trial. Eur J Orthop Surg Traumatol. 2015;25(5):799–806.
16. Fabre-Aubrespy M, Ollivier M, Pesenti S, Parratte S, Argenson J-N. Unicompartmental knee arthroplasty in patients older than 75 results in better clinical outcomes and similar survivorship compared to total knee arthroplasty. A matched controlled study. J Arthroplast. 2016;31(12):2668–71.
17. Liddle AD, Judge A, Pandit H, Murray DW. Adverse outcomes after total and unicompartmental knee replacement in 101 330 matched patients: a study of data from the National Joint Registry for England and Wales. Lancet. 2014;384(9952):1437–45.

Permissions

All chapters in this book were first published by Springer; hereby published with permission under the Creative Commons Attribution License or equivalent. Every chapter published in this book has been scrutinized by our experts. Their significance has been extensively debated. The topics covered herein carry significant information for a comprehensive understanding. They may even be implemented as practical applications or may be referred to as a beginning point for further studies.

The contributors of this book come from diverse backgrounds, making this book a truly international effort. We would like to thank all the contributing authors for lending their expertise to make the book truly unique. They have played a crucial role in the development of this book. Without their invaluable contributions this book wouldn't have been possible. They have made vital efforts to compile up to date information on the varied aspects of this subject to make this book a valuable addition to the collection of many professionals and students.

This book was conceptualized with the vision of imparting up-to-date and integrated information in this field. To ensure the same, a matchless editorial board was set up. Every individual on the board went through rigorous rounds of assessment to prove their worth. After which they invested a large part of their time researching and compiling the most relevant data for our readers.

The editorial board has been involved in producing this book since its inception. They have spent rigorous hours researching and exploring the diverse topics which have resulted in the successful publishing of this book. They have passed on their knowledge of decades through this book. To expedite this challenging task, the publisher supported the team at every step. A small team of assistant editors was also appointed to further simplify the editing procedure and attain best results for the readers.

Apart from the editorial board, the designing team has also invested a significant amount of their time in understanding the subject and creating the most relevant covers. They scrutinized every image to scout for the most suitable representation of the subject and create an appropriate cover for the book.

The publishing team has been an ardent support to the editorial, designing and production team. Their endless efforts to recruit the best for this project, has resulted in the accomplishment of this book. They are a veteran in the field of academics and their pool of knowledge is as vast as their experience in printing. Their expertise and guidance has proved useful at every step. Their uncompromising quality standards have made this book an exceptional effort. Their encouragement from time to time has been an inspiration for everyone.

The publisher and the editorial board hope that this book will prove to be a valuable piece of knowledge for students, practitioners and scholars across the globe.

Index

www.ingramcontent.com/pod-product-compliance
Lightning Source LLC
LaVergne TN
LVHW062130200926
848484LV00007B/1797